Caitlin Harper,

" Anatomy TA 2014 "
Department of Anatomy, Mayo Clinic
With Compliments,

Nirusha Lachman
Wojciech Pawlina

A Practical Guide for
MEDICAL TEACHERS

Content Strategist: *Laurence Hunter*
Content Development Specialist: *Ailsa Laing*
Project Manager: *Lucía Pérez*
Designer: *Christian Bilbow*
Illustration Manager: *Jennifer Rose*

A Practical Guide for
MEDICAL TEACHERS
Fourth Edition

Edited by

John A Dent MMEd MD FHEA FRCS(Ed)
International Relations Officer, Association for Medical Education in Europe;
Honorary Reader in Medical Education and Orthopaedic Surgery, University of Dundee,
Dundee, UK

Ronald M Harden *OBE* MD FRCP(Glas) FRCPC FRCSEd
General Secretary, Association for Medical Education in Europe; Former Professor of
Medical Education, Director of the Centre for Medical Education and Teaching Dean,
University of Dundee, UK; Professor of Medical Education Al-Imam University,
Riyadh, Saudi Arabia

Foreword by

Brian D Hodges PhD MD FRCPC
Richard and Elizabeth Currie Chair in Health Professions Education Research, Wilson
Centre for Research in Education; Professor, Faculty of Medicine and Faculty of Education
(OISE/UT), University of Toronto; Vice-President Education, University Health Network,
Toronto, Ontario, Canada

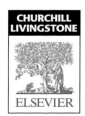

London   New York   Oxford   Philadelphia   St. Louis   Sydney   Toronto   2013

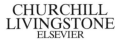

an imprint of Elsevier Limited

Fourth Edition © 2013, Elsevier Limited. All rights reserved.

First Edition 2001
Second Edition 2005
Third Edition 2009
Fourth Edition 2013
   Reprinted 2014

ISBN: 978-0-7020-4551-6

British Library Cataloguing in Publication Data
A catalogue record for this book is available from the British Library

Library of Congress Cataloging in Publication Data
A catalog record for this book is available from the Library of Congress

The chapter entitled 'Small group teaching' is in the public domain.

Notices
Knowledge and best practice in this field are constantly changing. As new research and experience broaden our understanding, changes in research methods, professional practices, or medical treatment may become necessary.

Practitioners and researchers must always rely on their own experience and knowledge in evaluating and using any information, methods, compounds, or experiments described herein. In using such information or methods they should be mindful of their own safety and the safety of others, including parties for whom they have a professional responsibility.

With respect to any drug or pharmaceutical products identified, readers are advised to check the most current information provided (i) on procedures featured or (ii) by the manufacturer of each product to be administered, to verify the recommended dose or formula, the method and duration of administration, and contraindications. It is the responsibility of practitioners, relying on their own experience and knowledge of their patients, to make diagnoses, to determine dosages and the best treatment for each individual patient, and to take all appropriate safety precautions.

To the fullest extent of the law, neither the Publisher nor the authors, contributors, or editors, assume any liability for any injury and/or damage to persons or property as a matter of products liability, negligence or otherwise, or from any use or operation of any methods, products, instructions, or ideas contained in the material herein.

ELSEVIER your source for books, journals and multimedia in the health sciences

www.elsevierhealth.com

Working together to grow libraries in developing countries

www.elsevier.com | www.bookaid.org | www.sabre.org

 ELSEVIER   BOOK AID International   Sabre Foundation

The publisher's policy is to use **paper manufactured from sustainable forests**

Printed in China

Contents

SECTION 3 EDUCATIONAL STRATEGIES

SECTION 4 TOOLS AND AIDS

SECTION 5 CURRICULUM THEMES

Foreword

It is an honour to pen the foreword to this fine book. Now in its fourth edition, *A Practical Guide for Medical Teachers* has become the go-to source for health professional educators. More than ever, trusted sources are required at a time when significant changes reshape what it means to be a learner, an educator or indeed to run a medical school. The rise of inter-professional, team-based education and practice, greater attention to institutional contexts and the 'hidden curriculum', ever increasing mobility of learners and teachers in a globalizing world and the rise of new technologies are just a few of the forces changing medical education rapidly and dramatically. The *Guide* is therefore a helpful companion in two ways. First it can be read in its entirety as a compendium of the issues facing health professions education today. The overarching design of the book facilitates such a comprehensive reading. Alternatively, the reader can dip in and out of concise, well-edited chapters to learn about new topics, to consult on best practices or to identify experts and resources for further learning. The design of the book makes it an ideal resource for educators to keep at close reach in the office, clinic or classroom.

The *Guide* is organized in seven sections, each designed with a focused, practical theme. The first section situates medical education in its context; across the continuum from the first days of medical school through to learning in clinical practice. Here, experts discuss curriculum design, and in this new edition, the emergent notion of a 'hidden curriculum' that is thought to have at least as much impact on students as the overt curriculum. The second section of the book addresses the many contexts in which medical education takes place. The chapters in this section remind us that one size does not fit all. Examining macro geographic contexts (rural, distance, community) and micro learning contexts (small groups, classrooms, bedside), the authors provide strategies to adapt and contextualize the overarching objectives introduced in section one.

The third section builds on the second, exploring a range of approaches to learning and teaching. Here, alongside well-established approaches such as problem-based learning, outcomes-oriented education and self-directed learning, we find an emphasis on team-based, integrated and interprofessional education. As healthcare delivery itself becomes more and more team-based and interprofessional these latter additions to the book are particularly valuable. The fourth section is designed to help educators grapple with the ever-widening scope of tools and technologies shaping medical education, while the fifth section takes up topics that no medical school can neglect. In this section, considerations for teaching communications, ethics and professionalism are enhanced with new writing about patient safety, something that will be particularly welcome to the educator confronted with increasing demands to demonstrate the clinical outcomes of educational processes. The sixth section provides a terrific reference for assessing students. No other area of medical education has undergone such profound evolution in recent years as assessment and this selection of experts has created a helpful resource that is right up-to-date. These chapters will surely help reduce the overwhelming sense that there are too many tools, approaches and controversies in the complex and burgeoning literature on assessment.

The seventh and final section is the capstone of the book. This section deals with the essence of what it means to be a medical educator. What do we want to achieve as educators? How do we choose the next generation? How will we support our students and each other while advancing academically our research, publications and leadership? In this part of the book, the reader is invited to join or reinforce their participation in the community of practice that is medical education.

The fourth edition of *A Practical Guide for Medical Teachers* contains a rich collection by the world's foremost experts on medical education. It is an essential resource for educators at all stages of their career, be they newly hired faculty members coming to grips with the challenges of a medical education career, midcareer faculty members tuning up on the best practices of curriculum, assessment or technology, or very experienced educators feeling a need to reflect on the latest challenges of our field. This marvelous book reminds us that, in the health professions, 'we are all teaching and we are all learning'.

Brian D. Hodges MD PhD FRCPC
Toronto 2013

Preface

The horizons of medical education are widening. Since the First Edition of *A Practical Guide for Medical Teachers* in 2001 there has been a steady rise of global interest in medical education, an increased awareness of the necessity for experience in education skills for all healthcare professionals and the need for some formal recognition of scholarship in medical education.

National and international conferences are attracting increasing numbers of delegates from developed countries as well as from those with emerging economies who previously may have been under-represented at international meetings. We are seeing a rise in the uptake of places on postgraduate courses in medical education, more frequent issues of medical education journals and the further development of e-journals and other new online resources. There is therefore a need to provide active support in medical education for a larger, international group of colleagues in all healthcare professions and at all stages of their personal professional development.

If we were to formulate a statement of intent to explain the purpose of this Fourth Edition, we might simply say that our aim is to help clinical colleagues to teach and to help students to learn. In general, healthcare professionals like to teach, and our desire through this book is to provide a practical guide to help each fulfil that role. A practical hands-on approach very much reflects our philosophy as much to teaching and learning as to innovation and development. Of course, we acknowledge that some may approach medical education from a different perspective, but we strongly believe in the importance of reaching out to help others in their teaching role, feeling that if we can do that, we will influence for good the learning and professional development of the next generation of students and trainees who will become the healthcare professionals of tomorrow. We were thrilled when the Third Edition of *A Practical Guide for Medical Teachers* was Highly Commended by the British Medical Association in 2010 in their annual Medical Book Awards in London.

As new trends in medical education continue to emerge, we have spotlighted seven this time which are discussed in the first chapter:

- Curriculum development and strategies
- Previously overlooked learning outcomes and how to assess them
- The importance of engagement with the curriculum by both teachers and students
- International accreditation and standardization in medical education
- The continuum of education from undergraduate to postgraduate training and continuing medical education
- Admission and selection procedures for medical education
- Leadership, scholarship and management in medical education.

This new edition has been significantly revised, and we are pleased that it has been possible to add seven new chapters without unduly expanding the total length of the book. In addition, a further 21 new contributors have brought a new perspective to existing chapters. A total of 77 colleagues from 14 countries have kindly contributed to this edition, making the book truly representative of international opinion on key topics in medical education. This international appeal has been highlighted by translations of recent editions into Chinese (for the People's Republic of China), Japanese, Vietnamese, Korean and Arabic.

We are grateful to all contributors for sharing their experience and expertise and would especially like to thank Dr Brian Hodges from the Wilson Centre for Research in Education at the University of Toronto for his generous comments in the Foreword. Dr Hodges has innovative theories on many topics in medical education and is a frequent speaker at international conferences.

Finally, having worked with the staff of Elsevier now for several years, we have become increasingly grateful to Laurence Hunter and his team for their support, patience and steady guidance during the preparation of each edition.

John A Dent
Ronald M Harden
Dundee, 2013

Contributors

Julie K Ash PhD BMBS BSc(Hons)
Lecturer, Health Professional Education,
School of Medicine, Flinders University,
Adelaide, Australia

Raja C Bandaranayake MBBS PhD
MSEd FRACS
Consultant in Medical Education; formerly
Professor of Anatomy, College of Medicine
and Medical Sciences, Arabian Gulf
University, Manama, Bahrain

John Bligh BSc MA MMEd MD FRCGP Hon FAcadMEd
Professor of Clinical Education and Dean of
Medical Education, Cardiff School of
Medicine, Cardiff, UK

Katharine Boursicot BSc, MBBS, MRCOG,
MAHPE, NTF
Reader in Medical Education and Deputy
Head, Centre for Medical and Healthcare
Education, St George's University of London,
London, UK

George Brown BSc DPhil HonDrOdont
Formerly Professor of Medical Education,
Medical Education Unit, University of
Nottingham, Nottingham, UK

Julie Browne BA(Hons) PGCE FAcadMEd
External Relations Manager, Wales Deanery,
University Hospital of Wales, Cardiff, UK

Alastair V Campbell MA BD ThD
Chen Su Lan Centennial Professor in Medical
Ethics; Director, Centre for Biomedical Ethics,
Yong Loo Lin School of Medicine, National
University of Singapore, Singapore

Mary Cantrell MA
Executive Director, Center for Clinical Skills
and Simulation Education, University of
Arkansas for Medical Sciences
Little Rock, Arkansas, USA

Jacqueline Chin BPhil DPhil(Oxon)
Assistant Professor, Centre for Biomedical
Ethics, Yong Loo Lin School of Medicine,
National University of Singapore, Singapore

Jennifer Cleland BSc(Hons) MSc PhD
DClinPsychol AFBPsS FHEA
John Simpson Chair of Medical Education,
School of Medicine and Dentistry; Chair,
Association for the Study of Medical Education
Research Group, Division of Medical and
Dental Education, University of Aberdeen,
Aberdeen, UK

Richard M Conran MD PhD JD
Professor and Second Year Medical Student
Program Course Director, Department of
Pathology, Uniformed Services University,
Bethesda, Maryland, USA

Ian D Couper BA MBBCh MFamMed
Professor of Rural Health, University of
Witwatersrand, Johannesburg, South Africa

Allan D Cumming BSc MBChB MD FRCPE
Professor of Medical Education and Dean of
Students, College of Medicine and Veterinary
Medicine, Queen's Medical Research Institute,
University of Edinburgh, Edinburgh, UK

David A Davis BA MD CCFP FCFP FRCPC(Hon)
Senior Director, Continuing Education and
Improvement, Association of American
Medical Colleges, Washington DC, USA;
Adjunct Professor, Family and Community
Medicine and Health Policy Management
and Evaluation, University of Toronto,
Toronto, Ontario, Canada

John A Dent MMEd MD FHEA FRCS(Ed)
International Relations Officer, Association for
Medical Education in Europe; Honorary Reader
in Medical Education and Orthopaedic Surgery,
University of Dundee, Dundee, UK

Peter Dieckmann PhD Dip-Psych
Danish Institute of Medical Simulation,
Capital Region of Denmark, Herlev
Hospital, Copenhagen, Denmark

Erik W Driessen PhD
Associate Professor in Medical Education,
Department of Educational Research and
Development, Faculty of Health, Medicine
and Life Sciences, Maastricht University,
Maastricht, The Netherlands

Itiel Dror PhD
Institute of Cognitive Neuroscience,
Department of Psychology, University
College London, London, UK

Steven J Durning MD PhD FACP
Professor of Medicine and Pathology and
Director, Introduction to Clinical Reasoning
Course, Uniformed Services University,
Bethesda, Maryland, USA

Robbert J Duvivier MD PhD
Student at Maastricht University, Maastricht,
The Netherlands

Sarah Edmunds BSc PhD CPsychol
Research Fellow, Department of Psychology,
University of Westminster, London, UK

Rachel H Ellaway BSc PhD
Assistant Dean, Curriculum and Planning,
and Associate Professor, Northern Ontario
School of Medicine, Sudbury, Ontario,
Canada

Luci Etheridge MBChB MRCPCH FHEA
Clinical Academic Teaching Fellow and
Honorary Paediatric Specialist Registrar,
University College London Medical School,
London, UK

Miriam Friedman Ben-David
(Deceased)

Gareth S Frith BA
Technology Enhanced Learning Manager,
Leeds Institute of Medical Education,
University of Leeds, Leeds, UK

Michael Frommer MB BS MPH
Adjunct Professor, Chair and Associate Dean,
Sydney Medical Program, School of Public
Health, University of Sydney, Sydney, Australia

Elizabeth Gaufberg MD MPH
Associate Professor of Medicine and Psychiatry,
Harvard Medical School; Director, Center for
Professional Development, The Cambridge
Health Alliance; Director, Arnold P. Gold
Foundation Research Institute, Cambridge,
Massachusetts, USA

Elizabeth A Gephardt MEd
Director, Pediatric Understanding and Learning
through Simulation Education (PULSE)
Center, Arkansas Children's Hospital, Little
Rock, Arkansas, USA

Trevor Gibbs MD SFHEA DA FAcadMEd MMedSc FRCGP
Professor and Consultant of Medical
Education, Primary Care and Adolescent
Health, Dundee; Development Officer,
Association for Medical Education in Europe,
Dundee, UK

Shiphra Ginsburg MD MEd FRCPC
Associate Professor, Internal Medicine
(Respirology); Scientist, Wilson Centre for
Research in Education, Faculty of Medicine,
University of Toronto and Mount Sinai
Hospital, Toronto, Ontario, Canada

Paul Glasziou MBBS PhD FRACGP
Professor of Evidence-Based Medicine and
Director of the Centre for Evidence-Based
Medicine, Department of Primary Health
Care, University of Oxford, Oxford, UK

Peter Gliatto MD FACP
Associate Dean, Undergraduate Medical
Education and Student Affairs, and Associate
Professor, Medical Education and Medicine,
Icahn School of Medicine at Mount Sinai,
New York, USA

Joanne Goldman MSc
Research Associate Continuing Education
and Professional Development, Faculty of
Medicine, University of Toronto, Toronto,
Ontario, Canada

Janet Grant MSc PhD MRCGP(Hon) FBPsS FRCP(Hon) MRCR(Hon)
Professor Emerita of Education in Medicine, The Open University; Honorary Professor, University College London Medical School; Director, Centre for Medical Education in Context [CenMEDIC] and FAIMER Centre for Distance Learning, UK

Larry Gruppen PhD
Professor and Chair, Department of Medical Education, University of Michigan Medical School, Ann Arbor, Michigan, USA

Frederic W Hafferty PhD
Professor of Medical Education; Associate Director, Program in Professionalism and Ethics, Mayo Clinic, Rochester, Minnesota, USA

Hossam Hamdy MBChB MCh FRCS FACS PhD(Edu)
Professor and Vice Chancellor for Medical & Health Sciences Colleges, University of Sharjah, United Arab Emirates

Ronald M Harden OBE MD FRCP(Glas) FRCPC FRCSEd
General Secretary, Association for Medical Education in Europe; Former Professor of Medical Education, Director of the Centre for Medical Education and Teaching Dean, University of Dundee, UK; Professor of Medical Education, Al-Imam University, Riyadh, Saudi Arabia

Sylvia Heeneman PhD
Associate Professor, Department of Pathology, Maastricht University, Maastricht, The Netherlands

Carl Heneghan MA MRCGP
Deputy Director, Centre for Evidence-Based Medicine, Department of Primary Health Care, University of Oxford, Oxford, UK

Patricia Hudes MSIT
Director of Faculty Development, Wright State University Boonshoft School of Medicine, Dayton, Ohio, USA

Jean S Ker BSc MD DRCOG FRCGP FRCPE FHEA
Professor, Medical Education, and Director, Clinical Skills Centre, Ninewells Hospital and Medical School, University of Dundee, Dundee; Clinical Skills Lead for Scottish Managed Education Network, UK

Sharon K Krackov EdD
Independent Consultant, Medical Education; Professor of Medical Education, Albany Medical College, Albany, New York, USA

Nirusha Lachman PhD
Associate Professor of Anatomy, Consultant, College of Medicine, Mayo Clinic, Rochester, Minnesota, USA

Sam Leinster BSc MD FRCS(Edin&Eng) SFHEA FAcadMEd
Emeritus Professor, Medical Education, and former Dean, Norwich Medical School, University of East Anglia, Norwich, UK

Susan J Lieff MD MEd MMan FRCPC
Professor of Psychiatry and Director, Academic Leadership Development, Centre for Faculty Development, Faculty of Medicine, University of Toronto; Vice-Chair, Education, Department of Psychiatry, University of Toronto, Ontario, Canada

Sean McAleer BSc DPhil
Course Director and Senior Lecturer, Medical Education, Centre for Medical Education, University of Dundee, Dundee, UK

Judy McKimm BA(Hons) MA(Ed) MBA DipHSW CertEd SFHEA FAcadMEd
Dean and Professor in Medical Education, College of Medicine, Swansea University; Visiting Professor in Healthcare Education and Leadership, University of Bedfordshire, UK

Danette W McKinley PhD
Director, Research and Data Resources, Foundation for Advancement of International Medical Education and Research (FAIMER), Philadelphia, Pennsylvania, USA

I Chris McManus MD PhD FRCP(Lond Edin) FMedSci
Professor of Psychology and Medical Education, Division of Psychology and Language Sciences, University College London, London, UK

Stewart P Mennin PhD
Emeritus Professor, University of New Mexico School of Medicine; Principal, Mennin Consulting & Associates Inc, Sao Paulo, Brazil

Larry K Michaelsen PhD
David Ross Boyd Professor Emeritus, University of Oklahoma; Professor of Management, University of Central Missouri, Warrensburg, Missouri, USA

John Norcini PhD
President and CEO, Foundation for Advancement of International Medical Education and Research, Philadelphia, Pennsylvania, USA

Doris Østergaard DMSc
Associate Professor, Danish Institute of Medical Simulation, Herlev Hospital, Capital Region of Denmark, Copenhagen University, Copenhagen, Denmark

Dean Parmelee MD FAPA FAACAP
Associate Dean for Academic Affairs, Wright State University Boonshoft School of Medicine, Dayton, Ohio, USA

Nivritti G Patil MBE BBBS MS FRCSEd FCSHK FHKAM(Surgery)
Honorary Clinical Professor, Senior Adviser, Department of Surgery and Institute of Medical and Health Sciences, Li Ka Shing Faculty of Medicine, University of Hong Kong, Hong Kong, China

Wojciech Pawlina MD
Chair and Professor of Anatomy and Medical Education, Department of Anatomy; Assistant Dean for Curriculum Development and Innovation Mayo Medical School, College of Medicine, Mayo Clinic, Rochester, Minnesota, USA

Laure Perrier MEd MLIS
Information Specialist, Continuing Education and Professional Development, Faculty of Medicine, University of Toronto; Li Ka Shing Knowledge Institute, St. Michael's Hospital, Toronto, Ontario, Canada

David Prideaux PhD MEd BA(Hons)
Emeritus Professor, Medical Education, School of Medicine, Flinders University, Adelaide, Australia

Subha Ramani MBBS MMEd MPH
Associate Professor of Medicine and Director, Faculty Development in Clinical Training, School of Medicine, Boston University, Boston, Massachusetts, USA

Trudie E Roberts BSc MB ChB PhD FRCP FHEA
Director, Leeds Institute of Medical Education, University of Leeds, Leeds, UK

Sue Roff BA(Hons) MA
External Tutor, Centre for Medical Education and Educational Consultant, formerly Centre for Medical Education, University of Dundee, Dundee, UK

Michael T Ross BSc MBChB DRCOG MRCGP EdD
Programme Co-Director, MSc Clinical Education, Centre for Medical Education, University of Edinburgh, Edinburgh; General Practitioner, NHS Fife, UK

James Rourke MD CCFP(EM) MClinSci FCFP LLD
Dean, Faculty of Medicine, and Professor of Family Medicine, Memorial University of Newfoundland, St John's, Canada

Leslie Rourke MD CCFP MClinSci FCFP
Associate Professor of Family Medicine, Faculty of Medicine, Memorial University of Newfoundland, St John's, Canada

John E Sandars MD MSc MRCP FRCGP FAcadMEd FHEA CertEd
Associate Professor, Academic Lead for e-Learning, Leeds Institute of Medical Education, School of Medicine, University of Leeds, Leeds, UK

Lambert W T Schuwirth MD PhD
Professor of Medical Education, Flinders
Innovation in Clinical Education, Health
Professions Education, School of Medicine,
Flinders University, Adelaide, Australia

Ann E Sefton MBBS BSc PhD DSc
Emeritus Professor; Former Associate Dean,
Faculties of Medicine and Dentistry, University
of Sydney, Sydney, Australia

Ivan L Silver MD MEd FRCP(C)
Professor of Psychiatry and Vice President,
Education, Centre for Addiction and Mental
Health, Faculty of Medicine, University of
Toronto, Toronto, Ontario, Canada

John R Skelton BA MA RSA MRCGP
Professor of Clinical Communication, College
of Medical and Dental Sciences, University of
Birmingham, UK

Yvonne Steinert PhD
Professor of Family Medicine and Director,
Centre for Medical Education and Richard
and Sylvia Cruess Chair in Medical Education,
Faculty of Medicine, McGill University,
Montreal, Canada

David T Stern MD PhD
Vice Chair for Faculty Affairs, Professor of
Internal Medicine and Medical Education,
Icahn School of Medicine at Mount Sinai,
New York, USA

Jill E Thistlethwaite BSc MBBS PhD MMEd
FRCGP FRACGP
Professor of Medical Education, Director of
the Centre for Medical Education Research
and Scholarship, School of Medicine,
University of Queensland, Brisbane,
Queensland, Australia

Cees P M van der Vleuten PhD
Professor of Medical Education, Department
of Educational Development and Research,
Maastricht University, Maastricht,
The Netherlands

Jeroen J G van Merriënboer PhD
Professor of Learning and Instruction, Research
Program Director, Department of Educational
Development and Research and Graduate
School of Health Professions Education,
Maastricht University, Maastricht,
The Netherlands

Teck Chuan Voo MA BA
Research Associate, Centre for Biomedical
Ethics, Yong Loo Lin School of Medicine,
National University of Singapore, Singapore

David Wall MBChB MMEd PhD PGCE FRCP FRCGP
Deputy Regional Postgraduate Dean,
Professor of Medical Education, University
of Birmingham, Birmingham, UK

Paul S Worley MBBS PhD DipObst RANZCOG
FACRRM FRACGP MBA
Dean, School of Medicine, Flinders
University, Adelaide, Australia

Anand Zachariah MD DNB
Professor, Medicine Unit 1 and Infectious
Disease, Christian Medical College, Vellore,
Tamil Nadu, India

Section 1

Curriculum development

New horizons in medical education

J. A. Dent, R. M. Harden

Every few years, new ideas and new trends in medical education become apparent. This is not to say that previous ideas and trends have been abandoned, but rather that changes in current circumstances or expanding understanding call for the further development of recognized procedures or the emergence of new approaches.

Recent topics in medical education

In previous editions of this book, emerging topics in medical education were discussed. In the last edition six were identified:

1. The globalization of healthcare delivery and international dimensions of medical education
2. A reconceptualization of the role of the doctor and recognition of the importance of learning outcomes in defining the curriculum for training an appropriate workforce
3. The changing context in which clinical experience is gained
4. The continuing developments of new learning technologies and their influence on teaching and learning
5. An evolving conceptualization of assessment and its role in medical education
6. The recognition of professionalism and scholarship in medical education

As these topics have continued to be discussed in the literature and in conference proceedings, a number of comments can now be made on each of them.

GLOBALIZATION OF HEALTHCARE DELIVERY AND INTERNATIONAL DIMENSIONS OF MEDICAL EDUCATION

Countries in need of international support can be identified by their position on the spectrum of socio-economic development in relation to their child mortality, family size and economic growth. The associated healthcare problems (which can be compounded by physician migration to employment in westernized urban centres) may be helped by international agencies or resources committed to facilitating local opportunities for medical education. The Foundation for Advancement of International Medical Education and Research (FAIMER) and its regional institutes support medical teachers through their fellowship training scheme. The World Federation for Medical Education (WFME) and the Panamerican Federation of Associations of Medical Schools (PAFAMS) exert an international influence in needy areas and the Association for Medical Education in Europe (AMEE) provides a wealth of printed resources and an annual international conference attracting more than 3000 delegates from over 100 countries. At the AMEE 2009 conference in Malaga, Matthew Gwee led a symposium discussing the international role of medical education in seeking to inculcate and nurture the hitherto overlooked professional qualities of compassion, empathy and integrity and their contribution to developing a sense of social responsibility. 'New models of international collaboration' was the theme for a plenary session at AMEE 2011 in Vienna. A resource which seeks to promote this is the newly relaunched website MedEdWorld, which provides a transnational collaborative learning approach with access to an e-library, synchronous online webinars and asynchronous discussion groups.

"MedEdWorld is an international health professions community of individuals and educational organisations."

"It provides an international network through which organisations, medical schools, individual teachers and students across the world can share ideas, experiences and expertise and through which they can collaborate in the further development of medical education."

Symposium: 'The doctor we are educating for the future,' AMEE 2010 conference

RECONCEPTUALIZATION OF THE ROLE OF THE DOCTOR AND THE IMPORTANCE OF LEARNING OUTCOMES IN DEFINING THE CURRICULUM FOR TRAINING AN APPROPRIATE WORKFORCE

The success of outcome-based education (OBE) in defining a new medical school curriculum at the University of Wollongong was described by Elizabeth Farmer at the AMEE 2010 conference in Glasgow. At the same conference, Stefan Lindgren, President of WFME, described how OBE also provides a mechanism for directing the training of other healthcare professionals and for meeting the educational requirements perceived necessary for the future global doctor. Competence-based education was the theme of the August 2010 issue of *Medical Teacher*.

"Doctors may not need in the future to undertake all their traditional roles, while other new roles may emerge instead."

Symposium: 'The doctor we are educating for the future,' AMEE 2010 conference

"Competency based medical education offers great promise as a means of addressing the needs of society, assuring competent practitioners, and emphasising the acquisition of skills, attitudes, and knowledge and their application to real-world practice."

Snell & Frank 2010

THE CHANGING CONTEXT IN WHICH CLINICAL EXPERIENCE IS GAINED

The expanding implementation of rural and remote medical education (RRME) in the undergraduate curriculum has been reviewed in AMEE Guide 47 (Maley et al 2009). A review of the current literature on ambulatory care education looked at the research and scholarship in this area and commented on key challenges and examples of good practice (Williams et al 2012). A rare example of a developing ambulatory care teaching programme was presented from the University of Otago, New Zealand, at AMEE 2011 in Vienna.

"The goal of global equity in health care requires that the training of health-care professionals be better tuned to meet the needs of the communities they serve....medical education is being driven into isolated communities by factors including workforce undersupply, education pedagogy, medical practice and research

needs.... RRME harnesses the rich learning environment of communities such that students rapidly achieve competence and confidence in a primary care/generalist setting."

Maley et al 2009

*"When there's not much you can do, this is something you **can** do."*

Patient response; Ambulatory Medical Programme at the University of Otago, Dunedin, AMEE 2011 conference

NEW LEARNING TECHNOLOGIES

The popularity and availability of e-learning using both static and mobile devices has brought with it concern about the quality of the students' learning experience. To maximize learning there is a need for an informed faculty to guide students to the most profitable sites. E-learning was the theme of the April 2011 issue of *Medical Teacher*.

Patient-focused simulation by the use of hybrids, part simulators appropriately attached to a simulated patient, to create a realistic clinical situation has been reported by Roger Kneebone at AMEE 2009 in Malaga. At the same conference the role of distributed simulation whereby portable, lightweight and inexpensive equipment is used to recreate key elements of a clinical setting in a cost-effective way, was illustrated by the creation of a simulated operating theatre in the conference venue.

"It appeared to be a good idea at the time but...."
Sandars 2011

"After a decade of disruptive change we seem to be moving into a period of consolidating the use of the digital in medical education."

Ellaway 2011

THE DEVELOPMENT OF ASSESSMENT AND ITS ROLE IN MEDICAL EDUCATION

Current theories in assessment have been discussed by Lambert Schuwirth and Cees van der Vleuten (2011) in AMEE Guide No. 57. There is widening uptake of the American Board of Internal Medicine Mini-Clinical Evaluation Exercise (Mini-CEX) as a usable approach to performance assessment. A series of consensus statements relating to criteria for good assessment, assessment for selection, assessment of professionalism, performance assessment, technology-based assessment and research in assessment were developed at the 14th Ottawa Conference in 2010 in Miami and refined in 2012 at the 15th Ottawa Conference in Kuala Lumpur.

"The consensus statements and recommendations contained in the six reports would be viewed as an attempt to provide clarity and focus on several issues in assessment. They are intended to be challenged, rebuked, modified and will evolve over time......to respond to the significant pressures for change in medical and health science education and to contribute to the developments taking place in assessment philosophy and techniques."

Issenberg 2011

"Assessment of medical competence and medical expertise is not an easy task, and is often dominated by tradition and intuition."

Schuwirth & van der Vlueten 2011

PROFESSIONALISM AND SCHOLARSHIP IN MEDICAL EDUCATION

Professional behaviour includes showing care and respect to patients and behaving with integrity, responsibility and accountability to all. Such professional behaviour needs to be explicitly integrated into the undergraduate curriculum in a structured approach, as discussed by Helen O'Sullivan in AMEE Guide No. 61 (2012). Demonstration of professional behaviour is equally important for postgraduates and medical teachers. A detailed set of learning outcomes related to professionalism is the subject of discussion.

"Professionalism for the twenty-first century raises challenges not only to adapting the course to changing societal values but also for instilling skills of ongoing self-directed continuous development in trainees for future revalidation."

O'Sullivan et al 2012

Current trends in medical education

In compiling this new edition we have reviewed recent publications and key presentations from international conferences. This has revealed new trends, of which the following are a selection:

- Curriculum development and strategies
- Previously overlooked learning outcomes and how to assess them

- The importance of engagement with the curriculum by both teachers and students
- International accreditation and standardization in medical education
- The continuum of education from undergraduate to postgraduate training and continuing medical education (CME)
- Admission and selection procedures for medical education
- Leadership, scholarship and management in medical education

CURRICULUM DEVELOPMENT AND STRATEGIES

The educational strategies as embodied in the SPICES model continue to evolve and are reviewed further by Ronald Harden in Chapter 2. Examples are an adaptive or personalized curriculum, problem-based learning enhanced through technology, interprofessional education and community-based education.

Changing social circumstances and careful consideration of fundamental principles and theory continue to influence curriculum development, as argued in the literature by Bleakley (2012). Underlying all our concepts of what a curriculum should be like, of course, is the existence of the 'hidden curriculum', which students actually follow and which is described further by Fred Haffery and Elizabeth Gaufberg in Chapter 7, one of the new chapters in this book.

PREVIOUSLY OVERLOOKED LEARNING OUTCOMES AND HOW TO ASSESS THEM

As student attitudes and professionalism become more integrated into the taught curriculum, the requirement for them to be assessed becomes more urgent, as highlighted at the 14th Ottawa Conference in Miami. Shiphra Ginsburg in Chapter 41 of this book outlines an approach.

Teamwork is another outcome which has attracted attention, and team-based learning is described by Dean Parmelee in AMEE Guide No. 65 (2012) and in Chapter 21. Finally, patient safety, why errors occur and how teaching and training in informed strategies can help to prevent them have been promoted by the WHO, were Itiel Dror's opening plenary of the AMEE 2010 conference in Glasgow and are described by him further in Chapter 34.

THE IMPORTANCE OF ENGAGEMENT WITH THE CURRICULUM BY BOTH TEACHERS AND STUDENTS

The symposium chaired by Matthew Gwee at AMEE 2010 in Glasgow looked at the student as a partner-in-learning with the teacher. In this model both the student and the teacher have a shared responsibility in the teaching–learning process. Strategies to enhance student engagement in medical school might include their involvement in the development of medical school curricula and support to develop extracurricular special interest groups, web-based learning sites or other student support resources. Student engagement has been identified in the 'ASPIRE to excellence' initiative as one of the domains where a school may demonstrate excellence in education. New strategies in faculty development to help teachers keep abreast of current teaching approaches was the subject of the First International Conference on Faculty Development in the Health Professions held in Toronto in 2011 (see Chapter 45).

INTERNATIONAL ACCREDITATION AND STANDARDIZATION IN MEDICAL EDUCATION

Faced with rapid changes in the practice of medicine, the ongoing development of regionally appropriate health systems and the uncontrolled proliferation of medical schools in some countries (some of which may have a strong commercial character), there is a need for some mechanism to ensure a degree of international standardization among medical schools. The Pan American Health Organization (PAHO), FAIMER, PAFAMS and the WFME are all involved in seeking to define appropriate standards and adapt them to local settings.

THE CONTINUUM OF EDUCATION FROM UNDERGRADUATE TO POSTGRADUATE TRAINING AND CME

The idea that the learning outcomes of the undergraduate curriculum can be equally appropriate, albeit at a more advanced level, in postgraduate studies and continuing professional development is probably a new thought to many. The concept of medical training as a continuum from undergraduate learning to CME was the theme of the AMEE 2012 conference in Lyon. This trend is explored further in Section 1 of this book.

ADMISSION AND SELECTION PROCEDURES FOR MEDICAL EDUCATION

There has been a growing interest in the methods adopted to select students for entry to medical studies. The multiple mini-interviews have become popular and are currently being evaluated and adapted from an international perspective. While this approach identifies a number of desirable traits in potential students, recent work is looking at mechanisms to identify undesirable traits as well. The whole question of student vocation in relation to suitability was discussed in a symposium at AMEE 2011 in Vienna chaired by Nicole Borges. Chris McManus discusses a range of selection processes in Chapter 43.

LEADERSHIP, SCHOLARSHIP AND MANAGEMENT IN MEDICAL EDUCATION

The question of leadership in medical education has usually been underrepresented in staff development programmes. Symposia on the topic in recent conferences have looked at questions such as why is leadership important, how can potential leaders be recognized, how can leadership be taught and what is the contribution of a postgraduate masters programme. The recent BEME Guide No. 19 by Steinert and colleagues (2012) discusses faculty development initiatives designed to promote leadership. These topics are reviewed by Yvonne Steinert in Chapter 45 and by Judy McKimm and Susan Lieff in Chapter 42.

Scholarship in medical education was the subject of AMEE Guide No. 43 by McGaghie (2009). Now an enhanced profile of scholarship in medical education is evidenced by the popularity of international conferences, the demand for postgraduate courses in medical education and the establishment of new online resources. In response to local needs, new national conferences are attracting audiences from all healthcare professions. International conferences are being regularly held in North America, the Middle East and Asia, with a biennial global conference attracting more than 1200 provided by the Ottawa group, and the annual AMEE conference in Europe attracting over 3000 delegates. An active interest in sharing and debate in medical education is now being shown by countries not previously able to participate fully in these opportunities.

Face-to-face courses in medical education continue to attract large groups of international participants, and the ESME-online basic and leadership courses launched in 2012 immediately attracted 60 participants from 24 countries. Global access to medical education websites, such as MedEdWorld, allows active participation in webinars, special interest groups and access to current journals or archived material anytime and almost anywhere.

Finally, the role of management in medical education is discussed further by Hossam Hamdy in Chapter 50.

Summary

Over the years what were new trends in medical education have developed into established topics and examples of best practice. At the same time, in response to both internal and external factors, further new trends evolve to meet new needs or to seek new answers to ongoing problems. A review of recent publications and of key presentations at international conferences has suggested the following current issues and trends:

- Curriculum development and strategies
- Previously overlooked learning outcomes and how to assess them
- The importance of engagement with the curriculum by both teachers and students
- International accreditation and standardization in medical education
- The continuum of education from undergraduate to postgraduate training and CME
- Admission and selection procedures for medical education
- Leadership, scholarship and management in medical education

We have begun to explore some of these in the following chapters along with more familiar topics of interest to all practising medical teachers.

References

AMEE 2009 Conference Archive. http://www.amee.org

AMEE 2010 Conference Archive. http://www.amee.org

AMEE 2011 Conference Archive. http://www.amee.org

AMEE 2012 Conference Archive. http://www.amee.org

ASPIRE. www.aspire-to-excellence.org

Bleakley A: The curriculum is dead! Long live the curriculum! Designing an undergraduate medicine and surgery curriculum for the future, *Medical Teacher* 34:543–547, 2012.

Ellaway R: E-learning: is the revolution over? *Medical Teacher* 33:297–302, 2011.

First International Conference in Faculty Development in the Health Professions. http://www.facultydevelopment2011.com

Harden RM, Sowden S, Dunn WR: Some educational strategies in curriculum development: The SPICES model, *Medical Education* 18:284–297, 1984

Issenberg SB: Ottawa 2012 Conference: consensus statements and recommendations, *Medical Teacher* 33:181–182, 2011.

McGaghie WC: Scholarship, publication, and career advancement in health professions education: AMEE Guide No. 43, *Medical Teacher* 31:574–590, 2009.

Maley M, Worley P, Dent J: Using rural and remote settings in the undergraduate medical curriculum: AMEE Guide No. 47, *Medical Teacher* 31:969–983, 2009.

O'Sullivan H, van Mook W, Fewtrell R, Wass V: Integrating professionalism into the curriculum: AMEE Guide No. 61, *Medical Teacher* 34:e64–e77, 2012.

Parmelee D, Michaelsen LK, Cook S, Hudes PD: Team-based learning: a practical guide: AMEE Guide No. 65, *Medical Teacher* 34:e275–e287, 2012.

Sandars J: It appeared to be a good idea at the time but... a few steps closer to understanding how technology can enhance teaching and learning in medical education, *Medical Teacher* 33:265–267, 2011.

Schuwirth LWT, van der Vleuten CPM: General overview of the theories used in assessment: AMEE Guide No. 57, *Medical Teacher* 33:783–797, 2011.

Snell LS, Frank JR: Competencies, the tea bag model and the end of time, *Medical Teacher* 32:629–630, 2010.

Steinert Y, Naismith L, Mann K: Faculty development initiatives designed to promote leadership in medical education. A BEME systematic review: BEME Guide No. 19, *Medical Teacher* 34:483–503, 2012.

Williams CK, Hui Y, Borschel D, Carnahan H: Scoping review of MD ambulatory education, *Medical Teacher* 0:1–10, 2012.

Curriculum planning and development

R. M. Harden

Introduction

Curriculum planning and development remains very much on the agenda for undergraduate, postgraduate and continuing medical education. The days are now past when the teacher produced a curriculum like a magician produced a rabbit out of a hat, when the lecturer taught whatever attracted his or her interest and when the students' clinical training was limited to the patients who happened to present during a clinical attachment. It is now accepted that careful planning is necessary if the programme of teaching and learning is to be successful.

 "Curriculum is in the air. No matter what the problem in medical education, curriculum is looked to as the solution."

Davidoff 1996

What is a curriculum?

A curriculum is more than just a syllabus or a statement of content. A curriculum is about what should happen in a teaching programme – about the intention of the teachers and about the way they make this happen. This extended vision of a curriculum is illustrated in Figure 2.1. Curriculum planning can be considered in 10 steps (Harden 1986b). This chapter looks at these steps and the changes in emphasis since the publication of the third edition of the text.

 The 10 steps described provide a useful checklist for planning and evaluating a curriculum.

IDENTIFYING THE NEED

The relevance or appropriateness of educational programmes has been questioned by Frenk et al (2010), Cooke et al (2010) and others. The need has been recognized to emphasize not only sickness salvaging, organic pathology and crisis care, but also health promotion and preventative medicine. Increasing attention is being paid to the social responsibility of a medical school and the extent to which it meets and equips its graduates to meet the needs of the population it serves.

 "Professional education has not kept pace with these challenges, largely because of the fragmented, outdated, and static curricula that produce ill-equipped graduates."

Frenk et al 2010

A range of approaches can be used to identify curriculum needs (Dunn et al 1985):

- *The 'wise men' approach.* Senior teachers and senior practitioners from different specialty backgrounds reach a consensus.
- *Consultation with stakeholders.* The views of members of the public, patients, government and other professions are sought.

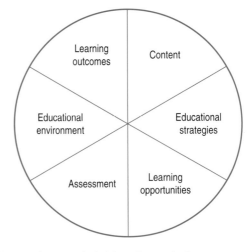

Fig. 2.1 An extended vision of a curriculum

- *A study of errors in practice.* Areas where the curriculum is deficient are identified.
- *Critical-incident studies.* Individuals are asked to describe key medical incidents in their experience which represent good or bad practice.
- *Task analysis.* The work undertaken by a doctor is studied.
- *Study of star performers.* Doctors recognized as 'star performers' are studied to identify their special qualities or competencies.

ESTABLISHING THE LEARNING OUTCOMES

 If you leave this book with only one idea, it should be the concept of outcome-based education.

One of the big ideas in medical education over the past decade has been the move to the use of learning outcomes as the driver for curriculum planning (Harden 2007). In an outcome-based approach to education, as discussed in Chapter 18, the learning outcomes are defined and the specified outcomes inform decisions about the curriculum. This represents a move away from a process model of curriculum planning, where the teaching and learning experiences and methods matter, to a product model, where what matters are the learning outcomes and the product.

 "A move from the 'How' and 'When' to the 'What' and 'Whether'"

Spady 1994

The idea of learning outcomes is not new. Since the work of Bloom, Mager and others in the 1960s and 1970s, the value of setting out the aims and objectives of a training programme has been recognized. In practice, however, long lists of aims and objectives have proved unworkable and have been ignored in planning and implementing a curriculum. But in recent years, the move to an outcome- or competency-based approach to the curriculum with outcome frameworks has gained momentum and is increasingly dominating education thinking.

AGREEING ON THE CONTENT

The content of a textbook is outlined in the content pages and in the index. The content of a curriculum is found in the syllabus and in the topics covered in lectures and other learning opportunities. Traditionally, there has been an emphasis on knowledge, and this has been reflected in student assessment. Content relating to skills and attitudes is now recognized also as important. Increasing emphasis has been placed on an authentic curriculum – a curriculum where the

content is more closely related to the work of the practising doctor. Basic science content, for example, is considered in the context of clinical medicine.

The content of the curriculum can be presented from a number of perspectives:

- subjects or disciplines (a traditional curriculum)
- body systems, e.g. the cardiovascular system (an integrated curriculum)
- the life cycle, e.g. childhood, adulthood, old age
- problems (a problem-based curriculum)
- clinical presentations or tasks (a scenario-based, case-based or task-based curriculum).

These are not mutually exclusive; grids can be prepared which look at the content of a curriculum from two or more of these perspectives.

No account of curriculum content would be complete without reference to 'the hidden curriculum'. The 'declared' curriculum is the curriculum as set out in the institution's documents. The 'taught' curriculum is what happens in practice. The 'learned' curriculum is what is learned by the student. The 'hidden' curriculum is the students' informal learning that is different from what is taught (Fig. 2.2 and see Chapter 7).

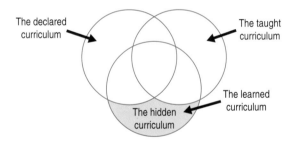

Fig. 2.2 The hidden curriculum

ORGANIZING THE CONTENT

An assumption in a traditional medical curriculum was that students should first master the basic and then the applied medical sciences before moving on to study clinical medicine. Too often students failed to see the relevance of what was taught to their future career as doctors, and after they had passed examinations in the basic sciences, they tended to forget or ignore what they had learned.

 "Early experience helps medical students socialise to their chosen profession. It helps them acquire a range of subject matter and makes their learning more real and relevant. It can influence career choices."

Dornan et al 2006

It has been advocated that the curriculum should be turned on its head, with students starting to think like a health professional from the day they enter medical school. Students at Hofstra Medical School, New York spend their first 8 weeks working as paramedics. In a vertically integrated curriculum, students are introduced to clinical medicine alongside the basic sciences in the early years of the programme. The need for students to continue their studies of the basic sciences as applied to clinical medicine in the later years is now recognized. In a final portfolio assessment, students at Dundee Medical School, for example, are expected to interpret the clinical cases they document in the context of an understanding of the basic sciences.

A spiral curriculum (Fig. 2.3) offers a useful approach to the organization of content (Harden & Stamper 1999). In a spiral curriculum:

- there is iterative revisiting of topics throughout the course
- topics are revisited at different levels of difficulty
- new learning is related to previous learning
- the competence of students increases with each visit to a topic.

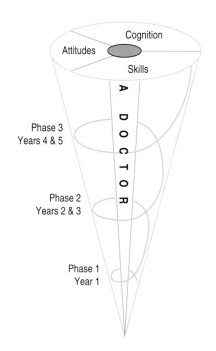

Fig. 2.3 A spiral curriculum

DECIDING THE EDUCATIONAL STRATEGY

 In planning a curriculum, ask teachers to identify where they think they are at present on each continuum in the SPICES model and where they would like to go.

Much discussion and controversy in medical education has related to education strategies. The SPICES model (Fig. 2.4) offers a useful tool for planning a new curriculum or evaluating an existing one (Harden et al 1984). It represents each strategy as a continuum, avoiding the polarizing of opinion and acknowledging that schools may vary in their approach.

Student-centred	Teacher-centred
Problem-based	Information-oriented
Integrated or interprofessional	Subject or discipline-based
Community-based	Hospital-based
Elective-driven	Uniform
Systematic	Opportunistic

Fig. 2.4 SPICES model of educational strategies

Student-centred learning

In student-centred learning, students are given more responsibility for their own education. What the student learns matters, rather than what is taught. This is discussed further in Chapter 19 on independent learning. It is now appreciated that the teacher has an important role as facilitator of learning and that the student should not be abandoned and needs some sort of guidance and support.

With a greater understanding of how students learn and with advances in learning techniques we will see a move to an adaptive curriculum, where the content and the teaching and learning methods and strategies are tailored to the personal needs of the individual learner. Students will spend different amounts of time studying a unit depending on their learning needs. Each student's mastery of the learning outcomes should be assessed before the end of the course, and at a time when further study can be arranged depending on the student's needs.

Problem-based learning (PBL)

PBL is a seductive approach to medical education which, as described in Chapter 20, continues to attract attention. Digital technologies can be used to present the problem or as a source of information to guide the student's learning. PBL is used not only with students working in small groups but also in the context of large groups, in individualized learning or with students working at a distance. Eleven steps can be recognized in the PBL continuum between information-orientated and problem-based/task-based learning (Harden & Davis 1998).

In task-based learning (TBL) the learning is focused on a series of tasks which the doctor may be expected to undertake, such as the management of a patient with abdominal pain. TBL is a useful approach to integration and PBL in clinical clerkships (Harden et al 2000).

 "TBL offers an attractive combination of pragmatism and idealism: pragmatism in the sense that learning with an explicit sense of purpose is seen as an important source of student motivation and satisfaction; idealism in that it is consonant with current theories of education."

Harden et al 1996

Integration and interprofessional learning

During the last two decades there has been a move away from structuring the curriculum around basic sciences and medical disciplines. Integrated teaching is now a standard feature of many curricula. It is discussed further in Chapter 22. Eleven steps on a continuum between discipline-based and integrated teaching have been described (Harden 2000).

There is a move to interprofessional teaching where integrated teaching and learning involving the different healthcare professions occur and where students look at a subject from the perspective of other professions as well as their own (Hammick et al 2007). This is discussed further in Chapter 23.

Community-based learning

 "Clinical learning sites may include mental health services, long-term care facilities and family practice clinics, as well as hospitals and health services in remote, rural and urban communities."

Kelly 2011

There are strong educational and logistical arguments for placing less emphasis on a hospital-based programme and more emphasis on the community as a context for student learning. Many curricula are now community orientated, with students spending 10% or more of their time in the community. This is discussed further in Chapters 13 and 14.

 Consider when planning the curriculum which learning outcomes can be achieved more readily in a community-based attachment. Examples may be coping with uncertainty and health promotion.

Community-based clerkships are now more closely integrated into the curriculum as a planned learning experience.

Electives

 "The elective is a traditional and much enjoyed part of most medical courses."

Bullimore 1998

Electives and student selected components (SSCs) are now firmly established as a valued component of the curriculum in many medical schools. They have moved from being a fringe event to an important educational activity that contributes to the expected exit learning outcomes.

It is no longer possible for students to study in depth all topics in a curriculum. Electives or SSCs provide students with the opportunity to study areas of interest to them, while at the same time developing skills in critical appraisal, self-assessment and time management.

Systematic approach

An opportunistic approach, where in the classroom teachers teach what is of interest to them and in the clinical setting students focus their learning on the patients that happen to be available, is no longer appropriate.

A more systematic approach to curriculum planning is necessary to ensure that students have learning experiences that match the expected learning outcomes and that the core curriculum includes the competences essential for medical practice.

 Think of the curriculum as a planned educational experience.

A range of paper and electronic methods can be used to record encounters students have with patients, and the records can then be analysed to see if there are gaps or deficiencies in the students' experiences.

The future will see greater use made of curriculum maps, where the students' progress through the curriculum is charted across the learning experiences, the assessments and the learning outcomes.

CHOOSING THE TEACHING METHODS

There is no panacea, no magic answer to teaching. A good teacher facilitates the students' learning by making use of a range of methods and applying each method for the use to which it is most appropriate. Chapters in this book describe the tools available in the teacher's toolkit:

- The lecture and whole-class teaching remain powerful tools if used properly. They need not be passive, and their role is more than one of information transfer.
- Small-group work facilitates interaction between students and makes possible cooperative learning, with students learning from each other. Small-group work is usually an important element in problem-based learning.
- Independent learning can make an important contribution. Students master the area being studied, while at the same time they develop the ability to work on their own and to take responsibility for their own learning.

 There is no holy grail of instructional wizardry which will provide a solution to all teaching problems. The teacher's toolkit should contain a variety of approaches, each with its strengths and weaknesses.

A significant development in recent years has been the application of new learning technologies including simulation and e-learning (Ellaway & Masters 2008). Computers may be used as a source of information, to present interactive patient simulations, to facilitate and manage learning and to support collaborative or peer-to-peer learning.

 "The move from desktop PCs to laptops, smart phones and tablets has increased the possibilities of learning closer to clinical patient experience, so called 'near patient learning' where students can access learning resources just prior to, or just after seeing and interacting with patients."

Roberts 2012

Teaching and learning experiences can be rated in terms of:

- authenticity, with theoretical approaches at one end of the spectrum and real-life ones at the other
- formality, with different levels of formality and informality.

Teaching situations can be located in each quadrant of the formality/authenticity grid (see Fig. 2.5).

PREPARING THE ASSESSMENT

Student assessment is a key component of the curriculum and is addressed in Section 6 of this book.

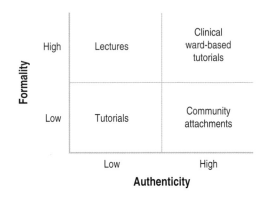

Fig. 2.5 Teaching situations

The significant effect that examinations have on student learning is well documented.

 "I believe that teaching without testing is like cooking without tasting."

Ian Lang, former Scottish Secretary

Issues that should be addressed in assessment include:

- What should be assessed?
  - A grid or blueprint should be prepared relating the assessment to the specific learning outcomes. This should include knowledge, skills and attitudes.
- How should it be assessed?
  Methods should include:
  - a written approach such as multiple-choice questions (MCQs) or constructed response questions
  - a performance assessment such as an Objective Structured Clinical Examination (OSCE)
  - a collection of evidence such as in a portfolio.
- What are the aims of the assessment process?
  Aims may include:
  - to pass or fail the student
  - to grade the student
  - to provide the student and teacher with feedback
  - to motivate the student
  - to support the learning. There is a move from 'assessment of learning' to 'assessment for learning' and 'assessment as learning'.
- When should students be assessed?
  Students can be assessed:
  - at the beginning of the course to assess what they already know or can do

○ during the course as formative assessment

○ at the end of the course to assess their achievement of the expected learning outcomes.

- Who should assess the student?

  ○ Depending on the context, the responsibility may rest with a national or international body, the medical school, the teachers or student peers

  ○ Increasing attention should be paid to self-assessment, with students encouraged to assess their own competence.

COMMUNICATION ABOUT THE CURRICULUM

Failure of communication between teacher and student is a common problem in medical education (Fig. 2.6).

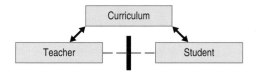

Fig. 2.6 Failure in communication

Teachers have the responsibility to ensure that students have a clear understanding of:

- what they should be learning – the learning outcomes
- their access to the range of learning experiences and opportunities available
- how they can match the available learning experiences to their own personal needs
- whether they have mastered the topic or not, and if not, what further studies and experiences are required.

 Failure to keep staff and students informed about the curriculum is a common recipe for failure.

Communication can be improved by providing students with:

- a clear statement of the learning outcomes expected at each stage of the curriculum
- a curriculum map which matches the learning outcomes to the learning experiences and the assessment
- an electronic or print-based study guide which helps the students to manage their learning and make the best use of their time.

PROMOTING AN APPROPRIATE EDUCATIONAL ENVIRONMENT

The educational environment or 'climate' is a key aspect of the curriculum (Genn 2001). It is less tangible than the content studied, the teaching methods used or the examinations. It is nonetheless of equal importance.

 Measurement of the education environment should be part of a curriculum evaluation

There is little point in developing a curriculum where an aim is to orientate the student to medicine in the community and to health promotion if the students perceive that what is valued by the senior teachers is hospital practice, curative medicine and research. In the same way, it is difficult to develop in students a spirit of teamwork and collaboration if the environment in the medical school is a competitive rather than a collaborative one.

Tools to assess the educational environment such as the Dundee Ready Education Environment Measure (DREEM) are available.

 "The educational climate is the soul and spirit of the medical curriculum."

Genn 2001

MANAGING THE CURRICULUM

Attention to curriculum management has become more important with

- increasing complexity of the curriculum including integrated and interdisciplinary teaching
- increasing pressures on staff with regard to their clinical duties, teaching responsibilities and research commitments
- distributed learning on different sites
- increased demands and increased student numbers at a time of financial constraints
- changes in the healthcare system and medical practice
- increasing demands for accountability.

In the context of undergraduate medical schools, it is likely that:

- responsibilities and resources for teaching will be at a faculty rather than departmental level
- an undergraduate medical education committee will be responsible for planning and implementing the curriculum
- a teaching dean or director of undergraduate medical education will be appointed who has a

commitment to curriculum development and implementation

- staff will be appointed with particular expertise in curriculum planning, teaching methods and assessment to support work on the curriculum
- time and contributions made by staff to teaching will be recognized
- a staff development programme will be a requirement for all staff
- an independent group will have responsibility for academic standards and quality assurance.

There are similar requirements with respect to postgraduate education.

 Consider which of the approaches to curriculum design described is dominant in your curriculum.

A number of approaches to the management of curriculum development can be recognized (Harden 1986):

- *The architect approach.* The emphasis is on the plans, with a clear statement of expected learning outcomes.
- *The mechanic approach.* The emphasis is on the teaching methods and educational strategies. There is more concern about how the curriculum is working than where it is going. The educational strategy may itself become the goal of the curriculum rather than a means to an end.
- *The cookbook approach.* Consideration is given to the details of the content and how much of each component or ingredient is included. The emphasis is on the individual components rather than on the overall curriculum, where the whole should be greater than the sum of the parts.
- *The railway timetable approach.* The emphasis is on the timetable, what courses are held and when, and the duration of each course. This simplistic view of curriculum planning ignores many of the real challenges facing medical education.

A final word: in any major curriculum revision, don't expect to get it right first time. The curriculum will continue to evolve and will need to change in response to local circumstances and to changes in medicine.

 "A little known fact is that the Apollo moon missions were on course less than 1% of the time. The mission was composed of almost constant mid-course corrections."

Belasco 1996

Summary

The development of a teaching programme can no longer be left to chance. A curriculum must be carefully planned. Ten questions need to be addressed. These relate to the following:

1. The needs the training programme is intended to fulfil
2. The expected student learning outcomes
3. The content included
4. The organization of the content including the sequence in which it is covered
5. The educational strategies adopted – integrated teaching is an example
6. The teaching methods used, including large-group teaching, small-group teaching and the use of new learning technologies
7. Assessment of the students' progress
8. Communication about the curriculum to all the stakeholders including the students
9. The educational environment
10. Management of the curriculum.

References

Cooke M, Irby DM, O'Brien BC: *Educating Physicians: A Call for Reform of Medical Schools and Residency*, San Francisco, 2010, Jossey-Bass.

Dornan T, Littlewood S, Margolis SA, et al: How can experience in clinical and community settings contribute to early medical education? A BEME systematic review. BEME Guide No 6, *Medical Teacher* 28:3–18, 2006.

Dunn WR, Hamilton DD, Harden RM: Techniques of identifying competencies needed by doctors, *Medical Teacher* 7(1):15–25, 1985.

Ellaway R, Masters K: AMEE Guide 32: e-Learning in medical education Part 1: Learning, teaching and assessment, *Medical Teacher* 30:455–473, 2008.

Frenk J, Chen L, Bhutta ZA, et al: Health professionals for a new century: transforming education to strengthen health systems in an interdependent world, *The Lancet* 376:1923–1958, 2010.

Genn JM: *AMEE Medical Education Guide no. 23. Curriculum, environment, climate, quality and change in medical education – a unifying perspective*, Dundee, 2001, AMEE.

Hammick M, Freeth D, Koppel I, et al: A best evidence systematic review of inter-professional education: BEME Guide no. 9, *Medical Teacher* 29:735–751, 2007.

Harden RM: Approaches to curriculum planning. ASME Medical Education Booklet no 21, *Medical Education* 20:458–466, 1986a.

Harden RM: Ten questions to ask when planning a course or curriculum, *Medical Education* 20:356–365, 1986b.

Harden RM: The integration ladder: a tool for curriculum planning and evaluation, *Medical Education* 34:551–557, 2000.

Harden RM: Outcome-based education: the future is today, *Medical Teacher* 29:625–629, 2007.

Harden RM, Crosby JR, Davis MH, et al: Task-based learning: the answer to integration and problem-based learning in the clinical years, *Medical Education* 34:391–397, 2000.

Harden RM, Davis MH: The continuum of problem-based learning, *Medical Teacher* 20(4):301–306, 1998.

Harden RM, Sowden S, Dunn WR: Some educational strategies in curriculum development: the SPICES model, *Medical Education* 18:284–297, 1984.

Harden RM, Stamper N: What is a spiral curriculum? *Medical Teacher* 21(2):141–143, 1999.

The undergraduate curriculum and clinical teaching in the early years

S. Leinster

Introduction

The aim of the undergraduate medical curriculum according to the General Medical Council is to produce graduates who

> ... will make the care of patients their first concern, applying their knowledge and skills in a competent and ethical manner and using their ability to provide leadership and to analyse complex and uncertain situations.
>
> GMC 2009, paragraph 7

The challenge for the medical teacher is designing and implementing a curriculum that will achieve this aim in the limited time that is available for the undergraduate component of medical studies. A narrow focus on the knowledge content of the course will fail to instil the attitudes and skills that are essential for an effective professional. While there is a correlation between knowledge and clinical performance, the two are not identical. It is now recognized that the ability to apply knowledge appropriately is the important measure. The emphasis should be on 'what can the student do?' rather than 'what does the student know?' (Corbett & Whitcomb 2004).

Following the Flexner Report in 1910, the conventional medical undergraduate curriculum had two distinct phases. In the preclinical phase the students learnt the basic science underlying medical practice and had little contact with patients. During the clinical phase, most learning took place in clinical placements or clerkships with little input from the basic sciences. Over the last 20 years there has been increasing emphasis on early clinical experience (Dornan et al 2006). The proponents of clinical teaching in the early years suggest at least three benefits from the early encounters with patients.

The first is motivation of the students (von Below et al 2008). Meeting patients and clinical practitioners reinforces the students' underlying ambition to become a doctor (Dyrbye et al 2007). This intrinsic motivation will lead to more effective learning than the extrinsic motivation that arises from the need to pass examinations in order to progress to the next stage of training (Williams et al 1999).

The second benefit is the provision of a clinical context for the learning of basic science. This contextualization of knowledge is important for the future retrieval and application of that knowledge (Schmidt 1983). Vertical integration leads to deep rather than superficial learning (Dahle et al 2002). The third benefit is that early clinical experience can increase the time that is available for students to practise their clinical and communication skills. Areas that the students find challenging (such as taking a history from a patient with communication difficulties) can be revisited. Since facility with any skill is related to the amount of purposeful practice that is undertaken (Ericsson 2004), the students should graduate with a greater level of proficiency in their basic interactions with patients.

In addition, clinical teaching in the early years plays an important part in the socialization of students into the medical profession (Dornan & Bundy 2004). It provides early acclimatization to a clinical setting and may avoid the problems associated with transition into the clinical years (Prince et al 2000). It may allow identification of those few students who are unsuited to clinical medicine at a much earlier stage.

However, while clinical teaching in the early years appears to benefit students, it can cause stress for staff who encounter it for the first time (von Below et al 2008).

Early clinical experience can take place within a wide variety of settings. While the majority takes place in community health settings, some is based in hospitals. A few involve nonclinical settings such as schools, voluntary organizations or community groups. The setting depends on the specific learning outcomes that are intended from the experience. There is no evidence from the literature that any one approach is best.

Any form of integration within the curriculum raises challenges as to who owns the curriculum.

Traditionally, each discipline or department was responsible for the selection of material and the delivery of teaching within its own domain. This can lead to a number of abuses including overloading of the curriculum, the teaching of irrelevant material and uncoordinated rather than planned repetition. For this reason, there has been a move towards centralization of curriculum planning with a single body being responsible for the final product, albeit in consultation with the relevant discipline experts.

Centralized curriculum planning can lead to the disengagement of most teachers, who may feel that what they are being asked to teach conveys at best an inadequate, and at worst an inaccurate, picture of their discipline. It is important that the teachers who are to deliver the curriculum should feel that they have a stake in it. This is one reason why it is less than ideal to import a curriculum that has been developed elsewhere.

Consensus planning allows the wider community of teachers to be involved. A multidisciplinary group agrees on the content of the curriculum through a process of discussion and compromise. The level at which the content is pitched is more likely to be realistic as the specialists' views are immediately tested against those of their colleagues. The wider community of potential teachers should comment on the results of these discussions. The process of discussion and review should continue until a broad consensus is reached. It is particularly important that generalists should be included in the review process, as they are best placed to assess the utility of the decisions.

At this stage it is helpful to have input from the public and from future employers. The roles of health professionals are undergoing rapid change and the competencies expected of a doctor in the future are unpredictable. Medicine exists to meet community needs for healthcare. Discussion with the community will inform the planning.

Curriculum planning

The curriculum encompasses learning methods, assessment methods, resources and timetabling in addition to content. Traditionally, much effort has gone into identifying the content while the learning methods have been assumed. As the awareness of different learning approaches has grown, the temptation has been to concentrate on learning methods to the relative detriment of content. Medical schools are labelled by their predominant teaching methods, for example, as problem based, systems based, community based or traditional. However, medical education is a preparation for practice rather than a purely intellectual exercise, and it is arguable that there must be a minimum essential content. If an effective

Table 3.1 The scope of curriculum planning	
Content	What knowledge, skills and attitudes should the course cover? What are the learning outcomes of the course?
Delivery	How will the learning be delivered? What teaching or learning methods will be used?
Assessment	How will the students' learning be tested?
Structure	How will the content be organized? How will learning and teaching be scheduled?
Resources	What staff, learning materials, equipment and accommodation are needed?
Evaluation	How will the organizers know that the course has been effective in delivering the learning outcomes?

curriculum is to be created, all areas must receive careful attention (Table 3.1).

Defining the content

AIMS AND OBJECTIVES

When approaching curriculum planning there is a temptation to assume that there is a shared understanding of the aims of the programme, but unless the meaning of the aims is made explicit misunderstandings will arise. The terms that are employed must be defined and must be specific. It is unhelpful to have the stated aim of 'producing a good doctor'. This begs the question of how a good doctor is to be defined.

 The curriculum needs to define the learning outcome, the setting in which it should be performed and the standard to which it should be performed.

CORE MATERIAL

Given the continuing expansion of medical knowledge, it is clearly impossible for students to learn all that there is to know. It is now widely accepted that there should be a core of knowledge that all students must acquire while encouraging them to develop deeper knowledge in selected areas that are of interest to them as individuals. The challenge has been how to identify the core knowledge.

 The core curriculum should reflect the consensus views of specialists and generalists. Specialists should not be permitted to determine the core curriculum in their own discipline.

Table 3.2 Cognitive processes in Bloom's revised taxonomy for knowledge and descriptors of outcome

Bloom's taxonomy	Meaning	Outcome descriptors
Remember	Retrieving relevant material from long-term memory	Recognize, recall
Understand	Determining the meaning of instructional messages, including oral, written and graphic communications	Interpret, exemplify, classify, summarize, infer, compare, explain
Apply	Carrying out or using a procedure in a given situation	Execute, implement
Analyse	Breaking material into its constituent parts and detecting how the parts relate to one another and to an overall structure or purpose	Differentiate, organize, attribute
Evaluate	Making judgements based on criteria and standards	Check, critique
Create	Putting elements together to form a novel, coherent whole or make an original product	Generate, plan, produce

After Krathwohl 2001.

There are a number of possible solutions. Some specialties could be considered optional. There are problems with this, as some common or important conditions may fall within the province of 'optional' specialties. The opposite approach is to ask each specialty to identify its own core material. This gives rise to practical problems, as the core identified in this way is too large to fit into a standard undergraduate programme. An approach that has been adopted by a number of medical schools is the identification of index cases or presentations that are based on the different ways in which the population comes into contact with healthcare professionals. The core knowledge that students need within each discipline is determined by what they need to know in order to understand and manage these core clinical problems. The cases may be identified from published health statistics or may be based on consensus among experienced practitioners. The list may vary from school to school depending on the patterns of practice around that school, but there is considerable overlap among the lists, suggesting that a realistic core is being identified (Bligh 1995, Mandin et al 1995, O'Neill 1999).

LEARNING OUTCOMES

The core defines the scope of the curriculum. The next step is to define what it is that the student needs to learn about the core. The most effective way to do this is to define learning outcomes for the course. These clearly express what the student will be able to do at the end of the course. When an entire course of 4–6 years is being considered the outcomes will, necessarily, be very broad. As smaller and smaller components of the course are considered, the outcomes become more and more focused and specific. The detailed outcomes for each component should map on to the overall outcomes (GMC 2009, Simpson et al 2002).

DOMAINS OF LEARNING

The Quality Assurance Agency recognizes four domains in higher education in which outcomes should be defined: knowledge and understanding, generic skills, cognitive skills and subject-specific skills (QAA 2004). In medical education a fifth domain is important, that of attitudes and professional development.

Within the knowledge and skills domains there is a hierarchy of outcomes which map on to the 'cognitive process' dimension in Bloom's revised taxonomy (Table 3.2; Krathwohl 2001). The attainment of each level assumes the attainment of the lower levels. The level which the students are expected to attain is specified by the descriptors used in the outcome. It is generally accepted that an adequate curriculum will be defined in terms of the higher levels of the taxonomy; there are few situations where remembering would be regarded as an adequate outcome.

Although Bloom recognized the psychomotor domain in addition to the cognitive and affective domains, he did not produce a taxonomy for it. However, a similar grid can be produced that can be used to define the learning outcomes in relation to skills that the student must acquire. This grid is commonly expressed in the form of Miller's triangle (Fig. 3.1) with the outcome levels ranging from 'knows how' to 'mastery'.

 The specificity of the learning outcome depends on the component of the course to which it applies. For the whole course, the learning outcome on prescription might be 'Write safe prescriptions for different types of drugs'. For an individual teaching session on the control of pain in chronic musculoskeletal disease, it might be 'Write a safe prescription for a common nonsteroidal anti-inflammatory drug in an elderly patient'.

The curriculum planner must specify which skills are necessary and to what level each should be displayed.

FURTHER ELEMENTS OF LEARNING OUTCOMES

So far, we have considered learning outcomes in terms of what the student can do. It is equally important to define the conditions in which the student can be expected to perform the task. Students qualifying from a medical school in the UK are required by law to start work in a closely supervised environment as Foundation Year 1 doctors. It is reasonable to define some of their learning outcomes as the ability to perform the task under close supervision. However, some tasks (such as emergency resuscitation) require the doctor to act independently, as he or she may be the first on the scene. The learning outcomes for resuscitation should specify that the student will perform competently without direct supervision. The conditions may also include the setting in which the student should be able to perform. The ability to manage a patient with a specific illness in a hospital ward may be different from the ability to manage the same condition in the community or presenting as an emergency in the accident and emergency department.

A third element is the standard to which the student will fulfil the learning outcome. This is the most difficult part of setting learning outcomes and the area where there is the most controversy. *Tomorrow's Doctors* (GMC 2009) specifies learning outcomes such as 'Be able to perform clinical and practical skills safely'. There is still enormous scope for debate on how this should be interpreted.

In practical terms this decision is taken by defining the nature and standard of the assessments that are set.

Delivery of the curriculum

In parallel with determining the content of the curriculum, decisions must be taken about how it will be delivered. While there is debate over which learning methods are the most effective and efficient, there are some established principles that should be taken into account. It is clear that knowledge is applied most effectively when it is learnt in the context in which it is to be applied. It is also accepted that active learning is more effective than passive learning (Schmidt 1983). However, a wide range of learning methods can meet these conditions.

Both traditional lecture-based courses and courses based on small-group, problem-based learning (PBL) produce effective medical practitioners (Schmidt et al 2006). The evidence for any difference in knowledge outcomes between traditional and problem-based courses is weak (Hartling et al 2010). However, there are differences in other outcomes (Albanese & Xakellis 2001, O'Neill et al 2003, Watmough et al 2006). The choice of methods for a given curriculum will depend on the range of outcomes that have been chosen. It is important that the outcomes determine the methods and not the other way round. In general, the use of a mixture of methods is likely to be more efficient than a doctrinaire adherence to a single method.

 The learning methods to be employed should be determined by the desired outcomes.

Assessment

Whatever the stated aims and objectives of the course, the students' perceptions of what is important will be determined by what is assessed and how the assessment is carried out (Newble & Jaeger 1983). The assessment policy and the detailed methods should form an important part of the curriculum planning process. A good case can be made for beginning the planning process by planning the assessment before planning the teaching. Certainly, the assessment should not be an afterthought.

Outcomes are defined in terms of actions. It follows that an outcome is valid only if the action can be observed and therefore assessed. Although 'knowledge' and 'understanding' are major levels in Bloom's taxonomy, 'know' and 'understand' are not useful terms as outcomes. The outcome descriptors in Table 3.2 are much more useful, as they define how the outcome could be tested. Thus knowledge can be tested by asking the student to recall something, and understanding can be tested by asking the student to explain or compare something.

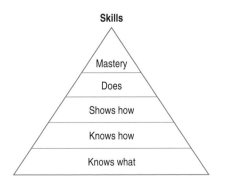

Fig. 3.1 Miller's skills triangle

The outcomes relating to skills are measured against Miller's classification. While the highest level of outcome is 'mastery', the highest level that it is practicable to assess is 'showing how'. Some argue that examinations conducted using simulated patients are equivalent to 'doing', but they do not measure how the candidate behaves when not being observed. For undergraduate training this is probably adequate, but for postgraduate training and continuing education it is not. Evidence that an individual has attained mastery or even that he or she regularly 'does' the relevant skill can only be inferred indirectly from such things as clinical records and audits (see Chapter 38, Performance and workplace assessment).

Outcomes relating to attitudes are even more difficult to assess. The use of self-reporting questionnaires may be biased by students giving the 'correct' or 'expected' answer rather than revealing what they really feel. Observed behaviour can act as a surrogate for attitude. For this reason, attitudinal outcomes may be written in terms of observed behaviour. Professionalism is increasingly seen as an essential component of assessment and is closely linked to assessment of behaviours. Longitudinal reports from a range of observers are more reliable than point observations.

 Planning the assessment should be an integral part of planning the curriculum.

Curriculum structure

The organization of students' learning is an important part of planning. Traditionally, teaching was organized according to disciplinary boundaries. There was usually a very marked divide between the subjects that were considered to be clinical and those that were preclinical. This made it very difficult to teach material in context and led to compartmentalization of knowledge, as illustrated in Fig. 3.2. Both horizontal and vertical integration are needed.

Horizontal integration has been achieved by replacing discipline-based teaching with system-based teaching. The focus has been moved from subjects such as anatomy or physiology to body systems such as the cardiovascular system or the digestive system. All of the relevant basic science is taught at the same time. This can take place with a preclinical/clinical divide or can be combined with vertical integration.

Vertical integration implies that clinical methods and science are taught at the same time as the basic science. This may be organized on the basis of body systems or as a number of 'vertical themes' that run through all the years of the curriculum. Often these vertical themes are related to generic professional skills and attitudes that are pertinent to all areas of medical practice such as clinical or communication

skills. The commonest form of vertical integration involves the early introduction of clinical contact in the course. As time goes on, the amount of clinical contact increases and the amount of basic science reduces. This has been described as an 'inverted triangles' curriculum (Fig. 3.3).

Some schools have gone further and have equal proportions of basic science and clinical contact throughout the course (Fig. 3.4).

Whatever the formal structure of the course, integration can only take place at the level of the students' experience of learning. Different approaches to achieving integration have been used with varying degrees of success. The most basic approach is to schedule within the same time frame lectures on the same system from the different disciplines. While this is relatively simple, any integration is largely a matter

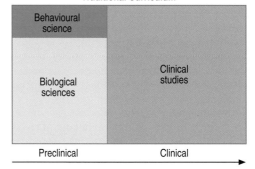

Fig. 3.2 The traditional curriculum

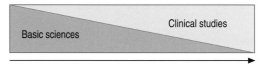

Fig. 3.3 The 'inverted triangles' curriculum model

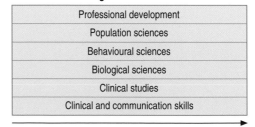

Fig. 3.4 The total integration model

of chance. For integration to occur, the scope and content of the lectures must be coordinated by an overseeing committee. Attempts have been made to have totally integrated lectures delivered by two or more individuals from different disciplines. These can be very effective if sufficient effort is put into planning and preparation. They do not work if the teachers prepare independently and meet up only to deliver the session.

Case-based curricula attempt to overcome the problems of integration by focusing learning around a series of clinical cases. As the students develop an understanding of the range of material relevant to the case, they are led to integrate this knowledge for themselves.

ORDERING

An important part of curriculum planning is determination of the order in which the learning outcomes will be delivered. There is no absolutely correct order, but there should be a transparent logic behind the arrangement. This will enable students to appreciate the relevance of particular learning outcomes and diminish the tendency to learn inefficiently by rote just because the topic has been placed in the curriculum and will be assessed.

 The curriculum should have a logical and transparent structure.

An effective structure will avoid needless duplication of material but will allow revisiting and reinforcement. Topics are first introduced at a simple level. Later in the course they will be studied in more depth and breadth. A common approach is to start with normality then move on to abnormality. Subjects may be revisited on several occasions. Harden and colleagues (1997) have described this as a 'spiral curriculum'. This spiral approach can take place within any of the previous models of curricular structure.

RESOURCES

Curriculum planning must consider the resources needed to deliver the curriculum. A lecture-based curriculum will need lecture halls large enough to hold an entire class at one time. Laboratory-based practicals will need teaching laboratory space. A curriculum based on small-group work will need a sufficient number of tutorial rooms.

Clinical placements are often a major constraint on curriculum planning. The number of patients willing to participate in teaching and suitable for the purpose is limited and will inevitably affect the structure of the planned course.

The greatest resource constraint is associated with the teaching staff. PBL and other small-group teaching results in greater staff–student contact time, and from this it has been deduced that this form of teaching must be more expensive. On the other hand, many forms of PBL do not use expert tutors and teaching staff can be deployed with greater efficiency, as they are not restricted to delivering a comparatively few teaching sessions on their own discipline. Whatever the theoretical considerations, a number of medical schools have introduced PBL without any increase in resources.

Any innovation within the curriculum will require preparation of the teachers, especially when any form of integration is involved. It is important that teachers are well informed about the curriculum, the educational rationale for it and their own role within it.

Evaluation

Every educational endeavour should be evaluated. Designing the evaluation strategy is an important part of overall curriculum planning. The evaluation should cover outcome as well as process, although evaluation of the latter is easier to achieve. The process evaluation should encompass the views of the students, the teachers and the administrative staff and should take place in such a way that rapid intervention and correction of faults can take place. Outcome evaluation is by necessity a much slower undertaking. There is likely to be a close relationship between the assessment process and the evaluation of outcomes. It is important that this linkage is prospective and incorporated in the overall design of the curriculum rather than being an afterthought.

 The plans for evaluation should be made while the curriculum is being planned.

Summary

Planning is essential for the development of any successful curriculum. The first stage is to define the aims and objectives of the programme. The core content is then specified in terms of learning outcomes. Once the content is defined, the modes of delivery have to be decided. A mixture of methods is likely to be better than adherence on principle to a single approach. Assessment is a major component of the curriculum, and the approach to assessment should be developed in parallel with the other aspects of the curriculum. A clear structure should be developed which ideally should include early clinical teaching. The necessary resources need to be identified and the staff thoroughly inducted into the rationale and implementation of the proposed curriculum. Finally, evaluation of the curriculum should be planned prospectively.

References

Albanese MA, Xakellis GC: Building collegiality: the real value of problem-based learning, *Medical Education* 35:1143, 2001.

Bligh J: Identifying the core curriculum: the Liverpool approach, *Medical Teacher* 17:383–390, 1995.

Corbett EC, Whitcomb ME: *The AAMC project on the clinical education of medical students: Clinical Skills Education*, AAMC, Washington DC, 2004.

Dahle LO, Brynhildsen J, Behrbohm Fallsberg M, et al: Pros and cons of vertical integration between clinical medicine and basic science within a problem-based undergraduate medical curriculum: examples and experiences from Linköping, *Sweden Medical Teacher* 24:280–285, 2002.

Dornan T, Bundy C: What can experience add to early medical education? Consensus survey, *BMJ* 329:834–837, 2004.

Dornan T, Littlewood S, Margolis S, et al: How can experience in clinical and community settings contribute to early medical education? A BEME Systematic Review, *Medical Teacher* 28:3–18, 2006.

Dyrbye LN, Harris I, Rohren CH: Early clinical experiences from students' perspectives: a qualitative study of narratives, *Academic Medicine* 82:979–988, 2007.

Ericsson KA: Deliberate practice and the acquisition and maintenance of expert performance in medicine and related domains, *Academic Medicine* 79:S70–S81, 2004.

General Medical Council: *Tomorrow's doctors*, ed 3, London, 2009, General Medical Council.

Harden RM, Davis MH, Crosby JR: The new Dundee medical curriculum: a whole that is greater than the sum of its parts, *Medical Education* 31:264–271, 1997.

Hartling L, Spooner C, Tjosvold L, Oswald A: Problem-based learning in pre-clinical medical education: 22 years of outcome research, *Medical Teacher* 32:28–35 ,2010.

Krathwohl DR. 2001. In Anderson LW, Krathwohl DR, editors: *A taxonomy for learning, teaching and assessing: a revision of Bloom's taxonomy for educational objectives*, New York, 2001, Addison Wesley.

Mandin H, Harasym P, Eagle C, Watanabe M: Developing a 'clinical presentation' curriculum at the University of Calgary, *Academic Medicine* 70:186–193, 1995.

Newble DI, Jaeger K: The effect of assessment and examinations on the learning of medical students, *Medical Education* 17:165–171, 1983.

O'Neill PA: The core content of the undergraduate curriculum in Manchester, *Medical Education* 33:121–129, 1999.

O'Neill PA, Jones A, Willis SC, McArdle PJ: Does a new undergraduate curriculum based on Tomorrow's Doctors prepare house officers better for their first post? A qualitative study of the views of pre-registration house officers using critical incidents, *Medical Education* 37:1100–1108, 2003.

Prince KJAH, van de Wiel M, Scherpbler AJJA, et al: A qualitative analysis of the transition from theory to practice in undergraduate training in a PBL medical school, *Advances in Health Sciences Education* 5:105–116, 2000.

Quality Assurance Agency for Higher Education: 2004 Online: http://www.qaa.ac.uk.

Schmidt HG: Problem-based learning: rationale and description, *Medical Education* 17:11–16, 1983.

Schmidt HG, Vermeulen L, van der Molen HT: Longterm effects of problem-based learning: a comparison of competencies acquired by graduates of a problem-based and a conventional medical school, *Medical Education* 40:562–567, 2006.

Simpson JG, Furnace J, Crosby J, et al: The Scottish doctor – learning outcomes for the medical undergraduate in Scotland: a foundation for competent and reflective practitioners, *Medical Education* 24:136–143, 2002.

von Below B, Hellquist G, Rödjer S, et al: Medical students' and facilitators' experiences of an Early Professional Contact course: active and motivated students, strained facilitators, *BMC Medical Education* 8:56, 2008.

Watmough S, Taylor D, Garden A: Educational supervisors evaluate the preparedness of graduates from a reformed UK curriculum to work as pre-registration house officers (PRHOs): a qualitative study, *Medical Education* 40:995–1001, 2006.

Williams GC, Saizow RB, Ryan RM: The importance of self determination theory for medical education, *Academic Medicine* 74:992–995, 1999.

Postgraduate training

D. Wall, N. G. Patil

This chapter is about postgraduate medical education and training, once the doctor has already qualified after a variable number of years at medical school and possesses a basic medical qualification. In many UK medical schools, this is a five-year course, although more recently some medical schools have developed a four-year graduate-only entry medical degree course, as is common in North America.

Introduction

TRAINING GRADES IN THE UK

In the UK doctors enter a first (intern) year now called Foundation Year 1. This year provides on-the-job training in a protected and structured environment with regular appraisals and assessments; often now in three posts each of 4 months duration. These are still usually in hospital specialties such as medicine, surgery, paediatrics, obstetrics and gynaecology. This is now followed by Foundation Year 2, with a further three posts of 4 months duration, including a wider range of specialties, including general practice. These general practice posts have proved a great success and are very popular with young doctors.

Following these 2 years, doctors enter specialty training. The time to complete such training varies, from 3 years for general practice to 8 years for some of the surgical specialties. Along the way there are annual assessments and postgraduate examinations to pass.

THE HISTORICAL PERSPECTIVE IN THE UK

In 1968, the Royal Commission on Medical Education (the Todd Report) commented that the organization of postgraduate medical education at that time could be described as 'chaotic'. The recommendations were for a pre-registration year, 3 years of general professional training and specialist training after that to reach career grade posts. The training grades were the pre-registration house officer, the senior house officer and the registrar and senior registrar in the specialist training posts.

In the 1990s, Sir Kenneth Calman proposed a reform of specialist training in the UK. This initiative established structured specialist training leading to a Certificate of Completion of Specialist Training (CCST) after a defined number of years of training (between 4 and 6 years), annual assessments and a final assessment. Such doctors were now to be called specialist registrars.

In 2003, The Department of Health began the *Modernising Medical Careers* movement and established Foundation Year 1 and Foundation Year 2 grades of doctor, and specialty registrars. A new UK-wide appointments process, the *Medical Training Application Scheme* (MTAS), was set up to go with it, and thus began one of the most disastrous episodes in UK medical education. The whole system did not work, and it left in its wake many thousands of disillusioned young doctors.

In 2007, following the MTAS debacle, Professor John Tooke was invited to report on the state of postgraduate medical education and make appropriate recommendations. He recommended that doctors should serve a 1-year pre-registration Foundation Year 1, then a period of core specialty training in a small number of specialty stems (medical, surgical, family medicine) and then further training in higher specialist training posts (and be called once again specialist registrars or GP registrars). His comments in the Tooke Reports of 2007 and 2008 sound remarkably like those of the earlier Todd Report of 1968.

UK medical and dental education has been regarded as one of the best systems in the world, but, with various changes recently, we have run into greater and greater difficulties. In 1996 the English Department of Health made a move to make postgraduate deans and regional advisers into civil servants and, later, NHS employees of the Strategic Health Authorities. This has led the Tooke Report to comment that '… the management and governance of the postgraduate deanery function in England is complex with little relationship to medical schools ...' (Tooke Report 2008). Strategic Health Authorities will be abolished in England in 2013, leaving the postgraduate deaneries with an uncertain future.

INTERNATIONAL PERSPECTIVE

Postgraduate medical education has become an issue of global significance, appeal and dimensions. While postgraduate educational opportunities in western countries are much sought after by doctors in the rest of the world, many doctors from western nations are equally eager to gain clinical experience working outside their countries. There is also increasing internationalization of the medical workforce following regional and international free trade agreements such as those implemented by the European Union (EU). The National Advice Centre for Postgraduate Medical Education (NACPME) at the British Council provides information to overseas-qualified doctors on postgraduate medical education and training in the UK.

In 2003, the World Federation for Medical Education (WFME) published a comprehensive document titled 'Postgraduate medical education – WFME global standards for quality improvement'. This publication provides a timely reminder in formulating the postgraduate medical curriculum; taking into account needs of individual countries, as well as of the region and the available human and material resources.

Fundamentals of postgraduate medical education

Doctors go on to develop their competencies and capabilities following the completion of their basic medical qualification. This phase of training is usually conducted in accordance with specified regulations and rules. Similarly to an apprenticeship, trainee doctors are placed in various clinical settings under the guidance of senior and experienced colleagues who take the responsibility for their instruction and supervision (WFME).

Postgraduate medical education initially involves a pre-registration (intern) year which provides on-the-job training in a protected environment. The aim of this 12-month programme is to ensure that the trainees possess the necessary practical knowledge and skills essential for safe medical practice. Successful completion of this internship allows a graduate to register as a medical practitioner with the relevant medical council or board. Graduates are also entitled to enrol for general practice or family medicine training, specialist and sub- or superspecialist training or for other formalized training programmes for defined expert functions. These are organized by the universities, specialist boards, medical societies and colleges or institutes for postgraduate medical education. This

further training typically lasts for a period of 6 to 8 years.

Internationally, there are considerable variations in the number of recognized specialties and expert functions in medicine as well as in the organization, structure, content and requirements of postgraduate medical education. For example, the Hong Kong Academy of Medicine, with its membership of 15 constituent professional colleges, offers postgraduate training in nearly 50 specialties (www.hkam.org.hk). The common curricular approach of all member colleges, of course, centres on the recognized clinical or practical placements, expert supervision, theoretical teaching, research experience, systematic assessments and evaluation of the training programmes.

Transition from medical student to doctor

In the UK the Foundation Year 1 house officer year is the first year of employment which junior hospital doctors undertake following their 5 years of medical undergraduate training. It is necessary to complete this year to obtain full registration with the General Medical Council.

However, this first year as a doctor is seen by many to be a stressful and difficult year, and people have often expressed the idea that they have been 'thrown in at the deep end' with little idea of what to expect in the working environment as a result of their undergraduate training. To this end, the General Medical Council has required undergraduate medical students to undertake a period of 'shadowing' with a pre-registration house officer as part of their final year. Ideally, this will be in the post in which they will later be working.

 The transition from medical student to doctor is a stressful and difficult transition for many.

In the medical education literature there are several studies which confirm these views. Looking at medical students and young first-year doctors from several medical schools, it appears to be a UK-wide problem. New doctors described their learning of clinical skills as 'haphazard and random' and wanted further training in practical skills and procedures, delegation of tasks and time management. Worryingly, 25% of these doctors were experiencing burnout, measured on the Maslach Burnout Inventory. Lack of preparation as an undergraduate was a problem, with only few competencies listed as showing that the young graduates were more than quite well prepared by their medical school education. Consultant education supervisors rated the young graduates as more than quite competent in only three areas: *awareness of own limitations, keeping accurate records* and *working in a team.* So the undergraduate course had only partially met its objectives in preparing the young graduates for their pre-registration house officer year.

Also, anecdotal evidence from consultants suggests that with the breakdown of the 'firm' structure within hospital practice, the reduction in working hours as a result of the requirements of the European Working Time Directive, and the Terms and Conditions of Service, there is less contact between pre-registration house officer and consultant, and the young doctors are often thought of as less experienced than their predecessors.

In the West Midlands, we studied the young pre-registration house officers and their consultant supervisors to see whether there were differences between how well prepared the pre-registration house officers felt they were and how well the consultants felt they were as a result of their undergraduate medical education. Both groups ranked communication skills areas highest (that is, best prepared) and ranked basic doctoring skills (such as prescribing, treatment, decision making and emergencies) lowest. House officers rated themselves significantly higher than did their consultant supervisors in 13 out of the 17 areas tested (Wall et al 2006).

 Young doctors consistently overestimate their abilities when compared with assessments made of them by their consultant supervisors.

It is not surprising, therefore, that some doctors experience difficulties and may struggle to cope.

CHARACTERISTICS OF POSTGRADUATE EDUCATION

As shown in Fig. 4.1, postgraduate medical training may be summarized as education, exposure and experience leading to expertise, evidence-based practice and excellence.

Postgraduate medicine is a high-stakes education and practice. The ultimate goal in postgraduate medical education has to be that the trainees will, progressively, receive the appropriate clinical exposure to gain the necessary experience required in achieving expertise that allows them to provide a high standard of care in their respective fields. Another chief aim of postgraduate medical education is that the trainee eventually becomes the trainer and goes on to participate in the training of his or her juniors and medical students. The principles of adult learning and the process of structured educational training are both vital in postgraduate medical education with respect to the development of clinical and practical skills. In specialties related to surgery, acquisition of

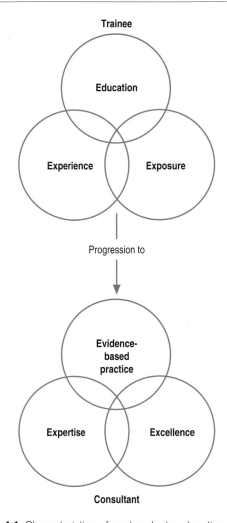

Fig. 4.1 Characteristics of postgraduate education.

practical or operative skills requires additional attention (Patil et al 2003).

 Compassion, communication, care and competence are essential ingredients of successful clinical practice.

The trainee is moving along the continuum from novice to expert, as described by Dreyfus and Dreyfus (2005). These five steps are as follows:

1. Novice
2. Advanced beginner
3. Competent
4. Proficient
5. Expert.

However, it may take some years as a career grade doctor (consultant or general practitioner principal) to achieve real mastery of one's subject. Few may ever reach the next level, after a lifetime's experience, which we have perhaps light-heartedly called the 7th dan.

Standards for training

In the UK, the General Medical Council sets standards for training posts and has required that there be an approved curriculum for the Foundation Programme and for all specialties. Such standards include approved training posts, a curriculum with end point assessments, a named educational supervisor, a protected teaching programme, an induction to the post, regular appraisals, assessments using a range of agreed assessment tools and a balance of appropriate clinical duties and study leave for courses.

CURRICULUM, TEACHING AND LEARNING AND ASSESSMENT – BLUEPRINTING

An important concept in medical education is that the curriculum outcomes should match what is taught and learned, and assessments should also closely match both the teaching and learning and the curriculum. This is what is called blueprinting.

NUTS AND BOLTS OF THE POSTGRADUATE CURRICULUM

Features of a postgraduate training include the following:

- a progressive syllabus that has both formal and informal elements
- a recognized trainer and training unit
- proactive supervision
- balance of clinical duties and educational activities
- protected time for education
- defined exit outcomes.

There has been a marked improvement in provision by the relevant bodies of structured syllabi for most postgraduate medical diploma or degree courses. This is in stark contrast to the days when the syllabus was a 'sea of uncertainty', and trainees felt that the sky was the limit when preparing for their examinations. Nowadays, the various authorities publish, both on their websites and as booklets, clear guidelines on core curriculum and assessment criteria for particular postgraduate specialties (Academy of Medical Royal Colleges, Royal College of Physicians and Surgeons of Canada).

Clinical placements, known as residencies in the United States and as specialty registrar posts in the UK, and other postgraduate training programmes provide trainees with a comprehensive exposure to all areas of clinical practice. Trainees also actively participate in the teaching of medical students and junior colleagues. This contributes significantly to the enhancement of their clinical maturity.

Clinical training lasts for 6–8 years with rotations to a different discipline every 4–6 months. This usually suffices to meet the stipulations of individual colleges with regard to adequate exposure and experience in particular disciplines. The training is further divided into basic and higher specialty training attachments. In most programmes a segment of training, in continuity with clinical attachments or as a dedicated rotation, is devoted to research.

Protected time, to attend structured educational activities such as protected teaching days, case presentations, X-ray meetings or workshops, is regarded as mandatory for all trainees. In practice, however, protected time for educational activities may be encroached upon by clinical commitments unless conscientious efforts are made by trainers and departments to make such time truly protected.

 Conscientious efforts must be made by trainers and programme directors to make 'protected time' truly protected.

Formative and summative assessment

FORMATIVE ASSESSMENT

This is provided in a variety of ways, including the following:

- presentations at ward rounds and grand rounds
- journal reviews
- performance at practical or surgical procedures
- audit of morbidity and mortality
- review of patient records
- mock examinations.

In the postgraduate curriculum, formative assessment to assist trainees in monitoring their progress may not be structured or appreciated as it is in undergraduate medical education. This is mainly because postgraduates are believed to be mature learners who do not need such close scrutiny. This is not always the case! In addition, consultants may consider this commitment as an extra burden in their supervisory roles.

The provision of commentary on the trainee's performance at journal reviews, ward rounds, morbidity and mortality meetings and procedure-related activities is a very useful practical measure. One structured approach that can be used to assess the trainee, the supervisor and the teaching quality of the unit or department is to hold in-house 'mock examinations'.

Here, constructive feedback on performance is given in a nonthreatening manner. These mock examinations also help candidates to prepare for their summative examinations.

 In-house 'mock examinations' are useful for evaluating the effectiveness of the training programme in individual departments or units.

Effective modalities for formative assessment of trainees include the *Objective Structured Assessment of Technical Skills* (OSATS) developed at the University of Toronto (see Chapter 38). This evaluation makes use of an operation-specific checklist involving direct observation of trainees performing various structured tasks. Another useful tool is the *Imperial College Surgical Assessment Device* (ICSAD), which utilizes computer-based assessment techniques to track the number of movements and the total time taken for a trainee to complete a set task (Patil et al 2003). Like the OSATS, The *Procedure Based Assessment*, developed by the Royal Colleges of Surgeons in the UK, has good reliability and validity and assesses the trainee performing various key operations in their chosen specialty.

Interaction between trainer and trainee

The quality of consultant supervision is the single most important factor in determining whether a trainee is satisfied with his or her training post. There are various opportunities for interaction between trainer and trainee:

- induction and orientation of trainee prior to commencing the rotation
- interactive clinical supervision
- formative logbook review
- trainee and supervisor consultative meetings at regular intervals
- constructive and supportive feedback
- career counselling.

 Consultant supervision is the single most important factor in determining whether a trainee is satisfied with a training post

Paice & Ginsberg 2003

The trainee's portfolio (now usually an electronic *e-portfolio*) constitutes a record of all the training postings, work experience, training activities with clinical supervisors, structured educational programmes attended, certified checklists of knowledge and skills, reflection on learning and other educational activities. It will include trainers' comments and assessments: both formative and summative (see Chapter 39).

Training for the role is essential, and these 'training the trainer' or faculty development courses have been shown to benefit the trainers and the doctors in training. Topics such as giving constructive feedback, teaching and learning, assessment, appraisal and managing poor performance are key in helping develop trainers' knowledge and skills in the role. Many Deaneries and Royal Colleges now provide such courses. In addition, many universities, pioneered by the University of Dundee in Scotland and the University of Cardiff in Wales, run certificates, diplomas and Master's degrees in medical education for those doctors and dentists who wish to develop their knowledge and skills further still.

Giving feedback constructively is one of the key skills for the trainer to understand and to use effectively. Encouragement and positive comment work far better than the methods of bullying, harassment and teaching by humiliation.

 Giving feedback constructively was the top theme in setting the key objectives for consultant teachers' faculty development.

This was the top theme in setting the key objectives for consultant trainers (Wall & McAleer 2000) in a study of consultants and doctors in training in three hospitals within the West Midlands. There are several methods, but two which work really well are presented below. These are *Pendleton's rules* and *The One-minute teacher*.

Pendleton's rules

1. Learner goes first and does the activity
2. Questions on facts of points for clarification only
3. Learner says what they thought they did well
4. Teacher then says what they thought they did well
5. Learner then says what they thought they did not so well
6. Teacher then says what they thought they did not so well and in discussion gives constructive advice on how to improve

Pendleton's rules (Pendleton et al 1984) were developed originally for looking at video recordings of doctors' consultations in a general practice setting. However, the format does work in other situations as well.

The one-minute teacher

- Get a commitment: what do you think is going on here?
- Probe for supporting evidence: what led you to that conclusion?

- Teach general rules and principles: when this happens, do this ....

- Reinforce what was right: specifically you did well on ....

- Correct mistakes: next time this happens, try this instead.

The one-minute teacher works well on a ward round, in a clinic and in the surgery and is a fairly quick and effective way of getting the doctors in training to give a view and then receive constructive feedback.

SUMMATIVE EXAMINATIONS

Postgraduate examinations are conducted by professional bodies such as colleges (e.g. for the Royal Colleges of various specialties in the UK, Australia, New Zealand, Canada and Thailand) or boards (e.g. the specialty boards in the United States), or by universities (e.g. in India, Malaysia and Papua New Guinea), following completion of the stipulated period of clinical experience and training. The award of diploma or degree may be as a fellowship (e.g. Fellowship of the Royal College of Physicians and Surgeons of Canada), a membership (e.g. Membership of the Royal College of Obstetricians and Gynaecologists), or a master's degree (e.g. Master of Medicine as in Singapore and Sudan, or Master of Surgery as in India).

In addition to these examinations at or near the end of training, all trainees will undergo an annual summative assessment, in the UK now called the Annual Review of Competency Progression (ARCP). This will review the trainee's progress for the year, taking information from their e-portfolio and often a face-to-face formal oral examination as well. It is pass or fail, and unsatisfactory performance will lead to targeted training, repeat of part of the programme or even, in serious cases, removal from the training programme altogether.

Examination format

Examinations are of four types:

- Written tests: multiple-choice questions (MCQs), extended matching questions (EMQs), short-answer questions (SAQs) and essays

- Oral examinations (vivas)

- Clinical examinations: short cases, long cases, objective structured clinical examinations (OSCEs)

- Logbook assessment.

Most written tests are now presented as MCQs, EMQs and SAQs (see Chapter 37). Traditional long essay questions are being reduced or abandoned altogether. The majority of examining bodies include an oral examination (viva voce) on topics related to applied basic sciences, critical care, evidence-based practice and the logbook. As for clinical examinations, there is a welcome trend in all specialties to structure these in the format of an objective assessment of the clinical, communication, practical management and procedural skills of each candidate. This is achieved by conducting the examination in an OSCE setting or in a real clinical environment (e.g. wards, ambulatory care units, intensive care units) using a checklist of items to be tested.

The Foundation Curriculum in the UK

There is an outcomes-based curriculum for the UK Foundation Curriculum. The 14 outcomes of the August 2011 curriculum are the following:

- Professionalism

- Good clinical care

- Recognition and management of the acutely ill patient

- Resuscitation

- Discharge and planning for chronic disease management

- Relationship with patients and communication skills

- Patient safety within clinical governance

- Infection control

- Nutritional care

- Health promotion, patient education and public health

- Ethical and legal issues

- Maintaining good medical practice

- Teaching and training

- Working with colleagues.

Teaching and learning, appraisals and assessments should all be based on these same outcomes. Assessment tools used to demonstrate progress have included the Mini Clinical Examination (Mini-CEX) for history taking and examination, case-based discussions (CBDs) for record keeping and decision making, direct observation of procedural skills for practical procedures (DOPS), and 360-degree assessment using Team Assessment of Behaviours (TAB) for attitudes and behaviours. TAB measures communication with patients, communication with colleagues, team working and accessibility (i.e. turning up on time, among other attributes).

Because of the poor perceptions by trainers and trainees of the Mini-CEX, CBD and DOPS as merely tick box exercises (Bindal et al 2011) these will only be used as supervised learning events and not as summative assessments in the future.

Using 360-degree assessment we can reliably measure trainees' attitudes and behaviours.

Evidence of all these will be kept in an e-portfolio by the Foundation doctor.

Doctors in training in difficulty

A full account of this area is outside the scope and capacity of this chapter. However, some pointers will help the educational supervisor and others in being aware of the possible problems and knowing some general principles of where to go to ask for further help, such as postgraduate Deaneries, medical charities, the National Clinical Assessment Service or even the regulatory bodies.

It has been recognized for some time that the transition from medical student to first-year doctor is a stressful and difficult one. Some of these doctors, up to 1–2%, need to undergo remedial training and repeat all or part of the year. In addition, doctors at the end of postgraduate training sometimes have great difficulty in passing their exit examinations, for a variety of reasons. Most of these doctors in difficulty can be helped and can get back on track to achieve a successful career.

How could a doctor in difficulty come to the notice of others in the service? The National Clinical Assessment Authority (NCAA 2004) highlighted several early signs of doctors in difficulty in terms of their education. These included the following:

- The disappearing act: not answering bleeps, disappearing, frequent sick leave
- Low work rate: slow when doing procedures, clerking patients, dictating letters
- Ward rage: shouting at the nurses or other colleagues
- Rigidity: poor tolerance of uncertainty, difficulty making priority decisions
- Bypass syndrome: nurses and other colleagues avoid asking the doctor to do anything
- Career problems: examination difficulty, disillusionment with medicine
- Insight failure: rejection of constructive feedback, defensiveness, counter challenge.

In order to conceptualize these, the various problems can be categorized into four main areas. These are as follows:

- Personal conduct
- Professional conduct
- Competence and performance issues
- Health.

In addition, adverse life events can play a part in any or all of the above.

Often people will not volunteer such information, so they can be asked about issues such as bereavements, severe illness, accidents, change of job, move of house, lack of family support and so on. A list produced by the University of Birmingham details some of these main stressors and gives some measure of how severe each may be (www.as.bham.ac.uk/study/support/sscs/counsell/stress.shtml). A score of 50 in a 6-month period is considered to be stressful enough to cause illness. You might want to work out your own score for the past 6 months (see Table 4.1).

Personal conduct issues (not related to being a doctor) can include theft, fraud, assault, vandalism, rudeness, bullying, racial and sexual harassment, child pornography and serious traffic offences.

Professional conduct issues (related to being a doctor) can include inappropriate breast examinations, claiming qualifications the doctor does not have, research misconduct, improper relationships with patients and breaches of confidentiality.

Competence and performance issues can include serious clinical errors, persistent poor timekeeping, poor communication skills and repeated failure to attend educational events. Behavioural problems may include the macho type of behaviour, not recognizing

Table 4.1 Main stressors and their severity

Event	Score
Death of a parent	50
Death of a close relative	40
Loss of a parent through divorce	35
Death of a close friend	30
Parents having rows or in financial trouble	28
Serious health problems, surgery, pregnancy	25
Engagement or marriage	25
In trouble with the law	22
Unemployed, financial trouble	19
Breakup with boy- or girlfriend	19
Interviews or starting a new job	18
Sexual difficulties	18
Not part of the crowd	16
Lack of privacy	15
Driving test	15
College pressures, exams, deadlines	14
Concern about appearance, weight, identity	13
Recent move, home, school, college	11
Lack of recognition	9
General feelings of frustration	6

one's limitations, not calling for help when heading for problems, authoritarianism and inappropriate behaviour.

Health and sickness issues can include various physical and mental illnesses, cognitive impairment and adverse life events which can cause serious problems. One common problem in doctors in training is postnatal depression, which is treatable but sadly not often diagnosed until late.

 Remember to consider postnatal depression as a cause of poor performance.

Other important areas to consider include cognitive impairment in the doctor (possibly after head injury or neurological diseases), the organizational culture and climate (what it is like to work in the organization) and workload. Although hours worked have declined since the 1970s, when 120 hours per week was common, the intensity and complexity of medical practice have greatly increased. Heavy workload, a long-hours culture, lack of sleep and shift work can cause problems.

Helping the doctor in difficulty is an expert task. The information here is merely to raise awareness of how and why these problems may arise and the need for referral. Thankfully, the prognosis is good for the vast majority who get into difficulty.

 In trying to help doctors in difficulty, always ask about adverse life events, as if you do not, they will probably never tell you.

Exit outcomes

Exit outcomes for postgraduate training include the following:

- Progression to independent responsibility
- Recognized postgraduate degree
- Certificate of Completion of Training (CCT) in the UK
- Registration as a specialist
- Eligibility for appointment as a consultant or general practitioner.

In the UK, the CCT is awarded to those trainees who have satisfactorily completed the designated period of training (6–8 years), have satisfactory assessments at the end of each year and have passed the specialty examination of the appropriate college. In the UK such trainees will apply to the General Medical Council for inclusion in the Specialist Register or General Practice Register. Those who are qualified outside the UK will have to be assessed by the General Medical Council for inclusion on its specialist register. Successful registrants are regarded as fully trained and are eligible to apply for a consultant or general practice post in the National Health Service (NHS).

Evaluation of training

A definition of evaluation is measuring the teaching or any aspect of the educational process. Evaluation in medical education is "… a systematic approach to the collection, analysis and interpretation of information about any aspect of the conceptualisation, design, implementation and utility of educational programmes. Evaluation measures the teaching …" (Mohanna et al 2010).

Evaluation questions we might ask are as follows:

- What did the GP registrars think of the cross-cultural communication skills course?
- What is the educational climate like for specialist trainees in the operating theatre?
- Was the 6-day faculty development course effective, and did people go on to put the lessons into practice?
- How reliable was our short listing and interviewing for paediatrics trainees?
- What do junior doctors think about career advice?

Evaluation is not merely about handing out questionnaires to doctors in training at the end of our teaching sessions. It is much more than this. There are many methods to use. Berk (2006) commented that student ratings have dominated as the primary measure of the evaluation of teaching effectiveness for the past 30 years. It is important to broaden and deepen the evidence base with other sources of evidence, so that in any one evaluation decision, multiple sources of evidence can be used.

 When evaluating a course or programme, try to use at least three sources of evidence so that the strengths of one method may compensate for the weaknesses of another.

Berk suggested drawing on at least three sources of evidence, so that the strengths of one may compensate for the weaknesses of others (for example, the different biases of peer ratings and student ratings). He suggested a total of 13 sources of evidence, using a wide range of methods of evaluation (see Table 4.2).

Summary

It should be a privilege to work with doctors in training and to bring them into what Lave and Wenger (1991) have described as communities of practice and an apprenticeship type of model where novices (the

Table 4.2 Thirteen types of evaluation

	Method used	Performed by	Outcome effect
Student (learner) ratings	Rating scale	Students	Formative and summative
Peer ratings	Rating scale	Peers	Formative and summative
External expert ratings	Rating scale	Experts	Formative and summative
Self ratings	Rating scale	Self	Formative and summative
Video recording of teaching	Rating scale	Self and peers	Formative and summative
Student interviews	Rating scale	Students	Formative and summative
Exit and alumni ratings	Rating scale	Graduates	Formative and programme
Employer ratings	Rating scale	Graduates' employers	Programme
Administrator ratings	Rating scale	Administrator	Summative
Teaching scholarship	Review	Administrator	Summative
Teaching awards	Review	Administrator	Summative
Learning outcome measures	Exams	Administrator	Formative
Teaching portfolios	All above	Students, peers, administrator	Summative

After Berk RA. Thirteen strategies to measure college teaching. Sterling, VA, 2006, Stylus Publishing LLC, with permission.

young doctors) were introduced into a particular community of practice, working with and learning from the experienced old-timers. The old-timers instilled into the youngsters the knowledge, skills, attitudes and professionalism of their craft. They described how we speak about crucial relations between newcomers and old-timers and about their activities, identities, artefacts, knowledge and practice. Much of British medicine and dentistry has been taught and learned like this.

 Remember that the apprenticeship model has served us well for many years.

We must be careful not to lose this in the rush to more structured curricula, teaching and assessments of the doctors in the early years. There is still the extremely important apprenticeship relationship between the trainee and the experienced trainer, who is able to pass on his or her long acquired experience to the next generation.

References

Berk RA: *Thirteen strategies to measure college teaching*, Sterling, VA, 2006, Stylus Publishing LLC.

Bindal T, Wall D, Goodyear H: Trainee doctors' views on workplace based assessments: Are they just a tick box exercise? *Medical Teacher* 33:919–927, 2011.

Dreyfus HL, Dreyfus SE: Expertise in real world contexts, *Organisational Studies* 26:779–792, 2005.

Lave J, Wenger E: *Situated learning legitimate peripheral participation*, Cambridge, 1991, Cambridge University Press.

Mohanna K, Cottrell E, Wall D, Chambers R: *Teaching made easy. A manual for health professionals*, ed 3, Oxford, 2010, Radcliffe Publishing Ltd.

National Clinical Assessment Authority: *Understanding performance difficulties in doctors. An NCAA Report*, London, 2004, National Clinical Assessment Authority.

Paice E, Ginsburg R: Specialist registrar training: What still needs to be improved? *Hospital Medicine* 64:173–175, 2003.

Patil NG, Cheng SW, Wong J: Surgical competence, *World Journal of Surgery* 27:943–947, 2003.

Pendleton D, Schofield T, Tate P, Havelock P: *The consultation. An approach to teaching and learning*, Oxford, 1984, Oxford Medical Publications.

Tooke Report: 2008 Aspiring to excellence. Final report of the independent inquiry into modernising medical careers. MMC Inquiry London. http://www.mmcinquiry.org.uk/MMC_FINAL_REPORT_REVD_4jan.pdf (accessed 30 January 2008).

Wall D, Bolshaw A, Carolan J: From undergraduate medical education to pre-registration house officer year: How prepared are students? *Medical Teacher* 28:435–439, 2006.

Wall D, McAleer S: Teaching the consultant teachers: Identifying the core content, *Medical Education* 34:131–138, 2000.

5 Continuing professional development

D. A. Davis, J. Goldman, L. Perrier, I. L. Silver

Introduction

Consider the two scenarios presented below.

Scenario 1. You have been invited to make a presentation on the broad topic of cardiology at Norfolk University's annual generalist programme: a large, primary care refresher course run by the University's School of Medicine for nearly two decades. In this very popular, lecture-based programme, you have 2 hours to lecture to over 350 participants. The title of your lecture is 'An update on heart disease: What the generalist needs to know'. You ask the course organizer, 'How can I make this more interesting, relevant and informative? How can I possibly fill 2 hours?'

Scenario 2. You are the coordinator of your hospital's grand rounds series. Your department chief and the hospital's chief executive officer note that rounds attendance has declined in recent years. Even visiting professors' presentations have disappointingly small participation. When you ask your colleagues why this is the case, they claim practice busyness, overbooked surgical suites and offices and other competing interests. You also sit on the hospital quality committee and observe that its performance indicators in several areas, such as asthma management and congestive heart failure, fall significantly behind comparable hospitals in the region. You have a feeling that changing rounds, perhaps by improving the presentations and format of the sessions and incorporating a quality improvement focus, might be an answer; however, you are unsure how to proceed.

These are not uncommon scenarios; many physician-teachers and course organizers are confronted with the challenge of making presentations to colleagues, to other health professional audiences, even to the public and, when given the opportunity to reflect, have a strong desire to improve this 'product', to make it more effective. From a personal perspective, doing a 'good job' brings the satisfaction of having accomplished a task well, most often recognized by the audience to which you are presenting. There is, however, another perspective, sizably different from the case in undergraduate teaching or residency training. Like the work

of clinicians themselves, teaching by well-prepared faculty and the effective educational intervention itself can bring about practice change and affect healthcare outcomes (Davis et al 1995) on a more immediate and possibly rewarding basis than undergraduate teaching and residency training. Further, while the steps to improving continuing professional development (CPD) are important, perhaps even self-evident in any teaching exercise, they assume far greater importance in the realm of practice. Here, one is engaged in a process of communication with peers: colleagues with their own practice needs, styles and requirements, and, moreover, their own areas of expertise.

This chapter outlines a four-step process to making CPD more effective for the teacher (Scenario 1) and the programme provider or organizer (Scenario 2). They are captured here as 'knowing' steps:

- Know the audience
- Know the topic
- Know the format
- Know the outcome.

 For effective CPD, the teacher, workshop leader or other faculty members should:

- Know the audience
- Know the topic
- Know the format
- Know the outcome.

Know the audience

It is a truism in CPD that one needs to know one's learners or students: 'Who is the target audience?' is a favourite planning phrase in continuing education. The answer is not so simple, and, apart from needs assessment (the second step in this process), truly knowing the audience may be the most important step in the process of providing CPD.

Consider the first scenario. In the Canadian context, 'primary care clinicians' can imply many types of practitioners, from semi-autonomous physician assistants or nurse practitioners to independent, self-regulating physicians who may be general practitioners (neither trained in family medicine nor certified by the national body) or family physicians, often with two or more years of specialty training in this complex discipline. In the United States, primary care is more eclectic in its mix: paediatricians, obstetricians, general internists, physician assistants, nurse practitioners and family physicians (general practitioners) may comprise the audience. 'Primary care clinicians' might also comprise teams, given the increasing emphasis on interprofessional collaboration as a means to improve healthcare and patient outcomes, and the role of interprofessional education in fostering the skills and behaviours necessary for effective collaboration (Health Canada Interprofessional Collaboration 2011). Thus, the primary care 'team' may consist of a range of healthcare professionals, such as physicians, nurses, social workers, dieticians and pharmacists, each bringing a particular role and perspective to the primary care setting (Goldman et al 2010, Meuser et al 2006).

 There is also reason embedded in [the findings of well designed, longitudinal studies] for optimism about the effect a carefully planned and implemented methodology on patient outcomes. [Such studies allow] many observations about evidence, physician practice, and the roles that an effective continuing education presence can occupy in health care and its quality and reform efforts, arenas in which this presence is often invisible, unconsidered, and neglected.

Davis 2011

Other participants' attributes that may be relevant are methods of payment and practice types or settings since these affect learners' abilities to maintain or deliver practice competencies. In the second scenario, declining rounds attendance may imply a strict fee-for-service environment, a frequent occurrence in the North American setting, in which time away from practice settings is not reimbursed. It may also imply that grand rounds activities frequently address only the resident case of the week or research project, or highlight a visiting speaker, and are often not related to the daily activities of most attendees. In some instances, physicians may receive incentives for attending CPD activities. For example, physician practices enrolled in the Practice Incentives Program in Australia may receive payment for participating in Quality Prescribing Incentive activities (such as clinical audits, case studies, practice visits) (Australian Government Department of Human Services 2012).

 'Know the audience' means, among other things, knowing the discipline, training, practice environment and continuing education or CPD requirements of the physician-learner involved in the event.

On the other hand, there are countervailing forces in the form of professional and regulatory guidelines that may compel physicians to participate in such events. In regards to licensure, there are guidelines that suggest a minimum number of hours of formal continuing education or CPD for a wide variety of physician groups. It is useful to know what these are for each jurisdiction and, where possible, to tailor interventions to meet them. For example, in the case of the Royal College of Physicians and Surgeons of Canada, additional CPD 'points' may be gained by asking physicians to perform pre-workshop chart audits, post-lecture structured reading and reflection exercises, or personal learning projects resulting from participation in a CPD activity (Royal College of Physicians and Surgeons of Canada). Similarly, in the United States, there are programmes based on recertification or maintenance of certification (American Board of Family Medicine, American Board of Internal Medicine, American Board of Medical Specialties). Further, the Accreditation Council for CME (ACCME) increasingly requires proof of competence, such as pre-/post-multiple choice tests, or performance, such as hospital measures, in addition to attendance at such activities (Accreditation Council for Continuing Medical Education). Some states in the United States have required CME topics such as human sexuality and risk management; tailoring the message to these issues where appropriate and relevant might increase attendance and participation (American Medical Association 2010).

Know the topic

The consulting cardiologist in Scenario 1 might believe, quite correctly, that he or she knows the subject area to be addressed; why else would an invitation to present be made? Why should the topic of needs assessment even be raised? The answer here, however, lies not just in knowledge of the subject area, but knowledge of how to tailor the information to meet needs and expectations at two levels: the practice needs expressed by the learner (the micro perspective) and the needs of patients, populations, healthcare systems, or regions (the larger, macro perspective). This twofold theme reflects and builds on that of a subjective/objective dilemma. This section presents tools, useful in both scenarios, in which CPD providers/teachers can determine the needs of their audiences and their patient populations.

SUBJECTIVE NEEDS ASSESSMENT: LEARNING AND CHANGE IN THE LIVES OF PHYSICIANS

Subjective needs are those that are identified and expressed by the learner. These needs are based on the learners' abilities to reflect and examine their own knowledge and practices.

 Examples of subjective needs assessment tools:

- Practice reflection
- Diaries or learning/question logs
- Questionnaires
- Focus groups
- Informal comments.

Subjective needs assessments reflect physicians' perceptions of problems and their experiences and learning styles and provide insight into their priority learning areas. These assessments can stimulate participation in CPD since physicians may be motivated to acquire additional knowledge in these identified areas (Moore 2003). Although self-assessment may seem straightforward, evidence suggests that physicians have difficulties performing accurate assessments by themselves, uninformed by external observations or data (Davis et al 2006). Given that self-assessment has been criticized for the lack of abilities in 'self-reporting' (Lockyer 1998), objective information and data on which to base judgments are also required.

The work of Fox and his colleagues (1989) is enlightening (and possibly humbling) to the CPD provider: it reveals that multiple factors affect practice changes and the diverse types of practice changes. In this qualitative study, over 300 North American physicians were asked, 'What did you most recently change in your practice? What caused that change? How did you acquire your learning in order to make that change?' Answers to each of these questions may help the CPD provider, whether teacher or organizer, prepare for this audience. First, physicians undertaking any change disclosed that they had an image of what that change was going to look like, such as a surgeon envisaging competently performing a new laparoscopic technique. Second, the forces for change in this study were widespread: while some drew from educational and CPD experiences, many more were intrapersonal (e.g. a recent experience with a dying relative, a life or career transition) or arose from changing patient demographics (e.g. ageing or changing populations and patient demands). Third, the changes varied from smaller 'adjustments' or accommodations (e.g. adding a new drug to a therapeutic armamentarium within a class of drugs already known and prescribed) to much larger changes characterized as 'redirections' (e.g. adopting an entirely new way or method of practice, or adding a nursing home to a practice population which previously included few

elders). Smaller modifications in practice might be accomplished with a brief CPD presentation, or even a didactic lecture; however, larger changes require a much richer CPD experience, perhaps encompassing a combination of a highly interactive session such as a hands-on workshop, and possibly a refresher or practical experience in the work setting.

A useful question to ask when preparing a presentation is 'What do audience members know or believe in regards to this particular issue?' A valuable model to use to address this question is that of Pathman et al (1996). In this model, Pathman outlines a continuum from awareness to agreement to adoption to adherence in regard to new information or clinical knowledge. The agreement stage is important in the case of clinical practice guidelines: for example, in the adoption stage a practice is picked up and implemented, though not uniformly or regularly, and in the adherence stage the clinical knowledge is consistently applied effectively and appropriately. Which CPD format is used at which stage depends on the particular stage along the continuum being targeted (Davis et al 2003). For example, didactic lectures may be chosen to promote awareness of an issue, while peer input and small group learning would be more appropriate for the agreement stage.

OBJECTIVE NEEDS ASSESSMENTS AND THE CLINICAL CARE GAP

Objective needs are practice gaps or areas in which clinical evidence has not been readily translated into practice. Examples of such gaps are not difficult to find. The Institute of Medicine's 2011 report titled 'Relieving Pain in America' points to large gaps in knowledge and skills among American physicians and other health professionals in pain diagnosis and management (IOM Report 2011). There are many other examples of clinical care gaps, varying only by country, clinical area, healthcare setting and other variables. There are also many tools available to measure these gaps; they are presented in the following.

 Examples of objective needs assessment tools:

- Chart audits
- Peer review
- Standardized patients to rate task performance
- Observation of physician practices
- Electronic health records that provide individual physician performance data
- Government publications
- Health services reports
- Quality metrics and continuous quality improvement reports
- Research literature.

Each needs assessment strategy enables the collection of different types of information and has an extensive body of literature on methods and effectiveness. The purpose of the needs assessment should determine the strategies used; a combined approach provides a more comprehensive understanding of the situation (Grant 2002).

Thus the creation of an effective CPD intervention presents, rather than a simple and straightforward process, a tricky minefield. To optimize learning, the truly effective CPD provider must weave a path through the learners' trainings and settings, learning styles and experiences, and subjectively and objectively determined practice and performance gaps.

 "Formal needs assessment can identify only a narrow range of needs and might miss needs not looked for, so breadth and flexibility of needs assessment methods should be embraced."

Grant 2002

Know the format

It is useful to think of the format or educational process in CPD less as a lecture or presentation and more as an intervention. In this manner one broadens the scope and possible perception of the educational encounter and makes the provider/teacher think more creatively about ways in which he or she can affect performance change in the learner and improve practice outcomes. Green's PRECEED model (Green et al 1980), which incorporates the elements of predisposing, enabling and reinforcing, helps with this concept. This chapter has already dealt with much of the preparatory work for the CPD intervention. In contrast, this section will deal with two key concepts: making the presentation (rounds, lecture, refresher programme, update or other conference) as effective as possible and using other methods to enable the transfer of information into the practice setting.

OVERVIEW: ENABLING LEARNING: THE CPD 'INTERVENTION'

Many years ago Miller (1967) described the classical learning experience as 'rows of lecture desks, laden with pitchers of water', with a speaker at the front communicating in a one-way manner. Although research regarding formal CPD methods (Davis et al 1999) has moved us forward, there are still many gaps in the practice of effective CPD. Further, while there are many elements to the theories of adult education (Knowles et al 1998), two key concepts, derived from Steinert and Snell (1999), stand out as crucial to the provision of effective CPD: engagement in the learning experience and relevance to the practice setting or needs of the learner. Interactivity and relevance can

be increased by improving teaching delivery methods and by providing case-based material.

Not all learning takes place in the classroom or conference centre, of course. Advances in Internet-based technology have made it possible to engage with learners before, during, and after a face-to-face education activity. A recent systematic review by the U.S. Department of Education (2010) showed better outcomes for learners participating in blended learning, combining online and face-to-face instruction. It is possible that the additional learning time and instructional elements, rather than merely the mode of learning, play a role in the enhanced outcomes (U.S. Department of Education 2010), and therefore programme planners are encouraged to consider strategies to extend the learning beyond the particular face-to-face programme. 'Advance organizers', whereby information is provided in preparation for the formal programme, is one strategy that can also be used to engage learners (Ausubel 1960, Kiewra et al 1997). Such an advance organizer can take the form of an e-mail message directing participants to a website where they can sign in, access materials and begin interacting with each other. Another strategy is to request that participants complete learning tasks prior to attending a conference. For example, in situations in which cases might be employed at the conference, learners might be encouraged to complete a short patient-audit form of five similar cases of a particular disorder to post online or bring to the conference.

Interactivity with one's experiences and setting

 Saying 'think about a case' may be made a little more powerful by providing time in the lecture to do so.

Schön (1990) has articulated the concept of reflection as a key element in learning. In this section, we provide several instances in which reflection-on-action can be enhanced by interactivity. For example, the effective lecture may begin with or include a suggestion to think about the last patient case that was difficult to manage, the earliest onset of Alzheimer's disease seen by the clinician-learner, or the case that caused the most ethically difficult decision making. One strategy is to ask participants to write down a clinical problem, or three questions they have, before the presentation. Alternatively, brainstorming questions before the presentation begins can provide instructors with cues as to where the audience is starting with the subject and can help the instructor focus on aspects of the topic the audience is really interested in.

Interactivity with learning materials

Handout material is often prized by learners as takeaway reminders of lecture notes, slides, references and management tips. Often, however, the lecturer fails to use the material during the presentation. This is a deficit that can be easily corrected, for example, by providing a multiple choice or similar quiz to be completed before, after or during a lecture or by developing a small paper case with prompts for diagnosis or management or with blank spaces left for the participant to fill in, for example, with points of history, new-start insulin orders, or other clinically relevant material.

Other methods include the use of clinical stories and live patient interviews. Patient-centred videos called Digital Stories that highlight the personal stories of patients' experiences of their illness have been effectively used in medical education (D'Alessandro et al 2004).

At the end of a lecture, the use of a 'one-minute paper' and commitment to change strategies can also help consolidate a participant's learning. For the one-minute paper, participants write down the key points or 'pearls' from a lecture or topics they might want to follow up after a conference (Angelo & Cross 1993). A commitment to change strategy involves asking participants to write down their commitment to change an aspect of their clinical practice following a conference (Purkis 1982).

Interactivity with the speaker/presenter

The most frequently used and easiest strategy by which to improve interactivity with the lecturer is the question and answer (Q&A) session. In a CPD experience similar to the first scenario described at the beginning of the chapter, planners found that a large, 2-hour block of lecture time could be effectively broken up into sequential 10+-minute periods of lecture and Q&A (Allen & Tanner 2005). Other Q&A methods include the audience response system (Miller et al 2003), a computerized vote-counting device that polls the audience for responses to projected multiple choice questions and provides the speaker with an instantaneous read on the uptake of his or her presentation. A somewhat less sophisticated system is one in which participants are given colour-coded cards and asked to hold up the one which corresponds to a particular answer. This method, while not affording the anonymity of the computerized system, is often deemed just as effective by presenters and enjoyable by participants.

 Methods for increasing interactivity with the speaker or presenter:
- Debates
- Panels
- Questions written on cards, handed to presenters
- Mandatory question periods
- Taking questions at the beginning of the presentation.

Interactivity with other learners

The notion of interactivity between learners has been advocated for decades by our adult education colleagues and is the goal of much faculty development activity (Hewson 2000). This type of interactivity builds on the ideas of reflection articulated above and addresses the principles of Knowles and colleagues (1998) and others (Fox et al 1989) about the intelligence and experience of the audience and the notion of translating knowledge into useful practical or tacit intelligence. Based on a relatively large literature (Forsetlund et al 2009, Silver & Rath 2002, Steinert & Snell 1999), a brief outline of some methods for promoting interactivity between learners follows:

- *Buzz groups:* Named for the noise such activity makes in a normally quiet conference or meeting, this method allows participants to engage neighbouring audience members in conversation about a case presentation, possible diagnoses, personal experiences, etc.

- *Write-pair-share:* This method starts with practice reflection (a quiet moment for participants to think of a particular case or an answer to a question and then write this information in a notepad), then participants discuss it with a neighbouring audience member, then share it with the larger audience (with facilitation from the presenter/ moderator).

- *Pyramiding (or snowballing):* This method builds from pairs of participants, moves to slightly bigger groups of four or six, and finally involves the entire audience in a case discussion or similar exercise.

- *Stand up and be counted:* This is a novel teaching method meant to capture diverse viewpoints. The process begins by the presenter articulating a simple if faintly provocative statement, such as 'Hormone replacement therapy for women over 60 years of age is never indicated'. Placed across one dimension of the lecture hall are signs indicating the five points often seen in Likerd questionnaire design ('strongly agree–agree–can't decide–disagree–strongly disagree'), and audience members are asked to stand up and position themselves under the point in the scale that most closely resembles their position with regard to the statement. The moderator then moves from group to group (often starting with the 'can't decide' group to determine their perspectives) to explore the reasons for their position. To conclude the session the moderator asks participants to return to their seats and summarizes the key concepts of the discussion (Tiberius & Silver 2001).

INCREASING RELEVANCE: THE CLINICAL SCENARIO

The addition of patient scenarios or vignettes that reflect actual clinical cases, frequently modified to protect patient privacy and to exemplify details of history, diagnosis or management, may enhance the relevance of CPD by promoting reflection and interaction.

'Standardized patients', about whom much has been written from the perspectives of teaching undergraduates and residents and assessing competence, are relatively less common in the CPD setting but are of potential value (Davis et al 1997, Kantrowitz 1991, Zabar et al 2010; see Chapter 26, Simulated/standardized patients). More ubiquitous and less expensive, the written case is relatively simple to construct and may be distributed before or during a lecture or presentation to stimulate discussion and problem solving, or can be used as a part of a slide presentation. A further addition to the field of CME has been the use of simulations, ranging from the simple printed, video or audio case simulation to much more complex technologies, represented by anaesthesia or resuscitation simulations (Marinopoulos et al 2007, Morrow et al 2007).

Following a conference or course, engagement and interactivity with the learners can continue in the form of online post-conference communication. This can take the form of electronic reminders, online discussion boards and data collection and sharing. The latter activity can involve the completion of a patient audit form in which participants describe how they have applied their new knowledge to the care of their next 5–10 patients with that condition.

The ultimate goal of engaging learners in ways that are relevant to their practice setting and needs, before, during and after an education event, is to encourage changes in clinical practice and patient outcome. The next section outlines some of these evidence-based learning strategies that help enable this process.

 Ways to add case-based material to presentations:

- Video/audio presentations
- Standardized patients, families
- Live operating-room links
- Real patients
- Case materials, e.g. X-rays, ECGs.

ENABLING CHANGE THROUGH KNOWLEDGE TRANSLATION AND PRACTICE-BASED LEARNING

There is increasing emphasis on the practical research field, and studying those methods geared to closing the gaps from knowledge to practice (Straus et al 2009) of which CPD is an important, even essential, component. Many terms are used to describe this process, including knowledge translation (Canada), implementation and dissemination (United States), and implementation science (United Kingdom and Europe) (McKibbon et al 2010). They share common elements; perhaps the decade-old definition of knowledge translation by the Canadian Institutes of Health Research is as representative as any: 'the exchange, synthesis and ethically-sound application of knowledge – within a complex system of interactions among researchers and users – to accelerate the capture of the benefits of research [for the public] through improved health, more effective services and products, and a strengthened health care system' (Canadian Institutes of Health Research. Instituts de Recherche en Santé du Canada 2008).

 "Knowledge translation involves a complex set of interactions between producers and users of new knowledge. Improved application of research findings occurs when health researchers move beyond a reliance on academic publication as a primary mechanism for disseminating results. Instead, more dynamic mechanisms that engage players whose decision-making would be informed by the research have been shown to increase uptake and application of research."

Canadian Institutes of Health Research 2008

Research has shown that health professionals require information and knowledge that are accessible and can be integrated into their practices, and that desired changes should be supported by appropriate reinforcements (Davis et al 2003). In order to incorporate elements of the results of research findings from the field of knowledge translation, the teacher or course organizer can draw upon the rich literature on reminders, protocols, flow sheets and algorithms for care, more often found in the health services research literature than that related to CPD (Jamtvedt et al 2006, O'Brien et al 2007), to facilitate the translation of knowledge into practice. Below is a short list of such activities and recent reviews which describe them and highlight their impact on physician performance or healthcare outcome.

- Academic detailing (O'Brien et al 2007)
- Opinion leader/educational influential (Flodgren et al 2007)
- Print materials (Marinopoulos et al 2007)
- Reminders (Shojania et al 2009)
- Audit and feedback (Jamtvedt et al 2006).

Of particular interest in the area of innovations in CPD has been the advent of small group longitudinal learning (De Villiers et al 2003). Here it appears that such groups lend themselves more to a 'competence' model of CPD and act as an alternative model to lecture-based CPD.

Know the outcome

There are many reasons for knowing the outcomes of CPD activities. These follow the outline provided by Dixon in her landmark article on the evaluation of CPD activities (Dixon 1978) that suggests a relatively linear, though perhaps overly simplistic, model of expected outcomes: perception of the educational activity, competency (knowledge, skill or attitude), performance change, and healthcare outcomes. Older models of change may be equally useful (Miller 1967), as are other more modern constructs such as that of Moore (2003) and Moore et al (2009). In many ways these steps mirror those of needs assessment.

PERCEPTION OF THE LEARNING EVENT

For Scenario 1, outcomes may include knowing the audience's perception of the presentation or lecture. The classical 'happiness index' need not be confined to an overall rating of quality of presentation; it may expand to incorporate a number of features such as match with learning objectives, use of audiovisual materials, quality of handouts, degree to which interactivity was achieved, relevance and other topics (Rothman & Sibbald 2002).

COMPETENCE

At least for the purposes of this chapter, a consideration of competence includes the acquisition of knowledge, skills and attitudes, the classic triumvirate of this dimension of impact on the learner. Tests for each of these are widely available and may include (Hays et al 2002, Schuwirth & van der Vleuten 2003, Scoles

et al 2003, Shaw & Wright 1967, Southgate et al 2001):

- knowledge: multiple choice examinations, true-false tests
- skills: performance simulators (e.g. advanced cardiac life support systems or anaesthesia mannequins), interviews with standardized patients
- attitudes: global rating scores.

PERFORMANCE AND HEALTHCARE OUTCOME CHANGES

While it might be difficult to demonstrate performance or healthcare change as the result of a lecture or presentation (for example, Scenario 1), Scenario 2 and other interventions like it offer an opportunity to demonstrate such outcomes. For Scenario 2, a post-intervention questionnaire might ask, 'Has the intervention (or series of interventions, like rounds) made any difference in how you practise or to patient outcomes?' Hospital and other records may be scanned for improved measures following a series of rounds to decrease complications. Office chart audits may be used to look for an increase in screening measures in primary care. Utilization data can be employed in a managed care setting to demonstrate decreased utilization of unnecessary tests.

 "Knowledge is a necessary but not sufficient condition for performance change to occur."

Anonymous

Summary

This chapter has outlined four steps in making the CPD experience more effective: from both the perspective of the individual CPD teacher and the broader viewpoint of the provider/organizer of such experiences. Captured as brief, take-home points, they include the following four principles:

- Know the audience: its composition, background, practice milieu and, most of all, its expertise
- Know the topic: the subject area and the objectives and goals of the session
- Know the format: choosing the educational process from a broad and wide range of interactive and relevant methods, adding pre-/post-intervention enabling and reinforcing materials and methods
- Know the outcome: and wherever possible, measure it.

This last step then becomes, in an attempt to make all such CPD experiences iterative, integral to further planning. Taken together, all four steps should help address the many questions stirred by a consideration of Scenarios 1 and 2.

Acknowledgements

We would like to thank Nathan Johnson, BSc, for his assistance in this chapter.

References

Accreditation Council for Continuing Medical Education: Available at: http://www.accme.org. Accessed July 8, 2011.

Allen D, Tanner K: Infusing active learning into the large-enrollment biology class: seven strategies, from the simple to complex, *Cell Biology Education* 4(4):262–268, 2005.

American Board of Family Medicine: Maintenance of Certification for Family Physicians. Available at: https://www.theabfm.org/moc/index.aspx. Accessed March 1, 2013.

American Board of Internal Medicine: Details and policies for maintenance of certification. Available at: http://www.abim.org/moc/policies.aspx. Accessed July 8, 2011.

American Board of Medical Specialties: Maintenance of certification. Available at: http://www.abms.org/Maintenance_of_Certification. Accessed July 8, 2011.

American Medical Association: State medical licensure requirements and statistics, 2010. Table 16: Continuing medical education for licensure reregistration. Available at: http://www.ama-assn.org/ama1/pub/upload/mm/40/table16.pdf. Accessed July 8, 2011.

Angelo TA, Cross KP: *Classroom Assessment Techniques*, ed 2, San Francisco, 1993, Jossey-Bass, 148–153.

Australian Government Department of Human Services: 2012 Practice incentives program. Quality prescribing incentive. Available at: http://www.medicareaustralia.gov.au/provider/incentives/pip/index.jsp. Accessed March 1, 2013.

Ausubel DP: The use of advance organizers in the learning and retention of meaningful material, *Journal of Educational Psychology* 51:267–272, 1960.

Canadian Institutes of Health Research. Instituts de Recherche en Santé du Canada: 2008 Defining and framing knowledge translation. Available at: http://www.cihr-irsc.gc.ca/e/26574.html#defining. Accessed July 8, 2011.

Canadian Interprofessional Health Collaboration: 2010 A national interprofessional competency framework. Available at: www.cihc.ca/files/CIHC_IPCompetencies_Feb1210.pdf. Accessed March 1, 2013.

Davis D: Can CME save lives? The results of a Swedish, evidence-based continuing education intervention, *Annals of Family Medicine* 9(3):198–200, 2011.

Davis D, O'Brien MA, Freemantle N, et al: Impact of formal continuing medical education: do conferences, workshops, rounds, and other traditional continuing education activities change physician behavior or health care outcomes? *Journal of the American Medical Association* 282(9):867–874, 1999.

Davis D, Evans M, Jadad A, et al: The case for knowledge translation: shortening the journey from evidence to effect, *BMJ* 327(7405):33–35, 2003.

Davis DA, Thomson MA, Oxman AD, Haynes RB: Changing physician performance. A systematic review of the effect of continuing medical education strategies, *Journal of the American Medical Association* 274(9):700–705, 1995.

Davis DA, Mazmanian PE, Fordis M, et al: Accuracy of physician self-assessment compared with observed measures of competence: a systematic review, *Journal of the American Medical Association* 296(9):1094–1102, 2006.

Davis P, Russell AS, Skeith KJ: The use of standardized patients in the performance of a needs assessment and development of a CME intervention in rheumatology for primary care physicians, *Journal of Rheumatology* 24(10):1995–1999, 1997.

D'Alessandro DM, Lewis TE, D'Alessandro MP: A pediatric digital storytelling system for third year medical students: the virtual pediatric patients, *BMC Medical Education* 4:10, 2004.

De Villiers M, Bresick G, Mash B: The value of small group learning: an evaluation of an innovative CPD programme for primary care medical practitioners, *Medical Education* 37(9):815–821, 2003.

Dixon J: Evaluation criteria in studies of continuing education in the health professions: A critical review and a suggested strategy, *Evaluation and the Health Professions* 1:47–65, 1978.

Flodgren G, Parmelli E, Doumit G, et al: Local opinion leaders: effects on professional practice and health care outcomes, *Cochrane Database of Systematic Reviews* 1:CD000125. DOI: 10.1002/14651858. CD000125.pub3, 2007.

Forsetlund L, Bjørndal A, Rashidian A, et al: Continuing education meetings and workshops: effects on professional practice and health care outcomes, *Cochrane Database of Systematic Reviews* (2):CD003030, 2009.

Fox RD, Mazmanian PE, Putnam RW: *Changing and Learning in the Lives of Physicians*, New York, 1989, Praeger Publications.

Goldman J, Meuser J, Lawrie L, et al: Interprofessional collaboration in family health teams: an Ontario-based study, *Canadian Family Physician* 56:368–374, 2010.

Grant J: Learning needs assessment: assessing the need, *British Medical Journal* 324(7330):156–159, 2002.

Green LW, Kreuter M, Deeds S, Partridge K: *Health Education Planning: A Diagnostic Approach*, Palo Alto, 1980, Mayfield Press.

Hays RB, Davies HA, Beard JD, et al: Selecting performance assessment methods for experienced physicians, *Medical Education* 36(10):910–917, 2002.

Health Canada Interprofessional Collaboration: Available at: http://www.hc-sc.gc.ca/hcs-sss/hhr-rhs/strateg/p3/index-eng.php. Accessed July 9, 2011.

Hewson MG: A theory-based faculty development program for clinician-educators, *Academic Medicine* 75(5):498–501, 2000.

Institute of Medicine: *Relieving Pain in America: A Blueprint for Transforming Prevention, Care, Education, and Research*, Washington DC, 2011, National Academy of Sciences.

Interprofessional Education Collaborative Expert Panel: 2011 Core competencies for interprofessional collaborative practice: Report of an expert panel. Available at: www.aacp.org/resources/education/Documents/10-242IPECFullReportfinal.pdf. Accessed March 1, 2013.

Jamtvedt G, Young JM, Kristoffersen DT, et al: Audit and feedback: effects on professional practice and health care outcomes, *Cochrane Database of Systematic Reviews* 2:CD000259, 2006.

Kantrowitz MP: Problem-based learning in continuing medical education: some critical issues, *Journal of Continuing Education in the Health Professions* 11(1):11–18, 1991.

Kiewra KA, Mayer RE, DuBois NF: Effects of advance organizers and repeated presentations on students' learning, *The Journal of Experimental Education* 65:147–159, 1997.

Knowles MS, Holton EF, Swanson RA, Holton E: *The Adult Learner: The Definitive Classic in Adult Education and Human Resource Development*, Houston, 1998,Gulf Publishing.

Lockyer J: Needs assessment: lessons learned, *Journal of Continuing Education in the Health Professions* 18(3):190–192, 1998.

Marinopoulos SS, Dorman T, Ratanawongsa N, et al: *Effectiveness of continuing medical education. Evidence Report/Technology Assessment No. 149. (Prepared by the Johns Hopkins Evidence-Based Practice Center, under Contract No. 290-02-0018.) AHRQ Publication No. 07-E006*, Rockville, MD, 2007, Agency for Healthcare Research and Quality.

McKibbon KA, Lokker C, Wilczynski NL, et al: A cross-sectional study of the number and frequency of terms used to refer to knowledge translation in a body of health literature in 2006: a Tower of Babel?,*Implementation Science* 5:16, 2010.

Meuser J, Bean T, Goldman J, Reeves S: Family health teams: a new Canadian interprofessional initiative, *Journal of Interprofessional Care* 20(4):436–438, 2006.

Miller GE: Continuing medical education for what? *Medical Education* 42(4):320–326, 1967.

Miller RG, Ashar BH, Getz KJ: Evaluation of an audience response system for the continuing education of health professionals, *Journal of Continuing Education in the Health Professions* 23(2):109–115, 2003.

Moore DE: A framework for outcomes evaluation in the continuing professional development of physicians. In Davis D, Barnes BE, Fox R, editors: *The Continuing Professional Development of Physicians: From Research to Practice*, 2003, AMA Press.

Moore DE Jr, Green JS, Gallis HA: Achieving desired results and improved outcomes: integrating planning and assessment throughout learning activities, *Journal of Continuing Education in the Health Professions* 29(1):1–15, 2009.

Morrow R, Fletcher J, Mulvihill M, Park H: The asthma dialogues: a model of interactive education for skills, *Journal of Continuing Education in the Health Professions* 27(1):49–58, 2007.

O'Brien MA, Rogers S, Jamtvedt G, et al: Educational outreach visits: effects on professional practice and health care outcomes, *Cochrane Database of Systematic Reviews* 4:CD000409, 2007.

Ontario Medical Association: 2008 CME Program for Rural and Isolated Physicians, Available at: http://www.oma.org/cme. Accessed April 16, 2008.

Pathman DE, Konrad TR, Freed GL, et al: The awareness-to-adherence model of the steps to clinical guideline compliance. The case of pediatric vaccine recommendations, *Medical Care* 34(9):873–889, 1996.

Purkis IE: Commitment for change: an instrument for evaluating CME courses, *Journal of Medical Education* 57(1):61–63, 1982.

Rothman AI, Sibbald G: Evaluating medical grand rounds, *Journal of Continuing Education in the Health Professions* 22(2):77–83, 2002.

Royal College of Physicians and Surgeons of Canada: Maintenance of certification program. Available at:

http://www.royalcollege.ca/portal/page/portal/rc/members/moc. Accessed March 1, 2013.

Schön D: *Educating the Reflective Practitioner: Toward a New Design for Teaching and Learning in the Professions*, San Francisco, 1990, Jossey-Bass.

Schuwirth LW, van der Vleuten CP: The use of clinical simulations in assessment, *Medical Education* 37 Suppl 1:65–71, 2003.

Scoles PV, Hawkins RE, LaDuca A: Assessment of clinical skills in medical practice, *Journal of Continuing Education in the Health Professions* 23(3):182–190, 2003.

Shaw ME, Wright JM: *Scales for the Measurement of Attitudes*, New York, 1967, McGraw-Hill.

Shojania KG, Jennings A, Mayhew A, et al: The effects of on-screen, point of care computer reminders on processes and outcomes of care, *Cochrane Database of Systematic Reviews* 3:CD001096. DOI: 10.1002/14651858.CD001096.pub2, 2009.

Silver I, Rath D: Making the formal lecture more interactive, *Intercom* 15(3):6–8, 2002.

Southgate L, Hays RB, Norcini J, et al: Setting performance standards for medical practice: a theoretical framework, *Medical Education* 35(5):474–481, 2001.

Steinert Y, Snell LS: Interactive lecturing: strategies for increasing participation in large group presentations, *Medical Teacher* 21(1):37–42, 1999.

Straus SE, Tetroe J, Graham I: Defining knowledge translation, *Canadian Medical Association Journal* 181(3-4):165–168, 2009.

Tiberius RG, Silver L: 2001 Guidelines for conducting workshops. Available at: http://www.siumed.edu/resaffairs/documents/Conductingworkshops.doc. Accessed July 9, 2011.

US Department of Education, Office of Planning, Evaluation and Policy Development: *Evaluation of Evidence-Based Practices in Online Learning: A Meta-Analysis and Review of Online Learning Studies*, Washington, DC, 2010.

Zabar S, Hanley K, Stevens DL, et al: Can interactive skills-based seminars with standardized patients enhance clinicians' prevention skills? Measuring the impact of a CME program, *Patient Education and Counseling* 80(2):248–252, 2010.

Preparing for general practice

T. Gibbs

Introduction

It is Monday morning. You are getting towards the end of your morning surgery. So far today you have seen 12 cases, including a child with an ear infection, a woman with high blood pressure, a man with depression, a painter and decorator with backache, two people with chest infections and a man with a possible stomach cancer. You have injected a painful shoulder joint and arranged an urgent hospital admission.

The door opens and 12-year-old Andrew comes in. When he first joined your list his asthma was badly out of control. If he tried to run anywhere he would cough and wheeze almost straight away. You and your team have spent the past few months teaching him about asthma, and gradually adjusting his medication. He seems much better and today he was full of smiles. After all, he has just been selected for the school football team – something he thought he could never achieve in a million years. As he leaves your consulting room he turns to you, 'Thank you doctor', he says, 'You really have changed my life.'

Haslam 2007

 "By learning you will teach; by teaching you will learn."

Latin proverb

General practice education must be of high quality; not only does GP training generally supply 50% of the hospital trainee workforce, good general practice reduces healthcare inequalities and morbidity in the population (Howard et al 2011). General practice is an important specialty, and nothing quite captures the specialty of general practice more than this statement and the quote above from Professor David Haslam, a leading general practitioner (GP) and past President of the Royal College of General Practitioners, UK.

General practice composes a specialty which is a complex mixture of holistic medical management in a primary healthcare setting, enhanced by evidence-based preventative care, teamwork and managerial administration, all facilitated by excellent communication and up-to-date clinical skills.

Within such a complex arena it is hardly surprising that the 'medical education' surrounding general practice has taken many significant and different courses over the last few years; some of its innovations have formed the basis of standard educational practice, and GP educators have played a significant part in healthcare educational reform.

This chapter will bring to the readers' notice some of the new changes that have occurred in teaching, learning and assessment in general practice. Cognisance is given to the fact that there are many variations of its definition; most of what appears in this chapter will apply to the UK model. However, readers should be aware that preparing for general practice is specific to the country within which the practice occurs, refined by that country's definition and the impact of specific cultural, religious and healthcare needs.

 "Never continue in a job you don't enjoy. If you are happy in what you're doing, you'll like yourself, you'll have inner peace. And if you have that, along with physical health, you will have had more success than you could possibly have managed."

Johnny Carson (1925–2005), U.S. comedian

Background

It is not possible to outline the whole history of general practice and how it developed in this chapter; readers are referred to the further reading list at the end. However, it is important to look at some of the milestones in the development of general practice which have inextricably bound together the specialty with teaching and learning.

In the UK, as early as 1776, it was Professor Andrew Duncan who proposed the building of a Peoples Dispensary in Edinburgh (UK) for the 'unfortunates of the city' who could not afford medical care. This building, finally built in 1783, was probably the first example of something akin to a general practice surgery. In its early description of purpose there was a significant paragraph in which Professor Duncan highlighted the importance and need for teaching and community-based research within the building, in order to give the doctors of the future an insight into the realities of caring for all: a truly life-altering statement in the early days of institution-dominated education.

Somewhat later, in 1878, and again in Edinburgh, graduated Sir James Mackenzie, one of the future doyens of general practice teaching and international research. He subsequently inspired Dr Richard Scott, who developed and built the first unit of general practice, specifically built for teaching, and in the same year that the National Health Service was formed (1948). Scott also opened the first academic Department of General Practice in 1956 and eventually took up the world's first post of Professor of General Practice in 1963.

The Royal College of General Practitioners (RCGP) was founded in 1952; it was the first officially recognized College specific to the specialty of general practice. The College became the main academic body for the subject and a key player in the educational development of all GPs through its key objective:

> ... to encourage, foster and maintain the highest possible standards in general medical practice ... through effective teaching and ongoing professional development.

Involving its local faculties, its devolved councils in Scotland, Ireland and Wales and its internal organization, the RCGP in 2005 was one of the first in the UK to be given an unconditional approval of its training programme by the Postgraduate Medical Education and Training Board (PMETB), the body responsible for validating all postgraduate medical education training in the UK. The RCGP is now the parent organization through which the postgraduate programmes for general practice are governed.

Recent years have seen the expansion of general practice: greater variation in activities providing a varied approach to healthcare and the daily activities of its practitioners. These years have seen the emergence of different models of employment (salaried, sessional and portfolio practitioners) and contracts (Personal Medical Services); different patterns of teamwork (group practice, health centres); geographical variation (rural and inner city practice);

an arena for a combination of skills and interests (police surgeon, occupational health, media doctor) and the development and accreditation of special interests which enhance patient care (GPs with special interests, e.g. gastroenterology, gynaecology, ophthalmology).

These recent changes not only have brought a new perspective into general practice and potentially an enhanced service, but also have made it one of the most potentially varied specialties in healthcare. This variation also creates a greater opportunity to look at the teaching, learning and assessment procedures within the specialty, creating opportunity for exciting educational innovations and educational research.

From an international perspective, many countries have 'adopted' the specialty of general practice. Frequently known as family practice, this branch of healthcare now follows many different patterns, each carrying its own training programmes, assessment and accreditation models and place within the hierarchical world of medicine and healthcare provision. Not all of these models provide diversity of healthcare. Not all provide equally comprehensive services, or the recognition of general practice as a specialty. Many countries follow the 'inverse-care law of general practice': those countries that would benefit from the advantages of effective general practice are often those that have a poorly developed or absent system of general practice.

What remains at the heart of general practice (be it the established and proven effective models found in the UK, United States and Australasia; the more refined models in Europe, sub-Saharan Africa and India; or the evolving models in the Far East, Eastern Europe and Middle East), apart from its diversity, is its reliance upon effective teaching and learning. It remains at the heart of the unique patient consultation and in the development of the specialty.

"An understanding heart is everything in a teacher, and cannot be esteemed highly enough. One looks back with appreciation to the brilliant teachers, but with gratitude to those that touched the human feeling. The curriculum is so much necessary raw material, but warmth is the vital element for the growing plant and for the soul of the child."

Carl Jung (1875–1961)

Undergraduate education and general practice

The seminal document *Tomorrow's Doctors* (GMC 1993) placed great emphasis upon the need both for undergraduate medical curricula to teach within a community setting (community-based education) and for programmes to encompass a community orientation towards healthcare (community-orientated education).

 "Clinical teaching should adapt to changing patterns in health care and should provide experience of primary care and of community medical services as well as of hospital-based services."

GMC 1993

When the General Medical Council (GMC) revised this document in 2003 and 2009, their statement regarding the use of general practice by universities expanded to include the wider variety of community placements, to be able to capture the demographic diversity of the community and for all students to contextualize their learning through the use of these community placements for early clinical exposure.

 "Clinical education must reflect the changing patterns of healthcare and provide experience in a variety of environments including hospitals, general practices and community medical services ... From the start, students must have opportunities to interact with people from a range of social, cultural and ethnic backgrounds and with a range of disability, illness and conditions."

GMC 2009

As a result of these directives, the majority of medical schools in the UK use general practice to greatly facilitate student learning, and comparative models exist in undergraduate education throughout the world.

Although the percentage of time that students are placed within the community and at what stage in the programme varies greatly among medical schools and countries, it is important to realise that general practice and the community can be used for two types of learning:

- Learning medicine in the community
- Learning about community-orientated medicine.

LEARNING MEDICINE IN THE COMMUNITY

Drawing specifically from the experience of UK medical care, the move towards a community approach to healthcare and an economics-induced reduction in patients' stay in hospital has meant that the majority of clinical material necessary for teaching and learning is within the community and accessed by and through GPs. It has been demonstrated that students can learn clinical medicine in the community (Murray et al 1999) and learn appropriate clinical skills in an

effective manner (Murray et al 1997) outwith the hospital environment. GPs make for effective teachers of medicine (Howe 2002). General practice and its immediate community provide an excellent clinical environment for students to contextualize their early learning (applied medical sciences and basic clinical skills) whilst providing a large and varied amount of clinical material for students to learn an holistic approach to healthcare during their more senior years.

LEARNING ABOUT COMMUNITY-ORIENTATED MEDICINE

It was Habbick and Leeder in 1996 who proposed that community oriented programmes can create:

... more appropriate knowledge, skills, and attitudes; deepen understanding of the whole range of health, illness, and the workings of health and social services; deepen the understanding of social and environmental factors to the causation and prevention of illness; make better use of expertise and availability of staff and patients who are in primary care settings; enhance multidisciplinary working; offer a broad range of learning opportunities; and increase recruitment to primary care and generalist specialisations.

Habbick & Leeder 1996

Many objectives, all appropriate for the new learner, were captured in one clinical environment, hence the appropriateness of general practice attachments within the clinical years.

The inclusion of community-based and community-orientated education in the undergraduate curriculum provides a great opportunity to consolidate the standard and explore new methods of teaching and learning, as well as developing the GP of the future. The community provides an ideal environment for students to learn from a diverse population of patients and illness; a true mixture of acute and chronic conditions; real-time clinical experience that reflects the true demography and public health of the environment and the ability for students to practise holistic healthcare, within a relaxed teaching environment with low student teacher ratios and student-centred learning. Community-based education provides advantages to the teaching organization through enhanced university teaching status, a potential for structured professional development and financial benefits and improved patient care through evidence-based practice. An increase in the number of patients for teaching, an enhanced collaboration between primary and secondary care and curriculum enhancement through contextual learning also give advantages to the university and medical school.

However, it does have its disadvantages, amongst them being the large numbers of community teachers needed, the conflict between service and teaching, issues of quality management and equity, transportation and the overall finance required. The true reflection lies in trying to find a balance between hospital and community-based learning in the real world of whatever country the student is domiciled.

From an international perspective, the balance between the advantages and disadvantages varies greatly, and all medical students do not experience similar clinical situations, nor do they have equal opportunities to learn in general practice or community environments. Very often the community is disregarded as a potential teaching resource, due to either a historical lack of respect for the community or a reflection of the quality of care that the community service can provide.

However, wherever medical students graduate they probably now have some sort of opportunity to increase and enrich their experience and knowledge of healthcare through some model of general practice, family medicine or community attachment.

 "Nothing seems more challenging than including basic science instruction in the process of moving medical education to the community."

Rothman et al 1995

Learning for general practice: Postgraduate vocational training

The very essence of general practice lies in its generality and diversity: the generality of the specialty, its patients, its environment and its holistic approach to healthcare; its diversity reflected by its cultural, religious and geographical variation as well as the ability to expand its services. Although these qualities bring excitement, they also bring complexity to its training process. The need to provide comprehensive teaching and learning for such a wide topic, whilst recognizing that the process of healthcare is dependent upon the health needs of the community and the clinical material available, requires a quality and very purposive training programme. Many countries throughout the world have had to produce training programmes for its doctors who wish to become GPs; these programmes are diverse and varied, and it is not possible, within the scope of this chapter, to provide a comprehensive coverage of them all. To provide a general background for discussion, the vocational training programme for general practice in the UK will be used and some of the effective innovations in that scheme described.

A GENERIC APPROACH TO GENERAL PRACTICE

This chapter has already alluded to the opportunities given in undergraduate curricula to use general practice and its community to learn medicine and understand the specialty of general practice and community medicine. Whereabouts within the curricula and for what length of time vary from medical school to medical school and country to country, but all should provide a sound basis for GP training.

At the present time within the UK, increased opportunity has now been developed in the new Foundation Programmes (Internships) that replaced the previous pre-registration year. Its expansion into a 2-year programme and the acceptance that general practice can provide a credible part of the pre-registration programme has allowed this (Table 6.1).

The process of specialty training for practice now resides firmly within the RCGP in the UK and through its links with the PMETB and its training structures found within the Postgraduate Deaneries. The RCGP has developed the first national training curriculum for general practice (RCGP 2007), structured and applied through recognized training practices and approved hospital posts, which culminates with the trainee in post receiving a Certificate of Completion of Training (CCT), entitling them to practise as a GP. (Although the term trainee has now been replaced by

Table 6.1 Pathway for general practice in the UK

Medical school	Average 5-year programme (graduate entry – 4 years) Uses general practice for integrated, contextualized learning and understanding community care
Foundation Year 1	Builds upon undergraduate training, learning objectives set by the General Medical Council (GMC) Uses general medicine and general surgery to provide specific competencies required for registration
Foundation Year 2	Training focused upon assessment and management of acutely ill patient, whilst creating opportunity to work in general practice, various clinical departments and research and academic organizations
Specialty (vocational) training for general practice	Defined programme of training and experience in an approved training practice plus experience in secondary care relevant to general practice

the terms registrar, specialist registrar in training or associate in training, recognition is given to the adoption and understanding of this term internationally and its use for international readers. Similarly, the term trainer is used rather than educational supervisor.)

Quality control of entry requirements to the training schemes has also been introduced through the National General Practice Recruitment Office, whereby a central clearing house vets and allocates appropriate trainees to selected posts (Patterson et al 2005, National Recruitment Office for General Practice Training 2011).

At present, the training takes 3 years; however, the forthcoming years could see the possibility of expansion to 5 years. Until 2008, general practice trainees could apply to be members of the RCGP, but it was not a requirement to become a practising GP. However, because of the intrinsic relationship between the College and the training programme, its curriculum and assessment process, all future accredited GPs must achieve membership of the College; indeed, satisfactory completion of the assessment process for general practice will be the same examination as for College membership.

"One of the first duties of the physician is to educate the masses not to take medicine."

Sir William Osler, Physician (1849–1919)

As a GP educator and frontline clinician, I am well aware of the major challenges – and opportunities – facing modern general practice.

Prof. Steve Field, Chairman RCGP, 2007

A CURRICULUM FOR GENERAL PRACTICE

The year 2007 saw the emergence of a curriculum for specialty training for general practice, a dynamic curriculum responsive to change dependent upon need. Previously, the monitoring of design, development and training for general practice had been delegated to the various local deaneries, and although the final outcomes were probably the same, there was the inevitable variation in content and standards of programmes. Although there is still some necessary and appropriate variation in teaching and learning methods, the development of this specific curriculum brings about a higher degree of conformity and quality management, necessary for such a varied specialty.

The RCGP curriculum is built upon six independent domains of core competences, formulated into *Being a General Practitioner* (RCGP 2008) and underpinned by the features of the discipline described in the European definition of general practice (WONCA 2005). This describes the learning outcomes for the discipline of general practice and the skills required to practise.

The six domains of competence that define general practice as a specialty are stated as the following:

1. Primary care management
2. Person-centred care
3. Specific problem-solving skills
4. A comprehensive approach
5. Community orientation
6. A holistic approach.

Within each of these competency areas are specific learning outcomes categorized under the learning domains of knowledge, skills and attitudes. Recognition is given to the fact that these six competency areas are not independent; a large amount of overlap is frequently observed. A more detailed description of how the curriculum is further structured is beyond the scope of this chapter but readers are referred to the RCGP website (www.rcgp.org) or the RCGP curriculum document (RCGP 2008).

These core competencies that have evolved into a complex curriculum structure are delivered in specific accredited training practices by trained GPs and their team, usually over a period of 1 continuous year (in Scotland, 18 months). Although it is often the practice that is accredited for training, learning is through learner-centred, needs-driven, one-to-one or team-based learning, and each trainee in practice having a dedicated trainer. It is this trainer's responsibility to not only organize the teaching programme but also organize and have responsibility for the trainee's assessment; all trainers having been accredited through a locally organized teaching and learning programme that equips them to facilitate the learning of trainees in practice. The curriculum is further complimented by 2 years of rotations through clinical/hospital specialties where the trainees learn about the specialty subject as it relates to general practice.

Further and more detailed information regarding the content and teaching methods applied can be obtained through the RCGP website (www.rcgp.org.uk).

E-PORTFOLIO IN GENERAL PRACTICE

The development of a curriculum for general practice has seen the parallel development of modern methods of assessment. To bring the curriculum and assessment together, the RCGP has developed an electronic portfolio, the e-portfolio.

Although still dynamic in its development, it presently provides an electronic educational vehicle that records the individual achievements, the learning

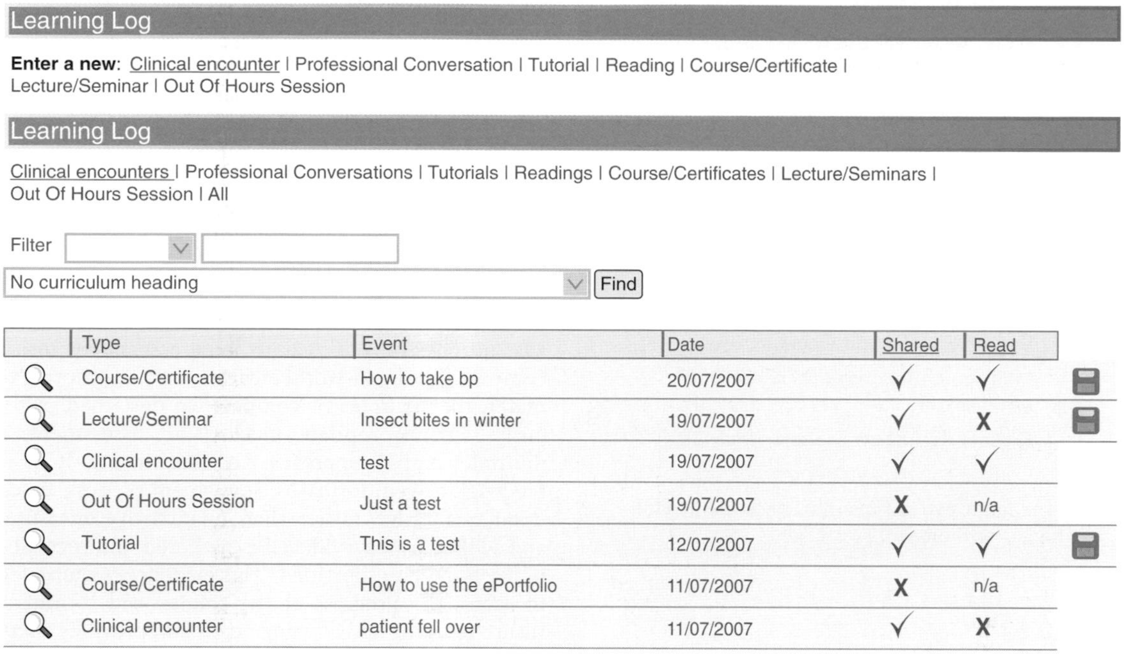

Learning Log

Enter a new: <u>Clinical encounter</u> | Professional Conversation | Tutorial | Reading | Course/Certificate | Lecture/Seminar | Out Of Hours Session

Learning Log

<u>Clinical encounters</u> | Professional Conversations | Tutorials | Readings | Course/Certificates | Lecture/Seminars | Out Of Hours Session | All

Filter

No curriculum heading   [Find]

	Type	Event	Date	Shared	Read	
🔍	Course/Certificate	How to take bp	20/07/2007	✓	✓	💾
🔍	Lecture/Seminar	Insect bites in winter	19/07/2007	✓	X	💾
🔍	Clinical encounter	test	19/07/2007	✓	✓	
🔍	Out Of Hours Session	Just a test	19/07/2007	X	n/a	
🔍	Tutorial	This is a test	12/07/2007	✓	✓	💾
🔍	Course/Certificate	How to use the ePortfolio	11/07/2007	X	n/a	
🔍	Clinical encounter	patient fell over	11/07/2007	✓	X	

Fig. 6.1 Example of a page in an e-portfolio for general practice training.

programmes and records of assessments (formative and summative) of the individual trainee. As such, it becomes a very personalized document that trainees take with them through training, including hospital-based training, and that specifically shows evidence of progression or non-progression, action taken through feedback and evidence of responses on behalf of all parties. Since a record of personal development, capturing experience, any difficulties encountered and their remediation is becoming mandatory for all future doctors, the e-portfolio becomes a potential educational tool to capture such information. It has the potential to become a clear statement of training and progression at whatever level and to give structure to personal development plans.

An example of one of the pages found within an e-portfolio for general practice training is seen in Fig. 6.1.

Assessment for general practice

Previous comments within this chapter have drawn attention to the diversity of general practice, which has led to wide, diverse but purposeful, objective-driven curriculum content, requiring appropriate structure and close supervision of the teaching and learning programme. Almost by definition this has meant that the assessment for general practice has similarly had to undergo reorganization, making its methods appropriate both for the learning content

and teaching methodology, whilst using newer methods to explore necessary competency and real life events.

Although the following methods are pertinent to the new UK-based curriculum, many of the methods are drawn from experience in international programmes and are applied in many international arenas that develop general practice.

The purpose of any assessment process for general practice is the development of an outcomes or competency-based system, which covers the whole of the learning process and is set to a standard that reflects the requirements of the practitioner of the future. It needs to also reflect the definition of the practitioner, as applied within the country of origin. Of interest in the global world is the degree of commonality in generic competencies practitioners need to have and how they reflect present global issues and ease of travel.

The models of assessment used in the RCGP curriculum for general practice are listed (Box 6.1). Each will be separately described below.

APPLIED KNOWLEDGE TEST (AKT)

The AKT is a summative test that assesses the knowledge required for modern day practice, and although it can be sat at any time within the programme, it is most appropriately taken at the end of training.

The test consists of a 3-hour, multiple choice test, sat at several dedicated centres for security reasons.

> **Box 6.1 Assessment methods used by RCGP-UK**
>
> - Applied Knowledge Test (AKT)
> - Clinical Skills Assessment (CSA)
> - Workplace-based assessment (WPBA) methods
>   - Case-based discussion (CbD)
>   - Direct observation of procedural skills (DOPS)
>   - Consultation Observation Tool (COT)
>   - Patient Satisfaction Questionnaire
>   - Multisource feedback (MSF) or 360° assessment
>   - Clinical Evaluation Exercise (Mini-CEX)
>   - Clinical supervisor's report
>
> (The latter two are used mainly in a hospital-based environment.)

It is IT-based and electronically marked and expects the trainee to answer 200 multiple choice questions (MCQs), made up of 80% clinical medicine, 10% critical reasoning and 10% health informatics and administration questions, all set at a higher level in the cognitive domain rather than the simple recollection of factual data. Candidates are allowed to resit the test in the event of a failure. The questions set are subject to standard assessment review and test item analysis.

CLINICAL SKILLS ASSESSMENT (CSA)

This assessment is designed to be:

> *... an assessment of a doctor's ability to integrate and apply clinical, professional, communication and practical skills appropriate for general practice.*
>
> RCGP 2007

Trainees are expected to take this assessment 12 months prior to qualifying as a GP. It consists of 13 simulated consultations (12 marked, 1 as a practice station), all assessed by trained assessors and similar to the well-known Objective Structured Clinical Examination (OSCE). Each consultation is a true reflection of the daily clinical encounters expected in practice, and each is assessed as a Clear Fail, Marginal Fail, Marginal Pass and Clear Pass. The areas covered are:

- primary care management
- problem-solving skills
- comprehensive approach, using a bio-psychosocial approach

- attitudinal aspects, practising ethically and professionally
- person-centred care.

The CSA also covers clinical practical skills necessary within the consultation environment.

Consultations are often videotaped for training purposes. Again, candidates who fail can resit the assessment, but need to note that extension to their training programme may be necessary.

WORKPLACE-BASED ASSESSMENT (WBPA)

The purpose of WBPA is to bring assessment into a contextualized real-world environment, attempting to match the six areas of competence described previously with appropriate methods of assessment, a multiple biopsy approach to assessment. It is a feedback-driven, formative assessment process, based upon qualitative rather than quantitative measures and within which evidence is gathered and recorded in the trainee's e-portfolio. This evidence is then used to assess the progress of the trainee and formulate future teaching and learning needs and provides documentary evidence of competence. WBPA is thought to triangulate teaching, learning and assessment, whilst offering real-world authentic assessment. It also assesses competencies not assessable by conventional methods of clinical assessment. WBPA consists of the following.

Case-based discussion (CbD)

Assessment is through a face-to-face, trainee–trainer discussion of a case seen within the practice setting. Cases are selected by the trainee; discussion and then assessment are based upon the template of the six competency areas. An average of eight assessments per year is at present expected by the RCGP. The advantage of this assessment method lies in its purposeful structure, rather than the ad hoc approach to exploration of a clinical case.

Direct observation of procedural skills (DOPS)

The trainee is asked to perform 8 mandatory and 11 optional procedures (Box 6.2) under direct observation, usually with different observers drawn from the practice team for different procedures. The trainee is marked against a template of competency, from which effective feedback is structured. The process should be iterative and reassessed if necessary.

Consultation Observation Tool (COT) and Clinical Evaluation Exercise (Mini-CEX)

With the COT being performed in general practice and the Mini-CEX carried out in the hospital environment, these two assessments both tend towards a

Box 6.2 Direct observation of procedural skills (DOPS)

Eight compulsory procedures:

- Application of simple dressing
- Breast examination
- Cervical cytology
- Female genital examination
- Male genital examination
- Prostate examination
- Rectal examination
- Testing for blood glucose

Some of these procedures may be combined, e.g. prostate and rectal examinations.

Eleven optional procedures:

- Aspiration of effusion
- Cauterization
- Cryotherapy
- Curettage/shave excision
- Excision of skin lesions
- Incision and drainage of abscess
- Joint and peri-articular injections
- Hormone replacement implant insertion
- Proctoscopy
- Suturing of skin wound
- Taking skin surface specimens for mycology

more summative assessment, using a marking template against a defined list of competencies. Each activity draws upon a specific clinical encounter from which the GP trainer or hospital-based clinical supervisor constructs or generates discussion designed to explore the trainees' approach to the management of patients. In general practice, the consultation is videotaped and used later, whilst in the secondary care sector the supervisor usually observes the interaction. In general practice, it is hoped that a varied clinical exposure is provided, and usually inclusive of three main areas:

- children aged under 10 years
- older patients, older than 75 years
- patients with mental health problems.

Over the 3 years of training, an average of eight observations are made per year.

Patient Satisfaction Questionnaire (PSQ)

The PSQ provides feedback to trainees by providing a measure of the patient's opinion of the trainee practitioner's relationship and empathy during the consultation. The evidence provided is useful in helping formulate the patient's future needs (PUNs) and facilitate the practitioner's educational development (DENs). It is usually required only once during the training period within practice, but it must address all the ethical and managerial problems encountered during such a specific exercise.

Multisource feedback (MSF)

The MSF or 360-degree feedback is designed to provide a clinical performance measure as well as an attitudinal and a professional behaviour assessment of the trainee. The essence of this assessment is the use of members of the larger team and patients to provide their individual assessments. It gives a perception of how these working colleagues see the trainee and how the trainee responds to healthcare in their environment. It is essential to collect data from as varied a cross-section of working colleagues as possible, usually a combination of clinical and nonclinical members of the healthcare team. Colleagues enter their opinions (anonymously) on the trainee's e-portfolio, using a seven-point rating scale covering specific areas of competency; this is then used formatively by the trainee and trainer. At least three such activities are expected during the 3-year training period.

Clinical supervisor's report (CSR) and trainers report

These reports allow the clinical supervisor in secondary care and the GP trainer to write a short structured report at the end of each hospital post and GP attachment. The report should cover trainee competency in three specific areas and link to the six core competency areas:

- The knowledge base required for the post
- The practical skills relevant for the post and transferable to general practice
- The professional competences required for quality care within the post.

General practice for the future

No clinical specialty should stop at the attainment of the competencies required for the post; each specialty must develop a programme of continuing professional development (CPD) which allows the practitioner to remain professional in the post (re-licensing) and up to date (re-certification).

As general practice has produced a major change in teaching, learning and assessment, so it has in the area of CPD. The RCGP has developed a number of initiatives designed to provide opportunity for structured CPD; these are beyond the scope of this chapter, but can be found on the RCGP website (www.rcgp.org.uk)

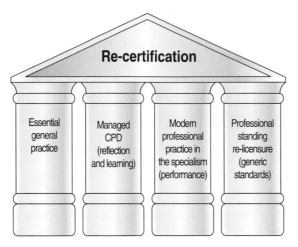

Fig. 6.2 The four pillars of re-certification. (From *Being a General Practitioner: A Curriculum for Specialty Training in General Practice.* 2007, RCGP, London with permission of the Royal College of General Practitioners).

and in specific papers from the RCGP (Sparrow 2007).

What is unique and important for the reader of this chapter and book is the RCGP's attempt to bring CPD under one 'roof', linking re-accreditation with re-certification, individual learning needs with improved patient care and quality-assured CPD with the concepts of trust, assurance and patient safety (Fig. 6.2) (see also Box 6.2).

Summary

There are very few who would disagree that general practice has made tremendous strides to establish itself as a clinical specialty amongst its peers. To do this, its training programmes, its methods of teaching, learning and assessment and its ability to support re-accreditation and re-certification procedures have been very carefully examined.

The specialty of general practice has provided an ideal environment for the development of modern medical education. It has learned lessons from around the world through experience and research and applied these in innovative ways.

Although considerable variation still exists throughout the world in the definition, management and development of general practice, and in certain areas the specialty does not yet exist, such innovations are fine examples of how healthcare professionals of the future should develop.

References

General Medical Council: *Tomorrow's doctors: Recommendations on undergraduate medical education*, London, 1993, General Medical Council.

General Medical Council: *Tomorrow's doctors: Recommendations on undergraduate medical education*, London, 2003, General Medical Council.

General Medical Council: *Tomorrow's doctors: Outcomes and standards for undergraduate medical education*, London, 2009, General Medical Council.

Habbick BF, Leeder SR: Orienting medical education to community need: a review, *Medical Education* 30:163–171, 1996.

Howard J, Gibbs T, Walsh K: Cost and quality of education for general practice, *Education for Primary Care* 22(2):70–73, 2011.

Howe A: Twelve tips for community-based education, *Medical Teacher* 24(1): 9–12, 2002.

Murray E, Jolly B, Modell M: Can students learn clinical method in general practice? A randomised crossover trial based on objective structured clinical examinations, *British Medical Journal* 315:920–923, 1997.

Murray E, Jolly B, Modell M: A comparison of the educational opportunities on junior medical attachments in general practice and in a teaching hospital: a questionnaire survey, *Medical Education* 33(3):170–176, 1999.

National Recruitment Office for General Practice Training. http://www.gprecruitment.org.uk. Accessed July 2011.

Patterson F, Ferguson E, Norfolk T, Lane P: A new selection system to recruit general practice registrars: preliminary findings from a validation study, *British Medical Journal* 330:711–714, 2005.

Rothman AI, Hays RB, Mann KV: Curriculum development. In Davis WK, Jolly BC, Page GC, et al, editors: *Moving medical education from the hospital to the community. Report of the Seventh Cambridge Conference on Medical Education*, Ann Arbor, 1995, University of Michigan Medical School.

Royal College of General Practitioners (RCGP): *Teaching, Mentoring and Clinical Supervision, Curriculum statement 3.7*, London, 2007, RCGP.

Royal College of General Practitioners (RCGP): *The Teaching and Learning Guide version 3.2*, London, 2008, RCGP.

Sparrow N: 2007. Good CPD for general practitioners. http://www.rcgp.org.uk. Accessed July 2011.

WONCA Europe: The European Definition of General Practice/Family Medicine, London, 2005, WONCA.

Further reading

Baker M, Chambers RA: *Guide to general practice careers*, UK, 2000, Royal College of General Practitioners.

Carter Y: *Guide to education and training for primary care*, Oxford, 2001, Oxford University Press.

Royal College of General Practitioners (RCGP): *Being a general practitioner: a curriculum for specialty training in general practice*, London, 2007, RCGP.

Simon C: Oxford Handbook of General Practice, Oxford, 2002, Oxford University Press.

Chapter

7

Section 1:
Curriculum development

The hidden curriculum

F. W. Hafferty, E. Gaufberg

"The real voyage of discovery consists of not in seeking new landscapes but in having new eyes."

Marcel Proust

The hidden curriculum (HC) is a theoretical construct for exploring the continuities and disconnects of educational life. At its most basic level, HC theory highlights the *potential* for conflicts between what faculty intended to deliver (the formal curriculum) and what learners take away from those formal lessons; all operating within a system's framework that emphasizes context and the interconnections and interdependencies of system elements. Examples of key influences include pedagogical context (the 'what' of what is being taught), the relational context (interactions among faculty and students, including factors such as power and hierarchy), physical context (space, layout, noise) and the context of organizational culture and group values. Building on this conceptual foundation, HC theory also recognizes that much of social life, including what happens in educational settings, takes place 'beneath the radar' because of its essentially routinized and everyday nature. Fundamental to the idea of a HC is the notion that becoming a physician involves a process of professional socialization within the culture and subcultures of medicine and medical practice.

"We (faculty) are teaching far more than we know. Every word we speak, every action we perform, every time we choose not to speak or act, every smile, every curse, every sigh is a lesson in the hidden curriculum."

Gofton & Regehr 2006

Any attempt to penetrate and ultimately to exert an influence on the HC begins by dissecting the formal curriculum, and thus what is *supposed* to be going on, at least according to those in power. With this as our foundation, we then proceed to explore 'what else might be happening.' The space between the official and unofficial, the formal and the informal, the intended and the perceived, then becomes our primary workspace. In doing this work, it is important to remember that the HC is not a 'thing' that one finds, fixes and then puts aside. There *always* is a hidden counterpart to the formal and intended curriculum. Context *always* exerts an influence. There *always* are unseen, unrecognized and un- or underappreciated factors that influence social life, and there *always* are things that become so routine and taken for granted that they become invisible over time. Purposeful inquiry may uncover and intentionally address pieces of these influences, but no discovery is ever complete and no discovery is ever permanent. There is a constant cycling and recycling between the formal and other-than-formal aspects of social life. Furthermore, the HC system's perspective requires us to acknowledge that any change in context and situation generates a new set of dynamics and thus new sets of influences which, in turn, help to construct new (overall) sets of relationships between the formal and hidden dimensions of social life.

We begin the chapter by tracing the historical roots of the HC within both sociology and education and how it came to surface within medical education during the 1990s. Next, we will explore how the concept has been used within healthcare and medical education over the past twenty-odd years. We also will note how this framework can be used to link many of the concepts and themes covered in other chapters of this book (e.g. assessment, role modelling, faculty development).

From there, we will turn to applications of HC theory to particular settings within medical education. We will highlight several domains of learning (e.g. classroom, rounds) as we become more specific about things to think about as we (as faculty) create learning opportunities for our students. This will be the most 'hands-on' section of the chapter as we introduce examples for decoding the HC at both the student and faculty levels.

Relevance

HC theory has deep conceptual roots within two academic disciplines: sociology and education. Philosopher and educational reformer John Dewey, for example, wrote on the importance of 'collateral learning' and the prevailing importance of indirect versus direct classroom instruction (Dewey 1938). For Dewey, the incidental learning that accompanies school and classroom life has an even more profound effect on learners than the formal or intended lesson plan. Dewey may not have used the term 'hidden,' but he clearly was concerned with the unintended, unnoticed and unconscious dimensions of learning.

Sociology, in turn, has had its own set of conceptual precursors, particularly its long tradition of differentiating between the formal and the informal aspects of social life. For example, sociology differentiates between social norms, which often function on an informal level, and laws, which are codified. Furthermore, sociology recognizes that there are many examples where norms have a more profound effect on social practices than laws: think highway speed limits and the difference between the posted speed limit (formal) and the more informal limits that govern the actions of both drivers and law enforcement. Sociology is joined by the academic literatures of business and management studies with its own rich history of differentiating between the formal and informal aspects of work and how tacit learning is a critical part of learning 'on the job.'

Since the 1990s, there has been a steady stream of articles in medical education literature drawing on the HC as a conceptual tool for examining medical training. Topics have included work on professionalism, ethics instruction, faculty development, gender issues, examination policies, identity formation and socialization, summative assessment, reflection, resource allocation, cultural competency, the impact of block rotations on student development, longitudinal training, messages conveyed in case studies, the training of international medical graduates, relations among specialty groups, the HC of scientific research and tools to measure the HC. The concept has been used to explore issues in palliative medicine, emergency medicine, orthopaedics and psychotherapy as well as in undergraduate courses such as anatomy and physiology, in residency training, and in continuing medical education. The HC has been examined in countries including the United States, UK, Australia, Canada, New Zealand, Europe and Scandinavia, Japan, India, Saudi Arabia, Sri Lanka and Qatar.

There also is a 'hidden' HC literature. There are many studies that draw upon the conceptual framework of HC theory without ever using key terms such as 'hidden' or 'informal'. These articles will not be identified using keyword searches in databases such as PubMed or ISI Web of Science. One example is Campbell and colleagues' examination of physician values regarding professionalism (largely quite positive and affirming) and the gulf that exists between these values and physician behaviours (Campbell et al 2007). The authors never reference the HC, but their article clearly highlights the difference that can exist between what physicians say and what they do and thus indirectly how students may be subjected to countervailing messages during their socialization into the physician's role.

Definitions and metaphors

 "Lessons from the hidden curriculum are taught implicitly, through role models, institutional leadership, peers, or during the course of practice...."
Fryer-Edwards 2002

In spite of a rather extensive literature on the HC, and in some cases because of this literature, there continues to be some confusion about what does, and does not, fall under the HC marquee. A few examples appear in Table 7.1, where they are roughly dichotomized into the formal (column one) and the other-than-formal (column two) dimensions of trainee and faculty learning.

In this table, we can see the variety of terms that denote the formal (e.g. 'official', 'stated') and the other-than-formal (e.g. 'actual', 'experienced') curriculum. It is, however, important to note that the terms in column one essentially are treated as equivalent within the medical education literature. The same is not true for the other-than-formal list. These terms are similar only in that they stand in some contrast to the formal curriculum. As we will see shortly, there are some important differences here.

Table 7.1 Terms and concepts

Formal	Other-than-formal
The codified curriculum	The actual curriculum
The curriculum on paper	The curriculum in action
The manifest curriculum	The experienced curriculum
The official curriculum	The hidden curriculum
The planned curriculum	The informal curriculum
The stated curriculum	The latent curriculum
	The null curriculum
	The peripheral curriculum
	The unintended curriculum

DEFINITIONS

The formal curriculum is the stated and the intended curriculum. This is what the school or the teacher says is being taught. As you will note in Table 7.1, the formal curriculum has at least two dimensions. The first is that it is stated: be that in writing (course catalogue, website, course syllabus) or orally by a teacher. A second dimension is intentionality. What does the instructor intend to teach or convey to students?

Working 'outward' from the formal, we quickly enter a myriad of distinctions and derivations within the other-than-formal aspects of social learning. These dimensions may be tacit, indirect, informal, unintended or otherwise invisible to the participants. What they share in common is that they are neither formally announced nor intended.

Educators often employ a simple dichotomy to differentiate between the formal curriculum and everything else that may be going on within the educational environment. In doing so, some use the terms 'hidden' or 'informal' as synonyms. There is nothing intrinsically wrong with such an approach just so long as everyone (investigators, subjects and readers) understands that what is being shoehorned into this latter category often can be quite different in terms of structural properties and impact. For example, the null curriculum covers what students learn via what is not taught, highlighted or presented. A literary analogy from a famous Sherlock Homes case is of the behaviour of a dog on the night of a murder.

 Gregory (Scotland Yard detective): "Is there any other point to which you would wish to draw my attention?"

Holmes: "To the curious incident of the dog in the night-time."

Gregory: "The dog did nothing in the night-time."

Holmes: "That was the curious incident."

Sir Arthur Conan Doyle, 1892

While students certainly garner a great deal from what faculty omit, fail to emphasize or do not evaluate/test, this is quite a different source and type of learning than the more informal rules students tacitly acquire, for example, how to communicate with a difficult patient as they go about their daily work activities.

Given that a simple dichotomy may obfuscate more than illuminate, we argue here for a basic three (formal, informal, hidden) or four (null) category approach to exploring the HC. In addition to the formal, important learning takes place via the relationships and interactions within the workplace (as one source of the informal curriculum) along with the less visible and/or obvious sources such as organizational culture (as one source of the hidden curriculum). The actual lessons may be similar, but it is important to maintain a conceptual distinction between informal norms that are widely shared and openly recognized versus those social influences that are less obvious to or less recognized by participants.

METAPHORS

 "Leopards break into the temple and drink the sacrificial chalices dry; this occurs repeatedly, again and again; finally it can be reckoned upon beforehand and becomes part of the ceremony."

Franz Kafka, 1917

While definitional distinctions can be critical in understanding the HC, they also can be limiting. This is particularly in the case of phenomena as highly fluid and enigmatic as learning: where influences may be hidden one day, formalized the next, only to have these new formal rules gradually slip beneath conscious reflection and scrutiny over time. For these reasons, using metaphors to capture the HC often can be quite illuminating and liberating in their potential to suggest new ways of thinking about the HC. Thus, we might employ the somewhat obvious metaphor of the iceberg, with its above-the-surface/visible versus its below-the-water-line/invisible dimensions to remind ourselves that the less-than-visible aspects of educational life may be more consequential than that which sits above the surface. Alternatively, we might embrace the more enigmatic metaphor of physics with its alternative realities or the fact that most of the universe is made up of something (dark matter) that is invisible to observers and therefore must be ascertained indirectly. The claim that much of organizational life is shaped by invisible or hidden forces may sound like hyperbole until one realizes how many different areas of science are rooted in a similar contention. After all, we know that most communication is nonverbal, that approximately 80% of mental processing takes place at an unconscious level, that approximately 80% of the universe is composed of invisible forces, and that approximately 80% of effects come from 20% of the causes (e.g. the Pareto 80-20 principle). These realities should at least give us some pause in wondering how much of learning meaningfully can be attributed solely to the formal curriculum.

The hidden curriculum in this book

The HC has both an explicit and implicit presence throughout this book. The term appears in Ross and

Cumming's (Chapter 16) observations on how peer-assisted learning (PAL) functions as a vehicle for transmitting the HC; in Campbell, Chin and Voo's (Chapter 31) material on the role of hierarchy and power in identity formation, the role of the HC in devaluing relationship-centred patient care and the importance of faculty development in countering the effects of the HC; in Harden's (Chapter 2) differentiation among the 'declared' (e.g. formal), the 'taught' ('what happens in practice') and the 'learned' (by students) curricula and finally in Gliatto and Stern's (Chapter 32) material on the HC and professionalism and the role of reflection in converting the HC to a more explicit vehicle for student learning.

 "...the chief barrier to medical professionalism education is unprofessional conduct by medical educators, which is protected by an established hierarchy of academic authority. Students feel no such protection...."

Brainard & Brislen 2007

The HC also can be tied to virtually every topic and issue covered in this book. Any attempt to develop a new and/or reform a pre-existing curriculum (Section 1) is doomed to failure unless educators are willing to tap into the other-than-formal dimensions of student learning. Likewise, learning venues and situations (Section 2) contains a myriad of opportunities to address HC issues. For example, mentoring can be viewed as an attempt to formalize some of the informal and tacit dimensions of role modelling, while the decline in bedside teaching transmits a myriad of potentially countervailing lessons to students on the importance (or lack thereof) of patient-centred medicine and the need for patient-centred learning. Similar arguments can be framed for educational strategies (Section 3), tools and aids (Section 4), curriculum themes (Section 5), assessment (Section 6) and staff and students (Section 7). For example, the selection process (Chapter 43) that governs student admissions is a wonderful place to study the HC since admissions often is the first place students encounter formal statements by the schools as to things like mission, values, focus and curriculum. The potential for rifts between these statements and actual school practices, including messages tacitly sent by the types of students admitted, represents an early wave of HC issues. Assessment practices tell students with far greater clarity than any handbook or course outline what faculty and the school really consider to be important. Even venues such as e-learning and simulation have been examined from an HC perspective (Taylor 2011).

Applications: Exploring/assessing the hidden curriculum

Applying the HC to issues of student learning and faculty development is not an easy or risk-free endeavour. It can involve considerable time and effort, and because it stands in contrast to a 'pure' teaching model (where students are empty vessels eagerly waiting to be filled by the knowledge, skills, behaviours and values possessed by their faculty), framing issues from a HC perspective may be quite disruptive and often will engender resistance. Nonetheless, by exploring the interface between the formal and the other-than-formal aspects of your own learning environments, you may come to more deeply appreciate what is really going on among students and faculty, between faculty and students, and between faculty/students and the broader sociocultural environment within which organizations are located. In this section, we outline practical methods to explore the other-than-formal aspects of learning environments. This is an essential step in aligning what we intend to teach with what is actually learned by our trainees.

1. *Getting started:* Learners (faculty and students) should be familiar with the overall conceptual framework as well as key terms (e.g. formal, informal, hidden, null). Help learners tune into the unintended learning moments that exist within the educational environment. For example, you might ask students to identify the messages or learning points embedded in common scenarios:

   a. You (the third-year medical student) are expected to do all sorts of nonmedical tasks such as picking up food for team members.

   b. Your attending physician stays at work until very late most nights. He often misses family events, most recently his wife's birthday. Residents who stay late are lauded as 'heroes' or 'champs'.

   c. Your resident pronounces your 16-year-old patient with cystic fibrosis dead and sits down with you to reflect on the event and to mourn the loss of the patient you cared for together.

   d. Your attending talks about the patient's diagnosis and poor prognosis to the ward team in front of the patient and without including the patient in the conversation or asking if he has any questions.

   e. Your grade on a particular rotation is determined largely by your score on a multiple-choice content exam.

   f. You observe a morbidly obese patient repeatedly being referred to as a hippopotamus by the intern and resident on your team.

g. You never observe a resident or attending take a sexual history.

A second exercise useful in highlighting the differences between formal and informal curricula is asking learners to identify the 'top ten things I learned in medical school that I wasn't supposed to' (Dosani 2010). Similarly, learners can create two lists and differentiate between what they are being taught versus what they are learning, where they are learning the latter (situations and circumstances) and examples of where the latter reinforces and/or undermines the former. Correspondingly, you can ask faculty to differentiate between what they are teaching and what students are learning. Similarly, learners can examine their own contribution to the educational environment. In order to bring home the notion that we all contribute to the HC, the educator might ask learners to identify and reflect on 'times I taught within the hidden curriculum'.

2. *Participant-observer inquiry:* Learners can take on the role of an amateur 'anthropologist of medical culture' (Harvard Macy Faculty 2011). A brief overview of basic ethnographic methods such as mapping the educational space and objective methods of data collection can be very useful here. Trainees may be asked to describe how people are dressed, the tools they equip themselves with, how they introduce themselves, where they stand or sit when they are in a group, who speaks first and the language that is used or the roles assumed by different members of the healthcare team. Faculty can be asked to do the same exercise. Comparing these two lists can be quite revealing. This method can be used in preclinical and clinical settings. In the pre-clinical setting, one may explore the relative participation (e.g. 'airtime') of faculty versus students in different learning environments. In addition, one can examine the use of technology such as laptops or hand-held devices, attendance rates and late arrivals and the content of pre- and postclass conversations. In clinical settings, such as rounds, a volunteer can time approximately how many minutes are devoted to patients' social/emotional needs versus a range of other topics such as health insurance, other 'business' considerations, joking or non-patient-related conversations. Asking trainees to write their anthropological observations in the third person, as if they are an outsider assigned to 'look in' to a strange new world, can help with the cultivation of 'HC eyes'.

3. *Share stories from the hidden curriculum.*

   a. Provide scheduled time and space, protected from other responsibilities, for sharing, listening and reflecting on student experiences. The use of triggers from the humanities (art, poetry, literature, film) can provide the learner critical distance and a safe opening to the sharing of personal experiences. Such opportunity for reflection is an important aspect of professional development, may stem negative effects of the emotional suppression experienced by many medical students, and ultimately may help prevent ethical erosion.

   b. Sharing learner stories with a wider medical school or hospital audience can have a transformative effect, as often more senior clinicians and educators have simply become desensitized to negative aspects of our learning environments.

   c. The following writing exercise has proved useful at one medical school (Gaufberg et al 2010). After familiarizing students with the concept of the HC, assign a brief reflection paper in which students tell a story from the HC and reflect on it. Use these stories to start a discussion. Stories may also be used as a form of feedback to faculty and others in educational (grand rounds, workshop) settings, with the opportunity for discussion. Dramatic enactment of the stories in the form of Readers' Theatre can be particularly powerful as a starting place (Bell et al 2010). On a larger scale, the sharing of humanizing examples from the informal curriculum ('appreciative inquiry') can be an effective means to effect positive institutional change (Suchman et al 2004).

4. *Focus attention and reflect upon workarounds.* Workarounds are the other-than-formal/unsanctioned ways of getting work done where the official or 'right' way is seen as inefficient, dysfunctional, out-of-date, or otherwise not appropriate. Workarounds can be found in the classroom or in the clinic or wards. Although there are no printed rulebooks for workarounds, initiates soon learn their critical role in getting things done. They also learn that there are right and wrong ways to perform these off-the-books practices. Ask students to come up with one example of a workaround they have engaged in or observed. Ask: 'How did you learn the rules of this particular workaround (observation, role modelling, clues from an insider)?' Encourage students to explore why we even have workarounds, particularly in the face of an ever more highly structured work environment.

5. *Focus on micro-ethical challenges.* Some authors and educators have argued that focusing on day-to-day micro-ethical challenges (Is it okay to 'practise' on patients? What do I do if my resident asks me to falsify a chart? Do I laugh at this dehumanizing joke?) are more developmentally appropriate for medical students than teaching about ethical challenges they will face only as full-fledged clinicians.

Micro-ethical challenges often occur within a hierarchy of evaluation in which students believe that the process or outcome of their decisions may have an impact on their grade.

Researchers at one medical school are using online technology (Qstream) to help students collaboratively probe the micro-ethical challenges they face in their day-to-day learning environments (Bell et al 2011). In this method, students receive an email every few days containing a brief case/scenario that poses a challenging professionalism dilemma in their learning environment. Learners 'tweet' a response, spending no more than 5 minutes on any case. Participants then see how their response compares to what peers say, creating an online collaborative community. Learners also receive scripted course feedback about topical literature-based considerations. Two weeks later, students are re-presented with the case/scenario, asked to vote for the best tweet submitted, see a tally of votes and receive further scripted course feedback. This round provides valuable reinforcement of course concepts and challenges. Such methods can be stand-alone, enabling student-centred exploration and learning with peer guidance, but also can be used as a springboard for discussion in a group reflective practice session.

6. *Turn your attention to the null curriculum.* Review teaching objectives and/or content with an eye towards things that have been left out. Correspondingly, what might your patients be concerned about that you fail to discuss or teach? Review your formal curricular offerings and explore how 'missing topics' might communicate messages to both faculty and students about what is and what is not within the scope of the doctor's concern. This can be a particularly difficult exercise. After all, how does one know when something is missing? Nonetheless, this kind of exercise can have a profound impact in reshaping how one does things in the future.

7. *Inventory and take stock of your physical surroundings.* How much and what kind of space does your school devote to clinical learning versus other organizational objectives such as administration or research? A school dominated by lecture rooms but with few spaces for small group learning more than likely will stress didactic over interactive learning processes. What about student and faculty awards? Where do you post them, if at all? There is a substantial 'meaning difference' between schools that post awards in highly trafficked areas and those that use a back hallway. Sometimes physical artefacts can be hiding in plain sight. Over the course of several days and during his normal work activities, one clinician conscientiously inventoried items

as he encountered them (Hafferty & O'Donnell 2006). He was dumfounded by what he 'newly saw.'

Conclusions

 "The relational processes of the hidden curriculum assure the perpetuation of its content."
Haidet & Stern 2006

While no single theme can subsume all of the concepts and framings covered above, there are a few particulars worthy of final comment. First, the HC is a versatile tool. The concept can be applied to a broad number of health education issues. Medical schools 'teach' far more to both faculty and students than they commonly take credit for: or perhaps would want to take credit for. Similarly, faculty and students are perpetually interactive and mutually influential co-participants in creating the normative soup that fuels the formal, informal and hidden curricula of medical education and medical practice. Second, the HC has an incessant and ubiquitous presence within educational settings. There is no learning environment without a HC. Its presence and its impact may be pivotal or relatively insignificant, but it is there nonetheless. Third, and related, the HC is universal. Whatever else links physicians trained in different countries, and whatever constitutes the shared values that allow us to talk about an authentic and international 'medical culture', there is a HC weaving its way through the particulars of that country and its training. Fourth, working with the HC is a reflective act and thus a form of pedagogical reflexivity. It is just as important to think about and probe into medical education than it is to deliver it. Finally, the HC is relational. The HC, like social life, is built in and around, and nourished by, relationships among participants and between participants and the surrounding environment. While the HC is fundamentally about probing the difference between the stated and the received, it is also about context and about situating some 'piece' within a larger relational whole. Regardless of what things look like 'on the surface', the HC is all about subterrestrial context and its connections.

References

Bell SK, Gaufberg E, Kerfoot BP: *Qstream: Harvard Medical School patient-doctor III pilot. Personal communication*, 2011.

Bell SK, Wideroff M, Gaufberg E: Student voices in readers' theater: Exploring communication in the hidden curriculum, *Patient Education and Counseling* 80:354–357, 2010.

Brainard AH, Brislen HC: Viewpoint: Learning professionalism: A view from the trenches, *Academic Medicine* 82:1010–1014, 2007.

Campbell EG, Regan S, Gruen RL, et al: Professionalism in medicine: Results of a national survey of physicians, *Annals of Internal Medicine* 147:795–802, 2007.

Dewey J: *Experience and Education*, New York, 1938, Collier Books.

Dosani N: *The top 10 things I learned in medical school (but wasn't supposed to!): Plenary Session: The hidden curriculum exposed: perspectives of learners and educators*, Canada, May 4, 2010, St. John's Newfoundland.

Gaufberg E, Batalden M, Sands R, Bell S: The hidden curriculum: What can we learn from third-year medical student narrative reflections? *Academic Medicine* 85:1709–1711, 2010.

Gofton W, Regehr G: What we don't know we are teaching: unveiling the hidden curriculum, *Clinical Orthopaedics and Related Research* 449:20–27, 2006.

Hafferty FW, O'Donnell JE: It's time to clean house: the commercial brandscaping of medical education, *Academic Physician & Scientist* 7:9, 2006.

Haidet P, Stein HF: The role of the student-teacher relationship in the formation of physicians: The hidden curriculum as process, *Journal of General Internal Medicine* 21(Supplement 1):S16–S20, 2006.

Harvard Macy Faculty: *Learning to Look: A Hidden Curriculum Exercise*, Boston, MA, 2011, Harvard Macy Institute.

Fryer-Edwards K: Addressing the hidden curriculum in scientific research, *American Journal of Bioethics* 2:58–59, 2002.

Suchman AL, Williamson PR, Litzelman DK, et al: The relationship-centered care initiative discovery team: Toward an informal curriculum that teaches professionalism: transforming the social environment of a medical school, *Journal of General Internal Medicine* 19(Part 2):501–504, 2004.

Taylor JS: The moral aesthetics of simulated suffering in standardized patient performances, *Culture, Medicine and Psychiatry* 35:134–162, 2011

Section 2

Learning situations

Lectures

G. Brown, S. Edmunds

The ubiquity of lectures

Lectures are the oldest and most ubiquitous method of learning in medicine and allied subjects. They are economical and at least as effective as other methods of teaching at conveying knowledge (Bligh 2001). Given the usefulness and universal usage of lectures it is important that all medical teachers develop and refresh their expertise in lecturing. This chapter provides a brief guide to improving student learning from lectures. It considers briefly the strengths and limitations of lectures, the processes of learning from lectures, the core skills and structures of lectures and some ways in which the efficacy of lectures may be evaluated.

 Merely reading this chapter is not sufficient to improve one's lectures: just as reading a text on clinical diagnosis may not be sufficient to make one a better clinician

Purposes, strengths and limitations of lectures

The main purposes of lectures are *coverage* of a topic or theme, *understanding* of processes and phenomena and *motivating* students to learn. Of these broad purposes, coverage is the most common, and the most common weakness (Brown & Manogue 2001). Understanding, the creation of new connections in the minds of the learners, and motivating students to learn are twin priorities. Beneath these priorities is a hidden purpose of developing one's own understanding of a subject and of the way students learn. *Docemur docemus:* we learn as we teach.

Lectures *can* provide an entrée into a difficult topic, overviews of a topic or theme, different perspectives on a subject, up-to-date résumés of research and accounts of relevant personal, clinical or laboratory experience. They *can* be used to provoke thought, to deepen understanding and to enhance scientific and clinical thinking. They *can* provide hints and guidelines on how to learn a topic or procedure as well as what to learn and thereby help students to revise and to develop into independent, thinking professionals. Lectures can, in short, bring a subject alive and make it more meaningful. Alternatively, they can kill it.

For lectures, like all methods of teaching, have limitations.

 'A superfluity of lectures can lead to ischial bursitis (pain in the buttock).'

Osler

Lectures can be boring and, worse, useless. If they are merely recitations of standard texts, then they are not fulfilling adequately their functions of developing understanding and motivating students to learn. If the lecture is used only to provide detailed coverage of facts and findings, then the students would gain more from reading a good textbook. If lectures are the only method of teaching used, then the students are not being well prepared for their future roles. Finally, lectures can induce passivity and compliance. But they are not necessarily passive modes of learning or authoritarian modes of teaching. Passivity and authoritarianism are not dependent on the learning method so much as on how that learning method is used by the lecturer or clinician.

 'The decrying of wholesale lecturing is certainly justified. The wholesale decrying of lectures is just as certainly not justified.'

Brown & Manogue 2001

Processes of lecturing and learning from lectures

AN EXPLANATORY MODEL

There is an old adage that states, 'Lectures are a method of transferring the notes of a teacher to the notes of a student without passing through the heads of either.' The germ of truth beneath this witticism is that lecturing should be concerned with *active* transfer of knowledge, understanding, skills and attitudes. Actions are required by both lecturers and students for the transfer to be successful. The lecturer needs to plan, structure, communicate clearly and interestingly and monitor the reactions of the students. The students need to listen, observe, summarize, note-take and subsequently study and apply the knowledge gained.

These actions can be summarized as a series of processes which are expressed in the following apparently simple explanatory model of lecturing derived from social and cognitive psychology (Brown & Manogue 2001) (see Fig. 8.1).

Amongst the many hints that can be adduced from the model are:

Articulate your intentions. If you use intended learning outcomes, use only a few. A brief statement of the structure and content of the lecture may be more meaningful to students than a list of learning outcomes. Ascertain what the students know, including their experiences and interests. Match your content and structure to your intentions.

Prepare the lecture and prepare particularly the opening phase of the lecture so it gains the attention of students. Ask yourself (and answer!) how can you make the lecture clear and interesting.

Bear in mind that transmission includes verbal messages, extra-verbal messages (emphatics, expressiveness, hesitations, stumbles) and nonverbal messages (eye contact, gestures, movement). These can convey your interest in the topic and favourable attitudes to students. Alternatively, they can convey boredom, disinterest, arrogance and hostility. In the lecture, use examples, give students time to copy diagrams, vary activities, speak clearly and use eye contact and gestures.

Use educational media effectively. Lectures can be enriched by educational media, such as PowerPoint, whiteboards, interactive whiteboards, slides, overhead transparencies, videos, sound recordings, models and simulations. 'Blackboard' or similar tools such as 'LEARN' can be useful. Electronic voting systems (EVS) can increase interaction in lectures and provide feedback to both the lecturer and the students. All of these can improve the quality of lectures, but they can also distract, confuse or produce mental dazzle. To be effective, educational media need to be designed for their purpose *and* the students.

Monitor the students' reactions and change accordingly. These reactions are the basis of lecturer responsiveness, and it is these features which account for student preferences for live rather than recorded lectures (Bligh 2001). Looking at students in different parts of the lecture theatre

Lecturer: Intentions–Transmission–Monitoring

Student: Intentions–Reception–Embedding–Retrieval–Application

Fig. 8.1 Explanatory model of lecturing.

enables the lecturer to gauge the reactions of interest, puzzlement or boredom of the students. Students who sit near the front tend to be the more interested; students who sit near the back tend to be the less interested or troublemakers (Brown & Atkins 1988). Monitoring can reduce the probability of disruption as well as help anticipate other reactions.

Bear in mind the limited capacity of the sensory and working memory, so do not talk too quickly and do chunk the information provided into meaningful and relatively brief sentences. Presentations that are too fast or too distracting cannot be processed by the working memory.

Remember that attention in lectures usually declines after about 20 minutes, so vary activities or switch the focus of the lecture.

The use of analogies, metaphors and similes will create new connections rapidly with existing schemata (networks of knowledge in the long-term memory).

The use of frequent summaries, guiding statements and cognitive maps can help students to change their schemata which can then be elaborated upon by the students after the lecture.

Personal narratives interwoven with concepts and findings can trigger the episodic memory (memories of events and experiences) and the semantic memory (memories of knowledge, ideas, skills) and so aid storage and retrieval. For example, explaining aspects of disease in relation to a patient or recounting one's initial attempts at performing a colonoscopy can assist students or trainees to learn, remember and understand.

The skills of lecturing

The processes of lecturing are effected through the skills shown in Table 8.1. Of these skills, the preparation of lectures, explaining and the use of educational media are the most important. A more detailed description of the skills and subskills involved in lecturing may be found in Brown and Atkins (1988), Brown and Manogue (2001) and Hargie (2006).

Table 8.1 The skills of lecturing. What are your strongest and weakest skills?

Skill	Comments
Preparation	Takes account of knowledge of learners. Specifies purposes or outcomes and provides structure and sequence. Undue specificity and very loose structures not recommended.
Opening	Gains attention, establishes rapport and provides framework of lecture.
Explaining	The key skill. Creates understanding in the learners. Clarity and generating interest are its key components. Embraces many of the skills of lecturing such as preparation, openings, use of audio-visual aids/IT, summarizing.
Presenting information	An important but lower level skill than explaining. It is concerned with coverage of the essential facts or theories. Danger of providing too much detail and inducing boredom.
Narrating	Telling a story of a patient, case or experience that captures the imagination of the students and deepens their understanding. A powerful but neglected skill.
Comparing and contrasting	Easy to do badly. Requires a clear outline of what is to be compared and contrasted and careful framing of the comparisons. 2×2 matrices are useful for paired comparisons.
Design and use of educational media	Important in medicine and health but sometimes produces mental dazzle or sleep rather than intellectual enlightenment.
Responsiveness to audience	A neglected skill. Includes monitoring audience, reading reactions of audience and responding accordingly.
Varying student activity	Necessary to keep them awake! Can improve learning and heighten interest. Ensure, if possible, that the changes in activity are relevant.
Summarizing	Should be used during a lecture as well as at the end of a lecture. Should emphasize the key points, show the links within the lecture topic and between the topic and cognate topics.

PREPARING LECTURES

The maxim 'know your subject, know your students' is the basis of good preparation. Its essential ingredients are purposes, content, organization and preparation of the lecture.

As indicated, the purposes of lectures are often stated as intended learning outcomes. Too detailed a set of outcomes becomes a straitjacket rather than a guide. It is equally dangerous to have no clear purposes. The purposes can be expressed in the form of statements (signposts) or questions. Questions can act as advanced organizers for note-taking by the students and can evoke curiosity. For example, at the beginning of a lecture in oral biochemistry, the lecturer could pose the question, 'Does eating carrots help you to see in the dark? To answer this question we need to consider the following questions…'

Too much content militates against learning in lectures. Students recall and understand presentations that are based on essential principles and a little detail better than those containing much detail (Bligh 2001). It is more important to provide understanding than to report detailed findings.

Structures of lectures will be outlined in a later section. Here we emphasize these points:

- Allow time for distributing materials.
- State and show the organization of the lecture to students.
- Do not overload with information.
- Occasionally include some small group activities in lectures.
- Provide summaries during the lecture.
- Use the conclusion to summarize and raise questions.
- Occasionally, invite the students to review, summarize and compare their summaries.

SOME SUGGESTIONS FOR PREPARING LECTURES

A method that has been found useful by new lecturers in Dundee and Nottingham is given in Box 8.1. In practice, lecturers often zigzag and backtrack rather than prepare lectures in a linear fashion.

Most lecturers speak at about 100–120 words per minute in lectures. This is the equivalent of about 15 pages of full lecture notes for an hour's lecture. This approach is not recommended except in the very early stages of learning to lecture or for lectures which are to be published as papers.

 For most lectures, if you must read aloud, rather than talk, then write the lecture as you would speak it, rather than speak the lecture as you would normally write it. Prose (the written word) is difficult to process aurally.

Box 8.1 Preparing a lecture

1. **Choose topic**
   It may have been given to you.

2. **Free associate**
   Write down whatever comes to you about the topic, facts, ideas, questions. Ring the things you are going to use.

3. **Produce a working title**
   Base this on the ideas you have ringed. Use the title to specify the objectives and structure of the lecture.

4. **Set out a structure**
   Produce a rough structure of the lecture.

5. **Read**
   Read for specific ideas and facts. Don't read too much. Reading can become a delaying tactic for the serious business of…

6. **Setting out the lecture**
   Set out the lecture, any educational media and any student activities. Prepare a summary sheet of the lecture. Check that the order of subtopics is okay. If not, change it.

7. **Prepare the opening**
   Think of a good way of opening the lecture which will gain interest and provide the framework of the lecture.

8. **Give the lecture**
   Rehearse it privately if you are worried about it. About 40 minutes in private is equivalent to 55 in the lecture theatre.

9. **Reflect and note**
   Make a note of any corrections you need to make, particularly if it is the first time you have given this lecture.

EXPLAINING

Explaining is concerned with giving understanding to others. Understanding consists of creating new connections in the schemata of the learners or creating new schemata. Three types of common explanations are the descriptive, the procedural (sometimes known as the interpretive) and the reason-giving, which includes causes. These types of explanation correspond roughly to 'What?', 'How?' and 'Why?' questions. (Together with the questions 'When?' and 'Where?' they can provide a quick way of preparing a lecture.) For example, a lecture on underperformance in medicine might address these questions: What is underperformance? How is it best measured? Why is it an important topic? When is it likely to occur? Where is it likely to occur?

 'Some people explain aptly, getting to the heart of the matter with just the right terminology, examples, and organization of ideas. Other explainers, on the contrary, get us and themselves all mixed up, use terms beyond our level of comprehension, draw inept analogies, and even employ concepts and principles that cannot be understood without an understanding of the very thing being explained.'

Brown & Manogue 2001

Two key variables of explaining are interest and clarity. These are valued characteristics by medical undergraduates, trainees and attendees at medical conferences (Brown 2006, Copeland et al 2000). The latter report that interest in an explanation is generated by expressiveness, the use of examples, cases, analogies, metaphors and appeals to the experience of the learners. As indicated in the model of lecturing, these features are conveyed verbally, extraverbally, nonverbally and through the use of educational media.

Clear explanations usually contain four structuring moves: signposts, frames, foci and links. 'Signposts' indicate the structure and direction of an explanation.

Today, I wish to outline for you four approaches to the management of cancer patients: surgical methods, radiotherapy, chemotherapy and psychotherapeutic methods.

'Frames' indicate the beginning and end of a section of the explanation.

That ends my summary of surgical methods; now let's look at the methods of radiotherapy, their strengths and limitations.

'Foci' emphasize the key points of an explanation.

So the important and neglected feature of cancer management is the role of counselling and support of patients in the preoperative and postoperative phases.

'Links' refers to links between the topics of the explanation and links between the explanation and the knowledge of the learner:

You can see that the use of psychological methods can aid the recovery of patients, whatever form of invasive treatment they undergo.
Some of you may have had a grandparent or a parent who experienced the side effects of chemotherapy. So you will know that some psychological support would have helped.

Common errors which make an explanation unclear are too elaborate or too brief a signpost; frames not provided consistently; key points not emphasized and neglecting links. The latter often occurs if the lecturer is trying to cover too much material.

 The message to be taken from this summary of explaining is plain: 'Be clear, be interesting.' Translating the message into practice is a challenge…

DESIGNING AND USING EDUCATIONAL MEDIA

At the risk of overgeneralizing, most medical and healthcare students are visual learners, and much of medical and healthcare practice relies on visual cues. Ideas and procedures that are linked through visualization are more likely to be stored and retrieved from the long-term memories of the students. And, as many lecturers know, designing a visual representation can deepen one's own understanding as well as providing deeper understanding to one's students.

Common advice on the use of educational media

Illustrations, diagrams, bullet points and summaries should be simple, brief and readable from the back of the class. Do not merely recite the list of bullet points on the slide: link the bullet points in a meaningful way. If the illustrations are important, give the students time to look at them and, if necessary, copy them. If the illustrations are available in a book, on the web or on an intranet give the reference. There is no need to always speak whilst the students are looking at illustrations; indeed, if you want them to look intensively, tell them what to look for and shut up.

When using video recordings, indicate which features should be attended to. Make sure they are audible. If possible, one should pose questions (advanced organizers) for the students to answer whilst watching the audio-visual materials, give them an opportunity to discuss briefly the materials and then summarize the main points and link them to the relevant parts of the lecture.

If you use handouts then decide on their purpose and design them accordingly:

Interactive handouts contain skeletal notes and diagrams which the students have to complete during the lecture. These can be reduced versions of the slides with space for the students to write their own notes. These are better than full handouts for recall and understanding (Bligh 2001, Brown & Manogue 2001). Students often request or expect handouts of the full lecture slides, but perhaps lecturers should resist this request and make the decision to use one of these other methods instead.

Outlines provide a one-page summary of the lecture and some annotated key references.

Key information handouts provide complex diagrams, references, quotations, formulae, proofs, etc.

Full handouts are virtually a transcript of the lecture.

Tasks and problems handouts state the tasks or problems that are to be used in the lecture so that students do not have to refer to the slide that the lecturer is using. Useful advice on the use of media may be found in Exley and Dennick (2004).

 Some students assume if they have the handouts in their files, they have the knowledge in their heads

Varying student activity

There is nothing wrong with someone with expert knowledge explaining ideas and procedures to someone less knowledgeable. But it does not follow that because one has a lecture class for 1 hour or more that one has to talk for the whole time. By varying student activities during a lecture one can renew students' attention, generate interest, provide opportunities for students to think and obtain some feedback of their understanding. But there is a cost: The lecturer has less time to talk. So there is a question that one has to ask oneself: Which is more important, that I cover all the material or the students learn more?

Ways of making lectures more interactive were mentioned in the explanatory model. Other ways are the use of handsets so the class's total responses to a Motivations for Reading Question (MRQ) can be obtained (Exley & Dennick 2004). One can also divide the lecture class into groups of three or four and set brief tasks such as studies, problems, interpretations of data or the advantages of a clinical procedure. Use these activities, but do not overuse them. Like all methods of teaching, overuse reduces their effect.

Structures of lectures

The structure of a lecture affects student note-taking and learning. Five common methods of structuring lectures are the following:

1. *The classical*, in which a lecture is divided into broad areas and then subdivided. This is the easiest method of structuring a lecture. An extension of this method is the *iterative* classical, in which a set procedure is applied to each topic. For example, signs, symptoms, diagnoses, management and prognosis may be applied to a set of related diseases. The iterative method is relatively easy to take notes from.

2. *The problem-centred*, in which a problem is outlined and various solutions are offered. When handled well, this method can play on the curiosity and clinical interests of the students.

3. *The sequential*, in which a problem or question is presented and followed by a chain of reasoning which leads to a solution or conclusion. It is easy to lose the students' attention when using this method, so the use of periodic summaries is recommended.

4. *The comparative*, in which two or more perspectives, methods or models are compared. It is better done visually rather than orally. A common error is to assume that the audience knows the perspective or methods under review. If in doubt, first outline each of the perspectives.

5. *The thesis*, in which an assertion is made and then proved or disproved through a mixture of argument and perhaps speculation. Potentially this is an interesting approach for students but, like the sequential approach, it can sometimes be difficult to follow.

Some lectures are based on a mixture of the above approaches, but usually one structure predominates. It is advisable to prepare a summary sheet of your lecture so you can identify its structure and ways of improving it. Often a simple change in the order or structure of a lecture can make the lecture more meaningful and interesting to an audience. Indicating the structure at the beginning of a lecture, preferably visually, helps the students to take notes.

An example of the structure of an iterative lecture is shown in Box 8.2. Other examples may be found in Bligh (2001), Brown and Manogue (2001), Cantillon (2003) and Dent (2001).

Evaluating lectures

Lectures are evaluated for judgemental purposes such as tenure, promotion and quality procedures and for developmental purposes such as improving expertise and student learning.

Common sources of evaluation are student opinion (satisfaction), student achievement and peer views. The methods of evaluation are focus groups, analyses of students' performance, individual interviews and questionnaires (open-ended and rating schedules). Methods based on small groups may provide valuable insights, but small groups may be dominated by vociferous students who may persuade others of their viewpoints. Discussions and open-ended questionnaires can provide insights which rating schedules cannot reveal, but they are more time-consuming to analyse. Nonetheless, they can provide a good basis for reflection. Rating schedules may tell you what is

---

> **Box 8.2** **An example based on the iterative/classical approach**
>
> **Introduction: Children's minor illnesses**
> - What they are; brief epidemiology
> - Trends in UK and Europe
> - Only minor if we keep them that way
> - Structure of lecture (iterative)
>
> **Measles**
> - Symptoms
> - Signs
> - Definition
> - Prognosis
> - Management
> - Prevention
>
> **Repeat iteration for mumps and rubella with slides**
> **Current controversy on MMR vaccinations**
> **Summary**

---

good or bad but not how to improve. Their value is limited by the quality of the rating schedule, the personal characteristics of the raters, the intrinsic difficulty of the subject and the quality of the learning environment. Reviews suggest that student opinion did not improve lecturing unless the lecturer wanted to improve (Brown & Manogue 2001). Despite these weaknesses, student ratings are the most widespread method of evaluating lectures.

If one's main purpose in evaluating lectures is the improvement of lecturing then the sample questionnaire in Fig. 8.2 is worth using. The items are based on research on lecturing; the questionnaire is easy to complete and analyse. Inspect standard deviations as well as means of scores obtained, and remember that one cannot please all of one's students all of the time. Compile a list of their comments, and if you wish to be rigorous, do a thematic analysis of the comments. The questionnaire can be used at the end of a lecture. It can be shown on a slide, then the students can write down the number of the item, their ratings of it and their comments. The same questionnaire can be used by peers so the results can be compared.

Peer feedback is increasingly used to evaluate lectures (Siddiqui et al 2007), although the meaning of the term 'peer' is sometimes stretched to include senior professors as peer evaluators. In the early stages of establishing a peer evaluation system, it is useful to use paired peer observation: A observes B; B observes A. This approach is less threatening than using a team of appointed evaluators. Guard against a system being perceived as judgemental if it is intended to be

Please rate the lecture(s) on the following items

On the whole lectures were:

	Agree strongly	Agree slightly	Disagree slightly	Disagree strongly
	4	3	2	1
Clear				
Interesting				
Easy to take notes from				
Thought-provoking				
Relevant to course				

Comments

Thank you for your help

Fig. 8.2 A simple way of evaluating a lecture.

developmental. Bear in mind the question: 'Is this wrong or merely different from the way I would do it?'

Finally, reflection on practice is probably the most powerful form of evaluation for the purpose of change. It involves collecting information from various sources, including one's own self-assessment. But this is only the first phase. The next phase of changing one's practice requires knowledge of ways of improving lectures, insight and the will to change.

Summary

Lectures are the most common method of teaching and learning. An understanding of the processes of lecturing and learning from lectures can be derived from cognitive theory. The key variables in effective lecturing are clarity and generating interest. The key skills in effective lecturing are preparation, explanation and the design and use of educational media. Varying activities in lectures can sustain attention and perhaps improve learning. Learning is probably improved by teaching students to learn from lectures. Having a clear underlying structure to the lecture helps students take notes. Evaluations of lectures may be based on student or peer opinion and the achievements of students. Reflection based on data collected is an important method of improving lecturing. So too is extending one's knowledge of lecturing and the will to change.

References

Bligh DA: *What's the Use of Lectures?* San Francisco, 2001, Jossey-Bass.

Brown G: Explaining. In Hargie O, editor: *Handbook of Communication Skills*, London, 2006, Routledge, pp 195–228.

Brown GA, Atkins MJ: *Effective Teaching in Higher Education*, London, 1988, Methuen.

Brown GA, Manogue M: AMEE medical education guide No 22. Refreshing lecturing: a guide for lecturers, *Medical Teacher* 24:231–244, 2001.

Cantillon P: Teaching large groups, *BMJ* 326:437–440, 2003.

Copeland HL, Longworth DL, Hewson MG, Stoller JK: Successful lecturing: a prospective study to validate attributes of the effective medical lecture, *Journal of General Internal Medicine* 15(6):366–371, 2000.

Dent JA: Lecturing. In Dent JA, Harden RM, editors: *A Practical Guide for Medical Teachers*, Edinburgh, 2001, Churchill Livingstone, pp 65–73.

Exley K, Dennick R: *Giving a Lecture: From Presenting to Teaching. Key Guides for Effective Teaching in Higher Education*, London, 2004, Routledge Falmer.

Hargie O, editor: *Handbook of Communication Skills*, London, 2006, Routledge.

Siddiqui ZS, Jonas-Dwyer D, Carr SE: Twelve tips for peer observation of teaching, *Medical Teacher* 29:297–300, 2007.

Small-group teaching

S. J. Durning, R. M. Conran

Medical educators can use a number of instructional situations for teaching learners (see Chapters 8–17). Small groups represent a teaching situation or environment of growing importance in healthcare education.

Recent studies are beginning to unravel the reasons why small groups have a positive effect on learning performance (van Blankenstein et al 2011). These studies cite both socio-behavioural and cognitive benefits. Socio-behavioural benefits include promoting learner motivation, social cohesion and authenticity. Cognitive benefits include facilitating elaboration and reflection or recourse to prior knowledge and experiences. Additionally, emotional engagement theories stress that instructional authenticity enables the learner to more meaningfully engage with the material to enhance learning; small-group teaching enables the potential for more authentic instruction than that provided in the large-group setting.

The reader is encouraged to review the benefits of small-group teaching to maximize potential learning. Furthermore, recent work has shown that learning situations can be complementary: for example, combining small-group teaching with lectures (Chapter 8) can facilitate the potential benefits of instruction with each format.

What is a small group?

Small groups are instructional settings that better optimize the instructor-to-learner ratio. Small-group sessions often complement large-group (i.e. lecture-based) courses: lectures are the 'prototype' for large-group teaching. Typically, when small groups are used to complement large-group teaching, a primary purpose of the small-group sessions is to further explore the key concepts in the lectures and readings with a practical emphasis to help students with complicated material pertaining to the subject being presented and discussions that are difficult to conduct in a larger group setting. Additionally, small groups can

also help educators integrate material from multiple courses, such as a clinical reasoning small group on chest pain that could integrate anatomy, physiology and pathology concepts into the session.

The size of the small group can vary greatly in healthcare education. Prior studies suggest that groups of five to eight learners are optimal. However, the number of students in a group should not conform to any set rule.

 "The number of students in a small group should not conform to any set rule."

Indeed, the experienced small-group teacher may be able to effectively facilitate a much larger number of students than a less experienced instructor. The goal with determining small-group size should focus on effectiveness that will be dependent upon goals and objectives for the session and learner experience/expertise with the content being discussed (i.e. difficulty of the content). For example, if the group is too small or the material is very straightforward to learn, exchange of ideas can be limited so a balance should be struck in determining the number of students in a small group. The challenge for the healthcare educator is to construct a small-group size that will best facilitate exchange of ideas and concepts for the content being discussed, given the learning goals and objectives for the session.

Newble and Cannon (2001) discuss three signature characteristics of small-group teaching: *active participation*, *purposeful activity*, and *face-to-face contact*. We believe that consistently achieving these three characteristics is essential for small-group teaching effectiveness.

 Three signature characteristics of small-group teaching are active participation, purposeful activity, and face-to-face contact.

According to these authors, if the small group lacks *any* of these components, the teaching activity will likely be suboptimal. For example, active participation and purposeful activity are needed for the cognitive benefits of elaboration and reflection. Elaboration and reflection accompanied with face-to-face contact are needed to optimize motivation and emotional engagement with the content. Indeed, the size of the group is less important than fulfilling these three characteristics. For example, effective team-based learning (Chapter 21) allows for larger groups through the formation of smaller subgroups within the teaching setting and can capitalize on these three signature characteristics within each subgroup. Indeed, one of the most often cited reasons for combining lectures with small groups is that it is extremely difficult, if not impossible, to have active participation and purposeful activity in the typical large-group lecture setting.

When to use small groups?

The reason(s) for choosing to incorporate small-group teaching into a curriculum should be primarily guided by learning goals and objectives. A secondary reason is the difficulty of the content being presented (which is dependent upon the expertise of the learner with the content). As stated above, if the content presented in the small-group session is too straightforward, the three signature characteristics discussed above are unlikely to be met. Further, since small groups are one of the most resource-intensive teaching formats, the reason(s) for using this format should be carefully considered, weighing the pros and cons of this format with alternatives.

There are many advantages to teaching in small groups, and we have introduced some of the theoretical benefits of this teaching format at the outset of this chapter. Additional benefits include the fact that small-group instructors can become more familiar with learners' knowledge, skills and experiences with the content being discussed than in larger group teaching settings. Instruction can therefore be more customized or tailored to the learners' needs in small groups. This benefit may be particularly important with complicated material, where learners may have a variety of differences in knowledge, skills and experiences and difficulty with integrating the material to be learned. Also, in small groups, the teacher has more opportunity for individualized feedback, which has been shown to be important, especially for learning complex information. Further, peer evaluation and self-reflection can add to teacher-directed feedback to enhance the experience for learners. Additionally,

learners have the opportunity to get to know their classmates and may be more comfortable asking questions during a small-group session than in larger group settings; again, this benefit may be particularly relevant when the content to be learned is difficult for learners (due to their relative expertise with the content).

Another potential benefit of small-group teaching is that learners can become familiar with adult learning principles, which are something they will be encouraged to apply for the rest of their professional lives. For example, learners are encouraged to take responsibility for their own learning (self-directed learning or self-regulation, e.g. adequate preparation for the small group, asking questions during the session, follow-up readings after the small-group session has concluded), and learners are encouraged to use problem solving and reflection skills. In a similar vein, small-group learners have the opportunity to develop important interpersonal and communication skills that they will use in their future practice. Small-group teaching also offers the opportunity for teachers to model professionalism, respect for different opinions and time management. Finally, small-group teaching promotes engagement between the teacher, learner and content, enabling the instructor to reinforce concepts that move beyond recalling content and asking trainees to apply this content in a more meaningful manner than in larger group settings. Therefore, small-group sessions should challenge the learner to apply what is learned in larger settings and/ or from textbook readings.

These advantages come at the cost of needing additional faculty for instructional purposes, so medical schools in the United States and elsewhere typically include other teaching formats, such as lectures and seminars, to introduce content and use small-group teaching to reinforce key learning concepts. Finally, recent work from the cognitive load literature suggests that using small-group sessions for straightforward content can actually increase extraneous (not useful for learning) cognitive load in learners and potentially impair learning; therefore, careful construction of goals and objectives for the small-group session will help maximize chances of success.

 Careful construction of goals and objectives for the small-group session will help maximize chances of success.

Two additional questions that are relevant to determining when to use small-group teaching are *what format of small-group teaching* and *what type of instructional methods*.

WHAT FORMAT OF SMALL-GROUP TEACHING?

A number of small-group teaching formats exist. Formats of small-group teaching include problem-based learning (PBL), case-based learning (CBL) and team-based learning (TBL). This content is beyond the scope of this chapter. The reader is encouraged to review this content in other chapters of this book. A notable distinction between PBL, CBL and TBL is the role of the instructor. In PBL, the instructor is a facilitator; being a subject matter expert on the content is not required. In CBL, the instructor is a facilitator but also typically provides summative comments at the end of the session, sharing their subject matter expertise. In TBL, the instructor typically provides both facilitation and subject matter expertise, the latter often provided through both summative comments and/or pre- and post-session quizzes.

WHAT TYPE OF INSTRUCTIONAL METHODS?

Several instructional methods for small-group teaching exist, and the number of methods involving robust technology is emerging (Table 9.1). Importantly, the most successful methods have clear goals and objectives and are organized around a purposeful activity. In healthcare education, the case-based structured discussion is probably the most common approach. Learners read about and then present a patient case and work through a series of tasks which could include asking for additional history and physical examination information, constructing a problem list, generating a differential diagnosis, comparing and contrasting diagnoses and constructing a treatment plan. In the CBL and TBL formats, time is typically allocated for the small-group instructor to clarify important teaching points and answer additional questions. In the PBL method, emphasis is placed on asking questions, and the teacher may or may not provide summary or conclusion remarks. Skills such as the 'one-minute preceptor' (Neher et al 1992) can be particularly effective in small-group settings. In this method, the teacher probes for understanding and then evaluates (or comes to an educational diagnosis of) the learner and provides next steps for their improvement.

 Instructional methods for the small-group setting:

- Surrogate patient encounters (e.g. paper cases, DVD cases, standardized patients)
- Actual patients
- Journal articles (i.e. thought-provoking reading material)
- Internet-based materials (e.g. wiki, blog, discussion board)
- Role plays
- Multiple choice or open-ended questions
- Completing a worked example

Table 9.1 Tips for a successful small-group session

Define the problem and purposes of the session
Coordinate statements: clarify and relate statements versus lecturing
Seek information (request facts from learners) and opinions
Give information (fill in gaps in group knowledge)
Test feasibility (challenge practicality and correctness of suggested solutions)
Expect silence, lack of knowledge and uncertainty
Facilitate a positive learning environment
Give students positive feedback and don't ask 'read my mind' questions
Don't provide too much information (don't lecture, and encourage students to follow up on questions raised during the session to enhance their learning)
Probe thinking process: try to think out loud, providing explanations to help students with complex tasks like clinical reasoning; ask students to explain their underlying thought process as well as the concepts they are applying, assumptions they are making and approach to the problem
Encourage participation of all group members (and prevent monopolization of the session by one or two students)
Practise higher-order skills (interpretation, reflection, synthesis, transfer)
Think out loud (students can benefit from hearing thoughts and feelings of others)
Stress the value of diversity of opinions and respect for peers
Facilitate learner interaction (enhance understanding, promoting teamwork)
Stress how a question can be addressed from many different perspectives
Review and reinforce teaching goals and objectives
Keep time constraints (time management skills)
Provide regular and timely feedback

How to effectively conduct a small-group teaching session

PREPARING FOR THE SMALL-GROUP SESSION

Preparation for the small-group teaching session has many similarities to preparation for other teaching sessions, like larger group teaching sessions. First, determine the learning objectives for the session. Become familiar with students' experience (if any) with the content being discussed from other aspects of the curriculum. Know what 'success looks like' for the session.

 Know what 'success looks like' for the small-group session.

This can be done by completing the statement, 'By the end of the session, learners will be able to...', keeping in mind that small-group sessions are an optimal place to ask learners to demonstrate higher-order skills, such as problem-solving, reflection and clinical reasoning. The reader is encouraged to review materials (Huggett 2010) on constructing goals and objectives. Second, know your audience (the learners) and the curriculum. For example, what has been the learners' prior experience with the content to be discussed in the small-group session in the curriculum? What topic or concept(s) might be particularly challenging for the learners? Third, become familiar with the structure of the small-group teaching session to include time for the session, instructional materials and number of sessions. Think about the activities and methods needed to achieve success. For example, is a review of a pertinent case from the last session or beginning the session with one or more multiple choice or open-ended questions needed? Fourth, it can also be very helpful to develop an instructional 'agenda' for the small-group teaching session. This optimally will be provided by the course or clerkship director (e.g. key teaching points and students' strengths or difficulties with the content from other aspects of the course). We believe that providing instructors with key teaching points, particularly for CBL and TBL, is important to maximize the effectiveness of the session. These teaching points can also be used for examination purposes and should reflect what is essential: key elements for discussion in the session. We do not, however, believe that these key teaching points should require most or all of the time scheduled for the small-group session. Indeed, providing teachers with a comprehensive or highly time-consuming list for discussion can lead to mini-lectures and/or stifling discussion.

LEADING THE SMALL-GROUP SESSION

Experienced small-group instructors recognize that their teaching style and the dynamics of the group are important elements. The time that the instructor spends preparing in advance should improve the organization and flow of the session. The attitude and behaviour (both verbal and nonverbal) of the instructor is one of the most critical elements for small-group teaching success (Jaques 2003). In the actual session, the focus should be on the *learner*.

We believe that an effective approach is to introduce your role at the first session, and let learners know how and when they can reach you outside of the session if they have additional questions or concerns. Each small group can be different based on the dynamics of the group members and the content being covered, so careful attention to the group dynamics as well as your own teaching strengths and weaknesses is important for success. Emphasizing the learner-centred approach is necessary for effective small-group sessions. In this approach, the teacher seeks understanding and provides frequent feedback to help the individual learner and the group to improve.

CONDITIONS FOR AN EFFECTIVE SESSION

The beginning of the small-group session is very important. In effective sessions, the instructor will typically set the learning climate, state the goals and objectives and provide some basic 'ground rules' which outline what is acceptable and unacceptable behaviour (e.g. arriving late or holding 'sidebar' conversations). Ground rules are important because successful small groups rarely occur simply because there is the meeting of a talented teacher with highly motivated learners. Discuss expectations for preparation, participation and evaluation. This is important, as studies suggest that when learners are aware of evaluation criteria, they are likely to be more willing to participate. Try to generate a learning environment that is cooperative rather than competitive, as the latter can lead to lack of participation by all but the most dominant members. A cooperative as opposed to a competitive learning environment can be particularly challenging to balance: evaluating learners while fostering a cooperative learning environment.

 "The secret of education is respecting the pupil."
Ralph Waldo Emerson

Some ways to improve this balance include making small-group session grades formative, using an evaluation system that sets learners up for success and/or holding multiple small-group sessions with learners (e.g. they receive a grade at the very end instead of after each session).

In the adult learning model, the teacher as lecturer is replaced with the teacher as facilitator. We believe that in a highly effective small-group session it may at times be difficult to distinguish the teacher from the learners. For instructors brought up in the lecture format of teaching and learning, small-group teaching can be a difficult skill set to acquire. Some teachers who are highly effective in large-group settings (e.g. lectures) are not skilled at small-group teaching and will resort to mini-lectures if not provided with training in small-group teaching. Faculty development needs should be identified and addressed.

 Do not assume that a teacher's success in large-group teaching will equate to effective small-group teaching.

For example, highly effective lecturers may be uncomfortable with silence, unexpected discussion directions or how to convey key teaching points without using the podium with PowerPoint slides. Table 9.1 gives some general guidelines or tips for the small-group teacher.

We believe that small-group instructors need to understand group dynamics to be successful in this teaching format, particularly when the session is going in a less than optimal fashion. Scholtes et al (2000) describe stages that groups often undergo that can help the small-group teacher. These four stages are outlined below; characteristics of an effective small-group teacher at each stage are listed in parentheses.

Forming: group members feel excitement and anticipation; some experience anxiety (develop relationships and establish rules)

Storming: resistance to tasks or expressed concerns about too much work; arguments (aid resolution of issues)

Norming: demonstrate acceptance of others in group; cohesion; fosters discussion and feedback (promote collaboration)

Performing: group's ability to work through problems; understanding of strengths and weaknesses of group members (monitor progress and provide feedback)

Evaluating (assessing) the small-group session

Evaluation of the small-group session involves two components, evaluation of small-group members and evaluation of the teacher. The former is important to emphasize that the activity is a meaningful part of the curriculum, and the latter is important to help the instructor become even more effective in this role. Both foster communication skills (team member versus leader) that ultimately can affect patient care.

From a programme evaluation perspective, small-group evaluation, in large part, reflects the adequacy of the learning environment (infrastructure, resources and personnel).

EVALUATION OF SMALL-GROUP PARTICIPATION

It is important to make criteria for participation explicit to the learner. This may actually foster their participation. When possible, invite small-group learners to participate in determining criteria so they feel responsible for their learning and success of the group. Examples of criteria are available elsewhere. In establishing criteria for small-group evaluation, it is important to allow flexibility for small-group teacher style, provide clear guidelines that both teachers and learners can understand and not set up a summative environment, as this may detract from learners' participation.

EVALUATION OF SMALL-GROUP TEACHING

Teaching in small groups, just like teaching in other formats/venues, can benefit from evaluation from both learners and faculty. To do this, information needs to be collected in an accurate and timely manner. Also, just like evaluation of small-group participation and learning, evaluation of small-group teaching can be informal (formative) or formal (summative). Informal methods can include surveys for learners on teaching effectiveness or evaluation forms collected by course faculty at the end of each session. Timing is an important issue, as one does not want to collect the evaluation data too long after the actual teaching event.

Formal evaluation should optimally draw upon multiple sources and data should be reliable and valid. Many institutions have formal questionnaires given to students to evaluate the effectiveness of each teacher in a course or clerkship. Another important and perhaps underutilized source of data is peer evaluations. Resources for this include direct observation with a structured evaluation form or viewing a videotape of a prior teaching session. Importantly, direct observation by peers should seek to obtain adequate sampling (view the teacher on multiple occasions) to ensure reliability of the data. Providing small-group teachers with acknowledgments of excellence, such as teaching awards, can help motivate a climate accepting evaluation and continual improvement. The reader is encouraged to consult resources regarding this topic, which is beyond the scope of this chapter.

Encouraging faculty participation should be the goal of any academic institution. Faculty (instructors) can benefit in several ways. Most important is enhancing their own communication skills that ultimately enhance patient care. Encouraging faculty participation also serves as a means to expose learners to the various specialties in medicine. Exposure to different clinical specialties (e.g. internal medicine and surgery) of instructors may affect learners' career choices. Faculty participation also provides the learner with a potential mentor based on a mutual rapport that can continue throughout the curriculum. Institutional support through monetary bonuses, faculty appointments, continuing medical education credit and academic awards can also enhance involvement.

Summary

Small-group teaching can be a highly effective educational method. Benefits of this method can be maximized by carefully considering the goals and objectives of the session, providing materials in which the learners can meaningfully engage in the content, having awareness of small-group teaching benefits and incorporating a system of learner as well as teacher evaluation and feedback that is clear and explicit. The attitude of the teacher and rapport developed with the learner is also critical for success.

References

Huggett KN: Teaching in small groups. In Jeffries WB, Huggett KN, editors: *An Introduction to Medical Teaching*, London, 2010, Springer, pp 27–39.

Jaques D: Teaching small groups, *British Medical Journal* 326:492–494, 2003.

Neher JO, Gordon KC, Meyer B, Stevens N: A five-step "microskills" model of clinical teaching, *Clinical Teaching* 5:419–424, 1992.

Newble DI, Cannon RA, editors: *Handbook for Medical Teachers*, ed 4, The Netherlands, 2001, Kluwer Academic Publishers.

Scholtes PR, Joiner BL, Joiner BJ: *The TEAM Handbook*, Madison, WI, 2000, Oriel Inc.

van Blankenstein FM, Dolmans DHJM, van der Vleuten CPM, Schmidt HG: Which cognitive processes support learning during small-group discussion? The role of providing explanations and listening to others, *Instructional Science* 39:189–204, 2011.

Clinical skills centre teaching

J. S. Ker

Introduction

Teaching consistent high standards of clinical skills is core to both the development of safe healthcare practitioners and the delivery of quality care for patients.

A specialized skills teaching centre or facility, whether static or mobile, provides the ideal setting for facilitating practitioners' technical and nontechnical skills while also protecting patients. Any such facility should be built around a balance between the needs of the users and those of the organization (Seropian & Lavy 2010).

The last 15 years have seen enormous advances in our knowledge of why and how adverse events occur in clinical practice. The influential report *To Err is Human* from the Institute of Medicine in the United States (Kohn et al 2000) followed by *An Organization With a Memory* (DOH 2000) have highlighted the cost of adverse events in terms of finances and harm to patients, often as a result of inconsistent standards of clinical skills. These have led to strategies to transform healthcare, which include the Lucien Leape Foundation (2009) and the World Health Organization's patient safety curriculum (WHO 2010), both of which recognize the central role of clinical skills facilities and the use of simulation.

This chapter considers the following questions:

*   What are clinical skills facilities and why is there a need for them?
*   What should we teach in a clinical skills environment?
*   How should we teach in clinical skills facilities?
*   What are the practical approaches to clinical skills teaching?
*   What are the limitations/challenges of clinical skills facilities?

What are clinical skills facilities and why is there a need for them?

WHAT ARE THEY?

Clinical skills facilities provide specialist expertise for all those who deliver healthcare services to patients and communities (Dent 2001, Seropian & Lavy 2010). The success of a clinical skills facility relies on three key factors: geography of the facility, leadership and management, and financial infrastructure. They need to be accessible and provide standards of training to enable flexible movement of staff across geographical boundaries.

A clinical skills centre can be defined in terms of:

*   facilities
*   specialist equipment
*   specialist faculty.

Facilities

Facilities should be flexible to enable different simulations to be undertaken by different sizes of groups of learners for different levels of simulation. Most clinical skills can be best taught and learnt in a small-group setting, and so multipurpose small-group teaching rooms linked together both geographically and by audio-visual links provide maximum flexibility.

Facilities such as an outpatient, dedicated ward, theatre and laboratory area can provide contextual simulations for learners. Contextual fidelity supports the transfer of skills to the workplace and creates a suspension of disbelief to enhance learning (Ker et al 2006). Clinical skills facilities can be linked and therefore used more efficiently and effectively through a managed educational network which can be implemented at a regional or national level (Ker 2011). Every facility needs to be working in collaboration with the healthcare system to ensure that teaching and learning reflect the needs of both current and future healthcare practitioners.

A hub and satellite model is a useful concept for ensuring standards across regions and healthcare settings. IT support can enable standards of skills practice to be delivered at any level, regionally, nationally or internationally.

A mobile facility which has the standard features of fixed facilities can provide additional benefits in terms of travel time and team training in small healthcare units, providing an educational service in remote and rural areas without interrupting patient care (NES 2011).

Specialist equipment

Specialist equipment in the clinical skills centre should reflect the reality of practice in relation to medical equipment and consumables. Environmental cues are crucial for learner engagement in simulation events, whether as a novice or expert. Increasingly, clinical skills facilities are being used to test systems of change in patient care delivery, minimizing risk to patients and providing evidence of utility.

In addition, there is an increase in the use of technology to provide realistic simulations, especially of highly complex technical skills such as laparoscopic techniques. There is increasing evidence that these virtual reality simulators can enhance cognitive skills (Sedlack & Kolars 2004). A variety of low-fidelity and medium-fidelity simulators should be provided where appropriate for each of the clinical skills sessions (see Chapter 25). Simulation is a powerful learning tool which is often used to support teaching in clinical skills centres:

"A person, device or set of conditions that tries to present patient problems authentically. The learner is required to respond to the problem as he or she would under natural circumstances."

McGaghie 1999

Simulation is therefore dependent not only on the situation created but also on the involvement of the learner (Dieckmann et al 2007). In healthcare education it should be considered a tool to recreate clinical reality without compromising patient care. In creating a simulation, all domains of learning (cognitive, psychomotor and affective) need to be considered in the reconstruction.

Salas (2005) identified guidelines to effective simulation-based training which include creating scenarios based on learning outcomes and embedding objective measures of both technical and nontechnical skills in the skills scenario and ensuring feedback is integrated into the process.

Simulated and real patients (see Chapter 26) who support clinical skills centre teaching contribute to preparing students to develop their:

- Communication skills
- History and physical examination
- Noninvasive procedural skills
- Consultation skills.

Specialist faculty

Faculty expertise is a definite prerequisite for a successful clinical skills facility.

There are a number of different types of faculty in clinical skills:

- Clinical skills educators with expertise in the use of simulation
- Clinicians with expertise in communication skills
- Clinicians with an interest in teaching.

Faculty have to develop experience in how much of the simulation they need to prepare the learners for and how much they should participate in the event as a facilitator or assessor. They also need to be trained to be familiar with the use of simulators, in whatever form, as part of the simulation learning event. Faculty need to be supported by administrative, academic support and technical staff, the latter of whom have expertise in maintaining part task trainers and simulators. This type of team can ensure that the skills facility is used to its maximum capacity.

It is very useful though not mandatory to have faculty who have both educational and clinical expertise. Most skills faculty should be advised to retain their clinical expertise with a health service commitment, as they have a role even in a simulated setting as a professional role model.

Faculty also need to have shared understanding of what clinical skills are and what technical and nontechnical skills are so that they can develop appropriate learning outcomes.

"A clinical skill can be defined very broadly as: 'Any action by a health care practitioner involved in direct patient care which impacts on clinical outcome in a measurable way'."

NHS Education for Scotland, Scottish Clinical Skills Strategy, 2007

The description of a skill is also dependent on which level is being delivered:

- Level 1 – Task or skill component
- Level 2 – Skill as part of a patient care scenario (Kneebone et al 2002)

- Level 3 – Skill being delivered in different health-care setting or context.

The delivery of clinical skills involves cognitive, psychomotor and affective components.

A technical skill involves mainly procedural skills, e.g. suturing, blood pressure, basic life support (BLS). Nontechnical skills include communication, decision making and prioritization skills (Table 10.1). Different approaches are needed to facilitate the development of these human factors (Glavin & Maran 2003). There is evidence that nontechnical skills are often the first sign of a potential adverse event, and therefore teaching and learning opportunities are required to specifically develop and rehearse these skills in the clinical skills environment (Salas 2005). In linking both together, Kohls-Gatzoulis et al (2004) demonstrated that learning a technical skill in surgery teaching cognitive skills enhanced the learning of technical skills.

WHY IS THERE A NEED?

There are three main areas which have driven the development of clinical skills centres. An example of each area is outlined below.

Educational drivers

There is evidence that rehearsing skills (cognitive, psychomotor and affective) in preparation for practice reduces the evidence of adverse events (Leonard et al 2004). There is also increasing evidence that behaviours observed in a simulated clinical setting can predict how professionals will behave in the reality of practice (Weller et al 2003). This 'knowing how' can only be gained through professional clinical experience, which clinical skills centre teaching can enhance through preparation, deliberate practice and reflection. Clinical skills centres, through a focus on the learner rather than the patient, can prepare the novice clinician for the healthcare environment (Maran & Glavin 2003).

Clinical skills centres can be used to provide standard reliable evidence of competence to practise at all levels: undergraduate, postgraduate and as part of continuing professional development (Whelan 2000, DOH 2007): as part of more robust regulatory requirements.

Political drivers

Patients now have an expectation that healthcare practitioners will have been prepared to an agreed standard of competence prior to their participation in the reality of healthcare practice (Santen et al 2004, Sedlack & Kolars 2004). In addition, there has been a move towards developing national clinical skills strategies to enhance the quality of clinical skills and to increase their cost-effectiveness (NES 2007).

Table 10.1 Examples of technical and nontechnical skills

Technical skills	Nontechnical skills
History taking	Situational awareness
Physical examination	Task management
Communication skills (with patient)	Team communication
Procedural skills	Situational awareness
Information management	Decision making

Service drivers

Clinical skills facilities, both fixed and mobile units, have been developed as a result of changes in healthcare provision (Issenberg 2002). Most developed countries now follow a system of short inpatient admissions with shift-working and changing roles and skills within the healthcare team. Patients are therefore more reliant on robust chains of communication for their quality of care (Scherpbier et al 1997). This has affected both the quantity and quality of students' clinical experience (Thistlewaite & Jordan 1999).

What should we teach in a clinical skills environment?

Teaching is now a specific part of the profile of any professional practitioner. Teaching in a clinical skills setting can provide evidence for a portfolio and can develop teaching expertise in the use of simulation to prepare learners for practice.

Clinical skills and simulation can be used for many different purposes, a number of which are given below (Ker & Bradley 2007).

REHEARSAL

The use of simulation in the clinical skills environment enables novice or expert practitioners to rehearse new skills in their component parts and then to practise them together without compromising patient care, and with the support of a facilitator using a structured programme.

Example: Learning to do venepuncture as technical skill building up to consenting and preparing a patient and then carrying out the procedure on a simulator attached to a patient during a ward simulation exercise.

REINFORCEMENT

Reinforcement of clinical skills can be achieved through providing e-learning support in clinical skills, which enables learners in their own time to participate in an interactive patient scenario, thus linking both technical and nontechnical skills and providing feedback.

Example: Provision of an e-learning package which revises basic science knowledge, health and safety and professional and ethical considerations associated with venepuncture.

RENEWAL

Clinical skills provide opportunities for experts in practice to revisit their skills proficiencies and relearn skills which can fade when seldom used.

Example: Identification of complications in clinical practice in relation to venepuncture practice such as needlestick injury and lack of use of protective equipment; workshop to revisit and video practice.

REDESIGN

In developing new ways of working, the skills facilities provide the opportunity to safely try out new roles and develop new systems for their integration into clinical practice.

Example: Development of venepuncture training as part of a package for GP receptionists using standard approaches.

RISK REDUCTION

There is now a knowledge platform in relation to how and why adverse events in healthcare practice occur. Clinical skills and simulation provide an opportunity to re-enact critical incidents and also ensure there is no unwarranted variation in the way skills education is delivered to different healthcare practitioners.

Example: There is no point having three ways of learning venepuncture. Interprofessional skills learning through team exercises can impact on patient safety.

REGULATION

Clinical skills facilities and simulation are increasingly being used for assessment, as they provide objective evidence of ability. Regulation is of increasing importance in all health professional practice, as explicit evidence of competence is required. Increasingly peer assessment is being used in clinical skills assessment.

Example: Standards of competence can be clearly defined through assessment checklists for a simulation setting and global assessment measures for assessing performance in the simulated workplace.

RESEARCH

Clinical skills and the use of simulation are relatively new in the development of capable and proficient healthcare practitioners, and there is an opportunity to identify the most effective and efficient methods through research.

Example: Using a skills exercise to explore clinical reasoning of novice practitioners.

How should we teach clinical skills?

Gaba (2004) identified 11 dimensions which needed to be considered for developing a successful simulation event for teaching clinical skills. Ker and Bradley (2007) simplified these dimensions into three key elements:

- Purpose element: Refinement, rehearsal, research, regulation
- Process element: Reality/fidelity of the simulation-based event
- Participants' element: Individuals, teams, organization.

In the clinical skills environment how the teaching and learning are carried out is dependent on the learning outcomes for the session as part of the overall curricular programme.

There are a number of educational theories that underpin learning in clinical skills centres. These include behaviourism, cognitive constructivism and reflective learning, examples of which are given below.

LEARNING CARDIOPULMONARY RESUSCITATION SKILLS: BEHAVIOURISM

Behaviourism is based on a stimulus-response type of learning and is very useful for skills and drills simulations such as CPR training, whether for basic or advanced life support. This is the best approach for emergency skills which need to be over-rehearsed and automatic.

LEARNING PATIENT CONSULTATION SKILLS: COGNITIVE CONSTRUCTIVISM

Cognitive constructivism is a useful approach to developing expertise in consultation skills. This builds on prior knowledge and experience and enables the simulation event, with the facilitation of the tutor, to be linked to existing experience in the cognitive, psychomotor, or affective domain and for this then to be either assimilated or accommodated as a new learning event. This is useful in the early years of the novice practitioner, as it enables links between other components of the curriculum and the clinical skills simulation. E-learning is a useful approach for ensuring that standards of practice and knowledge are shared and can provide reinforcement and preparation opportunities.

LEARNING FROM A WARD SIMULATION EXERCISE: REFLECTION

Developing a ward simulation exercise can utilize reflective learning to enhance transfer of skills from the simulated environment to the workplace. This involves structuring the simulation event to include a short simulation exercise with a structured period of debriefing and feedback. This can include requiring learners to document their assessment of their performance.

What are the practical approaches to clinical skills centre teaching?

Learners need to be engaged in the clinical skills teaching process, whether it is learning a technical or nontechnical skill or participating in a patient scenario or healthcare context.

TEACHING A TECHNICAL SKILLS TASK

Gagne (1985) listed three phases in designing the teaching of technical skills:

1. Cognitive phase: Consciously develop a routine with cues from facilitator.
2. Associative phase: Deliberate practice to integrate component parts. Rest periods interspersed with practice have been shown to be most effective.
3. Autonomous phase: Skill automatic to enable cognitive activity.

Students should be increasingly involved in identifying how they would like to run the session, as it is their learning time. Tutoring the same group each week enables the tutor to identify those who volunteer and those who are more reticent and require practice.

A useful approach to structuring a technical skills learning session with a group of novices is the STEPS technique, which keeps the whole group involved as you give everyone different components of the STEPS to do.

S – Set the foundation of prior learning, the importance of the skill and the context in which it will be learned and applied.

T – Tutor demonstration in real time without commentary.

E – Explanation with repeat demonstration.

P – Practise under supervision with feedback from peer and tutor.

S – Subsequent deliberate practise encouraged.

TEACHING A NONTECHNICAL SKILLS TASK

A useful approach to structuring a nontechnical skills session with novices includes the SIS-FR method, which involves structured immersion and interventions:

S – Set the context and identify roles and outcomes.

I – Immerse in roles and practise for agreed time frame.

S – Intervention to summarize progress.

F – Feedback from self, peers and tutor.

R – Refine practice, building on feedback by re-immersion.

DEBRIEF AND FEEDBACK FROM A CLINICAL SKILLS TEACHING SESSION

At the completion of any skills teaching session event there are four stages to the feedback process:

- Preparation
- Disengagement
- Constructive feedback
- Contemplation.

Each stage is crucial to promote learning from the skills teaching session and to facilitate transfer of learning to the workplace. Disengagement is a crucial stage after a learner has immersed him- or herself in a skills learning event. This disengagement stage enables the learner to disassociate from the healthcare practitioner role taken as a learner. Feedback enables the learner to compare him- or herself to a standard and identify strengths and weaknesses. Video debriefing, where students are given time to review their performance with the use of a structured feedback sheet, can assist in the development of these skills. Different models of constructive feedback can be effective (see Chapter 40) (Table 10.2).

This part of the programme is vital to the success of the sessions and to students identifying the links between knowledge pathways. It is also important for tutors to debrief their role in the clinical skills teaching session. This can be achieved through reflective questioning.

 Question: Can I improve my teaching in any way? Peer observation of teaching and feedback can be a helpful way of developing your role.

Question: How can this benefit my clinical role? Teaching and clinical skills outside of clinical skills teaching can be of benefit to the clinical team. It can also provide evidence for appraisal/revalidation.

DREYFUS' MODEL OF SKILLS ACQUISITION

In considering any clinical skills teaching session it is also important to recognize the development of expertise. This will have an impact on any learning event. Expertise may be considered as the end point in a

Table 10.2 Effective feedback

Features of effective feedback	Barriers to effective feedback
• Timed as close to the simulation session as possible • Based on direct observation of the learner, i.e. descriptive • Phrased in nonjudgemental language • Specific, not generalized • Focused on actions; constructive • Not focused on too many different aspects at the same time • Given adequate time • Given in an appropriate setting	• Lack of planning • Defensive learner • Too generalized • Inconsistent from multiple sources • Lack of respect/ credibility • Anxiety • Personalization of comments

Table 10.3 Levels of expertise

Level 1	Novice	• Rigid adherence to taught rules or plans • Little situational perception • No discretionary judgment
Level 2	Advanced beginner	• Guidelines for action based on attributes and aspects of situation (recognize global characteristics after experience) • Situational perception limited • All attributes and aspects treated separately and given equal importance
Level 3	Competent	• Coping with crowdedness • Sees actions in terms of longer term goals • Conscious deliberate planning • Standard routine performance
Level 4	Proficient	• Sees situations holistically • Sees importance in situation • Perceives deviations from normal • Decision making less laboured • Uses guidance but recognizes variation
Level 5	Expert	• Intuitive grasp of situations based on tacit understanding • Analytical approach used only in novel situations • Vision of what is possible

stepwise development of cognitive, psychomotor and affective skills. The Dreyfus brothers (2005) described five levels of development of expertise (Table 10.3).

What are the current trends in clinical skills teaching?

There are a number of current trends in the use of clinical skills facilities which are shaping clinical education and will impact on the future of healthcare delivery. There has been an exponential growth in the development of skills facilities and in the publications about the use of simulation in these purpose-built facilities. However, there needs to be more robust research on the following developments to ensure clarity regarding their added value. Scotland has taken the lead in developing a national strategy for clinical skills linked to healthcare needs with principles of equality of access both professionally and geographically (NHS 2007).

Six trends in clinical skills teaching are summarized here.

EVIDENCE BASE FOR CLINICAL SKILLS PRACTICE

The advent of clinical skills facilities has created the opportunity for faculty to explore the evidence base around a lot of clinical skills practice. There has been a rise in the number of organizations pooling their evidence to create evidence based on line procedural skills resources. It is essential, given the changing skills profile of different healthcare professionals, that standards of skills practice are identified so that patients with complex conditions are given the same safe standards of skills irrespective of the healthcare professional delivering them.

INTERPROFESSIONAL TEAM TRAINING AND LEADERSHIP SKILLS

With our increased knowledge of how adverse events occur in healthcare practice, clinical skills centres provide safe learner-centred environments to practise the components of clinical practice so that they prepare novices for the workplace. The vital role played by teams in both controlled and uncontrolled healthcare environments has highlighted the need for team training in healthcare (Shapiro et al 2004). Several studies have identified behaviours which assess nontechnical skills in a complex healthcare environment (Fletcher et al 2003). Studies analysing the enhancement of teamwork in complex environments through team training have produced varying evidence as to its level of impact on patient safety, but this may be due to the fact that as yet we do not have the tools to measure the eight skill dimensions of teamwork (Stout & Salas 1997).

 Dimensions of teamwork:

- Adaptability
- Situational awareness
- Performance monitoring and feedback
- Leadership and team management
- Interpersonal relations
- Coordination
- Communication
- Decision making.

There is also a shift, particularly in medicine, towards the need to develop leadership skills both educationally and clinically to reengage the profession in strategic development of the organization.

PEER LEARNING IN CLINICAL SKILLS

Peer-assisted learning is being used more frequently in clinical skills teaching with the appropriate training and support in place (Field et al 2007). Students find peer tutors easier to question about aspects of their learning as clinical novices.

TECHNOLOGY

The development of technology has highlighted the opportunities for some clinical skills education to be supported in second life (the virtual 3D world) with virtual skills facilities or by interactive web-based tutorials which can deliver clinical skills learning in the workplace at the time it is required (Regan & Youn 2008). In addition, mobile skills facilities are a useful strategy for delivering efficient cost-effective skills education in remote and rural settings.

PERFORMANCE ASSESSMENT

There has been an increasing focus on performance assessment and how clinical skills facilities can provide audio-visual evidence of clinical practice that is valid and reliable and can discriminate between the competent and incompetent practitioner. There is a move towards sampling standards of professional practice in the simulated workplace using a variety of tools, but there is still reliance, especially at the undergraduate level, on the use of simulation in clinical skills facilities to assess competency (Boursicourt et al 2007). In relation to assessing doctors in difficulty, a ward simulation exercise (Hyslop et al 2007) has also been shown to provide evidence of performance by using contextual simulation.

PREDICTORS OF PERFORMANCE

With the increasing emphasis on the need to provide explicit evidence of competence for the purposes of revalidation and re-licensure, more research focusing on identifying predictors of performance, especially in relation to the effects of stress and fatigue with the use of simulation (Howard et al 2003).

What are the limitations?

There are a number of caveats related to the use of clinical skills facilities for teaching. Clinical skills facilities do not replace clinical practice: they enhance the learner's state of preparedness for practice. They provide a safe environment for deliberate practice. A major challenge remains the ability to predict performance or competence in the workplace from that in a simulated context. Learning in the clinical skills environment also needs to be integrated into the curricular programme. There is also a concern that such an environment may induce abnormal risk-taking behaviours, as it is not perceived as real by learners. There is also the dissonance of the conflict that arises, particularly for novice learners when they observe practices in their workplace that differ from the ideal standard taught in the skills and simulation setting. There are also considerable costs associated with the use of clinical skills facilities in relation to consumables as well as the personnel and physical facilities (Ker et al 2010).

Summary

Clinical skills facilities provide excellent opportunities for all healthcare practitioners to prepare themselves for the realities of practice in a complex, high-reliability organization like a health service. It is therefore essential that teachers as well as students develop their expertise in the use of these facilities, and the specialized environment that these dedicated facilities offer, to ensure that learning is both accurate and maximized before being transferred to the workplace. There are many approaches to learning in clinical skills facilities using underpinning educational theories which enhance what can be learnt in terms of technical and nontechnical skills. There is emerging evidence of the importance of clinical skills facilities in ensuring that the risk of adverse events to patients is minimized through rehearsal, redesign, renewal, research, reinforcement and regulation.

References

Boursicourt K, Roberts T, Burdick WP: *Structured assessment of clinical competence. Understanding*

Medical Education series, Edinburgh, 2007, Association of Medical Education.

Dent J: Current trends and future implications in the developing role of clinical skills centres, *Medical Teacher* 23:483–489, 2001.

Department of Health: *An organisation with a memory*, London, 2000, Stationery Office.

Department of Health: Trust Regulation and Safety. The regulation of health care professionals in the 21st century, 2007.

Dieckmann P, Gaba D, Rall M: Deepening the theoretical foundations of patient simulation as social practice, *Simulation in Health Care* 2(3): 183–193, 2007.

Dreyfus HL, Dreyfus SE: Expertise in real world contexts, *Organization Studies* 26(5):779–792, 2005.

Field M, Burke J, McAllister D, Lloyd D: Peer assisted learning: a novel approach to clinical skills learning for medical students, *Medical Education* 41: 411–418, 2007.

Fletcher G, Flin R, McGeorge P, et al: Anaesthetists' non-technical skills (ANTS): evaluation of a behavioural marker system, *British Journal of Anaesthesia* 90(5):580–588, 2003.

Gaba DM: The future vision of simulation in health care, *Quality & Safety in Health Care* 13(1), 2004.

Gagne RM: *The Conditions of Learning and Theory of Instruction*, ed 4, New York, 1985, Holt, Rinehart and Winston.

Glavin R, Maran N: Integrating human factors into the medical curriculum, *Medical Education* 37(Suppl 1):59–64, 2003.

Howard SK, Gaba DM, Smith BE, et al: Simulation study of rested versus sleep-deprived anesthesiologists, *Anesthesiology* 98(6):1345–1355, 2003.

Hyslop JM, Anderson F, Hesketh EA, et al: Assessing the validity and reliability of an assessment instrument to evaluate poorly performing Foundation Year One doctors during ward simulation exercises, *ASME* conference, presentation, 2007.

Issenberg SB: Clinical skills training – practice makes perfect, *Medical Education* 36:210–211, 2002.

Ker J: Delivering a quality skilled workforce. Report and Recommendations for Health Boards on Clinical skills Education by the National Clinical Skills Managed Education Network, 2011, NES.

Ker JS, Hesketh EA, Anderson F, Johnston DA: Can a ward simulation exercise achieve the realism that reflects the complexity of everyday practice junior doctors encounter? *Medical Teacher* 28(4):330–334, 2006.

Ker J, Bradley P: *Simulation in medical education*, 2007. Understanding Medical Education Series, ASME.

Ker J, Hogg G, Maran N: Cost effective simulation. In Walsh K, editor: Cost Effective Medical Education, BMJ 2010.

Kneebone R, Kidd J, Nestel D, et al: An innovative model for teaching and learning clinical procedures, *Medical Education* 36(7):628–634, 2002.

Kohls-Gatzoulis J, Glenn R, Hutchison C: Teaching cognitive skills improves learning in surgical skills course: a blinded prospective randomised study, *Canadian Journal of Surgery* 47(4):277, 2004.

Kohn LT, Corrigan JM, Donaldson MS: *To Err is Human: Building a Safer Health System*, Washington, DC, 2000, National Academy Press.

Leape L, Berwick D, Clancy C: Transforming healthcare: a safety imperative, *Quality & Safety in Health Care* 18:424–428, 2009.

Leonard M, Graham S, Bonacum D: The human factor: the critical importance of effective teamwork and communication in providing safe care, *Quality & Safety in Health Care* 13(S1):185–190, 2004.

Maran NJ, Glavin RJ: Low- to high-fidelity simulation – a continuum of medical education? *Medical Education* 37(s1):22–28, 2003.

McGaghie WC: Simulation in professional competence assessment: basic considerations. In Tekian A, McGuire CH, McGaghie WC, editors: *Innovative Simulations for Assessing Professional Competence. Department of Medical Education*, Chicago, IL, 1999, University of Illinois at Chicago.

NHS Education for Scotland: Partnerships for care – taking forward the Scottish clinical skills strategy, *Executive Summary* 2007.

NHS Education for Scotland: *Clinical skills managed education network. Evaluation of the pilot of the mobile clinical skills unit 2009–2011*, 2011.

Regan JC, Youn E: Past, present, and future trends in teaching clinical skills through web-based learning environments, *Journal of Social Work Education* 44(2):95–115, 2008.

Salas E: Using simulation based training to improve patient safety: what does it take? *Journal of Quality and Safety* 37:363–371, 2005.

Santen S, Hemphill R, McDonald M, Jo C: Patients' willingness to allow residents to learn to practice medical procedures, *Academic Medicine* 79(2):144–147, 2004.

Sedlack RE, Kolars JC: Computer simulator training enhances the competency of gastroenterology fellows at colonoscopy: Results of a pilot study, *The American Journal of Gastroenterology* 99(1):33–37, 2004.

Seropian M, Lavy R: Design considerations for healthcare simulation facilities, *Journal for the Society for Simulation in Healthcare* 5(6):338–339, 2010.

Scherpbier AJJA, van der Vleuten CPM, Rethans J, van der Steeg A: *Advances in Medical Education*, Dordrecht, 1997, Kluwer Academic.

Shapiro MJ, Morey JC, Small SD, et al: Simulation based teamwork training for emergency department staff: does it improve clinical team performance when added to an existing didactic teamwork curriculum? *Quality & Safety in Health Care* 13(6):417–421, 2004.

Stout RJ, Salas E: Enhancing teamwork in complex environments through team training, *Group Dynamics: Theory, Research and Practice* 1(2):169–182, 1997.

Thistlewaite J, Jordan JJ: Patient centred consultations: a comparison of student experience and understanding in two clinical environments, *Medical Education* 33:678–685, 1999.

Weller J, Wilson L, Robinson B: Survey of change in practice following simulation based training in crisis management, *Anaesthesia* 58:471–473, 2003.

Whelan G: High stakes medical performance testing: The clinical assessment program, *JAMA* 283(13):1748–1749, 2000.

World Health Organization (WHO): Patient safety curriculum for undergraduate medical students, 2010, WHO publications.

Bedside teaching

J. A. Dent

Introduction

Clinical teaching at the bedside epitomizes the classical view of medical training. Students are motivated by the stimulus of clinical contacts, but the traditional, consultant-teaching ward round has not been without its shortcomings. Students may feel academically unprepared or inexperienced in the learning style required in an unfamiliar environment (Seabrook 2004). Inappropriate comments, late starts and cancellations may discourage and alienate students so that the value of the experience is dissipated. Finally, today's teaching hospitals may paradoxically have fewer patients appropriate for bedside teaching despite there being larger student groups attending than before.

 "Most medical students are taught by a system of negative reinforcement in the form of sarcastic remarks and derogatory comments."

Newton 1987

Despite these problems, ward-based teaching provides an optimal opportunity for the demonstration and observation of physical examination, communication skills and interpersonal skills and for role modelling a holistic approach to patient care. Not surprisingly, bedside teaching and medical clerking have been rated the most valuable methods of teaching. Despite this, bedside teaching has been declining in medical schools since the early 1960s as clinical acumen becomes perceived as being of secondary importance to clinical imaging and hi-tech investigations (Ahmed 2002).

The 'learning triad' and its environment

Traditional clinical teaching brings together the 'learning triad' of patient, student and clinician/tutor in a particular clinical environment. When all works well, this recipe provides a magical mix for producing effective student learning. Direct contact with patients is important for the development of clinical reasoning, communication skills, professional attitudes and empathy (Spencer et al 2000). But for the mix to work, a degree of preparation is required from each party involved.

 "Bedside teaching is the only site where history taking, physical examination, empathy and a caring attitude can be taught and learnt by example."

Nair et al 1997

Preparation

PATIENTS

Patients should be invited to participate without coercion and have the opportunity to decline to take part without feeling intimidated. Some institutions may require formal documentation of informed consent before patients can participate. They should be adequately briefed so that they know what will be expected of them, feel a part of the discussion and feel empowered to participate in the teaching session. They may be required to give some simple feedback to students afterwards. Usually patients enjoy the experience and feel they have contributed to student learning.

Depending on the model of ward teaching used, a variety of patients will be required for varying lengths of time, but consideration should be given to patients' needs and the possibility that other healthcare staff and visitors may need to see them.

STUDENTS

It is initially valuable for junior students to have had access to simulated patients who provide valuable learning opportunities for the examination of normal anatomy and physiology. This prepares them well for seeing patients in clinical situations. Between two and five students is probably the optimal number for bedside teaching. Students should comply with the medical school's directives on appropriate appearance and behaviour and, if unaccompanied by a clinical tutor, should introduce themselves to staff and patients, clearly stating the purpose of their visit.

Some may feel intimidated by an unfamiliar environment and the proximity of nursing staff and be embarrassed when putting personal questions to a stranger. They may feel anxious if unsure of their knowledge base or clinical abilities and fearful of consultant criticism of any inadequacies. As a result, some students position themselves towards the back of the group round the bedside to avoid participation, while more confident colleagues monopolize conversations with patients and tutors. An observant tutor will be aware of this behaviour and be able to redress the balance and ensure that all students have the opportunity to participate and that anxieties are allayed.

TUTORS

Tutors for ward-based teaching may be consultant staff, junior hospital doctors (Busan et al 2003), nurses or student peers. Kilminster et al (2001) describe teaching by specialized, ward-based tutors as helpful in developing student history-taking and examination skills.

Whether they appreciate its significance or not, tutors are powerful role models for students, especially for those in the early years of the course, so it is most important that they demonstrate appropriate knowledge, skills and attitudes (Cruess et al 2008). Prideaux and colleagues (2000) describe good clinical teaching as providing role models for good practice, making good practice visible and explaining it to trainees.

The seven roles of a clinician/teacher useful for analysing good clinical teaching:

- medical expert
- communicator
- collaborator
- manager
- advocate
- scholar
- professional.

Prideaux et al 2000

Appropriate knowledge

Experienced clinical teachers are soon able to assess the patient's diagnosis and requirements as well as the students' level of understanding. This ability to link clinical reasoning with instructional reasoning enables them to quickly adapt the clinical teaching session to the needs of the students (Irby 1992).

Experienced tutors link clinical reasoning with instructional reasoning.

Six domains of knowledge have been described which an effectively functioning clinical tutor will apply (Irby 1994):

- Knowledge of medicine: integrating the patient's clinical problem with background knowledge of basic sciences, clinical sciences and clinical experience
- Knowledge of patients: a familiarity with disease and illness from experience of previous patients
- Knowledge of the context: an awareness of patients in their social context and at their stage of treatment
- Knowledge of learners: an understanding of the students' present stage in the course and of the curriculum requirements for that stage
- Knowledge of the general principles of teaching, including:
  - getting students involved in the learning process by indicating its relevance
  - asking questions, perhaps by using the patient as an example of a problem-solving approach to the condition
  - keeping students' attention by indicating the relevance of the topic to another situation
  - relating the case being presented to broader aspects of the curriculum
  - meeting individual needs by responding to specific questions and providing personal tuition
  - being realistic and selective so that relevant cases are chosen
  - providing feedback by critiquing case reports, presentations or examination technique
- Knowledge of case-based teaching scripts: the ability to present the patient as representative of a certain clinical problem; the specifics of the case are used but added to from other knowledge and experiences in order to make further generalized comments about the condition.

Appropriate skills

If demonstrating clinical tasks to students on the ward, tutors must ensure that they are competent in performing them in whatever uniform approach has been taught in the clinical skills centre. They should avoid demonstrating inappropriate 'shortcuts'.

Appropriate attitudes

 "The essential feature is enthusiasm on the part of the teacher."

Rees 1987

Tutors responsible for timetabled ward teaching must arrive punctually, introduce themselves to the students and demonstrate an enthusiastic approach to the session. A negative impression at this stage will have an immediate negative effect on the students' attitude and on the value of the session. Tutors must show a professional approach to the patients and interact appropriately with them and the students (Fig. 11.1).

Hospital ward

The educational environment of the ward may be affected by many factors which impact on student behaviour and satisfaction (Seabrook 2004). Often district general hospitals appear more valued than teaching hospitals (Parry et al 2002). However, with some thought, some simple problems can be avoided.

Ward teaching should not take place when meals, cleaners or visitors are expected. It helps if the staff and patients are expecting the teaching session at a certain time so that X-rays and case notes can be ready and patients do not have to be retrieved from the day room or X-ray department.

The use of a side room for pre- or post-ward round discussion provides a useful alternative venue for discussion once the patients have been seen. Occasionally, a member of the nursing staff may be present in the teaching session to add multiprofessional input to the patient care discussion. Stanley (1998) suggests that systematic planning and preparation, especially

with increased use of pre- and post-round meetings, would provide more effective and structured training for postgraduate hospital doctors.

A teaching ward round deals with patients, not diseases. It develops students' thinking processes and introduces an approach to patients that they will follow for the rest of their working lives as doctors.

Delivery strategies

COX'S CYCLE

A plan of two linked cycles has been described (Cox 1993) to maximize the students' learning from each patient contact.

The 'experience cycle' involves student preparation and briefing to ensure that they are aware of what they are going to see and the opportunities available for learning. Before beginning, students should be briefed so that they understand the purpose of the session and the goals to be achieved. Any warnings about the patient conditions to be seen should be given and checks made on students' level of initial understanding. This is followed by the clinical experience of interacting with their patient, which may include history taking and physical examination, discussing the illness and thinking about management.

After leaving the patient, the experience cycle concludes with debriefing, when the information

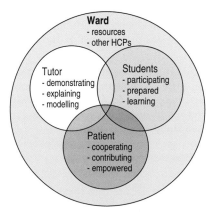

Fig. 11.1 The learning triad and its contribution.

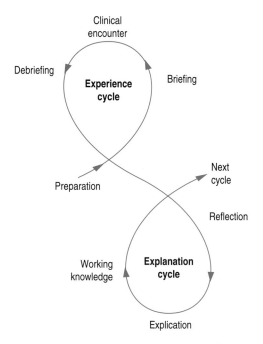

Fig. 11.2 Experience and explanation cycles (redrawn from Cox 1993, with modifications).

gathered is reviewed and interpreted and any misperceptions or misunderstandings are clarified. The experience cycle maximizes the value of the time spent with the patient.

The 'explanation cycle' begins with reflection, when students are encouraged to consider their recent clinical interaction in the light of previous experiences. Explication continues with the understanding of the clinical experiences at different levels according to the students' stage of learning and its integration into their previous learning experiences. Finally, a working knowledge is synthesized which prepares the students for seeing a subsequent patient (Fig. 11.2).

Tips to improve bedside teaching.
Ramani (2003) describes 12 tips to promote effective bedside teaching:

1. Preparation: revise your own skills, the learners' needs and the curriculum.
2. Planning: construct a road map of the activities and objectives of the session.
3. Orientation: orientate the learners to your plans for the session.
4. Introduction: introduce everyone present, including the patient!
5. Interaction: role-model a doctor–patient interaction.
6. Observation: watch how the students are proceeding.
7. Instruction: provide instruction.
8. Summary: tell the students what they have been taught.
9. Debriefing: answer questions and provide clarifications.
10. Feedback: give positive and constructive feedback to students.
11. Reflection: evaluate from your perspective what went well and what was less successful.
12. Preparation: prepare for your next bedside teaching session.

Outcome-based education

Many of the educational objectives of the medical curriculum can be experienced to different extents by students at any stage of the curriculum while they are working in the wards (Fig. 11.3).

- *Clinical skills.* For junior students there are opportunities to become proficient at normal physical examination while more senior students gain practice in eliciting abnormal physical signs.

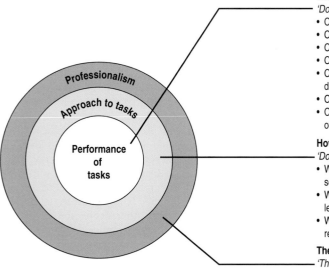

Fig. 11.3 The 12 learning outcomes.

- *Communication skills.* Many opportunities exist for students to practise communication skills.
- *Clinical reasoning.* Students can observe this in practice by junior and senior staff.
- *Practical procedures.* Venepuncture, cannulation of a peripheral vein, arterial blood gas sampling and bladder catheterization are procedures which are readily available on most wards for students to practise.
- *Patient investigation and management.* There are many opportunities for students to observe and discuss aspects of both of these.
- *Data interpretation and retrieval.* Interpretation of laboratory reports and accessing scientific papers for reference are examples.
- *Professional skills.* The observation of both junior and senior doctors in their working relationship with other healthcare professionals should help students develop appropriate professional behaviour.
- *Transferable skills.* Many of the abilities acquired in the ward setting will be of value in other doctor–patient situations.
- *Attitude and ethics.* Appropriate attitudes and ethical dilemmas can be observed by the students in their ward attachments.

All these aspects can be seen in the context of the patient as an individual rather than in the purely theoretical context presented in lectures. Students should be encouraged to return to the ward during private study time to practise clinical skills further.

TIME-EFFICIENT STRATEGIES FOR LEARNING AND PERFORMANCE

This approach is described by Irby and Bowen (2004). See Table 11.1.

Table 11.1 Teaching strategies for clinical teachers

Planning

- Direct/orientate learners
- Create a positive learning environment
- Pre-select patients
- Prime/brief learners

Teaching

- Teach from clinical cases
- Use questions to diagnose learners
- Ask advanced learners to participate in teaching
- Use 'illness scripts' and 'teaching scripts'

Evaluating and reflecting

- Evaluate learners
- Provide feedback
- Promote self-assessment and self-directed learning

LOGBOOKS AND PORTFOLIOS

The variety of clinical conditions available for a teaching session at any particular time will inevitably vary, so ward-based teaching will of necessity be opportunistic. Some form of documentation is required to ensure that all students see a comparable mix of patients. Logbooks or personal digital assistants (PDAs) can be used to document patients seen and to keep a record of the learning points (Davis & Dent 1994). These can be reviewed periodically and future sessions directed to making good any deficits.

TASK-BASED LEARNING

A list of tasks to be performed or procedures to be observed and carried out is usually a course requirement. Students' proficiency in any of these tasks is then scored in their clinical record book.

PROBLEM-BASED LEARNING

The patient's presenting complaint can be used as the focus of a problem-based learning exercise in which basic sciences and clinical sciences can be integrated.

STUDY GUIDES

A prescribed list of conditions to be seen in the ward may be laid out in the study guide with the learning points to be achieved documented for each.

Models for managing learning in the ward

APPRENTICESHIP/SHADOWING A JUNIOR DOCTOR MODEL

Shadowing a junior doctor on the unit where they will subsequently be working has become a required part of the final year programme for medical students in the UK. Students spend a number of weeks sharing the work and experiences of a junior doctor. Opportunities exist to share in carrying out ward tasks, formulating management plans and observing good practice. Confidence is increased by interaction with senior doctors and other professionals, by observing the working practice of junior doctors and by seeing patients individually. However, weaker students may feel they are ignored or that the only activities available to them are mundane ward chores.

PATIENT-CENTRED MODEL

Students attached to a ward for a period of time can be allocated a certain number of patients, each of whom they initially admit and then follow throughout their time in the hospital. They are made responsible for presenting them on ward rounds and should be able to comment on their current investigations, laboratory results and present status. Opportunities exist for practice in examination and communication skills. Patients can be followed for X-ray and to surgery and even visited at home on discharge so the student can assess the impact of illness and convalescence on the patient in the context of their home environment.

GRAND ROUNDS

Popular in some countries, this consultant-led ward round or side room presentation usually includes senior clinicians, trainees, junior doctors and other healthcare professionals. There are opportunities to observe multiprofessional interaction and possibly more complex patient problems. However, students often remain remote from the decision making and may not understand some of the complex issues being considered. There is likely to be little opportunity for interaction with clinicians or patients in this model.

BUSINESS WARD ROUND

This is a challenging activity for both clinicians and students. Little time is available for formal teaching, observing student performance or providing feedback. It may be necessary for the clinician to explain decisions being made in a variety of levels of complexity depending on the experience or seniority of others on the ward round. There may be little time for student teaching.

TEACHING WARD ROUND

This specially created ward round is aimed at taking students to a small number of selected patients to provide opportunities for them to see physical signs and hear aspects of the case history.

Reserved students may have little opportunity to interact with patients individually compared with more self-confident counterparts, but opportunities to ask and be asked questions exist to a varying degree. Where you position yourself at the patient's bedside influences how you will be able to conduct the bedside teaching session and allows different models of bedside teaching to be used:

- *Demonstrator model* (see Fig. 11.4). The clinical tutor demonstrates aspects of the case history and physical examination to the students.
- *Tutor model* (see Fig. 11.5). The clinical tutor stands to the side and critiques each student in turn as they enquire into aspects of the history and carry out aspects of the physical examination.
- *Observer model* (see Fig. 11.6). The clinical tutor distances him- or herself from the student–patient

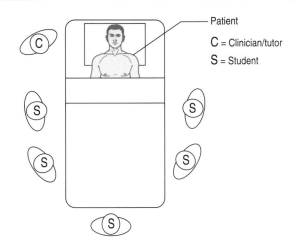

Fig. 11.4 The demonstrator model.

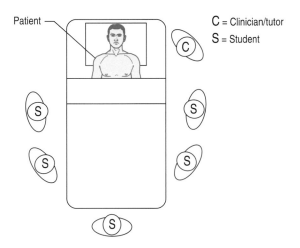

Fig. 11.5 The tutor model.

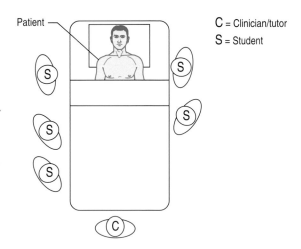

Fig. 11.6 The observer model.

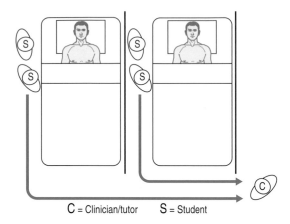

C = Clinician/tutor   S = Student

Fig. 11.7 The report-back model.

interaction and observes a single student or pair of students in a longer portion of history taking or examination, providing feedback to them all at the end as they discuss their findings and clinical interpretation.

- *Report-back model* (see Fig. 11.7). Working singly or in pairs, students take a history and examination without supervision and subsequently report back to the tutor in a tutorial room to present the case and receive feedback on content and delivery. Opportunities are given for students to practise their communication skills in their own time and to demonstrate their presentation skills and knowledge of the case, but their bedside technique has been unsupervised so no feedback on this can be given.

CLINICAL CONFERENCE

A patient from the ward is presented in a side room at a conference of senior clinicians which students attend. Diagnostic and management problems are discussed by the group once the patient has left. Students have the opportunity to observe the multifaceted management of difficult cases and the spectrum of professional input which may be required.

TRAINING WARD

A purpose-made training ward has been found to provide students with a useful opportunity to develop skills and knowledge in relation to patient management and interprofessional teamwork. (Reeves et al 2002).

Reflection and follow-up

STUDENTS

Students have found ward-based teaching the most valuable way of developing clinical skills. They should be encouraged to reflect on their experiences as described above and to complete their logbooks by reading round the patient problems they have seen.

PATIENTS

Remember to thank all who have taken part in the teaching session and identify any problems or difficulties that have arisen.

TUTORS

Ask yourself what went well and what was less satisfactory so that you can do better next time. The positive impact of teaching to the clinician-teacher has been reported by Wenrich et al (2011).

Student assessment

Assessment in the ward environment may take the form of a review of written material such as logbooks, task lists or reflective diaries (see Chapter 12, Ambulatory care teaching). Alternatively, students' clinical skills can be assessed by the Mini-CEX, a short, focused assessment followed by feedback, or by the direct observation of procedural skills (DOPS) (see Chapter 38, Performance and workplace assessment).

Staff development

The importance of training clinicians for their teaching role has been repeatedly emphasized by the GMC (2009). In 2001 Hesketh and colleagues described a comprehensive list of competencies for developing an 'effective teacher' based on the same three circle model and 12 learning outcomes of the undergraduate medical curriculum (Harden et al 1999, Simpson et al 2002). Ramani and Leinster (2008) have particularly applied this model for teachers in the clinical environment (Table 11.2).

All those involved in ward teaching bring a different perspective to patient care which is valuable for student learning. Sometimes they will have received no specific preparation for the teaching session and may not know how any particular session fits into the totality of the students' clinical experience at a particular stage of the course. Staff development courses and guides to teaching are important to help these enthusiastic clinicians in their teaching role. The GMC-commended series of booklets 'Getting started … a practical guide for clinical tutors' (Dent & Davis 2008) provide on-the-spot help for clinical teachers in a variety of teaching and learning venues. Tutors' individual approaches to clinical examination will also differ as examination technique may not be standardized within the medical school. While it may be of benefit for more confident students to observe a variety of different approaches to clinical skills,

Table 11.2 Applying the three-circle outcomes model for teachers in the clinical environment

Tasks of a clinical teacher: Doing the right thing	Approach to teaching: Doing the thing right	Teacher as a professional: The right person doing it
• Time efficient teaching • Inpatient teaching • Outpatient teaching • Teaching at the bedside • Work-based assessment of learners in clinical settings • Providing feedback	• Showing enthusiasm for teaching and towards learners • Understanding learning principles relevant to clinical teaching • Using appropriate teaching strategies for different levels of learners • Knowing and applying principles of effective feedback • Modelling good, professional behaviour, including evidence-based patient care • Grasping the unexpected teaching moment	• Soliciting feedback • Self-reflection on teaching strengths and weaknesses • Seeking professional development in teaching • Mentoring and seeking mentoring • Engaging in educational scholarship

weaker ones will find this lack of consistency confusing. Ideally, tutors should be briefed so that they are familiar with the approach to physical examination taught in the clinical skills centre and with the levels of expertise required of students at the various stages of the medical course.

Summary

Ward-based teaching offers unique opportunities for student learning which, for a variety of reasons, are becoming less efficiently utilized than they were. To attain maximum benefit from ward-based teaching, patients, students and tutors must each be appropriately prepared and the educational objectives must be understood. Various strategies can be used to advantage in both the planning and organization of ward teaching. Finally, a variety of styles of ward-based teaching can be utilized which provide a variety of learning opportunities for the students attending.

 "A good consultant is accessible, approachable and friendly, with the power of a god, the patience of a saint and the sense of humour of an undergraduate."

Lowry 1987

References

Ahmed MEK: What is happening to bedside clinical teaching? *Medical Education* 36:1185–1188, 2002.

Busan JO, Scherpbier AJJA, van der Vleuten CPM, Essed EGM: The perceptions of attending doctors of the role of residents as teachers of undergraduate clinical students, *Medical Education* 37:241–247, 2003.

Cox K: Planning bedside teaching, *Medical Journal of Australia* 158:493–495, 1993.

Cruess SR, Cruess RL, Steinert Y: Role modelling – making the most of a powerful teaching strategy, *British Medical Journal* 336:718–721, 2008.

Davis MH, Dent JA: Comparison of student learning in the out-patient clinic and ward round, *Medical Education* 28:208–212, 1994.

Dent J, Davis M: *"Getting Started …": A Practical Guide for Clinical Tutors*, Dundee, 2008, University of Dundee, Centre for Medical Education.

General Medical Council: *Tomorrow's Doctors*, London, 2009, General Medical Council.

Harden RM, Crosby JR, Davis MH, Friedman M: Outcome-based education; part 5. From competency to metacompetency; a model for the specification of learning outcomes, *AMEE Guide No. 14. Medical Teacher* 21:546–552, 1999.

Hesketh EA, Bagnall G, Buckley EG, et al: A framework for developing excellence as a clinical educator, *Medical Education* 35:555–564, 2001.

Irby DM: How attending physicians make instructional decisions when conducting teaching rounds, *Academic Medicine* 67:630–638, 1992.

Irby DM: What clinical teachers in medicine need to know, *Academic Medicine* 69:333–342, 1994.

Irby DM, Bowen JL: Time-efficient strategies for learning and performance, *The Clinical Teacher* 1:23–28, 2004.

Kilminster SM, Delmotte A, Frith H, et al: Teaching in the new NHS: the specialised ward based teacher, *Medical Education* 35:437–443, 2001.

Lowry S: What is a good consultant? As the junior doctor sees it, *British Medical Journal* 294:1601, 1987.

Nair BR, Coughlan JL, Hensley MJ: Student and patient perspectives on bedside teaching, *Medical Education* 31:341–346, 1997.

Newton DF: What is a good consultant? 'A worm's eye view'. *British Medical Journal* 295:106–107, 1987.

Parry J, Mathers J, Al-Fares A, et al: Hostile teaching hospitals and friendly district general hospitals: final-year students' views on clinical attachment locations, *Medical Education* 36:1131–1141, 2002.

Prideaux D, Alexander H, Bower A, et al: Clinical teaching: maintaining an educational role for doctors in the new health care environment, *Medical Education* 34:820–826, 2000.

Ramani S: Twelve tips to improve bedside teaching, *Medical Teacher* 25:112–115, 2003.

Ramani S, Leinster S: *Teaching in the clinical environment. AMEE Guide No. 34*, Dundee, UK, 2008, Association for Medical Education in Europe.

Rees J: How to do it: Take a teaching ward round, *British Medical Journal* 295:424–425, 1987.

Reeves S, Freeth D, McCrorie P, Perry D: "It teaches you what to expect in the future …":

interprofessional learning on a training ward for medical, nursing, occupational therapy and physiotherapy students, *Medical Education* 36: 337–344, 2002.

Seabrook MA: Clinical students' initial reports of the educational climate in a single medical school, *Medical Education* 38:659–669, 2004.

Simpson JG, Furnace J, Crosby J, et al: The Scottish doctor – learning outcomes for the medical undergraduate in Scotland: a foundation for competent and reflective practitioners, *Medical Teacher* 14:136–143, 2002.

Spencer J, Blackmore D, Heard S, et al: Patient-orientated learning: a review of the role of the patient in the education of medical students, *Medical Education* 34:851–857, 2000.

Stanley P: Structuring ward rounds for learning: can opportunities be created? *Medical Education* 31:425–429, 1998.

Wenrich MD, Jackson MB, Ajam KS, et al: Teachers as learners: the effect of bedside teaching on the clinical skills of clinician-teachers, *Academic Medicine* 86:846–852, 2011.

Ambulatory care teaching

J. A. Dent

Introduction

 Ambulatory care refers to any place where patients attend healthcare facilities without being admitted as inpatients.

One of the exciting challenges for today's medical teachers is the opportunity to develop ambulatory care clinical facilities for teaching purposes.

Advances in medical treatment and changing patterns of healthcare delivery have led to a move towards increased ambulatory and community care. Consequently, there is a change in the type of clinical problems being seen in teaching hospital wards. These patients are often acutely unwell, undergoing intense investigation/treatment or representing conditions which may be too advanced or too unusual for student learning requirements.

Medical teachers now have to look to different venues to find adequate numbers of patients with appropriate clinical problems suitable for undergraduate teaching.

This has led to a shift of focus and the development of teaching initiatives in a variety of ambulatory care venues (Bardgett & Dent 2011, Dent 2003, Dent 2005, Dent et al 2007).

 "More medicine is now practiced in the ambulatory setting, making the in-patient arena less representative of the actual practice of medicine and a less desirable place for students to glean the fundamentals of clinical care and problem solving than in the past."

Fincher & Albritton 1993

 "Placements should reflect the changing patterns of healthcare and must provide experience in a variety of environments including hospitals, general practices and community medical services."

General Medical Council 2009

Identifying new resources for ambulatory care teaching

In the teaching hospital, of course, a number of ambulatory care venues are present which are frequently used for teaching:

- outpatient clinics in a variety of specialties
- multiprofessional clinics where staff from a variety of disciplines see patients together, e.g. an oncology clinic, which may include surgery, radiotherapy and medical oncology
- sessions provided by other healthcare professionals, e.g. physiotherapy, occupational therapy.

But other venues in the hospital may be available to provide suitable opportunities:

- radiology and imaging suite
- clinical investigation unit, e.g. endoscopy suite
- nurse-led clinics, e.g. for pre-assessment of surgical admissions, audiology assessment, allergy testing
- dialysis unit
- child screening clinic
- day surgery unit.

However, finding a new, suitable venue is one thing; finding the budget to run a new programme in it is another. Finances may be required to support a new teaching programme, produce study guides or logbooks, provide clinical tutor sessions or reimburse patients' travelling expenses (Dent et al 2001b).

What can be taught and learned in ambulatory care settings?

Opportunities for student learning with inpatients in hospital wards is usually focused on:

- clinical skills
- clinical reasoning
- patient management

- investigations
- information handling.

In ambulatory care settings, however, patients are seen closer to their own social circumstances and environment, as their attendance in an ambulatory facility is part of a continuum in the management of their illness, often in the context of the contribution from other HCPs and community support services (Stearns & Glasser 1993).

Ambulatory care learning can therefore include opportunities for students to gain experience in:

- continuity of care
- context of care
- resource allocation
- health education
- patient responsibility
- a holistic approach to healthcare.

Practically all learning outcomes can be experienced in ambulatory care teaching venues (see Chapter 18, Outcome-based education).

Finally the ambulatory venue is more likely to provide opportunities for:

- reflection
- feedback
- formative assessment.

Role of a dedicated Ambulatory Care Teaching Centre (ACTC)

In addition to ambulatory care facilities already in place, a specific teaching area can be developed to provide a structured programme for teaching with ambulatory patients.

An ACTC (Dent et al 2001a) can give students the opportunity to meet selected patients with problems relevant to their stage of learning and with timetabled clinical tutors who are not at the same time being required to provide patient care.

The ACTC should have sufficient space for teaching with patients or clinical volunteers. Space is needed for small-group activities, for individual student–patient interviews (with or without supervision) and possibly for other healthcare colleagues to demonstrate particular aspects of patient care. Unlike a routine outpatient clinic, this protected environment helps students to feel comfortable to practise focused interview or examination skills free from embarrassment or time constraints.

Clinicians with an interest in teaching can be asked to take special teaching sessions in the ACTC, often

with the help of patients invited to attend from a 'bank' of patient volunteers.

A 'content expert' in the appropriate body-system is not necessarily required for much of the teaching; in fact, the ACTC is a good venue for peer-assisted learning programmes (see Chapter 16). Students may rotate among different tutors who can supervise different activities such as history taking, physical examination and procedural skills.

Supplementary resources can be made available in the ACTC such as summaries of case notes for the patients invited to attend from the patient bank. Laboratory reports, radiographs or revision material from basic sciences can be made available together with equipment for practising skills procedures such as ophthalmoscopy. A supply of video recordings that illustrate communication skills and clinical examination techniques provides a useful backup resource.

 Twelve tips for setting up an ACTC:

Design
1. Allow development time
2. Integrate curriculum needs and identify organisational constraints
3. Identify interested parties and their strategic role as a committee
4. Find suitable accommodation
5. Secure a budget
6. Acquire suitable resources and equipment

Implementation
7. Recruit and train enthusiastic staff
8. Evolve an implementation function for the steering group
9. Build up a bank of patients
10. Implement a teaching plan

Evaluation
11. Develop a multifaceted evaluation process
12. Develop a research and development function for the steering group

Dent et al 2001b

At the University of Otago, Dunedin, an ambulatory care teaching resource has been created to provide fourth-year students with the opportunity to see a variety of invited patients illustrating clinical conditions in particular organ systems. Students appreciated the dedicated and structured teaching time in a learner-friendly environment (Latta et al 2011).

Developing a teaching programme in ambulatory care requires:

- the identification of available venues
- the cooperation of enthusiastic staff
- a structured approach to teaching and learning
- a staff development programme

Table 12.1 The EPITOMISE acronym helps students to look for all learning outcomes in any patient encounter

E	ethics and enquiry (communications skills)
P	physical examination
I	investigations and interpretations of results
T	technical procedures
O	options of diagnosis, clinical judgement
M	management and multidisciplinary team
I	information handling
S	sciences, basic and clinical
E	education of the patient and yourself

When should ambulatory care teaching be provided?

Early clinical contact is a feature of innovative curricula (GMC 2009, Harden et al 1984). As hospital wards may no longer have patients with common clinical problems who are sufficiently well to see students, ambulatory care can offer a wide range of suitable clinical opportunities for undergraduate at all stages of learning. Less experienced students who are still developing their communication and examination skills can practise these in the dedicated teaching environment of the ACTC, which provides a 'bridge' between practising with simulated patients and manikins in the clinical skills centre and exposure to real patients in the busy environment of an everyday outpatient department.

In the later clinical years, when students have more extensive clinical experience, placement in routine clinics may be more appropriate. In these circumstances students can often learn as apprentices as part of the clinical team (Worley et al 2000).

Structured learning in ambulatory care venues

A structured approach is the key to maximizing the learning opportunities available to students in any ambulatory care venue. A variety of strategies have been described.

LOGBOOKS

It is important to organize the content of an ambulatory care session so that students can easily identify the educational opportunities available. The EPITOMISE logbook, based on the learning outcomes of the Scottish doctor (Simpson et al 2002), has been used to focus student learning on the learning opportunities related to the various patients seen. With every patient they meet, students are asked three questions:

- What did you see?
- What did you do?
- What did you learn?

They then document their experiences under each learning outcome point and reflect on what further learning needs they can now identify and how they will address these learning needs (Dent & Davis 1995) (Table 12.1 and Fig. 12.1).

Logbooks may also be used to assess the range of clinical conditions seen and identify omissions in student experience, but their primary role should be to help students reflect on their clinical experiences and provide a focus for periodic tutor review, mentoring and feedback.

TASK-BASED LEARNING

A list of prescribed tasks to be carried out in the ambulatory setting can be given to students. These may include:

- participate in consultation with the attending staff
- interview and examine patient
- review a number of new radiographs with the radiologist.

Additional tasks for future learning can then be built around each.

CASE STUDIES

'Focus scripts' described by Peltier and colleagues (2007) are used to facilitate the learning of history taking and physical examination skills. Similarly, using the patient journey as a model, students may be directed to follow a patient through a series of ambulatory care experiences from the outpatient department, through clinical investigations and pre-operative assessment, to the day surgery unit and follow-up clinic (Hannah & Dent 2006).

LEARNER-CENTRED APPROACH

Students present cases to their tutor in a structured way under the heading 'SNAPPS', which encourages a question and answer approach.

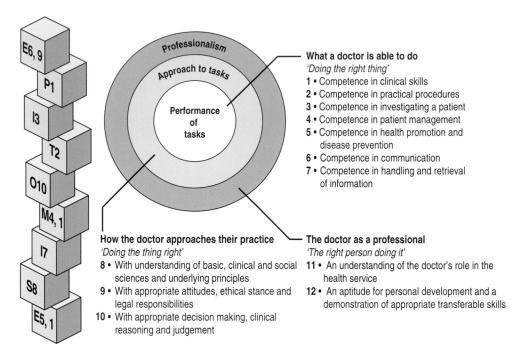

Fig. 12.1 EPITOMISE logbook links students' clinical experience in any venue to the curriculum learning outcomes of the Scottish doctor.

- Summarize the history and physical findings
- Narrow down the differential diagnosis
- Analyse the diagnosis by comparing possibilities
- Probe the preceptor with questions
- Plan patient management
- Select a case issue for self-directed learning

CONFERENCES AND INDEPENDENT STUDY

Higher-level thinking may be focussed by timetabled pre-and post-event discussions with the clinician (Da Rossa et al 1997).

MICROSKILLS FOR STUDENTS

Lipsky and colleagues (1999) describe how students can take the initiative both before and after the outpatient event to facilitate their own learning.

 Twelve tips for students to improve their learning in the ambulatory setting:

1. Orientate to the objectives of the session
2. Share their stage of clinical experience with the tutor
3. Orientate to the clinical location
4. Read around the clinical conditions to be seen

5. Review case notes or summaries provided
6. Be prepared to propose a diagnosis and management plan
7. Explain their reasons for these decisions
8. Seek self-assessment opportunities
9. Seek feedback time from the tutor
10. Generalize the learning experience
11. Reflect on their learning
12. Identify future learning issues.

Based on Lipsky et al 1999

Who can help with ambulatory care teaching?

STAFF

Sending students unannounced to a newly identified teaching venue, suitable though that might be for meeting undergraduate needs, is scarcely going to be welcomed if the staff working there feel themselves, with some justification, to be overburdened with current patient-care activities, underresourced in general and ill-prepared for an additional task.

Attempts should be made in advance to identify the most appropriate clinical staff who might be able to participate in the new teaching opportunity and how they could best be prepared for the job. It doesn't always have to be the senior clinician in the area who has to take the lead role (Ashley et al 2009). In the majority of ambulatory care settings, the delivery of enthusiastic clinical teaching depends on dedicated healthcare professionals teaching at the same time as they carry out their routine patient-care tasks. When developing a teaching programme in a new location it is important to be sensitive to the possible tensions this working/teaching role may generate.

Colleagues

In most cases doctors enjoy the stimulus of having students with them in their workplace provided that the demands of their service commitment can still be met. Additional clinical teachers or research fellows may be able to help occasionally.

Junior staff

Rather than having suddenly to take a clinical teaching session at short notice, junior staff can be helped to develop their teaching skills by having the opportunity to observe good teaching sessions given by a senior tutor. Preparatory briefing material can be used effectively to help them to learn more about medical education and to orientate them to the teaching role (see Staff development section in this chapter).

Other healthcare professionals

Other colleagues working in the ambulatory care setting can also contribute to the teaching programme:

- Nurse practitioners
- Occupational therapists
- Physiotherapists
- Dieticians
- Speech therapists
- Chiropodists
- Social workers.

PATIENTS

Most importantly, there are usually ample numbers of willing and available patients in ambulatory care venues.

Routine patients

"Many patients have actually enjoyed their interactions with students and have been glad to take part in their education."

Krackov et al 1993

However, unselected patients attending the ambulatory care venue may or may not match the requirements of the students present and learning may become opportunistic. It may be difficult for the tutor to utilize them efficiently and the value of the learning experience may be diminished.

Selected patients

Patients with appropriate clinical problems can be pre-selected for a specially provided teaching clinic. Patients are advised that they have been appointed to attend a teaching clinic and, although they will be seen and treated by a specialist, there will be students present and their appointment may take longer than usual. They should be asked to consent to this clinic arrangement before attending.

'Bank' patients model

It is possible to build a 'bank' of clinical volunteers with appropriate histories and stable clinical signs who will attend clinical teaching sessions when invited (Dent et al 2001a). These patients are not currently undergoing active treatment. In a systems-based course, patients with a history of a relevant condition can be invited at the appropriate time. In this model the patient's contribution can more readily be focussed on student learning needs. The tutor should be able to prepare the session for maximal educational advantage in advance and should help students to integrate the clinical experience to learning experiences encountered elsewhere.

OTHER STUDENTS

Junior students appreciate peer tutoring sessions in the ACTC from more senior students. These sessions provide supervised practice in history taking and physical examination and simple diagnostic procedures. Often senior students find that taking the role of tutor is a stimulus for their own learning (see Chapter 16).

Managing teaching in ambulatory care venues

IN THE OUTPATIENT DEPARTMENT

Depending on their experience, students may take part to different extents in a routine outpatient clinic ranging from observation to full participation (see Table 12.2). The choice of teaching model to be used depends on the number of staff present, the number of rooms available, the number and prior experience of the students and the busyness of the clinic (number of patients attending). Cooperation with the other healthcare professionals working in the clinic is vital. However, in any teaching model, students should be encouraged to take an active approach to learning.

Having one student joining you in a clinic can be a relatively straightforward experience, but a variety

Table 12.2 A variety of teaching models to engage students in outpatient clinics

	Junior students	Senior students
Single student	Sitting-in model Breakout model	Apprenticeship/ parallel consultations Report-back model
Several students	Grandstand model Breakout model	Supervised consultations

of models can be used depending on the student's experience.

Sitting-in model

One-to-one teaching is much appreciated by students who can observe the patient consultation and interact confidently with the clinician and patients, but they may not have the chance to see patients independently. Less confident students may feel vulnerable in this setting and may need encouragement to participate; more senior students may be able to function more fully.

Apprenticeship/parallel consultation model

A small number of senior students may be able to interview the patient either alone or under supervision. This involves active student–patient interaction, which reinforces learning. Some students may feel intimidated when performing under observation, but if a separate room is available they can interview and examine a patient without constraints before later presenting the case to the tutor. Regan-Smith and colleagues (2002) describe restructuring outpatient clinics to allow learners who have already had training to see patients who are booked in parallel sessions with the tutor's patients (see also Chapter 15). Walters and colleagues (2008) found that the overall consultation time was not increased when rural GPs supervised medical students in this model.

Report-back model

Students see patients without supervision and at an appointed time take them to present to the clinician in turn (see Fig. 12.4). Students have time and space to interview and examine their patient at their own pace. Meanwhile, the clinician will have been able to see other patients attending the clinic independently.

 Decide which model you are going to use in your clinic depending on how many rooms are available for you to use and how many members of staff are available to help with the clinic.

Don't be afraid to change models during the clinic to vary the session for the students and yourself.

Having a larger group of students with you in a routine clinic can be more difficult to organize.

Grandstand model

Frequently students are crowded into the consulting room attempting to observe and hear the consultation. Interaction with both patient and clinician is limited, and patients may feel threatened by the large audience. The clinician's interaction with the patient may also be inhibited. The use of a study guide or logbook to direct independent learning may be helpful for students here.

Breakout model

Students sit in with the clinician and observe a whole consultation with a patient. They then, individually or in pairs, take the patients to another room to go over parts of the interview or examination again at their own pace (Fig. 12.2).

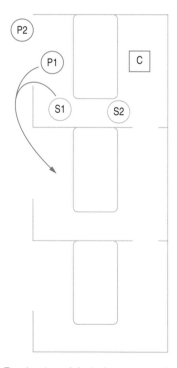

Fig. 12.2 Breakout model: students see patients independently after the consultation.

Supervising model

If several rooms are available the students may be divided into smaller groups to see selected patients independently in a separate room. After a suitable time the clinician can go to each room in turn to hear the students' report on their interview (see Fig. 12.3). The students have time and space to interview and examine their patient at their own pace and benefit from individual feedback on their performance (Fig. 12.4).

IN A TEACHING CLINIC

A selected group of patients is invited to the event which, although dealing with real patient problems, is announced in advance as being focused on student learning.

IN THE ACTC

Structured learning can be provided by invited patients and clinical tutors familiar with the learning outcomes of the curriculum, the objectives of the teaching session and the needs and expected level of performance of the students.

Student learning can be supported by a study guide, by a logbook and by having additional learning resources available to the tutor. The opportunity for self-reflection, peer critique and tutor feedback can be created by taking video recordings as students practise their performance of history taking or examination skills (Dent & Preece 2002).

Overall, there is probably a need for a programme director who will coordinate ambulatory care teaching across various venues and for an administrator, preferably with a background in healthcare, who will manage the patient bank, timetable tutors and student sessions and facilitate the provision of other resource material required.

IN A CLINICAL INVESTIGATIONS SUITE

Clinical investigations suites for radiology, endoscopy, clinical measurement and vascular assessment can be used if students are directed to the particular learning outcomes available in each and if staff are able to spend some time teaching. Students can follow a structured logbook and interact with a patient in activities which may include a pre-event interview for assessment and consent by medical or nursing staff, the imaging process itself with radiographers or endoscopists (either clinicians or specialist nurses) and an interpretation or reporting session with radiologists or other specialists. Additional resources which might be available to help students to integrate their learning around these cases might include case histories, flow

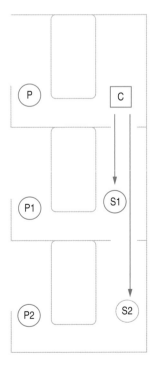

Fig. 12.3 Supervising model: students practise consultations under supervision.

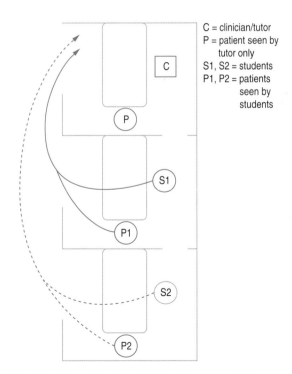

C = clinician/tutor
P = patient seen by tutor only
S1, S2 = students
P1, P2 = patients seen by students

Fig. 12.4 Report-back model: students see patients independently and report back with them to the tutor who has meanwhile been seeing other patients.

diagrams of management procedures, anatomical models or collections of radiographs.

Students should also be prompted by their logbook to integrate their learning by reference to material experienced elsewhere or by directions to other helpful resources or to the clinical skills centre to revise clinical skills.

IN THE DAY SURGERY UNIT

Although currently underutilized (Seabrook et al 1998), attachments to day surgery units (DSUs) can provide opportunities for structured teaching following the patient journey (Hannah & Dent 2006). Experience in pre-op assessment, diagnosis, theatre technique and postoperative care can be provided in a multiprofessional environment. As the number of patients attending is usually large, and patients are usually otherwise well, it is relatively easy to structure a teaching session to include a variety of learning objectives. Various programmes have been described (Hannah & Dent 2006, O'Driscoll et al 1998, Seabrook et al 1998) which may be implemented without compromise to patient care (Rudkin et al 1997). Twelve tips for developing a clinical teaching programme in a DSU have been described (Dent 2003).

 Twelve tips for developing a clinical teaching programme in a DSU:

Preparation
1. Identify the learning objectives that students can achieve in the DSU
2. Secure institutional support and form an implementation/steering group representing all parties involved
3. Discuss implications, expectations and limitations with DSU staff and tutors
4. Identify a method for selecting appropriate patients
5. Identify space for student–patient consultations
6. Reserve space in a skills training unit
7. Provide staff development opportunities

Delivery
8. Provide a study guide/logbook
9. Employ a DSU-based tutor/supervisor
10. Provide opportunities for student reflection, tuition and assessment

Evaluation
11. Evaluate feedback from students, tutors and DSU staff
12. Discuss research and development opportunities with all parties involved.

Dent 2003

IN A REGIONAL DIAGNOSTIC AND TREATMENT CENTRE (RDTC)

In some regions of the UK, community-situated hospitals have been redeveloped as regional diagnostic and treatment centres (RDTCs). In these facilities a wide range of healthcare activities take place on an ambulatory basis. These centres can provide students with ideal opportunities to experience outpatient consultations, clinical investigations and day case therapy and surgery. A four-week structured clinical attachment in the RDTC can provide new learning opportunities focussed on ambulatory and community care (Dent et al 2007). These experiences can be enhanced by subsequent placements with a local general practice.

Staff development for ambulatory care teaching

 Seven factors of effective teaching:

- Knowledge
- Organisation and clarity
- Enthusiasm
- Group instructional skills
- Clinical supervision skills
- Clinical competence
- Modelling professional characteristics.
Irby et al 1991

Irby and colleagues (1991) list the ideal requirements of teaching staff. Formal staff development sessions may be required to help colleagues unfamiliar with the medical school curriculum or student learning needs or with balancing service delivery with clinical teaching. Simple instructional brochures can be circulated in advance to brief tutors (Dent & Hesketh 2003), or a more interactive approach can be taken to encourage staff participation in teaching such as the GMC commended series of booklets, "Getting started …" (Dent & Davis 2008).

Assessment in ambulatory care

Assessment in ambulatory care may take the form of a review of written material (Denton et al 2006).

- Tutor review of a logbook or e-logbook can be done by the tutor in isolation but is more valuable for formative assessment if carried out together with the student.

- A task list or checklist review monitors tasks accomplished during the session, but descriptors should be used to guide the assessor to evaluate the level of student competency achieved more precisely.

- Reflective diaries are valuable for students for revision and reflection and also to identify any omissions in their learning.

Alternatively, students' clinical skills can be assessed (see Chapter 38, Performance and workplace assessment), but this may be more difficult given the time constraints of the ambulatory care setting,

- Mini-CEX (Norcini et al 2003). Multiple, short, focused assessments of clinical skills followed by feedback are carried out by a variety of assessors during the attachment.

- Direct observation of procedural skills (Norcini & Burch 2007). The student's or trainee's ability to carry out a wide range of procedures can be closely assessed using a structured score sheet and feedback then given.

- Microskills for students (Lipsky et al 1999). Students take the initiative to seek self-assessment opportunities and feedback.

Evaluation of ambulatory care teaching

Whatever venue or form of ambulatory care teaching is developed, it is important to evaluate it by seeking feedback from patients, staff and students. The results may be pleasantly surprising (Dent et al 2001a) and will help to refine the programme for future use.

 "Ambulatory education is timely and needed, and, to a large degree, ambulatory programmes are being rated highly by the students who participate in them."

Krackov et al 1993

Summary

The ward setting has become less suitable for clinical teaching as inpatients are now fewer in number and more often acutely ill. Transferring the emphasis of teaching to the ambulatory care setting opens a number of previously underutilized venues for student–patient interaction. The educational objectives to be achieved are different from those traditionally seen in ward-based teaching.

A teaching programme in ambulatory care can be facilitated by:

- the identification of available venues
- a structured approach to teaching and learning

- the development of an ACTC
- a staff development programme.

Strategies to facilitate learning include a structured logbook and a variety of models to manage student–patient interaction in various settings to maximum advantage.

The educational opportunities available in the ACTC can be developed further by a clinical director who can coordinate the patients attending, the 'bank' of invited volunteers and the most efficient use of colleagues from other healthcare professions.

There are advantages to medical schools in recognizing the increasing role ambulatory care teaching has to contribute to the undergraduate curriculum, and appropriate resource should be invested to develop it further.

References

Ashley P, Rhodes N, Sari-Kouzel H, et al: "They've all got to learn". Medical students learning from patients in ambulatory (outpatient and general practice) consultations, *Medical Teacher* 31:e24–31, 2009.

Bardgett RJM, Dent JA: Teaching and learning in outpatients and beyond: how ambulatory acre teaching can contribute to student learning in child health, *Archive of Disease in Childhood: Education and Practice* 96:148–152, 2011.

Da Rossa AD, Dunnington GL, Stearns J, et al: Ambulatory teaching "lite": less clinic time, more educationally fulfilling, *Academic Medicine* 72:358–361, 1997.

Dent JA: Twelve tips for developing a clinical teaching programme in a day surgery unit, *Medical Teacher* 25:364–367, 2003.

Dent JA: AMEE guide Number 26: Clinical teaching in ambulatory care settings – making the most of learning opportunities with outpatients, *Medical Teacher* 27:302–315, 2005.

Dent JA, Davis MH: Role of ambulatory are for student-patient interaction: the EPITOME model, *Medical Education* 29:58–60, 1995.

Dent JA, Angell-Preece HM, Ball HM-L, Ker JS: Using the ambulatory care teaching centre to develop opportunities for integrated learning, *Medical Teacher* 23:171–175, 2001a.

Dent JA, Ker JS, Angell-Preece HM, Preece PE: Twelve tips for setting up an ambulatory care (outpatient) teaching centre, *Medical Teacher* 23:345–350, 2001b.

Dent JA, Preece PE: What is the impact on participating students of real-time monitoring of their consultation skills? *British Journal of Educational Technology* 33:349–351, 2002.

Dent JA, Hesketh EA: Developing the teaching instinct: how to teach in an ambulatory (outpatient) teaching centre, *Medical Teacher* 25:488–491, 2003.

Dent J, Skene S, Nathwani D, et al: Design, implementation and evaluation of a medical education programme using the ambulatory diagnostic and treatment centre, *Medical Teacher* 29:341–345, 2007.

Dent JA, Davis MH (editors): *"Getting started …"* A practical Guide for Clinical Teachers. Centre for Medical Education, University of Dundee, 2008.

Denton GD, DeMott C, Pangaro LN, Hemmer PA: Narrative review: use of student-generated logbooks in undergraduate medical education, *Teaching and Learning in Medicine* 18(2):153–164, 2006.

Fincher RME, Albritton TA: The ambulatory experience for junior medical students at the Medical College of Georgia, *Teaching and Learning in Medicine* 5:210–213, 1993.

General Medical Council: *Tomorrow's Doctors*, London, 2009, General Medical Council.

Hannah A, Dent JA: Developing teaching opportunities in a day surgery unit, *The Clinical Teacher* 3:180–184, 2006.

Harden RM, Sowden S, Dunn WR: Some educational strategies in curriculum development: the SPICES model, *Medical Education* 18:284–297, 1984.

Irby DM, Ramsay PG, Gillmore GM, Schaad D: Characteristics of effective clinical teachers of ambulatory care medicine, *Academic Medicine* 66:54–55, 1991.

Krackov SK, Packman CH, Regan-Smith MG, et al: Perspectives on ambulatory programs: barriers and implementation strategies, *Teaching and Learning in Medicine* 5:243–250, 1993.

Latta L, Manning P, Tordoff D, Dent J: Teaching and learning in an integrated ambulatory medicine programme for undergraduate medical students in Dunedin, NZ. AMEE 2011, Vienna, Austria, Conference Abstracts, August 2011, 27–31.

Lipsky MS, Taylor CA, Schnuth R: Microskills for students: twelve tips for learning in the ambulatory care setting, *Medical Teacher* 21:469–472, 1999.

Norcini JJ, Black LL, Duffy FD, et al: The mini-CEX: a method for assessing clinical skills, *Annals of Internal Medicine* 138:476–481, 2003.

Norcini J, Burch V: *Workplace-based assessment as an educational tool. AMEE Guide 31*, Scotland, 2007, AMEE, Dundee.

O'Driscoll MCE, Rudkin GE, Carty VM: Day surgery: teaching the next generation, *Medical Education* 32:390–395, 1998.

Peltier D, Regan-Smith M, Wofford J, et al: Teaching focused histories and physical exams in ambulatory care: multi-institutional randomised trial, *Teaching and Learning in Medicine* 19:244–250, 2007.

Regan-Smith M, Young WW, Keller AM: An effective and efficient teaching model of ambulatory education, *Academic Medicine* 77:593–599, 2002.

Rudkin GE, O'Driscoll MCE, Carty VM: Does a teaching programme in day surgery impact on efficiency and quality care? *Australian and New Zealand Journal of Surgery* 67:883–887, 1997.

Seabrook MA, Lawson M, Malster M, et al: Teaching medical students in a day surgery unit: adapting medical education to changes in clinical practice, *Medical Teacher* 20:222–226, 1998.

Simpson JG, Furnace J, Crosby J, et al: The Scottish doctor – learning outcomes for the medical undergraduate in Scotland: a foundation for competent and reflective practitioners, *Medical Teacher* 14:136–143, 2002.

Stearns JA, Glasser M: How ambulatory care is different: a paradigm for teaching and practice, *Medical Education* 27:35–40, 1993.

Walters L, Worley P, Prideaux D, Lange K: Do consultations in rural general practice take more time when practitioners are precepting medical students? *Medical Education* 42:69–73, 2008.

Worley P, Silagy C, Prideaux D, et al: The parallel rural community curriculum: an integrated clinical curriculum based on rural general practice, *Medical Education* 34:558–565, 2000.

In the community

P. S. Worley, I. D. Couper

Introduction

Patient care is increasingly moving from hospital wards to community clinics. This contributes to the widening gap between the 'designed' broad-based curriculum advocated by professional bodies and the learning that can be delivered in a tertiary hospital-based course, causing medical schools to search for new sites in which to prepare the next generation of doctors. One solution, for many schools, is community-based medical education (CBME).

What is community-based medical education?

CBME usually refers to medical education that is based outside a tertiary or large secondary level hospital. Community-oriented medical education, on the other hand, describes curricula that are based on addressing the health needs of the local community and preparing graduates to work in that community.

Community-oriented education is often, quite sensibly, based in the community, but it is possible for large components of such a curriculum to be delivered in a tertiary centre. The medical course at Newcastle University New South Wales, Australia, is a good example of a community-oriented programme largely delivered in tertiary settings.

It may be argued that tertiary hospitals are also 'in the community'. Globally the health system has developed tertiary centres to cater for the high-technology elements of healthcare efficiently and to a high standard. This has resulted in a system that is primarily accountable internally, through processes of audit and peer review. It is not accountable to any one local community, as patients are admitted from many different communities, often over significant distances.

The tertiary centre requires highly developed referral filters to keep people 'out'. The two principal filters are the primary care system and community-based specialist services. The former incorporates a wide range of healthcare providers, clinics, health centres, practices, governmental and non-governmental organizations, district hospitals, etc. The latter may be consulting medical specialists and the outreach teams from tertiary centres, such as home-based palliative care services.

Thus CBME focuses on the care provided to patients both before the decision to refer to a tertiary hospital and after the decision to discharge the patient from such care. In many of these circumstances the traditional doctor–patient relationship will not apply and patients may be referred to as 'clients' or, even more appropriately, as members of defined local communities.

When discussing CBME in primary care, it is important to understand the difference between the uses of the terms 'primary care' and 'primary healthcare'. The former refers to the first point of contact for members of the community with the health system and will usually not require a referral.

Primary healthcare (PHC) concerns a philosophy of healthcare which emphasizes the need to address the priority health problems in the community by providing promotive, preventive, curative, rehabilitative and palliative services. Accordingly, PHC proposes broad-based approaches to health through collaboration between sectors and advocates strong participation of 'consumers' in healthcare planning. Most CBME curricula are based on a PHC philosophy and are conducted in a primary care setting, but it is possible for neither of these two elements to be present, for example, in a rotation based in the private clinic of a psychiatrist with the primary aim of learning advanced psychotherapy.

Common settings for CBME include:

- general practice/family medicine clinic
- village/community health centres
- specialist, consulting clinics
- patients' homes
- schools
- factories
- farms
- community fairs
- shopping centres.

 "It is possible to cut across the traditional clinical discipline boundaries so entrenched in medical education by teaching in rural general practice but not fundamentally about rural general practice."

Worley et al 2000

Uses for CBME

The setting and structure of CBME are principally determined by the aims of the particular component of the curriculum to be delivered. These can be divided into preclinical and clinical aims.

PRECLINICAL AIMS

CBME has been used to advantage for learning in such diverse areas as epidemiology, preventative health, public health principles, community development, the social impact of illness, the PHC approach, the healthcare team and understanding how patients interact with the healthcare system. It is also commonly used for learning basic clinical skills, especially communication skills, and for learning a variety of professional development skills through the mentorship of primary care doctors.

These latter aims could also be learned in a tertiary hospital with no particular disadvantage but are often taught in the community because the faculty who have a special interest in these areas, and have been delegated with the responsibility for teaching them, are often primary care practitioners.

CLINICAL

The curricular aims of clinical CBME courses fall into four categories, three of which have the hospital as the primary locus for training and a fourth which has the community as the primary locus.

To learn about general practice/family medicine

A primary care, general practice or family medicine rotation is the most common clinical CBME attachment and appears in most contemporary medical curricula. It occurs either in a short, discrete block of time or in a continuity rotation of perhaps a full or half day per week for a semester, a year or more. There are advantages and disadvantages with both models (Table 13.1).

Whichever structure is chosen, it is essential to have a well-planned orientation to the rotation, the practice and the community. This may also involve intensive instruction in relevant clinical skills and in the structure of healthcare delivery in the local community, especially if this is the first such exposure for students. Many additional useful tasks may be linked to these rotations, such as doing home visits, developing an ecomap of local resources or health facilities available to patients, meeting with community-based organizations or support groups, and visits to other health workers in the area. An opportunity to debrief and reflect on their experiences is also helpful to consolidate students' learning and conduct course evaluation. These suggestions are relevant to both undergraduate and postgraduate learning.

To learn about a particular specialty other than general practice/family medicine

There are a number of good examples of this type of CBME. At University College London, students spend 4 weeks in a tertiary hospital and 4 weeks based in a general practice with the specific aim of learning about internal medicine (Murray et al 1997). Evaluation of this model indicates that the student learning at both sites was complementary and students valued the CBME component highly. At the University of Pretoria in South Africa, students spend part of a 7-week community-based rotation specifically developing obstetric skills. In addition to such undergraduate models, postgraduate training programmes in disciplines traditionally taught in hospitals, for example, paediatrics, psychiatry and internal medicine, are creating CBME learning experiences as they seek to prepare their residents appropriately for current and future practice.

To learn about primary care

In this model, the tertiary hospital is still the primary learning area, but community sites are used to fill in the gaps in the curriculum, because of a mismatch between curriculum goals and what is achievable in the hospital context. Important areas covered may be in relation to learning about primary healthcare, community-based practice, team-based care and

Table 13.1 Community-based medical education (CBME) in general practice

Type of CBME	Advantages	Disadvantages
Discrete block	Immersion experience	Requires accommodation for student
	Allows student to focus entirely on general practice	Large variation in student experience at different times of the year
	Easy to timetable	School and public holidays impact have significant negative impact
	Intense mentorship relationship	Adverse effect on practice income or consulting time
	Often has a regenerative feeling for the student: 'a change is as good as a holiday'	Can be tiring for the preceptor
	Possibility of using rural and remote practices	
	Easy to conduct evaluation and assessment before and afterwards	
Continuity rotation	Can follow specific patients over time	May be conflicts with activities in the 'feeder' rotation
	Can see seasonal differences in practice	Available sites limited by recurring transport costs and time
	Usually no student accommodation required	May be seen by student as less important than the concurrent hospital-based discipline
	Can integrate learning with another hospital-based discipline	Preceptor may lose interest, leave, get unwell over the extended time period
	Student can develop a specific role in the practice over time	Evaluation often contaminated by variable concurrent learning in hospital
	Impact on practice income may be less apparent as only one session per week	
	May appear less tiring to the preceptor as effort is spread over a longer period	

working with communities. The primary care context can be used to integrate learning from a range of disciplines, for integrating clinical practice and public health and for interprofessional and multidisciplinary learning.

The Integrated Primary Care (IPC) block at the University of the Witwatersrand, Johannesburg is an example of this. Students complete a 6-week rotation in primary care clinics and community hospitals, applying the knowledge and skills acquired from the major specialties (from internal medicine to public health) to undifferentiated patients, their families and communities, in an integrated programme that is jointly managed and examined by representatives from the major disciplines, and are orientated to the importance of primary healthcare (Nyangairi et al 2010).

To learn multiple disciplines concurrently

In this case, the whole curriculum is based on community practice, whether this be for 1 year or for the entire period of training. This might be the orientation of a whole medical school, such as Walter Sisulu University in South Africa, University of Wollongong in Australia, Ateneo de Zamboanga University in the Philippines, and the Northern Ontario School of Medicine in Canada, or an option for a subgroup of students, such as the Flinders Parallel Rural Community Curriculum (PRCC) at Flinders University in Australia.

This concept takes advantage of the broad patient base in primary care and, with some exceptions, has mostly been situated in rural communities. There are two principal reasons for this that relate to educational opportunities and health policy agendas.

Rural practice, in most countries, has a broader range of patients, involves fewer referrals, and the clinicians are more likely to have significant roles in primary care, emergency medicine, obstetrics and inpatient care. Thus, it is relatively simple for the rural preceptor to give students access to continuity of care through initial diagnosis, investigation, initial management (including as an inpatient) and ongoing care of a range of patients.

Extended rotations of this type have also been shown to be associated with a high number of students choosing a career in rural practice (Worley et al 2008) and thus have been supported financially by government authorities as a significant long-term strategy with regard to the rural medical workforce.

Table 13.2 Comparison of extended CBME and tertiary rotations

Education factors	Sequential tertiary rotations	Extended CBME
Illness spectrum	Highly filtered case-mix; all of high severity and complexity	Greater access to common conditions; many different levels of severity and complexity
Contact with patients	Cross-sectional; snapshot of patients at similar points in their illness	Longitudinal; see improvement/relapse/further decision making over time
Role in patient care	Passive; students feel 'in the way'; as soon as the students have learnt the specific functioning of one team, they move to another ward and discipline with new supervisors and expectations	Active; valued extended time in a single setting with the same supervisor enables safe participation to increase over the year
Student attitude	Regard time on ward as 'study'	Regard time in practice as 'work'
Access to subspecialist expertise	Face to face, easy to organize	By planned visits, internet resources, or video-conferenced tutorials
Professional development	See supervising clinicians only in clinical context and role	See supervising clinicians in clinical and social/family contexts and roles
Delegation of teaching	Specialist supervisors delegate significant amount of teaching to junior medical staff	Primary care practitioner supervisors delegate some teaching to resident and visiting specialists
Modelling for future practice	Learning in a high-technology, high-cost environment	Learning in a low-technology, low-cost environment

Evaluation of this programme has shown that students in the Flinders PRCC perform better in examinations than their hospital-based peers (Worley et al 2004) and develop the skills and personal qualities required to practise in areas of need (Couper & Worley 2010). Based on the Flinders experience, the contrasts between this extended form of CBME and multiple tertiary hospital rotations, combining inpatient and ambulatory outpatient experience, are summarized in Table 13.2.

 "When they returned to the hospital environment, students did not feel themselves at a disadvantage compared with traditional students."

Oswald et al 2001

Practical principles for successful CBME

The latter two categories particularly share an understanding of the community as a context which is much greater than any particular discipline or level of care, and are underpinned by some important principles. Although advocates of CBME will talk in passionate terms about its advantages, experienced innovators will rightly point out that success is not guaranteed.

It is certainly possible to have poor quality CBME, and even in successful programmes, the issues of sustainability over time and quality control over numerous sites are important challenges that need to be recognized at the outset. Previous analysis of the literature on CBME, combined with authors' experience in CBME development and management, has led to the recognition of four key relationships that are crucial to success (Worley 2002).

THE CLINICIAN–PATIENT RELATIONSHIP

Enabling the student to participate, in a meaningful way, in the clinician–patient interaction is a key to medical education in any context. Although the primary care system emphasizes the importance of the doctor–patient relationship, successfully integrating the student into this privileged interaction requires explicit attention in CBME. It is not automatic and requires permission, planning and that the student acquires prerequisite skills, knowledge and attitudes. It also requires attention being paid to establishing effective working relationships with non-doctor clinicians, who in many contexts, particularly in Africa, are the primary clinical supervisors of medical students.

As clinical CBME usually occurs in pressurized, first-line consulting rooms, in practices or in clinics, it is more likely to be successful and sustainable if it can be structured in a way that enhances, rather than detracts from, the clinician's work and the patient's satisfaction with the care provided. Patient consent is a key first step. This is easier to manage if student teaching is seen as a 'norm' within the clinic, rather than an unusual occurrence. That is, the clinic is branded as a teaching site where it is expected that students will be part of the healthcare team.

Evaluations of patient satisfaction with student participation in such community settings have been extremely positive. In particular, there appears to be a certain 'status' attached by patients to their carer being an affiliated university teacher, a recognition of the importance of training the next generation of doctors well, and an appreciation of the extra time and interest a student may give to a patient. In the context of rural CBME, patients may see this as their opportunity to recruit a potential future doctor to their region.

Teaching takes time, and it is important to structure this teaching to have the least negative impact on the number of patients that can be seen. If this is not the case, the clinician may decide to discontinue involvement, require significant financial compensation or encourage purely passive observation by the student. All these are undesirable. Experience with extended CBME programmes indicates that it may even be possible to increase practice capacity by involving the students in useful components of the patient care (Walters et al 2008). It appears that this capacity increases as the student's time in a particular practice increases. At the same time, the student's role in contributing to patient care must not be abused; students need time to learn from each patient they see.

How can students become integrated in a meaningful and helpful way? The following practical suggestions have been found to be useful:

- Ensure there is a separate consulting room available for student use.
- Modify the appointment schedule, without reducing the total number of patients, so that patients are booked in simultaneous pairs, one for the student, and one for the doctor. The doctor sees her patient first, then moves to the other room to see the 'student's' patient.
- Encourage patients seen by the student to return when the student is consulting.
- Provide a quiet student study area in the health facility with internet access.
- Arrange a system for the student to be contacted for after-hours or emergency calls.
- Allow students choice in their practice sites.
- Involve the host facility or practice in student selection and matching.

- Provide training and academic recognition for local supervisors.
- Employ an administrator to timetable and coordinate the multiple learning sites/sessions for each student.
- Encourage academic staff to work clinically in the community selected for teaching.

It is recognized that these suggestions are easier to achieve in a resource-rich environment, but they provide useful principles for all CBME programmes, and many can be implemented with a minimum of resources. There are many tools that can be used as adjuncts to consulting room learning. These might include logbooks, self- and peer-assessment tasks, skills lists and specific activity requirements, such as home visits, working with other professionals, accompanying patients who are referred and attending support groups or local health service meetings. The basis for the success of these is student-directed learning, where students have flexibility to meet their own needs, measured against clear objectives. This is not simply a cost-effective strategy for resource-constrained environments, but a highly effective way of learning. Appointing appropriate mentors is also critical to success.

 "Rurally based students saw double the number of common medical conditions and assisted in, or performed, six times as many procedures
    as city-based students, with the result that the majority of the students were sure they had a better educational experience than their city counterparts."

Worley et al 2000

THE UNIVERSITY–HEALTH SERVICE RELATIONSHIP

In many tertiary centres today there is considerable tension between the research and education agenda of the university and the clinical service targets of the health service. In CBME contexts, the challenge is to enable the presence of medical students to enhance the objectives of both organizations and create a symbiotic relationship between the two.

How can this be achieved? What does the health service gain?

Bringing medical education to a health service can be seen as recognition of the quality of that service. A university presence may also bring with it expectations and expertise in audit, quality control and peer review that improve patient care and further validate this perceived higher status as a teaching centre. The presence of students can be a powerful motivator for local health service staff, many of whom describe a new sense of meaning in their work as a result of students' presence.

Students can also be given tasks which contribute to the health service beyond patient care. Health facility audits, quality improvement projects, creation of facility ecomaps and resource lists, and similar student activities, conducted with the support and guidance of health facility managers, can assist health service development and ensure that students are seen to be useful by these managers, not only by clinicians. Beyond that, these activities can be critical in developing students' ability both to contribute to and critique the performance of the health system in the context of a local community and a multiprofessional team, which are essential ingredients of 21st century medical education (Frenk et al 2010).

How does the university benefit?

In addition to the health service providing access to valuable clinical education opportunities for the university, the community setting can open up new avenues of clinical and health service research and with this the funds to undertake this work jointly. This perspective may be important when innovators seek to encourage tertiary academics to participate in community-based programmes.

There can be benefit to both organizations from shared resources. For example, students and staff in community settings require access to the latest and widest information sources available to supplement their clinical experiences. This may be through internet and university library access, tutorials from visiting academics, specifically developed CD-ROM materials or video-conferenced educational sessions. These same resources can be put to good use by the health service. This may lead to joint funding of the infrastructure required.

The principle of redundancy is important in relation to the use of distance education technology (David Badger, Flinders University, personal communication). Students have different learning styles. Some may enjoy searching the web, whilst others may prefer watching a videotape of a lecture. Still others may choose to read a textbook. Electronic resources and power supplies also have a habit of malfunctioning at inconvenient times, especially in remote communities. For high-stakes learning, students in the community must be provided with more than one way to learn coursework, to cater both to different learning styles and to unexpected malfunction.

Technology should also be used appropriately, rather than simply for the sake of using it; for example, teaching teleconferences (audio rather than video) provide a very useful, cost-effective tool for linking students from many sites to teachers at the university or located at one distant site.

 A new set of criteria for modern medical curricula:

- product-focused
- relevant to society
- interprofessional
- shorter
- multiple sites
- symbiotic.

Bligh et al 2001

 Shared ownership of curriculum development and student selection enhances commitment from clinicians and the community.

THE GOVERNMENT–COMMUNITY RELATIONSHIP

Thus far in this section we have been focusing particularly on clinical learning. However, medical curricula have broader aims than the one-to-one interaction with patients. Gaining an appreciation of the health needs of communities, and methods to address these through local initiative and government policy, are important aspects of most modern medical programmes. CBME can provide excellent opportunities for such learning. However, there are often tensions between national government policy and local community perceptions of health service priorities.

A further key notion that underpins successful CBME is the creation of a university presence in a local community that brings together national policy and local community needs. The first mechanism for this is through targeted research. Medical students, especially as part of their preclinical learning, can engage in locally driven research that can lead to changes in local understanding and practice. Examples of this may include understanding the occupational health risks of vineyard workers, or factors that improve the local uptake of chemically impregnated mosquito nets. This research may also provide data that enable access to further government funding sources.

Second, students can learn through participation in community development. This may involve local implementation of national priorities such as immunization, sanitation, food hygiene practices, antenatal care and agricultural safety. This is best undertaken whilst living in the community concerned.

Third, the effectiveness of CBME as a local medical recruitment tool is a powerful synergy of local workforce needs with national workforce policy. This can be both a means to access additional educational funding from national sources and a motivator for continued community participation. This is not, however, inevitable. It will only be effective if the student experience is a positive one. It will be facilitated if both the local community and the potential government funders have a sense of ownership and engagement with the CBME programme. This may be attained through an advisory committee, student selection, social introductions to community groups, support for student accommodation or transport subsidies.

In light of these potential benefits, it is important for universities to be diligent in collecting appropriate workforce data and maintaining a longitudinal database of their students' career paths. Thus, if students gain a sense of 'belonging' and appreciation from 'their' community, and an understanding of the relevant government policy agendas, they can become passionate and articulate advocates for the community and see immediate results from their learning at a population level.

Many medical schools are now recognizing this government–community relationship as they attempt to deliver socially accountable medical education. The Training for Health Equity Network (THEnet, www.thenetcommunity.org) is a small group of innovative medical schools that are committed to this approach and have developed an evaluation framework to guide its implementation.

THE PERSONAL–PROFESSIONAL RELATIONSHIP

The final relationship to consider in making the most of CBME is the tension that often exists between the personal values and priorities of the individual physician and the expectations of the profession. Education in primary care settings can result in students spending a relatively large amount of time with one supervisor. This can lead to the development of an effective mentor relationship that can assist the student in analysing their own personal values in the light of professional norms, but it requires vulnerability on behalf of both supervisor and student for this to happen. A well-developed mentor relationship may persist after the student leaves and prove influential in future career decisions.

Many clinical educators are concerned at the attrition of humanistic values that occurs in traditional medical school training. The continuity that extended CBME provides has been shown to mitigate against this attrition and enhance important values such as empathy and altruism. The Consortium for Longitudinal Integrated Clerkships (CLIC, www.clicmeded.com) is a network of medical schools that are committed to this continuity approach to medical education.

There are practical ways of encouraging this value-based learning to occur. First, it should be explicitly recognized in the curriculum. The best way to do this is to link it with specific assessment. This may involve interviews based on a reflective diary of the student's clinical experiences or written ethical or legal analysis of critical incidents observed by the student. Objective structured clinical examination (OSCE) stations can also be constructed to test this learning. For example, stations can be constructed around contraception advice to minors, requests for euthanasia or termination of pregnancy.

CBME is also an excellent opportunity for students to observe the role of clinicians outside the clinic, both in terms of further professional responsibilities, such as community health education, and in terms of how being a doctor impacts on their family and social life in that community. This is best learned if the student is a resident in the community. It is crucial to find accommodation for students that will support the experience as being a positive one. In this regard, curriculum planners should pay attention to the growing number of students who have partners and children. A community experience may be used by the whole family to determine the benefits and disadvantages of living and working in such a community after graduation, but this requires significant additional expense.

One factor that is important to be aware of is student safety. This may entail educating students about issues of safe travel, carefully managing physical risks to students in communities where violence is a significant issue, managing the risk to the student of exposure to communicable diseases such as HIV and assisting students to deal with relative isolation, cultural change and, for some, living away from home for the first time. Students must have clarity on insurance policies in terms of the extent of coverage and the responsibility expected from them. Students also, from time to time, become unwell, or have family or social crises. They need to have access to assistance independent of their teacher/assessor. Such resources should be arranged before any need arises and students should have written and verbal explanation of the arrangements.

CBME academic and administrative staff who support the personal and professional development of their students will find that the students not only gain cognitive and psychomotor knowledge and skills during their attachment, but also have the opportunity to gain affective skills and find themselves changed by the experience.

Community-based medical education, as an effective long-term workforce redistribution strategy, can provide a point of synergy between a local community's priorities and government policy.

"Innovations in clinical education may help inoculate medical students against the degradation of attitudes."

Krupat et al 2009

Summary

Community-based medical education is an increasingly popular tool in the medical educator's toolbox. Its use reflects the growing importance of community-based practice in the 21st century health system. There are many forms of CBME allied to the various curricular aims it is intended to deliver, and many curricula are developed through necessity or opportunity rather than being based on clear medical education research.

Moving medical education from tertiary centres into the community involves institutional change and requires proactive leadership and significant resources. CBME is not a cheaper alternative to traditional medical education. Teaching in the community may require additional time and person-power because of the low student–teacher ratio and the costs of supporting students at a distance, such as accommodation, travel for students and academic staff, and information and communication technology.

Whilst it is clear that further research is urgently required, it is hoped that the principles outlined in this chapter can help innovators to avoid major pitfalls and increase the likelihood of positive feedback from all the stakeholders involved. Successful change involves rethinking problems as opportunities and having the creativity to find practical solutions. Organizations such as the Network: Towards Unity for Health, THEnet and CLIC can provide a forum for exchange of ideas and support for change agents. Become aware of the CBME initiatives worldwide through the Network's and CLIC's regular international conferences: you will be inspired and invigorated.

 Pay as much attention to the students' learning of 'heart' knowledge as you do to their 'head' knowledge.

References

Bligh J, Prideaux D, Parsell G: PRISMS: new educational strategies for medical education, *Medical Education* 35:520–521, 2001.

Couper ID, Worley PS: Meeting the challenges of training more medical students: lessons from Flinders University's distributed medical education program, *Medical Journal of Australia* 193(1):34–36, 2010.

Frenk J, Chen L, Bhutta ZA, et al: Health professionals for a new century: transforming education to strengthen health systems in an interdependent world, *Lancet* 376(9756):1923–1958, 2010.

Krupat E, Pelletier S, Alexander E, et al: Can changes in the principal clinical year prevent the erosion of students' patient-centered beliefs? *Academic Medicine* 84(5):582–586, 2009.

Murray E, Jolly B, Modell M: Can students learn clinical method in general practice? A randomized crossover trial based on objective structured clinical examinations, *BMJ* 315:920–923, 1997.

Nyangairi B, Couper ID, Sondzaba NO: Exposure to primary healthcare for medical students: experiences of final-year medical students, *SA Family Practice* 52(5):467–470, 2010.

Oswald N, Alderson T, Jones S: Evaluating primary care as a base for medical education: the report of the Cambridge Community-based Clinical Course, *Medical Education* 35:782–788, 2001.

Walters L, Worley P, Prideaux D, Lange K: Do consultations in general practice take more time when practitioners are precepting medical students? *Medical Education* 42(1):69–73, 2008.

Worley P, Silagy C, Prideaux D, et al: The Parallel Rural Community Curriculum: an integrated clinical curriculum based in rural general practice, *Medical Education* 34:558–565, 2000.

Worley P: Relationships: A new way to analyse community-based medical education? *(Part one)* *Education for Health* 15:117–128, 2002.

Worley P, Esterman A, Prideaux D: Cohort study of examination performance of undergraduate medical students learning in community settings, *BMJ* 328:207–209, 2004.

Worley P, Martin A, Prideaux D, et al: Vocational career paths of graduate entry medical students at Flinders University: A comparison of rural, remote and tertiary tracks, *Medical Journal of Australia* 188(3):177–178, 2008.

Further reading

Boaden N, Bligh J: *Community-Based Medical Education*, London, 1999, Arnold.

Couper I, Worley PS, Strasser R: Rural longitudinal integrated clerkships: lessons from two programs on different continents, *Rural and Remote Health* 11:1665, 2011.

Hays R: *Practice-Based Teaching. A Guide for General Practitioners*, Emerald, Victoria, Australia, 1999, Eruditions Publishing.

Maley M, Worley P, Dent J: Using rural and remote settings in the undergraduate medical curriculum: AMEE Guide No. 47, *Medical Teacher* 31(11):969–983, 2009.

Palsdottir B, Neusy AJ: Transforming medical education: lessons learned from THEnet. Available at http://www.thenetcommunity.org/about-thenet.html. Accessed 1 December 2011.

Schmidt H, Magzoub M, Feletti G, et al: *Handbook of Community-Based Education: Theory and Practice*, 2000, Network Publications.

The Network: Towards Unity for Health, http://www.the networktufh.org

Worley PS, Prideaux DJ, Strasser RP, et al: Why we should teach undergraduate medical students in rural communities, *Medical Journal of Australia* 172:615–617, 2000.

Chapter

14

Rural and remote locations

J. Rourke, L. Rourke

 Learning in rural/remote locations can be an outstanding and sometimes life changing experience.

 Consistently positive rural/remote teaching and learning experiences combine good planning and excellent learning settings with interested learners and enthusiastic teachers.

Introduction

The rural/remote location is an ideal setting for practical community-based learning where medical learners can develop knowledge, skills and attitudes that are useful in any medical practice setting.

Rural medical education learning experiences play an important role in the training and recruitment of rural physicians (Curran & Rourke 2004, Rourke et al 2005, Maley et al 2010). Rural learning experiences have been found to have high educational value from junior medical students to senior trainees/residents (Zorzi et al 2005, Rourke 2005). There is substantial literature that shows that rural medical learners, at a variety of learning stages, do as well as or better than urban learners on medical examinations and other measures of performance (Schauer & Schieve 2006, Power et al 2006, Waters et al 2006, Worley et al 2004, Goertzen 2006, Bianchi et al 2008, Denz-Penhey & Murdoch 2010). A detailed critical review of North American studies identified 'evidence that placement in rural settings is a positive learning experience that students value and that preceptors find gratifying' (Barrett et al 2011).

Discovering the joys and challenges of rural/remote practice can lead some medical learners to choose rural/remote practice as a career (in this chapter, 'medical learners' refers to students, trainees and residents). As medical schools expand and address their social responsibility to train medical doctors for locations and in fields where they are most needed, increasing numbers of medical learners are experiencing training in a distributed medical education model (Rourke 2010, Eley et al 2008, Maley et al 2010). This provides the opportunity for rural general practitioners/family physicians, consultants, and other rural healthcare professionals to become more involved as medical teachers (sometimes called preceptors in the medical literature).

Many rural medical doctors are enthusiastic natural teachers with broad clinical skills managing a wide variety of patient care challenges within strong community–patient–physician relationships. This can facilitate excellent learning experiences for medical learners. As in any setting, however, rural teaching and learning experiences can be quite variable. A needs analysis study found that 'the majority of rural preceptors had no clear understanding of how what they taught fitted into the overall curriculum, their role as a clinical teacher had not been clearly defined … and that undergraduate students had little understanding of what they needed to learn during their attachment' (Baker et al 2003). In addition, evaluation of feedback from students found that 'while rural GP preceptors performed well overall in regards to providing quality teaching learning experiences, there was significant spread of scores across all criteria' (Baker et al 2003).

As much of the learning is centred around patient care, the rural medical teacher has a dual role, providing both patient care and teaching effectively and efficiently (Ferenchick et al 1997, Irby & Bowen 2004).

 A practical framework approach to teaching and learning in a rural and remote setting:

- before the learner arrives
- the first day
- during the rotation
- assessment and wrap-up.

Adapted from Rourke and Rourke (1996)

Before the learner arrives

Good planning and preparation prior to the arrival of the medical learner are essential to set the stage for a successful rural learning/teaching experience. Preceptor preparation, programme support, a well-prepared medical doctor's office and staff, engaged colleagues, helpful hospital and healthcare organizations and community partnerships are vital ingredients. Communication and clarity are essential ingredients at every step of the way.

PRECEPTOR PREPARATION

Teaching medical learners is like medical practice: no matter how much experience one has, there is always more to learn.

Interactive collegial workshops focused on teaching in a rural setting can be particularly helpful and enjoyable learning opportunities for rural medical doctors.

 Six attributes of community preceptors/rural medical teachers who were scored highly by medical students:

1. Welcoming learners as legitimate participants in a community of practice
2. Creating a central role for learners in patient care and teaching
3. Regularly engaging learners in self-reflection to monitor their progress
4. Helping learners discover learning opportunities in routine patient encounters
5. Using feedback to shape rather than evaluate learner performance
6. Creating an environment where learners felt comfortable practising new skills with patients.

Adapted from Manyon et al 2003

Ideally, rural medical doctors are part of a rural medical education network that includes faculty development to develop their skills as medical teachers.

Rural doctor associations are taking the lead around the world in providing workshops and developing resource materials. As well, some medical organizations and university faculties of medicine are increasingly providing faculty development and continuing medical education via distance learning, on-the-road learning, and other innovative formats ideal for rural medical teachers.

PROGRAMME SUPPORT

Successful teaching and learning in the rural setting require extensive support and communication with the programme responsible for the learners.

Programme support should include site development visits to the rural practice so that expectations, issues and concerns can be dealt with face-to-face and in a collegial constructive manner. Well-functioning programmes also provide extensive faculty

development that brings together the rural medical teachers in their regions for multidirectional information sharing, planning and faculty development sessions. Information technology providing access to the medical school's teaching and clinical resources should be made available to the rural site. Rural medical learners and teachers should be able to participate in relevant distance learning-supported educational and clinical rounds.

 There needs to be a clear understanding of the learner's, the rural medical teacher's and the programme's roles and responsibilities.

Many rural medical teachers take a variety of learners at a variety of knowledge and skill levels from a variety of programmes with many different expectations. For each learner placed with a rural medical teacher, the programme should provide clear information that outlines the programme's learning objectives and expected/required evaluation.

In addition, the programme should provide the rural medical teacher with a letter or other indication that the learner is in good standing. Any major outstanding concerns or issues should be communicated to the rural medical teacher prior to the learner's arrival, especially if they could add an undue element of risk to patient safety and the rural teacher's medical practice.

Programme financial support for learner travel, accommodation, information technology and other expenses should be clearly established before the rotation.

Rural medical teachers are an invaluable teaching resource and need to be recognized in a positive fashion. In the past, financial support for rural medical teachers has often been severely lacking. Programmes need to realize that teaching in the often busy rural clinical setting requires a significant time commitment, often at the expense of monetary remuneration and personal time.

A WELL-PREPARED MEDICAL DOCTOR'S OFFICE AND STAFF

Positive and supportive office staff members are key to a happy and successful practice. Similarly, their engagement is just as vital to the rural learning and teaching experience.

It is very helpful to involve the staff in planning how best to use the office space, organize scheduling and handle the communications with patients. Ideally, there will be enough examining rooms to accommodate the learner(s) and also a separate review and study space equipped with high-speed internet access.

The medical doctor's office staff members need to know the dates and plans before the learner arrives to anticipate and effectively schedule the patient care and other activities of both the learner and teacher. It is very important that all involved understand the skill level, roles and responsibilities of the learner and how to best integrate their involvement into the patient care and other activities of the office. The staff can contribute significantly to a positive teaching and learning experience by helping select and introduce the most appropriate patients for the learner and by responding positively to questions from both patients and the learner. Staff can be an invaluable source of feedback from themselves and from patients regarding their experience with the learner.

 Preparing a learner's manual can help consolidate the practice preparation and planning and is an invaluable guide to prepare and orient learners.

Ideally, the learner's manual will be made available on the web with links to a variety of relevant resources for learners to review prior to arrival. Useful features include information about the community and area including climate, travel information and social and recreational opportunities; accommodation arrangements; a description of the practice including schedules, location and key personnel; related community and hospital learning activities with other medical doctor colleagues and allied health personnel; and copies of office, hospital and other protocols for learners.

MAIN PRECEPTOR/RURAL MEDICAL TEACHER AND ENGAGED COLLEAGUES

It is important that there is a main preceptor/rural medical teacher with responsibility for organization, orientation, supervision and evaluation of the learner.

In the past, learners on rural rotations were often placed with solo rural medical doctors. Increasingly in the 21st century, rural medical doctors work with a small number of close colleagues, either in a group practice or in a shared patient care/call coverage arrangement within a community or hospital setting. In this setting, there may be one or several rural medical doctors who will periodically take on the main preceptor/medical teacher role.

Involvement of other colleagues provides a broader rural experience of different teachers' knowledge, skills and attitudes. This provides the opportunity for experienced rural teachers to help their colleagues in also becoming medical teachers. Care needs to be taken in the choice and role of colleagues to maximize the positive learning experience. Many rural medical doctors find that the questioning approach of learners provides reflection and stimulation for their own continuing medical education.

HELPFUL HOSPITAL AND HEALTHCARE ORGANIZATIONS

Hospital-based care is a much more active component for many rural general practitioners/family physicians than for their urban colleagues. Similarly, rural specialists may provide a much broader generalist approach to care than their urban colleagues. This can significantly broaden and enhance the learning opportunities on rural rotations.

The rural community hospital, with its smaller number of healthcare professionals who are accessible and working in close proximity, can be an ideal location to see collegial interdisciplinary team care functioning in practice. Team members can also provide valuable learning opportunities and feedback for the rural medical learner.

Before the rotation begins, the rural medical teacher should establish appropriate protocols with the approval of the hospital medical advisory committee to outline the level of activities and supervision for learners at different stages of education. A supportive hospital administration and staff and regional healthcare organization can be very helpful with enabling this process.

COMMUNITY PARTNERSHIPS

Rural communities increasingly see the value of rural medical learners as potential future recruits to help stabilize their long-term medical doctor workforce. Many rural communities are exceptional places to live and work, often in areas where urban people go for their holidays. Communities can facilitate the rural medical learner's welcome and involvement in social and recreational activities and thus spark the learner's interest in future practice in their own or another rural community. Positive community engagement reduces the potential for rural medical learners' sense of isolation and shifts some of the organizational burden away from the rural medical teacher.

 Ongoing communication with all these involved participants – colleagues, hospital, healthcare organizations and community – prior to each learner's arrival will pave the way for a positive learning experience.

The first day

 The main preceptor/rural medical teacher should set aside a block of time on the first day to welcome and orient the learner.

The first day is the most important time to establish a positive impression and set out clear roles and expectations. Some form of contracting to establish mutual expectations, roles and responsibilities should be done on the first day or shortly thereafter (Kelly 1997). Ideally, the learner will have individual goals in addition to those of the programme. Equally important is discussing potential problems, concerns or anticipated absences of the learner. The medical doctor's office staff, hospital staff and community members should play a key role in the orientation as well. A letter/notice displayed in the reception area and examining rooms signed by the preceptor introducing the learner can help connect the learner and patients. Patient care responsibilities should start slowly and be gradually ramped up to help avoid the whirlwind of information and responsibilities that can overwhelm learners at the start of rural rotations.

During the rotation

 Effective teaching behaviours of rural preceptors/rural medical teachers:

1. Actively involve the student, providing adequate supervision and appropriate independence

2. Develop and foster a supportive interpersonal relationship with the student to facilitate learning

3. Emphasise problem solving and the understanding of general principles

4. Balance clinical and teaching responsibilities

5. Demonstrate clinical and professional competence

6. Use an organised approach, including goal setting and summation

7. Provide the student with ongoing feedback, assessments and evaluations.

Goertzen et al 1995

A learner's role and contribution to patient care will be dependent on his or her level of education and knowledge, skills and attitudes. As the learner demonstrates competence and commitment to care, her or his level of responsibility can be increased within the range expected for the educational level in keeping with the concept of graded responsibility. The learner should be involved in the follow-up care of patients he or she has assessed, as continuity of care is a vital component of rural patient care, learning and teaching. This may include a variety of settings such as the medical doctor's office, the hospital, the nursing home and the patient's home. It can also involve following patients through specialist/consultant and allied healthcare investigations and treatments. Longitudinal integrated clerkships based on this principle are becoming a core component of

many medical schools (Walters et al 2003, Zink et al 2008, Couper et al 2011).

The rural patient care setting is ideal for case-based discussion and learning using a patient-centred approach (Stewart et al 1995). Patients, staff and medical doctors all appreciate good scheduling. Adding a learner to the patient care process will require a well planned and flexible schedule to accommodate patient care needs and to optimize the learning/teaching experience. Time is required for review and discussion both throughout and at the end of the day. Time-efficient strategies for clinical teaching are described elsewhere in this book.

In addition, it is advisable to set aside dedicated time for discussion of broader issues such as the doctor–patient relationship and social relationships in small communities. Learners can observe how professionalism and compartmentalization allow rural teachers to combine, yet keep separate, patient care responsibilities and social relationships in rural communities. The awareness of how to set appropriate and flexible personal/professional boundaries is of value in any socially interconnected setting, both rural and urban (Rourke & Rourke 1998, Rourke et al 1993).

Many rural medical teachers are also involved in local leadership roles. Rural communities, as smaller microcosms, often provide opportunities for rural medical doctors to 'make a difference', not only in individual patient's lives, but in the local health system and the community as a whole. Ideally, the learner will not only witness this community leadership, but will participate as well.

 The CanMEDS roles describe seven aspects of the ideal physician: medical expert, communicator, collaborator, manager, health advocate, scholar and professional.
Frank 2004, 2005

Learners in a rural setting can see these multiple roles lived on a daily basis (Box. 14.1).

 Rural medical teachers should never underestimate the role model and mentorship they provide to their learners.

Satisfaction of the rural medical teacher with his or her professional and personal life is almost always apparent to the learner. Similarly, the level of collegiality between rural medical teachers and their family physician, consultant and allied healthcare colleagues is evident.

 Enthusiasm or disillusion with rural practice or living can significantly affect a learner's view of rural practice and influence future career plans.

This can be challenging when rural teaching locations have a shortage of physicians and the medical teachers have heavier than optimal clinical loads.

Learners can also make an excellent contribution to learning/teaching by leading discussions and preparing presentations on topics of interest or importance to the learner, medical doctors, staff, patients and/or community.

OBSERVATION/DEMONSTRATION/FEEDBACK

There is no substitute for the direct observation of the learner, the direct demonstration of clinical skills by the teacher and the provision of effective feedback.

Direct observation at the start of the rotation can help provide the medical teacher with a clear understanding of the medical learner's knowledge, skills and attitudes that is vital to determining the graded responsibility that can be given. Direct observation helps both learner and teacher identify areas of strength and areas for improvement and can avoid the all too easy over- or underestimation of a learner's abilities and needs. The one-on-one learning/teaching in rural practice provides the ideal setting for rapid assessment and advancement of learning. Daily

---

Box 14.1 CanMEDS roles can be adapted into rural learning objectives

Medical/expert/clinical decision-maker: 'Know and do the right thing.'
Identify the knowledge and skills required for a rural/community-based practice and note how they differ from urban practice.
Identify limitations and demonstrate use of referral resources appropriately.
Demonstrate diagnostic and therapeutic skills for ethical and effective evidence-based patient care within the context and limitations of the rural/community environment.
Identify peer review, audit, and other methods of assessing one's practice and rural/community patient care.

Communicator: 'Communication is the key to success.'
Identify particular healthcare challenges and difficulties from a rural/community patient's cultural and geographic context.
Demonstrate good interviewing and communication skills with patients.
Demonstrate effective communication with all members of the rural/community healthcare team as member, coordinator and leader.

Collaborator: 'Work with others.'
Identify and use local community resources, programmes and distant referral resource and clinical-support networks.
Demonstrate collaboration with local family physicians, consultants, allied health professionals and tertiary care subspecialists.
Identify when and how to effectively transfer patients from smaller referring centres to tertiary care centres.

Manager: 'Be efficient and effective.'
Identify effective practice management appropriate for rural/community practice.
Identify strategies to develop referring and/or referral base.
Identify and discuss benefits and risks of investigations and treatments available locally, regionally and at tertiary care centres.

Health advocate: 'You can make a difference in your community!'
Demonstrate preventative healthcare and health promotion.
Advocate for accessible and appropriate rural healthcare.
Identify existing and potential resources to meet the unique needs of the patients and community.

Scholar: 'Yes, you can be a scholar in the country.'
Identify and develop strategies for self-directed, life-long learning strategies including use of distance education to maintain up-to-date and competent skills relevant to a rural/community setting.

Professional/personal: 'Remember yourself, your partner, and your children.'
Identify and experience the joys and challenges of rural/community medical practice and life.
Identify and develop strategies to balance personal, family and professional needs and demands.
Demonstrate positive attitude and working relationships with patients, staff, administration and colleagues.

Modified from CanMEDS and adapted from Rourke & Frank 2005

informal discussions, encouragement and advice should be part of the fabric of the rural rotation.

As with advanced skill development processes for musicians, athletes and others, demonstration of procedures and techniques by the teacher followed by the opportunity for deliberate practice can accelerate skills development and mastery in medical learners (Ericsson 2004).

Both learner and teacher can monitor progress by repeated direct observation. Some programmes provide video equipment to aid the direct observation process. This can be a very valuable teaching tool but does require additional consideration with regard to patient privacy, acceptance and consent.

 Providing effective feedback is a core skill for medical teachers and often requires significant faculty development.

The most helpful and appreciated feedback is frequent, timely, specific and constructive. Modified Pendleton's rules provide a useful framework that can be easily used in the rural setting (Pendleton et al 1984) (Table 14.1).

Providing feedback to and assessment of the rural learner may pose unique opportunities and challenges. The rural setting, with its close teacher–learner relationship and low number of learners, often provides the opportunity for in-depth understanding and identification not only of strengths, but also of weaknesses not yet identified in the larger training milieu. Good feedback that addresses these concerns is important for the learner's future progress. Giving negative feedback, however, can be particularly difficult in this setting for several reasons: fewer local teaching colleagues for support, distant programme support and the rural teacher–learner social connections. As with professional–personal patient boundaries, this situation requires teacher skill and compartmentalization. In these instances, programme support to the rural teacher is vital.

Assessment and wrap-up

In addition to the frequent informal feedback provided throughout the rotation, specific times for more formal assessment should be set aside during and at the end of the rural rotation. Ideally, the assessment is linked to the objectives for the rotation. The CanMEDS roles for physicians provide a broad framework that can be functionally adapted to emphasize the broad and important knowledge, skills and attitudes required for exemplary rural practice (Rourke & Frank 2005). See Box 14.1.

Rural medical education assessments should have multiple inputs and be multidirectional. Patients, staff

Table 14.1 Modified Pendleton's rules for direct observation and/or videotape review

1. **Clarify**
   Ask for clarification of information and feelings as necessary.
2. **Good points first**
   Ask the learner what he or she did well.
   Tell the learner what you observed that was done well.
3. **Areas to improve**
   Ask the learner to identify what he or she had difficulty with and what could be improved.
   Provide specific suggestions for improvement.
4. **Constructive summary**
   Mutually develop a constructive summary.

Adapted from Pendleton et al 1984.

and other physicians involved with the learner can provide valuable multisource feedback for both the formative and summative assessments (Davis et al 2006).

Rural medical teachers should understand the difference between formative and summative assessment. Formative assessment is ongoing and designed to teach and form future learning. Summative assessment is an evaluation of the learner and occurs at the end of the rotation.

 A mid-rotation formative assessment provides the opportunity for the learner and main preceptor to discuss progress, problems and planning for the remainder of the rotation.

A mid-rotation formative assessment helps set the stage so the end of rotation summative assessment does not come as a surprise. If a learner is showing major signs of difficulty by the mid-term assessment, the programme should be notified and involved in planning how best to address this in the remainder of the rotation or in remedial alternatives.

The summative end of rotation assessment should be done with the learner before he or she leaves the rotation. Any major concerns should be clearly outlined and discussed. The requisite paper or electronic forms should be sent immediately to the programme so that they can help shape the learner's future training.

In addition to assessment of the learner by the medical teacher, the medical teacher should be evaluated by the learner. Learners are often reluctant to give direct negative feedback to and provide assessments of a preceptor or a specific rotation, with concerns that it may affect future training or employment options. For this reason learner assessments of a training location and preceptors are often anonymized, and information is provided back to the medical teacher only when there are three or more learner assessments received. In addition to evaluating the medical teacher, the assessment should also include other aspects of the rural experience including accommodation, social/community aspects and information technology and programme support.

Troubled and troubling learners

Learners are not immune from illnesses and emotional stresses. The latter can be aggravated by a rural rotation that places the learner in a new location with new expectations and roles far away from the support of close friends and family. Learners belonging to minority groups may have difficulty finding people with similar interests, experiences or cultural norms in the rural community (Steinert & Walsh 2006). Despite the best of intentions, the close one-on-one nature of the rural rotation can potentially lead to conflict between the learner and medical teacher, staff or others. When isolation is a significant problem, consideration should be given to placing two learners at the same site. Pairing of learners at a rural site also provides leadership and teaching opportunities for the learners, particularly if they are at different stages in their learning.

The teacher and programme should be prepared to help learners with illnesses and stresses by arranging timely and appropriate medical care and counselling as required. While it is important that the rural medical teacher be empathic and supportive, the rural medical teacher should if possible avoid assuming the role of medical doctor or counsellor for the learner, as this blurring of boundaries may compromise the medical care or counselling needed by the learner, as well as the teaching/learning rotation and the evaluation. When a learner is ill, arrangements often need to be made for time off. Occasionally the illness has the potential to interfere with competence to provide patient care; particularly with psychiatric illness, the potential for suicide must not be ignored.

 In all cases of ill, troubled or troubling learners, involvement of physician colleagues and programme support personnel is vital.

Summary

Rural and remote locations are becoming an increasingly important setting for medical education. Good planning and effective communication before the learner arrives, on the first day, during the rotation and at assessment and wrap-up can help ensure the success of rural learning experiences.

Before the learner arrives, good preparation involving the rural medical teacher, office and staff,

colleagues, hospital and community and programme organization and support sets the stage for success.

Welcome and orientation on the first day followed closely by contracting regarding programme and individual learner goals, concerns, expectations, roles and responsibilities, and early direct observation of the learner establishes a strong foundation for progress through the rotation.

During the rotation, learning is facilitated by appropriate scheduling with case-based time-efficient strategies for clinical teaching including demonstration, observation and feedback. The rural and remote medical setting can also show a wide scope of medical care in various settings, interprofessional team care, role modelling and mentorship, and community involvement with personal/professional boundaries. The CanMEDS roles for medical doctors provide a broad framework to apply in the teaching setting. Faculty development can be a key to acquiring effective skills in providing feedback.

Assessment should be informal and formal, formative and summative, linked to the rotation objectives, and multisource and multidirectional. In cases of ill, troubled or troubling learners, additional support should always be sought.

It takes courage to welcome learners into one's rural practice and become a rural medical teacher, but the benefits are many. We have found that learners have stimulated us to demonstrate excellent medical care and to stay up to date. Learners have enriched our lives and those of our staff, our colleagues, our children and our community. It is a great joy to watch learners advancing in knowledge, skills and attitudes, while appreciating the joys and challenges of rural practice and rural life en route to becoming exemplary medical doctors, both rural and urban.

Acknowledgements

We would like to acknowledge the tremendous contribution of our teachers, learners, colleagues, staff and patients to our teaching and learning over the years.

References

Baker PG, Dalton L, Walker J: Rural general practitioner preceptors – how can effective undergraduate teaching be supported or improved? *Rural Remote Health* 3(1):107, 2003.

Barrett FA, Lipsky S, Lutfiyya MN: The impact of rural training experiences on medical students: a critical review, *Academic Medicine* 86:259–263, 2011.

Bianchi F, Stobbe K, Eva K: Comparing academic performance of medical students in distributed learning sites: the McMaster experience, *Medical Teacher* 30(1):67–71, 2008.

Couper I, Worley PS, Strasser R: Rural longitudinal integrated clerkships: lessons from two programs on different continents, *Rural and Remote Health* 11:1–11, 2011.

Curran V, Rourke J: The role of medical education in the recruitment and retention of rural physicians, *Medical Teacher* 26:265–272, 2004.

Davis DA, Mazmanian PE, Fordis M, et al: Accuracy of physician self-assessment compared with observed measures of competence: A systematic review, *American Medical Association* 296(9):1094–1102, 2006.

Denz-Penhey H, Murdoch JC: Is small beautiful? Student performance and perceptions of their experience at larger and smaller sites in rural and remote longitudinal integrated clerkships in the Rural Clinical School of Western Australia, *Rural and Remote Health* 10:1–7, 2010.

Eley DS, Young L, Wilkinson D, et al: Coping with increasing numbers of medical students in rural clinical schools: options and opportunities, *Medical Journal of Australia* 188:669–671, 2008.

Ericsson KA: Deliberate practice and the acquisition and maintenance of expert performance in medicine and related domains, *Academic Medicine* 79(10)Suppl:S70–S81, 2004.

Ferenchick G, Simpson D, Blackman J, et al: Strategies for efficient and effective teaching in the ambulatory care setting, *Academic Medicine* 72(4):277–280, 1997.

Frank JR: The CanMEDS Project: the Royal College of Physicians and Surgeons of Canada moves medical education into the 21st century, *Royal College Outlook* 1:27–29, 2004.

Frank JR, editor: *The CanMEDS 2005 Physician Competency Framework. Better Standards. Better Physicians. Better Care*, Ottawa, 2005, The Royal College of Physicians and Surgeons of Canada.

Goertzen J: Learning procedural skills in family medicine residency: comparison of rural and urban programmes, *Canadian Family Physician* 52:622–623, 2006.

Goertzen J, Stewart M, Weston W: Effective teaching behaviours of rural family medicine preceptors, *Canadian Medical Association Journal* 153(2): 161–168, 1995.

Irby DM, Bowen JL: Time-efficient strategies for learning and performance, *The Clinical Teacher* 1(1):23–28, 2004.

Kelly L: Integrating family medicine residents into a rural practice, *Canadian Family Physician* 43: 277–286, 1997.

Maley M, Worley P, Dent J: Using rural and remote settings in the undergraduate medical curriculum. AMEE Guide 47, *Medical Teacher* 31:969–983, 2010.

Manyon A, Shipengrover J, McGuigan D, et al: Defining differences in the instructional styles of community preceptors, *Family Medicine* 35(3): 181–186, 2003.

Pendleton D, Schofield T, Tate P, Havelock P: *An approach to learning and teaching. The consultation: an approach to learning and teaching*, Oxford, 1984, Oxford University Press, pp 68–72.

Power DV, Harris IB, Swentko W, et al: Comparing rural-trained medical students with their peers: performance in a primary care OSCE, *Teaching and Learning in Medicine* 18(3):196–202, 2006.

Rourke J: How can medical schools contribute to the education, recruitment and retention of rural physicians in their region? *Bulletin World Health Organization* 88(5):395–396, 2010.

Rourke J, Frank JR: Implementing the CanMEDS physician roles in rural specialist education: the multi-specialty community training network, *Education for Health* 18(3):368–378, 2005. Joint issue with Rural and Remote Health 5:406.

Rourke J, Rourke LL: Practical tips for rural family physicians teaching residents, *Canadian Journal of Rural Medicine* 1(2):63–69, 1996.

Rourke JTB: A rural and regional community multi-specialty residency training network developed by the university of western ontario, *Teaching and Learning in Medicine* 17(4):376, 2005.

Rourke JTB, Incitti F, Rourke LL, Kennard M: Relationship between practice location of Ontario family physicians and their rural background or amount of rural medical education experience, *Canadian Journal of Rural Medicine* 10(4): 231–239, 2005.

Rourke JTB, Smith LFP, Brown JB: Patients, friends, and relationship boundaries, *Canadian Family Physician* 39:2557–2564, 1993.

Rourke L, Rourke J: Close friends as patients in rural practice, *Canadian Family Physician* 44:1208–1210, 1998.

Schauer RW, Schieve D: Performance of medical students in a nontraditional rural clinical programme, 1998–99 through 2003–04, *Academic Medicine* 81(7):603–607, 2006.

Steinert Y, Walsh A, editors: *A faculty development program for teachers of international medical graduates*, Ontario, 2006, The Association of Faculties of Medicine of Canada Ottawa, Available at: http://www.afmc.ca.

Stewart M, Brown JB, Weston WW, et al: *Patient-Centered Medicine, Transforming the Clinical Method*. London, New Delhi, 1995, SAGE Publications.

Walters LK, Worley PS, Mugford BV: Parallel rural community curriculum: is it a transferable model? *Rural and Remote Health* 3:236, 2003.

Waters B, Hughes J, Forbes K, Wilkinson D: Comparative academic performance of medical students in rural and urban clinical settings, *Medical Education* 40(2):117–120, 2006.

Worley P, Esterman A, Prideaux D: Cohort study of examination performance of undergraduate medical students learning in community settings, *BMJ* 24:328(7433):207–209, 2004.

Zink T, Halaas GW, Finstad D, Brooks KD: The rural physician associate program: the value of immersion learning for third-year medical students, *Journal of Rural Health* 24:353–359, 2008.

Zorzi A, Rourke J, Kennard M, et al: Combined research and clinical learning make rural summer studentship programme a successful model, *Rural and Remote Health* 18(3):329–337, 2005.

Distance education

15

J. Grant, A. Zachariah

Before you begin …

This chapter looks different from the other chapters in this book. It is presented as a distance learning workbook. So you have the opportunity to experience distance learning, see how a distance learning course is constructed, experience different types of exercises and get feedback on your learning.

INTRODUCTION TO THE COURSE

Welcome to this short course on distance learning in medicine! It consists of a *workbook* which should take you about 1 hour to study.

Distance learning is one of the most needed modes of medical education given the rapid changes in medical practice, the large number of doctors requiring constant updating and the need to educate in remote and rural areas.

Learning activities

You will find a number of brief exercises called *learning activities*. These are one of the most important parts of the course. They give you the opportunity to think about, use, apply and understand more fully the content being presented. And each gives you feedback on your responses.

OBJECTIVES

After completion of this course, you should be able to:

- Define 'distance learning' and consider its advantages and disadvantages
- Outline how distance education courses may be designed for clinical medicine

- Identify the media and learning experiences that can be blended into a distance learning course for medicine
- Describe the structure of a distance learning text and the design of learning activities
- Describe how students learning at a distance can receive feedback
- Describe how distance learning courses are developed
- Describe the meaning of a wrap-around course and how this may be used in medical education
- Discuss quality assurance in distance learning.

CONTENTS

The following table will help you plan your study time.

Table 15.1

Table of Contents	Time for study	Page
1. **WHAT IS DISTANCE LEARNING?**	3 minutes	p. 123
Activity 1. What methods can be used to help a medical student or doctor learn at a distance?	3 minutes	p. 123
Activity 2. Advantages and disadvantages of distance learning in medical education	2 minutes	p. 124
2. **TECHNOLOGY AND DISTANCE LEARNING**	3 minutes	p. 125
Activity 3. Technology and print in distance learning	3 minutes	p. 125
3. **THE STRUCTURE OF A DISTANCE LEARNING TEXT**	3 minutes	p. 126
Activity 4. Features of distance learning texts	5 minutes	p. 126
Activity 5. Design of learning activities	5 minutes	p. 127
4. **FEEDBACK ON LEARNING**	2 minutes	p. 128
5. **BLENDING DIFFERENT ELEMENTS OF THE COURSE**	4 minutes	p. 128
6. **MANAGING CLINICAL ATTACHMENTS BY DISTANCE LEARNING**	3 minutes	p. 129
Activity 6. What are the principles of designing clinical experience on a distance learning course?	3 minutes	p. 129
7. **THE STUDENT'S LEARNING EXPERIENCE**	3 minutes	p. 130
8. **MANAGING DISTANCE LEARNING**	3 minutes	p. 130
9. **DEVELOPMENT OF DISTANCE LEARNING COURSES**	5 minutes	p. 131
10. **QUALITY ASSURANCE IN DISTANCE LEARNING**	3 minutes	p. 132
Activity 7. Quality assurance in distance learning	5 minutes	p. 132
11. **CONCLUSION**	2 minutes	p. 133
ESTIMATED TOTAL STUDY TIME FOR THIS WORKBOOK: 1 hour		

1. WHAT IS DISTANCE LEARNING?

Let's think about the various methods that are available to help people who are learning medicine at a distance (Tables 15.2 and 15.3).

Table 15.2		
Activity 1	**What methods can be used to help a medical student or doctor learn at a distance?**	**Allow 3 minutes**
Please jot down here your ideas about what methods can be used to help students and doctors learning at a distance. Do this before reading the feedback that follows!		

Table 15.3 Feedback. A number of people have tried the activity. They listed the following methods. Compare what you said with their list.

Printed workbooks	DVDs	Email
Learning packages	Video conferencing	Face-to-face tutorials
Guided texts	CDs	Web-based resources
Online library resources	Telephone tutorials and feedback	Computer conferencing
Telemedicine	Television	Radio programmes
Community/clinical work	Online teaching	E-learning courses
Readers and textbooks	Residential meetings/Skills labs	Student discussion groups (live, online)
Virtual and simulated environments, e.g. virtual microscope	Tutor-marked assignments and feedback	Assessments: computer-based, paper-based, practical

This activity shows that distance learning can comprise many components, blended together to make one well-planned course. The content of a distance learning course is limited only by the imagination of the teacher.

Given this, how shall we define distance learning? Grant (2008) defines 'distance learning' as:

> *Individual study of specially prepared learning materials, usually print and sometimes e-learning, supplemented by integrated learning resources, other learning experiences, including face-to-face teaching and practical experience, feedback on learning and student support.*

Distance learning provides a rich, planned experience for learners, quality assured, flexible and cost effective.

Given this, you should consider the advantages and disadvantages of distance learning for medical education by trying Activity 2 (Tables 15.4 and 15.5).

Table 15.4

Activity 2	Advantages and disadvantages of distance learning in medical education	Allow 2 minutes
What do you think are the advantages and disadvantages of using distance education in medical teaching? Jot down your thoughts in the following space.		

Advantages	Disadvantages

Table 15.5 Feedback

Advantages	Disadvantages
Makes quality-assured teaching available to all	Clinical skills development requires integrated face-to-face teaching
Is particularly useful for physicians who are working full time or have limited time available. Is an excellent method for knowledge development	Distance education courses require supervision of clinical experience and careful planning to ensure an appropriate blend of learning opportunities within limited time
Can reach out to doctors in remote locations and those who have not had the opportunity for postgraduate study	Distance learning takes initial skilled effort to design and produce
Can be cost-effective and uses teachers' time efficiently	

2. TECHNOLOGY AND DISTANCE LEARNING

Although many people equate e-learning and distance learning, you can see from Activity 1 that technology offers just one way of learning. It should be used when the curriculum demands it, and when it is feasible and cost-effective. Technology is simply another medium alongside all the others. The next activity asks you to think about this (Table 15.6).

Table 15.6			
Activity 3	**Technology and print in distance learning**		**Allow 3 minutes**
Complete the following chart to help you analyse the relative strengths and weaknesses of technology and print for distance learning.			
Technology		**Print**	
Strengths	**Weaknesses**	**Strengths**	**Weaknesses**

FEEDBACK

Technology

You might have said that technology offers rich, interactive visual images, immediate feedback, better illustrations, student–teacher communication and a more modern feel.

But you might have noted that technology is expensive to produce, requires access to hardware, broadband and regular electricity, is not portable, requires typing skills, does not allow scribbling, highlighting and note-taking, is more difficult to flick backwards and forwards, is harder on the eyes and tends to imply entertainment rather than teaching.

Print

Print is limited in visual presentation, seems more old-fashioned, is less flexible in giving feedback and offers no interpersonal communication.

But print is cost-effective, is easily updated, is flexible to use, requires no equipment or back-up, allows note-taking and highlighting, requires no technical skills, is portable and flexible and is the most familiar medium for learning. Teachers can reach out to students who do not have regular internet. Busy practising physicians can keep the text in hand and do small activities whenever they have time.

3. THE STRUCTURE OF A DISTANCE LEARNING TEXT

You will remember that the definition of distance learning given in Section 1 emphasizes that materials must be 'specially prepared'. The next two activities ask you to think about what this means (Tables 15.7 and 15.8).

Table 15.7		
Activity 4	**Features of distance learning texts**	**Allow 5 minutes**
Look through this chapter. Note down any features that make it different from a usual book chapter. Say what you think the function of each feature is in terms of helping the distance learner.		
Feature		**Function**

Table 15.8 Feedback. You might have noticed the following:	
Clear aims, instructions, timings	Ensures learners are clear about the task and can plan their time
Conversational style	Simulates a tutorial atmosphere
Short sections	So that the learner has a sense of progress and will not skip sections
Clear page layout	So that the learner does not get lost in a variety of boxes and options
In-text activities with timings	Ensures that the learner is active, thinking and applying learning within an appropriate amount of time
Feedback	So that the learner knows if he or she is on track and to offer new information

Whether the medium is print or technology, these design features are essential to supporting and retaining the interest of the learner. Distance learning texts must be written to encourage the learner to keep studying, give a sense of progress, stimulate active learning, give feedback and offer 'a tutorial in print'. Distance learning texts for medicine may be written to simulate a ward round, providing clinical information, asking and answering questions and emphasizing learning points.

Now let's turn to the design of learning activities which stimulate active learning and a sense of achievement and give feedback to the student (Table 15.9).

Table 15.9

Activity 5	Design of learning activities	Allow 5 minutes

Read the following activity taken from the module on 'Respiratory problems and HIV infection' from the Fellowship in HIV Medicine course at Christian Medical College [CMC], Vellore. The student would have studied a text beforehand. Then answer the two questions that follow.

Pneumonia

The following exercise will help you learn the approach to a patient with HIV infection and pneumonia.

A 30-year-old woman diagnosed with HIV infection 5 years ago presents with acute-onset fever with chills, cough and purulent blood-tinged sputum of 3 days duration. She complains of sharp pain on the right side of the chest which increases with deep breaths.

On examination: she appears ill and toxic, pulse rate 130/min, respiratory rate 26/min, temperature 103°F. She has flaring of alae nasi. Oral candidiasis present. Impaired resonance over axillary and infrascapular areas on the right side, bronchial breathing and increased vocal resonance over the same areas.

1. What is your clinical diagnosis?

2. What is the likely organism causing this infection?

3. Does this patient require admission?

4. What tests will you order immediately?

5. What treatment will you start?

Now answer these questions:

a. What are the design features of the above activity which foster clinical learning?

b. What other types and designs of activities might be appropriate for a clinical course?

FEEDBACK

a. Features in the design of this activity which facilitate learning in medicine:
   - The activity provides appropriate clinical information for a common clinical problem and simulates learning at the bedside
   - The questions focus on the important learning objectives relating to this clinical problem
   - The student studies relevant information beforehand and then applies it through the activity
   - Clear timings are given
   - The purpose of the exercise is clear.

b. Distance learning activities appropriate for a clinical course:
- Providing clinical, microbiology and X-ray images
- Sequencing case information in time as the case evolves
- Writing prescriptions
- Designing patient information sheets
- Preparing a local guideline
- Filling in blanks, matching items, extended matching activities
- Labelling diagrams.

Distance learning modules can be completely self-contained, where all the resources are provided in the module. Modules also may be designed as 'wrap-around' materials that complement a prescribed text. Such a module requires clear instructions regarding navigating through the prescribed text and attention to timing. In general, the wrap-around text would present activities and commentary to prepare students for readings from the text and then to help them to use or reflect on that reading. The distance learning modules for the CMC Fellowship in HIV Medicine course were completely self-contained, due to the absence of good texts in HIV care for the Indian setting. However, for another course for new junior doctors, we have developed wrap-around modules that complement standard undergraduate textbooks.

4. FEEDBACK ON LEARNING

Students need to know how well they are progressing and understanding, so feedback on learning is essential in distance learning, as it is for all learning. This is achieved in a number of ways, some of which you have already experienced here. Feedback to the student is offered in:

- in-text activities
- tutor-marked assignments
- tutorials
- student groups
- on-line support
- assessments.

If you reflect on your own education, you might wonder whether you received such consistent and deliberate comments and guidance!

5. BLENDING DIFFERENT ELEMENTS OF THE COURSE

The activities so far have shown that distance learning is made up of a rich variety of activities and is much more than a delivery medium. But this richness poses the challenge of integrating and blending the resources and experiences without losing the student along an insufficiently signposted path. The key to success is simple:

- Provide all learning resources so that they are available *at the time* the student needs them. Avoid, for example, asking the student to access patient records if they are likely to be studying in their room at night!
- Use one central learning guide: this can be, for example, the distance learning course in print, or a curriculum map in print or on a PDA (handheld computer) associated with a timetable and learning resources.
- In the central guidance, give clear instructions on what resources to access or activities to undertake and ensure that the student returns from these to the central guidance.

- Use clear icons alongside the text to indicate the type of resource to be accessed. For example:

 The student is directed to certain pages of supplied material and then asked to return to the workbook.

 Next, the student is directed to the relevant section of a CD to watch an interview with a patient.

 Finally, the student would be referred to the patient's notes provided and asked to read their history.

6. MANAGING CLINICAL ATTACHMENTS BY DISTANCE LEARNING

Distance learning methods can be used in conventional courses to support students who are distributed across the community. Clinical attachments everywhere can be supported by distance learning. This might involve:

- A *distance learning workbook* with supporting materials
- A paper or computer-based *curriculum map* of content to be covered
- A reflective *portfolio* submitted online to a mentor or peer group for comment
- Structured *preparatory and reflective exercises* and projects linked to clinical experience
- *Formative assessments*
- Ongoing *clinical assessments* with feedback linked to the curriculum map
- *Quality control* of the clinical attachment, to include support to teachers (Table 15.10).

Table 15.10

Activity 6	What are the principles of designing clinical experience on a distance course?	Allow 3 minutes
Consider here what principles you might follow in designing distance learning materials to support students on clinical attachments.		

FEEDBACK

- The clinical learning objectives should be clear.
- The student requires exposure to common clinical problems.
- Adequacy of the exposure and level of skill development should be monitored through case records, log books and formative assessments.
- The student should take the appropriate level of clinical responsibility necessary for their learning.
- The course should make maximum use of the clinical experience available.
- The distance learning guidance should prepare students for the clinical experience and enable them to reflect on it. The clinical teacher or supervisor should be aware of the distance learning component and support the students appropriately.

In some courses, clinical contacts are planned centrally. For the Fellowship in HIV Medicine course, students have three clinical contact periods, totalling 5 weeks, at the central training institute spread over the year. These are designed for progressive skill development and increasing responsibility. The students also improve their skills through clinical care projects at their local institutions. In other courses, clinical work may be planned carefully at the students' institutions or elsewhere supervised by local trained tutors. A portfolio or map of the clinical experience may assist the student.

7. THE STUDENT'S LEARNING EXPERIENCE

A wide variety of experiences are available to the distance learning student, just as they are to students in conventional programmes. A difference between the two will be the central learning guide, which might be the organizing vehicle for:

- Studying specially prepared course materials
- Undertaking learning activities and checking understanding
- Referring to web-based or CD-ROM resources
- Online conferencing with peers
- Participating in asynchronous online tutorial groups
- Participating in synchronous online 'expert' events
- Telephone or web-based tutorials
- Working within a virtual clinical environment
- Exercises to prepare for and reflect on clinical work
- Submitting electronic Tutor Marked Assignments, receiving and discussing feedback
- Discussion with a mentor about progress and integration of course components.

These activities might look suspiciously like a conventional course. But the main difference is the degree of organization, the central distance learning text, the style of those materials and the amount of planned support and feedback that the student receives.

8. MANAGING DISTANCE LEARNING

It will be clear by now that a distance learning course is carefully planned and highly managed. Ensuring that all the parts of the course are working and being presented and used in time; that all students are progressing properly; and that teachers are supported and students are active requires a learning management system (LMS). This can be paper-based, but is often a centralized, computer-based system, offering the following functions:

- Student registration
- Student records
- Teacher records, including appraisals and feedback
- Timetables
- Learning resources
- Assessments
- Assessment records
- Messaging
- Records of communications with students and teachers
- Evaluation and monitoring data.

Most of these functions can also be offered by an efficient office, if reliable technology is not available. Whatever system is used, whether high- or low-tech, the lesson is the same: records that track course development and implementation, student progress and teacher activity are fundamental to success in distance learning.

9. DEVELOPMENT OF DISTANCE LEARNING COURSES (TABLE 15.11)

Table 15.11 Distance learning courses require very careful preparation and development. They should all go through the following stages.

Needs assessment	Determines what content is required at what level
Feasibility study	The course design must fit the available funding, staffing, infrastructure and opportunities for teaching and learning
Multidisciplinary course team	The development team should have experts in distance learning, content experts, assessment experts and an administrator
Three drafts with piloting at draft two	To ensure that the student's journey through the course is as effective as possible, courses should go through stages of outlining the content of each element of the course, then a first draft which is discussed by the course team, and a second draft which is worked through by 'pretend' students to test timing and clarity, and reviewed by an external content expert, before preparing the third and final draft
Planning clinical experience	Careful planning of clinical experience at a local centre or main training centre
	Development of appropriate portfolios, log books and case records to record clinical exposure
Preparation and support of tutors	Teachers should be trained in supporting students in relation to: • course content and structure • giving written and verbal feedback • clinical supervision • project guidance • e-mentoring • spotting students in difficulties • student assessment
Preparation and support for students	All students require initial information about: • course structure and content • how to access and use the course elements and resources • organization of time • communication with other students and teachers sources of support • the assessment system • what feedback to expect • responsibilities as learners
Preparing assessment methods	Preparation of guidelines for all assessments, project work and final examination. Setting the pass standards
Evaluation and monitoring methods	Appropriate methods of gathering information are essential for trouble shooting and improvement
Maintenance course team for monitoring and updating	Once the course is up and running, a team is required to monitor its implementation, the activities of tutors and progress of students, to oversee the reliability and validity of the assessments and to decide when updating is required

10. QUALITY ASSURANCE IN DISTANCE LEARNING

Quality assurance is fundamental to the success of any distance learning course. Try the next activity (Table 15.12).

Table 15.12		
Activity 7	**Quality assurance in distance learning**	**Allow 5 minutes**
This activity will help you to review everything that you have learned in this course, as well as addressing a very important issue: quality.		
Look back over this course and see if you can spot all the elements of distance learning design and development that form part of the quality assurance strategy.		

FEEDBACK

You might have noticed the following quality assurance activities:

During course development:

- needs assessment and feasibility study
- careful course design and development to ensure relevance and usefulness
- team feedback to authors
- testing course materials in draft
- trying out activities to collect material for feedback
- external assessment of the course.

Of tutors:

- preparation of local tutors
- ongoing monitoring and support for tutors.

For learners:

- preparation of learners
- support and feedback for learners locally and centrally.

Of the course:

- evaluation and monitoring the course in use, tutor activity, student progress, assessment process and results
- updating as required.

11. CONCLUSION

In this short distance learning course, we have tried to provide you with some insight into the potential of using distance learning for medical education. Distance learning may be used for a small undergraduate clinical posting, for a complete postgraduate training programme or even for a whole medical school course. The example of the HIV course has shown that distance education can not only train doctors but also strengthen clinical services at the community level.

Whatever media you use, however, the same rules of development and design apply, as you have learned in this course. We hope you have enjoyed it.

References

Grant J: Using open and distance learning to develop clinical reasoning skills. In Higgs J, Jones MA, Loftus S, Christensen N, editors: *Clinical Reasoning in the Health Professions*. New York, 2008, Elsevier.

Further reading

Lentell H, Perraton H, editors: *Policy for Open and Distance Learning: World Review of Distance Education and Open Learning*, Vol. 4, Abingdon, 2003, Routledge.

Mills R, Tait A, editors: *Rethinking Learner Support in Distance Education: Change and Continuity in an International Context*. Abingdon, 2002, Routledge.

Salmon G: E-moderating. *The Key to Online Teaching and Learning*. Abingdon, 2004, Routledge.

Chapter
16

Peer-assisted learning

M. T. Ross, A. D. Cumming

Introduction

There has been a considerable increase in the number of medical schools incorporating various kinds of peer teaching, peer assessment and medical teacher-training into their undergraduate curricula in recent years. There has also been a noticeable increase in the number of teacher-training courses, qualifications and formalized teaching opportunities available to junior medical staff. These are reflected in the growing literature and supporting evidence for teaching and learning approaches that we will collectively refer to here as 'peer-assisted learning' (PAL). This chapter outlines the principles of PAL, the potential applications in medical education with examples from the literature, issues to consider when planning and developing new PAL initiatives and the relationship between PAL and so-called 'collaborative learning'.

Training-grade doctors and medical students have a long history of supporting and assisting the learning of their peers and colleagues. Examples in the literature can be traced as far back as Aristotle. However, this has tended to be informal, opportunistic and largely undocumented. The origins of the phrase 'See one, do one, teach one' are obscure, but the legacy lives on, although generally now with much more consideration of patient safety and quality assurance. Consultants and other experienced healthcare professionals have long been expected to take on teaching responsibilities, and this is increasingly reflected in professional standards for practice and contractual agreements. Only relatively recently, however, have medical undergraduates and junior doctors been required to learn about teaching and gain some practical teaching experience as part of their formal curriculum. Most learning outcome and competency frameworks for undergraduate and postgraduate medical training now include statements about learning to teach, and medical job applications at all levels enquire about teaching experience and training. PAL approaches represent practical and effective ways for medical students and postgraduate trainees to gain experience in teaching, to undertake focused teacher-training, and to receive constructive feedback on their teaching skills.

> *"One who has just acquired a subject is best fitted to teach it."*
>
> *Quintillian (c. 80 AD)*

Defining PAL

PAL can be defined as 'People from similar social groupings who are not professional teachers helping each other to learn and learning themselves by teaching' (Topping 1996). Using this definition, 'peers' share certain characteristics but are not necessarily from the same course or year of study, and may include students and trainees from different healthcare disciplines. Peers are not professional teachers or 'experts' in their subject areas, and should not be significantly different in status or qualification. The term 'near-peers' is sometimes used if there is a significant difference between otherwise similar groups, for example, junior doctors teaching senior medical students. The term PAL is a broad umbrella term, covering a wide range of teaching and learning situations. Because it has been developed in different ways across a spectrum of educational fields, the terminology is diverse and sometimes conflicting. PAL approaches are sometimes referred to as peer teaching or tutoring; near-peer teaching; peer-supported learning; peer-assisted study; peer assessment; cooperative or collaborative learning; peer group learning; students helping students; student tutoring or facilitation; student mentoring; study advisory schemes; teaching assistant schemes; supplemental instruction; parrainage and proctoring. Terminology is not standardized, and some of these terms are also used to describe learning and teaching situations which are not PAL. A confusing variety of terms have also been used to describe PAL participants, activities and learning and teaching situations depending upon local preference and context. For clarity in this chapter and elsewhere, we attempt to standardize terminology so that in any organized PAL 'project', 'tutors' assist the learning of 'tutees' through a variety of PAL 'interactions' or 'sessions'. It is recognized, however, that in some instances, as in the production of PAL learning resources, there may be no direct interaction between tutors and tutees. In 'reciprocal PAL' each participant may at different times be tutor and tutee.

Theoretical basis for PAL

Most PAL participants report the experience to be enjoyable and beneficial in a variety of ways. Feedback suggests that the nature of the interaction and relationship between PAL tutor and tutee may be qualitatively different than that between student or trainee and 'expert' teaching staff. Many educational, psychological, social and organizational theories have been proposed to explain the success and appeal of PAL. Topping and Ehly (2001) offer an accessible introduction to this literature, highlighting cognitive, communication, affective, social and organizational factors.

COGNITIVE FACTORS: CHALLENGE AND SUPPORT

PAL typically involves tutors and tutees being challenged in their understanding, beliefs and assumptions: leading to 'cognitive conflict', which Piaget and others consider crucial to learning. Topping and Ehly note that tutors derive less academic benefit from PAL if there is low cognitive challenge, although they suggest that the cognitive demands of monitoring learner performance and of detecting, diagnosing and correcting tutee errors in PAL are typically high (Topping & Ehly 2001). PAL tutors are closer to the academic level of tutees than 'expert' staff and so may be better able to understand their difficulties, sometimes referred to as 'cognitive congruence' (Ten Cate & Durning 2007). For tutees, supported or 'scaffolded' learning within Vygotsky's 'zone of proximal development' (the distance between what a learner can achieve independently and what he or she can achieve with more experienced assistance) through interaction with more experienced peers is thought to be very significant (Topping 1996). In a classic study, Bargh and Schul demonstrated that learning content in order to teach it results in better understanding and recall than learning the same content for a test (Bargh & Schul 1980). Such goal-orientated information processing, content learning and structuring are thought to offer significant cognitive benefits to PAL tutors (Ten Cate & Durning 2007).

COMMUNICATION FACTORS

All participants, whether tutor or tutee, may be called upon to recall, explain and structure their understanding of content, perhaps for the first time. Verbalization is considered to be of key importance to the success of PAL, with both tutors and tutees gaining significant benefit from listening, explaining, questioning, clarifying, simplifying, summarizing and hypothesizing during PAL interactions (Topping 1996).

"How do I know what I think until I see what I say?"

E. M. Forester

AFFECTIVE AND SOCIAL FACTORS

Tutor enthusiasm and competence are likely to motivate tutees and lead to role-modelling. Because of their similarity, PAL participants are likely to establish a relaxed relationship with their peers. Ten Cate and Durning (2007) outline current thought on the impact of this 'social congruence' in motivating and reducing anxiety in tutees and of PAL as a vehicle for transmitting the 'hidden curriculum'. They also discuss affective aspects of PAL for tutors including Maslow's need for esteem, role theory and self-determination theory. This suggests that by 'acting' as a relative expert, tutors are likely to feel, and then become, more like an expert in terms of competency, autonomy, esteem and motivation.

"The authority of those who teach is often an obstacle to those who want to learn."

Cicero

ORGANIZATIONAL FACTORS AND THE PAL PROCESS

PAL is often voluntary and supplemental to core programme learning activities. As such, it may result in increased time and engagement with content for tutors and tutees and may add variety and interest to their studies. In some cases tutors also receive additional teaching from staff as preparation for PAL interactions. Group sizes are often small, resulting in more individualized and immediate feedback for tutees than may be possible from staff. Intrinsic rewards from participating in PAL are thought to have a significant effect on tutor attitudes and motivation, as may extrinsic rewards such as payment, privilege and evidence of participation for their CV and job applications.

All the above factors feed into the PAL process in which participants may extend, modify and rebuild their knowledge and skills; develop shared understanding; rehearse and consolidate core skills; generalize specific concepts; and give and receive feedback and reinforcement. This may lead to increased self-awareness, metacognition and self-confidence in both tutors and tutees.

Evidence for PAL

The medical and healthcare education literature now contains a substantial body of project evaluations, discursive papers and research on PAL (Ross & Cameron 2007). Together with evidence from school and postcompulsory education in other disciplines (Topping 1996), there is much evidence to support and guide the use of PAL. It must be remembered, however, that PAL is not one single approach. Although there is evidence for the utility, acceptability and effectiveness of PAL with certain types of content in particular situations, it will not be appropriate in all situations. There is evidence that PAL can have disadvantages and unintended consequences, particularly if used indiscriminately or inappropriately. For example, it would probably be detrimental to PAL tutees for a tutor to give a didactic lecture on a topic about which they knew little, or teach them how to diagnose or manage complex cases. It may, however, be very effective to have a PAL tutor facilitate a discussion and question-generating session on such topics, lead a problem-based learning tutorial or teach specific well-defined clinical skills (such as shoulder ultrasound in Knobe et al 2010). Commonly cited advantages of PAL for tutors, tutees and the host institution, and potential disadvantages, are discussed below.

 "PAL strategies are very well researched, with a substantive evidential basis for effectiveness in terms of raising achievement, fostering social and emotional gains, and often also developing transferable interpersonal skills."

Topping & Ehly 2001

ADVANTAGES FOR TUTORS

Many PAL approaches encourage tutors to reflect upon and revise their own prior learning, to become more self-directed in identifying and addressing any learning needs they may have in relation to the topics being taught and to increase their self-confidence in content knowledge and skills. They may be motivated to learn new content and find new ways of thinking about and structuring content. They develop knowledge, skills and attitudes towards teaching and gain a greater sense of engagement with the educational programme. Development of skills in communication, verbalization, observation, assessment and the giving and receiving of feedback have all been reported from

PAL, as have team-working, responsibility, organizational skills and empathy. In follow-up surveys many years later, PAL tutors often report that the experience had a significant and lasting impact on their clinical practice, teaching skills and attitudes.

 "This course was a real confidence builder for me."

PAL tutor in Bibb & Lefever 2002

ADVANTAGES FOR TUTEES

If PAL is supplemental to the core curriculum, tutees effectively gain additional teaching; provided the content does not conflict with or take too much time away from core teaching. They also gain opportunities to ask questions and receive detailed feedback on their knowledge and skills. If PAL is used to deliver core teaching, as an alternative to professional teachers, then the question arises, how do PAL tutors compare to 'expert' teachers? In situations where tutees would be better served by core teaching from experts, it would be hard to justify replacing this with PAL. The small number of studies directly comparing PAL tutors with experts suggest that they can, in certain situations, achieve similar outcomes in terms of tutee evaluation (e.g. Perkins et al 2002) and examination scores (e.g. Knobe et al 2010). It has also been suggested that in certain situations PAL tutors may be more effective than expert teachers in helping tutees attain defined outcome measures, whilst in other situations they will be less effective. Selection of outcome measures and many other factors will affect such comparisons. Caution must therefore be exercised when interpreting sweeping generalizations such as 'peer tutors are as good as or better than staff', which are commonly seen in the literature. Peer and expert teaching do seem to result in qualitatively different learning experiences for tutees. PAL interactions are often relatively relaxed and informal, providing tutees with opportunities to formulate and ask even apparently 'silly' questions. They can disclose ignorance or misconception without intimidation or concern that this may affect their assessment. PAL tutors are felt to be more aware of problem areas than expert tutors, as they are, or have recently been, in the same situation themselves. PAL tutors can often help tutees by talking about their own strategies and study skills and can act as role-models and motivators for tutee learning.

 PAL may be particularly useful to ease the transition and cultural change when the context of learning changes acutely: for example, new students or those moving from a preclinical to a clinical environment.

ADVANTAGES FOR THE INSTITUTION

PAL approaches can also offer significant advantages to the institution. They can help address curricular outcomes and external requirements for students and trainees to gain experience in teaching. PAL may also be used to address other content gaps in core curricular teaching, to encourage a culture of collaborative learning rather than competitiveness between peers and to stimulate student engagement in the educational programme. From a quality assurance perspective, it has been observed that compared to staff it may be easier to train PAL tutors and standardize their teaching. PAL may result in cost savings when students deliver teaching which would otherwise be delivered by salaried staff. However, as many PAL projects are supplementary to the curriculum or require additional training, supervision or reward for tutors, PAL may in fact generate additional costs to the institution.

 "This model should not be seen as a method for reducing the teaching commitment of clinical staff but as a mechanism to allow their expertise to be focused more appropriately on other neglected areas in the curriculum."

Perkins et al 2002

Potential disadvantages and concerns about PAL

A number of authors have expressed concerns that PAL tutors may have inadequate depth of content knowledge and so may teach 'the wrong thing' or give incorrect information to tutees. They lack the experience of professional teachers and may not be able to teach the knowledge and skills that they possess adequately. They may lack experience in facilitating small groups and have difficulty retaining focus and discipline. They may overload tutees with information or present information in such a way that it leads to confusion or reduced confidence. There may be personality issues between students or boundary issues and personal relationships which interfere with the tutee–tutor interaction. If the PAL project involves peer physical examination (PPE) there may be increased potential for peer pressure, embarrassment and inappropriate behaviour. These are real and important issues, and they have been reported from various institutions. It should be noted, however, that similar issues have also been reported for staff teaching. Concerns have been raised about PAL tutors being used as 'cheap labour' to teach on established courses because there are insufficient staff, where there are limited benefits for tutors or where tutees would be better served by staff teaching. Concerns have also

been expressed about the time and effort required to organize supplemental PAL projects, train tutors and monitor outcomes, all of which may take resources and efforts away from 'core' teaching. When developing PAL it is worth considering how these potential disadvantages can be minimized and how advantages can be maximized. A number of general principles for successful PAL have been identified in the literature and are presented by theme in the next section.

Components and choices in PAL

PAL has been developed in many different ways for a wide variety of applications. Ross and Cameron synthesized much of this literature into a comprehensive framework of issues to address and decisions to be made when considering new PAL initiatives (Ross & Cameron 2007). This PAL planning and implementation framework consists of 24 questions arranged into eight themes (Table 16.1) and is discussed below.

BACKGROUND

PAL projects are developed within the context of wider educational programmes and should be considered in relation to programme learning outcomes, opportunities and progression. The opportunities and constraints, acceptability and potential applications of PAL will depend upon local institutional factors and the structure, processes and principles of the curriculum. PAL may be mandatory or supplemental to core teaching. Multiple PAL projects may be linked to provide teaching experience for all students in a particular year group. It is important to be clear about why PAL is being considered, to be aware of the context and to identify who will lead the PAL project. Sometimes PAL is entirely student-led or staff-led, although in most cases it is a combination of both.

AIMS

There are many reasons why PAL approaches may be considered, including educational, social, organizational and financial. It is helpful to consider these separately under aims for tutors, tutees and the institution. Aims often relate to the reported advantages of PAL detailed above. Ensuring that PAL projects have clear aims and learning objectives and well-defined and structured subject areas can increase tutor familiarity with material and also provide a structure and focus to sessions. It is also important to define aims so that the PAL project can be properly evaluated.

 Think carefully about programme learning outcomes and how to maximize benefits for both PAL tutors and tutees.

Table 16.1 PAL planning framework

Domain	Question
Background	What is the current situation and context in the curriculum?
	Why is this PAL project being considered now?
	Who is responsible for the project, and who will lead it?
Aims	What are the aims and objectives of the project for tutors?
	What are the aims and objectives of the project for tutees?
	What are the aims and objectives of the project for the institution?
Tutors	Who will be tutors, and how will they be recruited?
	What training will tutors require, and how will this be provided?
	How else will tutors prepare themselves and reflect afterwards?
Tutees	Who will be tutees, and how will they be recruited?
	What related prior knowledge and experience will tutees have already?
	What information and preparation will tutees require before the interaction?
Interaction	What will be the format of the interaction, and what resources are required?
	What would be a typical plan of activities during the PAL interaction?
	When and where will PAL interactions occur, and how will they be arranged?
Evaluation	What feedback will be collected from participants, and how will it be used?
	How else will the project be piloted and evaluated?
	What are the academic hypotheses, and how will they be tested?
Institution	Who are potential stakeholders in the project?
	What are the staff time and funding implications of the project?
	How could the project be developed, and how might it affect the curriculum?
Realization	What are the potential pitfalls or barriers to the success of this project?
	What are key points on the timeline for this project?
	What actions need to be taken to develop the project, and by whom?

From Ross MT, Cameron HS: AMEE Guide 30: Peer assisted learning: a planning and implementation framework. *Medical Teacher* 29:527–545, 2007.

TUTORS

Tutors can be recruited compulsorily as part of a course, on a voluntary basis or on the basis of high achievement. There are also a few reports from secondary education in which tutors are recruited on the basis of low achievement; in recognition of the potential cognitive benefits of tutoring. Tutors are usually drawn from the same year as tutees or from a more advanced year and so generally have a similar or more advanced level of ability compared to tutees in relation to the content. Very occasionally, tutors have even been drawn from a lower year. Some reciprocal PAL programmes involve tutors becoming tutees and vice versa. It is important that the tutors feel confident enough to undertake the task well and understand what is expected of them. Tutors may have to complete supplementary tutor training on content or educational approaches prior to PAL interaction. This might, for example, include learning how to facilitate a small group, teach practical skills or provide feedback. Tutors may also be required to research a topic, prepare learning materials or generate a lesson plan in advance of PAL sessions.

 Try to ensure that tutors know what is expected of them, ideally giving them an opportunity to practise and gain confidence in their teaching through simulation before the PAL interaction.

TUTEES

Most PAL projects are offered as supplemental teaching for all students in the target group on a voluntary basis. Less often PAL is used to deliver core compulsory teaching (e.g. Perkins et al 2002) or is only available to selected students, such as those with poor academic achievement. In all cases it is important to consider tutees' prior learning and experience. Most PAL projects involve no specific additional tutee preparation, although they may sometimes be asked to read preparatory material or even to participate in training prior to the PAL interaction.

INTERACTION

PAL sessions can be incorporated into the curriculum, timetabled outside normal working hours or held on an ad hoc basis depending upon the availability or needs of participants. There is wide variation in the frequency of sessions, where they are held, how long they last, how tutors and tutees are matched together and how many tutors are present (from one-to-one diads to large group lectures). Involving more than one tutor per session increases the breadth of tutor knowledge, reduces the effect of an individual tutor's personality and may minimize idiosyncratic teaching. Sessions can be organized by staff or by students themselves at a variety of locations. The commonest form of PAL in the medical education literature is the peer-led supplementary small-group tutorial, typically for revision (exam practice, past papers, discussion), remediation (help with content or study skills) or the practice of clinical skills (observed practice, review of videos, reflection). Some forms of PAL involve didactic lectures and tutorials in which new content is presented to tutees (e.g. Bibb & Lefever 2002). Other forms of PAL do not involve face-to-face contact at all, but rather involve online interaction using social networking tools such as blogs and asynchronous discussion (e.g. Shanks et al 2000) or the production of resources such as written summaries, revision aids and computer-aided learning programmes.

 You may want to explore different types of PAL to provide tutors with a variety of teaching experiences, including large-group, small-group and individual teaching, facilitation, giving feedback, creating resources, course organization and student support.

EVALUATION

Numerous approaches to evaluating and formally researching PAL can be found in the literature, from simple participant questionnaires to formal randomized controlled trials. PAL tutors and tutees are almost invariably positive about their experiences in feedback questionnaires. Interviews with participants, focus groups or observational studies by staff or simulated patients can be more revealing about how well PAL interactions have functioned. Studies of outcome measures such as assessment results, or comparisons between different types of PAL interaction or tutor training, are less common in the literature but are fertile ground for further research.

INSTITUTION

The administration and financial implications of PAL projects vary considerably depending upon the content being taught, the amount of training and support given

to tutors and whether sessions are timetabled and organized by members of staff or by students. Staff involvement and contribution to PAL initiatives will depend upon the content being taught, the PAL approach and the local context. As with planning any other teaching and learning initiative in higher or continuing education, it is recommended that PAL is undertaken in a considered, logical and reflective manner, aligning content and processes with learning outcomes for the educational programme and seeking approval and stakeholder engagement as appropriate.

 If tutees are to choose from a list of available PAL sessions, the administrative time required will be greatly reduced with the use of an online sign-up tool.

REALIZATION

A number of potential pitfalls and unintended consequences of PAL have already been highlighted in this chapter, most of which can be avoided with careful planning. Simply thinking in advance about these potential problems and early recognition may be all that is required to avoid them. A timeline and action points will also facilitate communication between different stakeholders and ensure that important deadlines are not missed.

Applications and examples of PAL in healthcare education

Many teaching modalities and strategies have been used in PAL including revision tutorials, PBL facilitation, student support, various types of summative and formative assessment, lectures and the production of learning resources. A number of practical illustrative examples of PAL projects in the healthcare literature are outlined below.

 "First-year students perceived a significant increase in their knowledge of dental anatomy as well as their confidence and enthusiasm to begin studying the material."

Bibb & Lefever 2002

SKILLS TRAINING IN SHOULDER ULTRASOUND (KNOBE ET AL 2010, GERMANY)

Nine willing medical students in Years 3 and 4 were selected and trained in shoulder ultrasound. The remaining students in their year groups were randomly assigned into two groups to be taught either by their trained peers or by experienced staff. There was no difference in scores between peer-taught or staff-taught groups in theoretical MCQs and practical OSCE assessments. Peer tutors scored significantly higher in both assessments. Peer tutors were rated lower than staff tutors in terms of evaluation of perceived competence and leaving tutee questions unanswered. Other examples can be found in the literature in which PAL is used to help students learn skills in communication, history-taking, physical examination, practical procedures, evidence-based medicine, X-ray and ECG interpretation and prescribing.

SHORT COURSE ORGANIZATION, DELIVERY AND ASSESSMENT (BIBB & LEFEVER 2002, USA)

Year 4 dental students participated in a student-selected elective course in which they created a 3-hour, 'Welcome to dental anatomy micro-course' under staff guidance for incoming students in the first week of Year 1. Tutor training included an introduction to learning theory, selecting and sequencing content, presentation skills, writing of test questions and assessment of outcomes. Staff tried to remain nondirective. The PAL course consisted of handout learning materials, a series of formal 20-minute lectures, a brief assessment of tutee knowledge and evaluation. Tutees reported afterwards that their knowledge had significantly increased and that they were more confident and enthusiastic about studying the core programme material. They still felt the course had been useful when surveyed after an anatomy exam 5 weeks later. PAL tutor feedback suggested that the experience was positive and rewarding and that it had increased their confidence, understanding of the educational process and presentation skills.

TRAINING IN BASIC LIFE SUPPORT (PERKINS ET AL 2002, UK)

Year 2 volunteer healthcare students delivered a compulsory core Basic Life Support (BLS) course to Year 1 medical, dental, nursing and physiotherapy students. Tutee learning outcomes were compared to those tutored by critical care and resuscitation training staff. Outcomes were measured using an external assessment of BLS skills, an MCQ test and tutee evaluation of teaching quality. There was no significant difference in MCQ results or tutee evaluation, but students taught by PAL tutors were more likely to pass the practical BLS assessment (98% versus 85%). PAL tutors were also more likely to attend planned sessions than staff (100% versus 75%).

ASSESSMENT OF PEERS IN AN OSCE (REITER ET AL 2004, CANADA)

Final-year medical students acted as peer examiners in lieu of staff or residents as examiners in an OSCE for 126 first-year medical students. The OSCE stations involved 8 minutes of interaction with a standardized patient, followed by 5 minutes of examiner feedback to the student and giving the student a completed assessment form. During rest stations, OSCE candidates completed a questionnaire about the feedback they had received during the previous OSCE station. Peer examiners received significantly higher 'quality of feedback' ratings from candidates than staff. After the OSCE most candidates were positive about being assessed by peers and reported being willing to undertake this role themselves. There was no significant difference in candidate performance in an OSCE led by staff one year later. PAL examiners assigned significantly higher marks than staff, which the authors felt could reduce reliability and may have led to reciprocity bias. Other studies suggest, however, that with appropriate training medical students can assess their peers as accurately and reliably as staff.

POSTGRADUATE PAL BASED ON REAL CLINICAL CASES (WONG ET AL 2004, USA)

'Resident' doctors in the third year of postgraduate hospital-based training participated in a 4-week daytime rotation in which they were required to research and answer clinical questions posed by their peers and themselves relating to inpatient care. They attended ward rounds and saw all patients under the care of the inpatient medical team, helping as required, and offered medical opinions for other inpatients on request. They logged all questions, answers and sources in a portfolio accessible to other residents, and once weekly selected and prepared patient cases for discussion at an educational meeting for their peers, liaising before and after with a staff member to discuss content and feedback. The 13 residents who undertook this rotation in the first year generated 86 formalized clinical questions, answering 93% of them. All found the rotation to be a valuable educational experience.

PAL and collaborative learning

Collaborative learning can be defined in many ways, the broadest of which is 'A situation in which two or more people learn or attempt to learn something together' (Dillenbourg 1999). Undergraduate medical students and postgraduate trainees commonly work, study and learn together in groups, share experiences and stories and offer mutual support and advice. Informal collaborative learning is very commonly seen in friendship or study groups, 'coffee room' discussions and team meetings. Formal collaborative learning includes small-group tutorial activities, problem-based learning and 'buddy' systems. Some types of PAL, particularly reciprocal forms, involve collaborative learning. However, PAL aims and learning outcomes are often very different for tutors and tutees. Depending upon the format and context, collaborative learning may be associated with some or all of the potential benefits and drawbacks of PAL.

Conclusions

There is increasing evidence in the literature to support the efficacy and acceptability of PAL for a variety of situations and applications. PAL is particularly useful for well-defined subject areas such as basic sciences or practical clinical skills, but has also been successfully applied to the more complex areas of training such as communication skills, facilitation of self-directed learning and short-course organization. The literature also suggests that PAL is less suitable for subjects where teachers need a broad general knowledge or considerable experience, such as advanced consultation skills and complex decisions about patient management. Development of a new PAL initiative should be undertaken with care, attention to detail, adequate resourcing and educational scholarship, similar to the development of any other component of an undergraduate or postgraduate curriculum. It is particularly important to ensure alignment with programme learning outcomes, to carefully plan the approach in consultation with all relevant stakeholders and to engage in ongoing evaluation and development.

Summary

PAL is a collective term for interactions between similar groups of people, who are not professional teachers or 'experts', helping each other to learn by teaching. The concept dates back to ancient times, but has come to the fore recently in medical education; particularly in countries where all graduates must have teaching skills and experience. There is a growing medical education literature on PAL. This includes using PAL to teach and assess knowledge-based subjects; training and reinforcement of clinical examination and communication skills; revision and help with study skills; course organization; resource preparation; and the facilitation of self-directed and problem-based learning. Many of these programmes report considerable benefits for both student tutors and tutees. There are potential pitfalls and drawbacks of PAL, but with careful planning these can be minimized.

References

Bargh JA, Schul Y: On the cognitive benefits of teaching, *Journal of Educational Psychology* 72(5):593–604, 1980.

Bibb CA, Lefever KH: Mentoring future dental educators through an apprentice teaching experience, *Journal of Dental Education* 66(6):703–709, 2002.

Dillenbourg P, editor: *Collaborative-Learning: Cognitive and Computational Approaches*, Oxford, 1999, Elsevier.

Knobe M, Münker R, Sellei RM, et al: Peer teaching: a randomized controlled trial using student-teachers to teach musculoskeletal ultrasound, *Medical Education* 44:148–155, 2010.

Perkins GD, Hulme J, Bion JF: Peer-led resuscitation training for healthcare students: a randomised controlled study, *Intensive Care Medicine* 28:698–700, 2002.

Reiter HI, Rosenfeld J, Nandagopal K, Eva KW: Do clinical clerks provide candidates with adequate formative assessment during objective structured clinical examinations? *Advances in Health Sciences Education* 9:189–199, 2004.

Ross MT, Cameron HS: AMEE Guide 30: Peer assisted learning: a planning and implementation framework, *Medical Teacher* 29:527–545, 2007.

Shanks JC, Silver RD, Harris IB: Use of web-based technology in a peer-teaching program, *Academic Medicine* 75(5):538–539, 2000.

Ten Cate O, Durning S: Dimensions and psychology of peer teaching in medical education, *Medical Teacher* 29:546–552, 2007.

Topping KJ: The effectiveness of peer tutoring in further and higher education: a typology and review of the literature, *Higher Education* 32(3):321–345, 1996.

Topping KJ, Ehly SW: Peer assisted learning: a framework for consultation, *Journal of Educational and Psychological Consultation* 12(2):113–132, 2001.

Wong JG, Holmboe ES, Huot SJ: Teaching and learning in an 80-hour work week: a novel day-float rotation for medical residents, *Journal of General Internal Medicine* 19(5 Pt 2):519–523, 2004.

Mentoring

S. Ramani, L. Gruppen

Introduction

The traditional mentoring relationship is described as one that develops between a senior professional, the 'mentor', and a younger colleague, the 'mentee' or 'protégé'. In *The Odyssey*, Ulysses' trusted friend, Mentor, was given the responsibility of educating Ulysses' son, Telemachus, when he set out for the Trojan War. From this epic arose the use of the word 'mentor' as a wise and faithful counsellor. In the modern world, a mentor is a counsellor and teacher who motivates and assists a junior colleague in attaining success.

An effective mentoring relationship is often viewed as an essential step for achieving success in politics, business and academia. Medical faculty who had mentors reported that mentoring positively influenced personal development, career guidance and overall productivity. Effective mentoring can increase career satisfaction and reduce faculty burnout as well as increase professional networking and collegiality. Yet a recent systematic review reported that fewer than 50% of medical students and 20% of faculty members reported having a mentor. Women seem to have more difficulty finding mentors than men.

At institutions where formal mentoring programmes exist, mentors rarely receive training on the mentoring process and are often ill-equipped to face challenges when taking on major mentoring responsibilities. Mentor–mentee relationships are also challenged by increased clinical, research and administrative demands on faculty. Moreover, there is a perception that mentorship is undervalued by academic institutions and does not contribute to career advancement.

It is therefore essential for medical institutions to implement formal mentoring programmes, provide staff development and support for mentors and overtly recognize and find ways to reward faculty who take on major mentoring responsibilities.

DEFINITIONS

Mentoring implies a two-way relationship between the mentor and the mentee. The mentor has a genuine interest in the professional growth of a mentee, and often the relationship is judged by the mentee's success. The mentor supplies information, gives advice and facilitates professional networking, but also offers critical support for the mentee during trying periods. A mentor is often confused with an advisor, role model or collaborator.

Advising involves supplying information in a neutral fashion. Although the advice or information is given in a friendly manner, a bond need not develop between the advisor and the advisee. An advising relationship can be terminated after one meeting or several meetings and usually focuses on a specific career goal, e.g. further specialization, research collaboration, clinical placement or learning plan.

A role model is one whose professional behaviours and academic values are emulated by junior faculty or trainees. There does not have to be an actual personal relationship between the one who incorporates these characteristics and the role model. A mentor can be a role model, but a role model need not be a mentor. A role model could be a historical figure such as Sir William Osler.

Collaboration is more often a partnership between peers with the mutual goal of increasing productivity, increasing resources or developing specific skills. Such relationships can be long-term, but are more usually short lived and end when the goals have been achieved.

 Mentoring does not need to be a lifelong or career-long relationship. It can be short and time-defined and still effective.

"The process whereby an experienced, highly regarded, empathic person (the mentor) guides another individual (the mentee) in the development and re-examination of his or her own ideas, learning, and personal and professional development. The mentor, who often, but not necessarily works in the same organization or field as the mentee, achieves this by listening, or talking in confidence to the mentee."

SCOPME 1998 (Standing Committee on Postgraduate Medical and Dental Education)

Benefits of mentoring

The benefits of a mentoring relationship are manifold. A successful partnership can lead to the professional development of both individuals. Mentors experience the satisfaction of nurturing and aiding the professional growth of a junior trainee or colleague. Institutions may recognize and reward successful mentors. More recently, the Association of American Medical Colleges consensus group on Educational Scholarship has urged institutions to add mentoring to their list of educational activities that can promote educational scholarship and academic advancement. Mentors often feel professionally stimulated and perhaps rejuvenated with a feeling that they are giving back to their professions. Their mentees, in turn, may continue their legacy by mentoring their own students and junior colleagues.

Mentees benefit by receiving support during their professional development and when facing professional problems. They have time to reflect on their goals and strategies and ideally should be supported while they solve their problems. They are able to orient themselves more quickly to the organizational structure, goals and policies and develop confidence in navigating the maze and politics of a medical organization. They are also able to turn to a senior person in a crisis and are challenged to reach for loftier goals in their career.

Challenges in mentoring

Although the benefits and advantages of mentoring are most often espoused in the literature, mentors should be aware that there are risks and problems associated with mentoring relationships. Mentors and mentees may not enter the relationship with common goals and expectations and levels of commitment. Mentees may make unreasonable demands of their mentors and even expect them to solve all their emotional and academic problems. Assigned mentors may be disinterested and unhelpful to their mentees, and such

relationships may be threatened by hierarchy, generational tensions or personality clashes. Mentors may try to propagate their own career interests in their mentees and fail to recognize that their mentees' professional aspirations and identity could be very different from their own. Mentors who are also their mentees' superiors and evaluators could threaten their mentees' growth by involving them in their own research or educational activities, and there could be conflicts in authorship of shared publications and presentations. Finally, both parties should be careful to avoid emotional overdependence or inappropriate personal feelings, all of which could damage irreparably the careers of both.

Approach to mentoring

BALANCING SUPPORT, CHALLENGE AND VISION

In 1986, Daloz described a mentor–protégé model which balances three elements: support, challenge and vision. Support refers to activities that boost self-esteem of the protégé such as showing respect, providing opportunities and resources and giving positive feedback. Challenge forces mentees to work actively towards their career goals and reflect on their skills and values; actions include listing tasks to achieve goals, setting timelines and providing constructive or negative feedback. Finally, mentors help mentees develop their professional vision by stimulating discussions about their long-term goals. Without challenge, there can be no professional growth in the careers of mentees. However, mentees need support if they are to venture out of their comfort zone and challenge themselves. Support will enable mentees to have a sense of belonging within their organization and continue to set lofty professional goals even if initial attempts are unsuccessful. Finally, professionals should be able to periodically set long-term career goals including how they would handle career transitions. Underlying all these values should be the realization that mentees have the freedom to completely change career paths during the course of their academic life and need support during these changes. This model has been validated by educators in the Department of Family Medicine at the University of Wisconsin.

Roles of a mentor

Several roles have been previously described for a physician researcher mentor, but these roles apply equally to non-researchers, educators, administrators and leaders who take on mentoring responsibilities in medical education.

Seven possible roles of a mentor:

1. Teacher
2. Sponsor
3. Advisor
4. Agent
5. Role model
6. Coach
7. Confidante.

As is evident from the roles listed above, a mentor has several functions in a mentoring relationship. We describe some important ones below:

- *Professional socialization*: mentors can help mentees who are new to an institution learn about institutional vision and goals, help them find their way around a large organization and refer them to peers or senior colleagues for further guidance or collaboration. This socialization also applies to the profession more generally, understanding its traditions, values, leaders and challenges.

- *Career development*: mentors can help mentees establish professional goals early in their career and guide them towards the resources needed to achieve these goals. These goals can relate to research, administrative or educational aspects of a medical educator's career but the goals could also relate to personal growth. Guidance is especially crucial during career transitions: from trainee to faculty, as well as faculty career transitions.

- *Networking*: mentors can help mentees network within and outside their own institution for further mentoring, collaboration in research or educational activities and skill development.

- *Feedback*: mentors can review periodically whether their mentees are proceeding in the right direction to accomplish their academic goals and redirect them when needed. In addition, they can review mentee evaluations by juniors, peers or seniors and provide feedback on their strengths and weaknesses.

- *Coaching*: mentors can provide coaching when their mentees have to learn new skills. If they themselves do not possess these skills, mentors must be proactive in referring mentees to others who could help their mentees gain these skills. Mentors should be able to see the potential in their mentees and actively groom them for future leadership positions.

- *Support*: mentees need support from mentors when they are exploring career paths, stretching their talents to make innovative contributions or facing failures or conflicts with other colleagues.

They may also seek their mentors' help when faced with personal challenges, and under these circumstances mentors need to be very aware of professional boundaries.

Attributes of an effective mentor

While reviewing the literature on mentoring, we found several studies that surveyed mentees about mentoring relationships and described key characteristics of successful mentors. The most effective mentors allow their mentees to take the initiative in making career decisions. They are available, approachable and good listeners. They are unselfish and take pride in seeing their mentees become even more successful than themselves. They are ready to provide positive and negative feedback in a nonjudgemental way. They are willing to go the extra mile to help mentees succeed professionally as well as personally. They prevent their mentees from taking on excessive academic and administrative duties, particularly career-killing initiatives. Mentees need help in navigating institutional politics and overcoming the negative aspects of the work environment. Mentors maintain confidentiality in their mentoring relationships and are sensitive to gender and ethnic differences between themselves and their mentees. An effective relationship is personal, professional and intimate, but nonsexual. They are well aware of professional boundaries and refer their mentees to the appropriate resources when they find themselves out of their depth. Such issues could be professional but are frequently personal or emotional. For example, a mentor should not take it upon him- or herself to help a mentee through personal trauma or depression or even substance abuse.

An analysis of mentee letters nominating their mentors for a prestigious award revealed the following traits of excellence in mentoring:

1. Exhibit admirable personal qualities, including enthusiasm, compassion and selflessness.

2. Act as a career guide, offering a vision but also tailoring support to each mentee.

3. Commit time to the mentoring relationship with regular, frequent and high-quality meetings.

4. Support personal and professional balance.

5. Leave a legacy of good mentoring through role modelling and institute policies to set global expectations and standards for mentorship.

 What mentees value in mentors:

Academic:

- Guidance in professional development
- Preparation for promotion

- Help with specific strategies to achieve professional goals
- Development of academic identities
- Assistance in networking
- Setting high standards and expectations
- Help with navigating institutional politics
- Help with academic socialization
- Using his or her influence to support mentees' academic advancement
- Directing mentees towards assignments that prepare them for higher positions

Psychosocial:

- Allowing mentees to formulate ideas and goals
- Being available
- Acting as an advocate
- Showing respect, empathy
- Being trustworthy, respecting confidentiality
- Giving nonjudgemental feedback
- Knowing the mentee as a person and a professional

Types of mentoring relationships

Mentoring relationships do not need to be face-to-face or one-on-one or even senior-to-junior. In the modern educational setting, several trainees and faculty enjoy long-distance mentoring relationships and group peer mentoring, which educators have reported as successful in promoting academic success of mentees.

- *Dyadic mentoring*: this is the most traditional form of mentoring between a senior mentor and a junior mentee. The notion of a senior professional promoting the career of a junior mentee has shaped mentoring in medical education, and senior physicians are expected to model desired behaviours and attitudes for their juniors.

- *Multiple*: frequently a mentee may choose one senior person as a primary mentor but have other secondary mentors who can be useful in specific areas of his or her career. More recently, group mentoring has been described where members of a peer group allow each member of the group to reflect on their goals and problems and mentor each other.

- *Formal*: many institutions have formal mentoring programmes and assign mentors for trainees or junior faculty similar to a 'blind date'. It has been reported that such formal mentoring relationships are characterized by power and status differentials and are less successful in the long run. However, it

has also been reported that the majority of medical trainees and faculty report they have no mentors; therefore, a formal programme could be a good starting point to provide mentees with opportunities to discover other mentors.

- *Informal*: informal mentoring occurs serendipitously when two individuals meet and discover mutual interests and goals. This type of mentoring has been described as the most successful and is characterized by a long-term, supportive, compatible and mutually satisfying relationship. However, only a minority of trainees or faculty are fortunate enough to develop these informal mentoring relationships. Women and those belonging to an ethnic minority often find it particularly difficult to find mentors informally.

- *Peer*: educators have reported that peer mentoring relationships can be very successful. With increased responsibilities of senior faculty as well as disproportionately low numbers of senior faculty, all junior faculty and trainees cannot be mentored by senior faculty effectively. Peer group mentoring can support relationship development, avoid the power issues that often accompany the use of senior mentors and compensate for the dearth of trained and willing senior mentors. It moves from a hierarchical mentoring relationship to a collaborative and mutually beneficial one.

- *Distance*: several professional organizations promote one-on-one long-distance mentoring relationships. Such mentoring usually focuses on research collaboration, but with the advent of electronic communication, it is easy for all medical educators to maintain distance relationships via telephone or email. These relationships sometimes begin when a mentor and mentee work at the same institution and continue after they move on to different organizations.

Stages of a mentoring relationship

1. Initiation phase: a mentoring relationship can be initiated spontaneously by the discovery of mutual interests or as a result of a formal mentoring programme. During this phase, the mentor and mentee should meet frequently and discuss shared goals, values and interests. This forms the settling-in period of the relationship and lets them evaluate whether there is a fit between their personalities. By the end of this period, the relationship ideally becomes open and relaxed.

2. Cultivation phase: during this phase, the work aspect of the relationship begins in earnest. Now that the mentor and mentee have a trusting relationship, it is time to set the ground rules for the

relationship. The mentor should encourage the mentee to establish career goals and list discrete tasks to achieve these goals. Together, they review these goals and activities and the mentor provides feedback, resources and networking. The mentor challenges the mentee to accomplish their academic goals and provides support for these efforts.

3. Separation phase: separation can be planned (end of training, retirement of the mentor) or unplanned (sudden departure of the mentor from an institution or illness). Planned separations are tinged with sadness, but there is time to adapt to the separation and there is also excitement about the future. Unplanned separations can lead to a sense of abandonment, anger or depression.

4. Redefining phase: a mentoring relationship can continue beyond the training period or after the mentee and mentor have moved on to different organizations. During this phase, the mentee becomes more of a peer and a successful mentoring relationship could promote lifelong friendship. Mentors who discover this stage find it most rewarding.

 All mentoring relationships go through phases 1 through 3. Phase 4 does not always happen, but when it does, it is very rewarding.

Designing mentoring programmes

The undeniable benefits of mentoring naturally lead many institutions to seek to promote it. A common strategy is to develop a mentoring programme in which faculty members are assigned to learners to serve as mentors. These 'arranged marriages' are necessary in such programmes because relying on the haphazard and unpredictable dynamic of the 'natural' development of a mentoring relationship would likely leave many learners without a mentor. Leaving mentoring relationships to develop naturally has become even more problematic with the increased pace of clinical and academic work and heightened demands on productivity. Fewer faculty members have time to mentor a learner or may see this as a luxury that will produce little institutional recognition.

Formal or planned mentoring programmes may be designed by an institution as a short-term means of attaining a specific goal and the mentor's role is defined by the goals of the programme. Unfortunately, assigned mentoring relationships can often result in a forced fit between learner and mentor that proves to be less effective than hoped for. Indeed, many of these relationships wither from neglect because they lack a foundation of shared experience or common interest.

Improving mentoring programmes

ALLOW MENTEES TO HAVE SOME INFLUENCE ON THE ASSIGNMENT OF THE MENTORS

Although it will be simplest for a programme to assign mentors, giving learners an opportunity to identify mentors from a pool of mentor candidates gives them greater input into the relationship and may improve the probabilities of a successful relationship. Giving up the control over mentor assignment requires greater flexibility on the part of the programme in recruiting an adequate pool of mentor candidates. However, doing so gives learners some opportunity to get to know the mentors. It also addresses the complication that some mentors are identified by multiple learners and others are not selected by anyone.

CLARIFY THE EXPECTATIONS OF THE RELATIONSHIP

Mentoring programmes may target differing outcomes, such as research productivity, career development, learning in a specific domain or advancement in a specific role, such as teaching. These different targets will influence the purpose and the structure of the programme and thus need to be made clear to mentors and learners.

ALLOW FOR CHANGES IN MENTORING ASSIGNMENTS

Because some assignments of mentors are likely to fail, it is important that a learner in such a relationship does not suffer as a consequence. Programmes should provide the opportunity to replace one mentor with another or even add a mentor to complement the assigned mentor's contributions.

MONITOR THE HEALTH OF THE RELATIONSHIPS

Mentoring programme administrators cannot assume that once the mentoring assignments have been made, all will turn out well. Periodic queries to both mentors and learners are essential to uncover problems in the relationship. These queries should be sensitive to the fragility of early mentoring relationships and the goals of the programme as well as those of the mentors and learners.

FOSTER COMMUNICATION

Programmes should support events and mechanisms that increase the amount and quality of communication between mentors and learners. These can include social events, scientific sessions, and periodic reminders to both mentor and learner about the importance of communication.

RECOGNIZE AND SUPPORT THE MENTORS

Too often, mentors are unsung heroes who receive little acknowledgement of their efforts. In part, this is because much of the mentor's efforts are invisible to anyone other than the mentee. Mentoring programme administrators must work diligently to ensure that mentors are recognized and rewarded appropriately, whether through public expressions of gratitude and recognition, compensation, or promotion or position. Such recognition may well require a change in the culture of the institution, which thus becomes a mandate for mentoring programme administrators.

PROVIDE STAFF DEVELOPMENT FOR MENTORS

Although some mentors are born and others are made, all can benefit from opportunities to develop their skills in aspects of the mentoring relationship. Mentoring, like many academic activities, requires a significant amount of effort, and there are those who perform this role effortlessly and effectively. But most mentors are not born with these skills and would benefit from staff development and mentoring themselves. The literature provides multiple examples of staff development initiatives for improving mentoring skills and the themes of these efforts can be described in the following 12 tips for developing mentors.

 Mentors need:

- clear expectations of their roles
- enhanced listening and feedback skills
- awareness of culture and gender issues
- to support their mentees but also challenge them
- a forum to express their uncertainties and problems
- to be aware of professional boundaries
- mentoring
- recognition
- to be rewarded
- protected time
- support
- opportunities for peer mentoring.

Evaluating mentoring and mentoring programmes

Mentoring programmes need to be evaluated frequently to ensure that they are meeting their goals and that the mentoring is successful. The same basic evaluation principles used in evaluating other educational programmes apply to mentoring programmes, and some specific issues are worth highlighting.

EVALUATING THE MENTORING PROCESS

Much of the evaluation will focus on the mentoring *process* rather than the *outcomes* of mentoring, simply because the outcomes (career success, publications, etc.) often take a very long time to manifest themselves. Some relatively simple measures of the process include frequency of meetings, length of the mentoring relationship and the number of mentors or learners who drop out of the programme. However, most process variables will reflect the perceptions, experiences and attitudes of the mentors and mentees. Questionnaires, interviews and focus groups are all appropriate methods for such data collection.

Important dimensions that could be derived from the participants include overall satisfaction with the mentoring relationship, understanding of the programme goals, expectations of the mentor or learner for the other party, identification of specific strengths and weaknesses in the relationship, suggestions for programme improvement and learner comfort in challenging the mentor or in sharing sensitive issues. The specific items included in the evaluation must reflect the goals of the programme and the fundamental characteristics of the mentoring relationship outlined earlier in this chapter.

EVALUATING THE MENTORING OUTCOMES

As noted before, the relevant outcomes to evaluate are a reflection of the purposes of the programme, but an overarching principle is that these outcomes need to be clearly identified in measurable terms. 'Achieving success in their chosen field' may be an appealing goal for a mentoring programme but is useless as an evaluation guide unless the programme can define what 'success' looks like and how it can be assessed.

That said, there are a number of common outcomes of mentoring programmes that can be mentioned. Career progression can be measured by the number of years between promotions or other landmarks, which can then be compared with other learners outside the programme. Scientific productivity as standard measures (publications, presentations, grants, etc.) can also be quantified and compared to a non-mentored group of similar learners. The development of a professional or collegial network is often a programme goal, and several innovative methods have been identified to quantify such networks and compare their development and change over time, as well as compare them to networks of non-mentored learners.

Summary

Faculty or trainees in effective mentoring relationships state that they find their professional identity and accomplish their goals faster than those without mentors. Balancing support, challenge and vision is one of the most important foundations of successful mentoring, and this should be emphasized in mentor development. Institutions should try to move away from inflexible, assigned mentoring and create an environment where spontaneous mentoring relationships can form and flourish. The traditional dyadic, senior mentor–junior protégé relationship is only one of the many types of mentoring relationships that are possible in the modern world of medical education. Mentors are not born and should be trained, supported and rewarded. Expectations of a mentoring relationship should be explicitly stated between mentors and mentees whether the focus is on research, educational or administrative areas. Lastly, mentoring programmes should be evaluated for both process and outcomes with the understanding that it may take several years to evaluate measurable outcomes.

Further reading

Balmer D, D'Alessandro D, Risko W, Gusic ME: How mentoring relationships evolve: A longitudinal study of academic pediatricians in a physician educator faculty development program, *Journal of Continuing Education in Health Professions* 31(2):81–86, 2011.

Berk RA, Berg J, Mortimer R, et al: Measuring the effectiveness of faculty mentoring relationships, *Academic Medicine* 80(1):66–71, 2005.

Bower DJ, Diehr S: Support–challenge–vision: a model for faculty mentoring, *Medical Teacher* 20:595–597, 1998.

Cho CS, Ramanan RA, Feldman MD: Defining the ideal qualities of mentorship: a qualitative analysis of the characteristics of outstanding mentors, *American Journal of Medicine* 124(5): 453–458, 2011.

Daloz L: *Effective Teaching and Mentoring: Realizing the Transformational Power of Adult Learning Experience*, San Francisco, 1996, Jossey-Bass.

Department of Health – Doctor's Forum: 2004. Mentoring for doctors: signposts to current practice for career grade doctors. Available at: http://www.academicmedicine.ac.uk/uploads/DH%20guidance.pdf

Feldman MD, Arean PA, Marshall SJ, et al: Does mentoring matter? Results from a survey of faculty mentees at a large health sciences university, *Medical Education Online* 23:15, 2010.

Hesketh EA, Laidlaw JM: Developing the teaching instinct 5: mentoring, *Medical Teacher* 25:9–12, 2003.

Omary MB: Mentoring the mentor: another tool to enhance mentorship, *Gastroenterology* 135:13–16, 2008.

Oxley J, Fleming B, Golding L, et al: 2003. Mentoring for doctors: enhancing the benefit. A working paper for the Doctors' Forum, Available at: http://www.academicmedicine.ac.uk/uploads/Mentor1.pdf

Pololi LH, Knight SM, Dennis K, Frankel RM: Helping medical school faculty realise their dreams: an innovative, collaborative mentoring program, *Academic Medicine* 77:377–384, 2002.

Sambunjak D, Straus SE, Marusic A: Mentoring in academic medicine: a systematic review, *JAMA* 296(9):1103–1115, 2006.

Sambunjak D, Straus SE, Marusic A: A systematic review of qualitative research on the meaning and characteristics of mentoring in academic medicine, *Journal of General Internal Medicine* 25:72–78, 2009.

SCOMPE (Standing Committee on Postgraduate Medical and Dental Education). Supporting doctors and dentists at work: An inquiry into mentoring, London, 1998, SCOPME.

Shea G: *Mentoring: A Practical Guide*, Normal, IL, 1997, Crisp Publications.

Tobin MJ: Mentoring: seven roles and some specifics, *American Journal of Respiratory and Critical Care Medicine* 170(2):114–117, 2004.

Section 3

Educational strategies

Outcome-based education

R. M. Harden

A move from process to product

Callahan suggested in 1998 that 'it is an odd fact of contemporary medicine that there is comparatively little discussion or debates on the goals of medicine.' Over the last 15 years there has been a dramatic change, with consideration of the competencies and abilities expected of a doctor high on the agenda. Indeed, it can be argued that the move to outcome-based education has been the most significant development in medical education in the past one or two decades: more important than the changes in educational strategies such as problem-based learning, in instructional methods such as the use of new learning technologies and in approaches to assessment including the use of portfolios. All of these are important. They are, however, a means to an end: what matters are the abilities gained by the doctor as a result of the educational experience.

 One of the most effective ways a teacher can facilitate students' learning is to discuss the expected learning outcomes with them on day one of the course.

A vision of the type of doctor to be graduated and the associated learning outcomes are the first two of the ten questions to be answered in the development of a curriculum as described in Chapter 2. Only when these have been specified can we consider the content of the curriculum, the teaching and learning methods, the educational strategies and the approach to student assessment to be adopted (Fig. 18.1).

There has been a change in emphasis from process, where what matters is the education approach, to the product, where the abilities and attitudes of the graduates are of key importance. This is the essence of outcome-based education (OBE). The use made of simulators and e-learning, team-based and interprofessional approaches to the curriculum and assessment techniques such as the OSCE and the Mini-CEX are important and are addressed in other chapters in this book. Their contribution to the education programme, however, must be guided by the expected learning outcomes.

 "A good archer is not known by his arrows but by his aim."

Thomas Fuller

The trend toward OBE

OBE is now at the cutting edge of curriculum development internationally. The 2011 and 2012 AMEE Conferences saw presentations on the topic from more than 10 countries in different regions around the world. The 4th Asia Pacific Medical Education Conference (APMEC) in Singapore had OBE as its theme. The Tuning Initiative in Europe sought to standardize learning outcomes across the different countries in Europe.

The UK General Medical Council (GMC) guidelines for medical schools, 'Tomorrow's Doctors', changed from an emphasis in 1993 on issues such as integration, problem-based learning and the abuse of lectures, to guidelines in 2003 and 2009 that highlighted the expected learning outcomes to be achieved on completion of the undergraduate course.

 "In line with current educational theory and research we (the UK General Medical Council) have adopted an outcomes-based model. This sets out what is to be achieved and assessed at the end of the medical course."

Rubin & Franchi-Christopher 2002

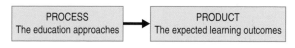

PROCESS	PRODUCT
The education approaches	The expected learning outcomes

Fig. 18.1 In OBE there is a move from an emphasis on process to an emphasis on product.

The Association of American Medical Colleges (AAMC) initiated a Medical Schools Objectives Project (MSOP) which encouraged educators to think about what was expected of medical students no matter which medical school in the United States they attended. In Canada, the CanMEDS recommendations from the Royal College of Physicians and Surgeons of Canada and in the United States, the Accreditation Council for Graduate Medical Education (ACGME) areas of competence set out the expected learning outcomes in postgraduate education.

 "… medical education is on the brink of a major paradigm shift from structure and process-based to competency-based education and measurement of outcomes."

Carraccio et al 2002

Why the move to OBE

OBE is not some passing fad that lacks an educational underpinning. While there has been some opposition to the approach, there are sound reasons for the position OBE now has at the forefront of education thinking. Here are some of the arguments for adopting OBE.

ATTENTION TO NEGLECTED AREAS OF COMPETENCE

Consideration of the expected learning outcomes for an educational programme leads to a questioning of the validity of what is currently taught, and thus possible omissions or neglected areas can be identified. These can include communication skills, clinical reasoning, decision making, self-assessment, creativity, patient safety and social responsibility: all important abilities for the practising doctor. The need to specify the abilities expected of our students on graduation and the delivery of a course of studies to achieve this is a message with which it is difficult to disagree.

THE PROBLEM OF INFORMATION OVERLOAD

Advances in medicine and the medical sciences, with the doubling of knowledge every 2 years, poses a significant problem for the medical curriculum. While the length of the course has remained relatively constant, what the student might be expected to learn has expanded hugely. No longer can we say to students, 'I cannot say precisely what I want you to learn from the course; just do your own thing.' We need to specify more clearly from the wide range of possibilities what it is we expect the student to learn.

ASSESSMENT OF THE LEARNER'S PROGRESS AND THE CONTINUUM OF EDUCATION

The need for a more seamless transition between the undergraduate, postgraduate and continuing phases of education is now accepted. Implicit in this is a clear statement of the learning outcomes expected of the student or trainee, for example, the required communication skills, prescribing skills or mastery of practical procedures, at the end of each stage before they move on to the next phase of their training. Clarity is also necessary with regard to the required achievements by learners as they progress through each phase of the training programme including the 4, 5 or 6 years of the undergraduate curriculum. It is useful to chart a student's progress towards each of the learning outcomes (Fig. 18.2).

 Learning outcomes provide a vocabulary to support the planning of the continuum of medical education across the different phases.

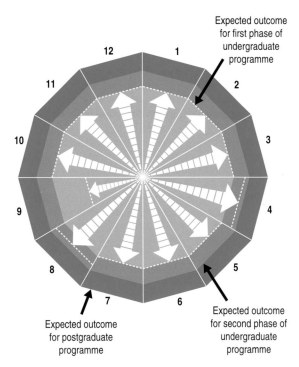

Fig. 18.2 A representation of progress by a first-phase student in relation to each of 12 learning outcome domains. The expected progress for each outcome is indicated by the inner target for the first phase of the programme, by the middle target for the second phase of the curriculum and by the outer target for postgraduate training (with permission from Harden RM: Learning outcomes as a tool to assess progression, *Medical Teacher* 29:678–682, 2007.)

The student's progress in each of the outcome domains can be looked at from different perspectives (Harden 2007):

- Increased breadth, e.g. extension to new topics or different practice contexts
- Increased difficulty, e.g. more advanced or in-depth consideration
- Increased utility and application to medical practice, e.g. a move from theory to practice and integration of what is learned into the work of a doctor
- Increased proficiency, e.g. more efficient performance with fewer errors and less need for supervision

STUDENT-CENTRED AND INDIVIDUALIZED LEARNING

 "When we talk about individualisation … we mean the ability of educational programs to adjust to meet students' and residents' learning needs and offer educational experiences that acknowledge differences in background, preparation, and rate of mastering concepts and skills, in contrast to the current one-size-fits-all approach."

Cooke et al 2010

As described in Chapters 2 and 19, there is a move to student-centred education and independent learning. A clear understanding of the required learning outcomes by the teacher and student is necessary if the student is expected to take more responsibility for his or her own learning. Standardization of learning outcomes and individualization of the learning process was one of four goals for medical education identified in the Carnegie Foundation for the Advancement of Teaching Report, Educating Physicians (Cooke et al 2010). Clearly stated learning outcomes, Cooke et al suggest, contribute to increased efficiency of education, tailoring the education to the needs of the individual learner and possibly reducing the duration of training time for a trainee.

ACCOUNTABILITY

The different stakeholders, including students, teachers, the profession, the public and government, now expect a clear statement of exit learning outcomes against which an education programme can be judged. No longer is it appropriate to see the programme as some form of 'Magical Mystery Tour' where the endpoint of training is uncertain. This is even more important at a time of financial constraint where resources may be limited.

 "There needs to be a clear definition of the end point of training and the competences which will need to be achieved."

Calman 2000

A clear statement of learning outcomes is essential to support the current emphasis on academic standards and the accreditation of the education programme of a school. Learning outcomes are also important in the recognition of excellence in education in a medical school through programmes such as the ASPIRE-to-excellence initiative (www.aspire-to-excellence.org).

Implementation of OBE

LEARNING OUTCOMES AND INSTRUCTIONAL OBJECTIVES

In OBE the learning outcomes are identified, made explicit and communicated to all concerned. Recognition of the need to provide the learner with information about the end point and direction of travel is not new. In the 1960s, promoting the use of instructional objectives, Mager asked, if one doesn't know where one is going, how can one decide how to get there? Learning outcomes differ from instructional objectives, and five important differences can be recognized (Harden 2002):

- Learning outcomes, if set out appropriately, are intuitive and user-friendly. They can be used easily in curriculum planning, in teaching and learning and in assessment.
- Learning outcomes are broad statements and are usually designed round a framework of 8–12 higher-order outcomes.
- The outcomes recognize the authentic interaction and integration in clinical practice of knowledge, skills and attitudes and the artificiality of separating these.
- Learning outcomes represent what is achieved and assessed at the end of a course of study and not only the aspirations or what is intended to be achieved.
- A design-down approach encourages ownership of the outcomes by teachers and students.

OUTCOME FRAMEWORKS

Learning outcomes are commonly presented as an agreed-upon set of domains within a framework that describes the larger picture of the abilities expected of a doctor. The move to competency-based education has much in common with outcome-based education, and competency frameworks may be similar to outcome frameworks (Albanese et al 2008).

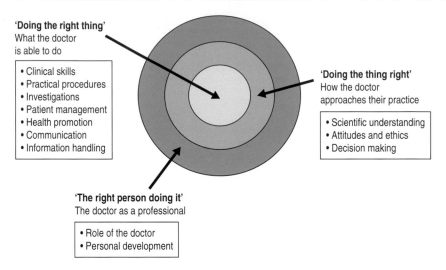

'Doing the right thing'
What the doctor
is able to do

- Clinical skills
- Practical procedures
- Investigations
- Patient management
- Health promotion
- Communication
- Information handling

'Doing the thing right'
How the doctor
approaches their practice

- Scientific understanding
- Attitudes and ethics
- Decision making

'The right person doing it'
The doctor as a professional

- Role of the doctor
- Personal development

Fig. 18.3 The Dundee three-circle framework as adopted in the Scottish Doctor with 12 learning outcome domains (from Scottish Deans' Medical Curriculum Group: *The Scottish Doctor*, 2008. AMEE, Dundee).

The Dundee three-circle model (Fig. 18.3) as adopted in the Scottish Doctor is an example of an outcome framework. It covers the following:

1. *In the inner circle (doing the right thing)*: the technical competencies – what a doctor should be able to do, as classified in seven domains, e.g. communication skills and practical skills and procedures.

2. *In the middle circle (doing the thing right)*: the intellectual, emotional and analytical competencies – how the doctor approaches his or her practice. This includes an understanding of basic and clinical sciences, appropriate attitudes and appropriate judgement and decision making.

3. *In the outer circle (the right person doing it)*: the personal intelligences – the doctor as a professional including the role of the doctor and the doctor's personal development.

The Global Minimum Essential Requirements (GMER) specification used a similar framework (Schwarz & Wojtczak 2002). The ACGME defined six general competencies thought to be common to physicians training in all specialties (Leach 2004). These are related to the Scottish Doctor outcomes in Fig. 18.4. The CanMEDS framework is based on the six physician roles: medical expert, communicator, collaborator, manager, health advocate, scholar and professional (Frank 2005). Each principal domain in an outcome or competency framework can be specified in more detail.

SELECTING OR PREPARING AN OUTCOME FRAMEWORK

When a set of learning outcomes is developed for the first time, there are the following possibilities with regard to the use of a framework:

- An existing framework, as described above, can be adopted.

- An existing framework can be modified to suit the specific needs of the education programme.

- A new framework can be developed. Any new framework should be checked against the criteria for an outcome framework as described in Table 18.1.

Table 18.1 Criteria for an outcome/competency framework

- The framework is clear, unambiguous and intuitive to the users.
- It reflects accepted and defined areas of competence.
- The vision and mission of the programme are reflected in the domains chosen.
- It is manageable in terms of the number of outcome domains (usually 6–12).
- It supports the development of enabling outcomes in each of the domains.
- The relationship between different outcomes is indicated.

	The Scottish Doctor Learning Outcomes	ACGME Outcome Project					
		a Patient Care	b Medical Knowledge	c Practice-based Learning and Improvement	d Interpersonal and Communication Skills	e Professionalism	f System-Based Practice
A	1 Clinical Skills						
	2 Practical Procedures						
	3 Patient Investigation						
	4 Patient Management						
	5 Health Promotion and Disease Prevention						
	6 Communication						
	7 Information Handling						
B	8 Scientific Basis						
	9 Attitude and Ethics						
	10 Decision Making						
C	11 Role of Doctor in Health System						
	12 Personal Development						

Fig. 18.4 THE ACGME and the Scottish Doctor learning outcomes (from Scottish Deans' Medical Curriculum Group: *The Scottish Doctor*, 2011, University of Edinburgh).

AN OUTCOME-BASED CURRICULUM

In OBE decisions about teaching and learning methods, curriculum content, educational strategies, assessment, the educational environment and even student selection should be based on the specified learning outcomes (Harden et al 2009a) (Fig. 18.5). To date, much of the attention in OBE has focussed on the specification of learning outcomes and less on the implementation of an OBE approach in practice. There are two requirements for OBE. The first is that learning outcomes are clearly defined and presented. The second is that decisions relating to the curriculum are based on the learning outcomes specified. One can infer that a programme is outcome-based only if both conditions are met (Spady 1994).

 Do not use learning outcomes as a window dressing for your courses or teaching programme. The learning outcomes need to inform the decisions you take as a teacher or trainee.

An outcome-based design sequence should be adopted in which the first step is the specification of the exit learning outcomes for the curriculum. The next step is to derive the outcomes for the different phases of the curriculum from these exit outcomes. A blueprint should then be developed relating each learning outcome for the phase to the learning opportunities and to the assessment. The process is repeated for the courses within each phase, the units within each course and the learning activities within each unit. In this 'design down' process, the outcomes for the phases, courses, units and learning activities should be aligned with and contribute to the exit outcomes.

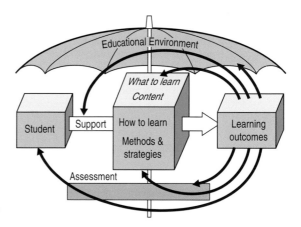

Fig. 18.5 A model for the curriculum emphasizing the importance of educational outcomes in curriculum planning (with permission from Harden et al: An introduction to outcome-based education, *Medical Teacher* 21(1):7–14, 1999).

"Teachers should be informed of and have easy access to written learning outcomes for their courses so that they can plan their teaching strategies and methods."

Subha Ramani 2006

In OBE there also has to be an acknowledgement that it is the teacher's responsibility to ensure that all students master the learning outcomes, and how this is achieved may vary from student to student.

Myths about OBE

If there is a problem with OBE, it does not rest with the principle but with how it is implemented in practice.

There are a number of misconceptions or misunderstandings about OBE:

- Some teachers are concerned that OBE is concerned with detail and that the big picture may be missed. While this may have been true with the objectives movement in the 1960s, OBE is concerned with broad parameters for competence and meta-competence (Harden et al 1999b).

- Some teachers see OBE as a threat, bringing loss of their freedom or autonomy. On the contrary, OBE does not dictate teaching methods: the existence of an agreed-upon set of outcomes empowers teachers to develop their own programme that they believe will help the student to achieve the required learning outcomes.

"There is a fine line between the competency framework that emancipates learners and that which prevents their 'expansive learning'."

Dornan 2010

- Others believe that OBE ignores trends in medical education and the move to student-centred learning. On the contrary, in OBE students are empowered and are more able to take responsibility for their own learning.

- Some teachers are concerned that OBE is about minimum competence. This need not be the situation. Learning outcomes can be specified at different levels of mastery as demonstrated in the Brown abilities (Smith & Dollase 1999).

Summary

OBE is a key development and a response to current challenges facing medical education that offers many advantages. A statement of learning outcomes pro-

vides a language or vocabulary that helps to chart the progress of students through the different phases of education and to identify a learning programme to meet their personal needs.

Only when the end point of the journey is determined can the best way to get there be decided.

Learning outcomes should be specified using an appropriate outcome framework. An existing framework can be adopted or modified or a new framework created. Using the learning framework, outcomes should be developed for each course and learning experience. Decisions about the curriculum content, teaching methods, educational strategies and assessment should be related to the agreed learning outcomes.

References

Albanese MA, Mejicano G, Mullan P, et al: Defining characteristics of educational competencies, *Medical Education* 42:248–255, 2008.

Cooke M, Irby DM, O'Brien BC: *Educating Physicians: A Call for Reform of Medical Schools and Residency*, San Francisco, 2010, Jossey-Bass.

Frank JR, editor: *The CanMEDS 2005 Physician Competency Framework. Better Standards. Better Physicians. Better Care*, Ottawa, 2005, Royal College of Physicians and Surgeons of Canada.

Harden RM: Learning outcomes and instructional objectives: is there a difference? *Medical Teacher* 24:151–155, 2002.

Harden RM: Learning outcomes as a tool to assess progression, *Medical Teacher* 29:678–682, 2007.

Harden RM, Crosby JR, Davis MH: An introduction to outcome-based education, *Medical Teacher* 21(1): 7–14, 1999a.

Harden RM, Crosby JR, Davis MH, Friedman M: From competency to meta-competency: a model for the specification of learning outcomes, *Medical Teacher* 21(6):546–552, 1999b.

Leach DC: A model for GME: shifting from process to outcomes. A progress report from the Accreditation Council for Graduate Medical Education, *Medical Education* 38(1):12–14, 2004.

Schwarz MR, Wojtczak A: Global minimum essential requirements: a road towards competency-oriented medical education, *Medical Teacher* 24:125–129, 2002.

Smith SR, Dollase R: Planning, implementing and evaluating a competency-based curriculum, *Medical Teacher* 21(1):15–22, 1999.

Spady WG: *Outcome-Based Education: Critical Issues and Answers*, Arlington, VA, 1994, The American Association of School Administrators.

Independent learning and study skills

R. C. Bandaranayake, R. M. Harden

Introduction

Other chapters in this book look at how students learn in large- and small-group settings and 'on the job' working with their colleagues. In all three phases of the continuum of medical education – undergraduate, postgraduate and continuing – learners spend a significant portion of their time learning on their own. The formal learning in the taught part of any educational programme may represent only a small part of the total learning of the student.

Independent learning may follow a lecture, precede or follow a small-group session and follow a clinical learning session. The intensity of independent learning is highest in the short period before a formal examination, in preparation for the latter. In distance learning programmes the predominant activity is independent learning.

> *"Self-instruction may be an alternative to other forms of teaching, but it can also be combined with them."*
>
> *Rowntree 1990*

The importance of the deliberate inculcation of the skills of independent learning is often not fully recognized in the undergraduate curriculum. In most instances the only recognition it is given is in the provision of a list of recommended textbooks.

In this chapter we will consider:

- what we mean by independent learning and study skills
- the important role they play in any curriculum
- component skills in self study
- the development of a study plan
- the effective use of learning resources for independent study
- the teacher's role in independent learning

- how the student can review prior learning effectively
- how the student can undertake self-assessment
- some trends in independent learning.

What are independent learning and study skills?

The concept of independent learning means different things to different people. It incorporates six key principles:

- Students learn on their own.
- Students have a measure of control over their own learning, in that they choose:
  - where to learn (deciding the context of learning)
  - what to learn (diagnosing personal learning needs)
  - how to learn (identifying methods and resources)
  - when to learn (deciding time and pacing).

Think about the extent to which student control of their learning would, in your subjects, be advantageous.

- Students may be encouraged to develop their personal study plans (Challis 2000).
- Differing needs of individual students are recognized and responded to appropriately.
- Learning is supported by learning resources and study guides prepared specifically for this purpose
- The role of the teacher changes from transmitter of information to manager of the learning process: a more demanding but a more rewarding role (Harden & Crosby 2000).

Many terms are used, often interchangeably, though different meanings may be implied, to describe this approach to learning:

- Independent learning: emphasizes that students work on their own to meet their own learning needs.
- Self-managed learning, self-directed learning or self-regulated learning: emphasizes that students have an element of control over their own learning, with responsibility for diagnosis of learning needs, identifying resources and assessing the degree of learning by themselves. Implicit in this approach is that students have a clear understanding of the intended learning outcomes.
- Resource-based learning: emphasizes the use of resource material in print or multimedia format as a basis for students' learning and the freedom this gives the students.
- 'Just-for-you' or flexible learning: emphasizes the wide range of learning opportunities offered to students and flexibility in responding to individual student needs and aspirations.

 "Flexible learning is a generic term that covers all these situations where learners have some say in how, where or when learning takes place."

Ellington 1997

- Open learning: is often used interchangeably with flexible learning. It emphasizes the provision of greater access for students to their choice of education.
- E-learning: learning is facilitated by information and communication technology.
- Distance learning: emphasizes that students work on their own at a distance from their teacher. Implicit in this approach is that the teacher interacts with students at a distance and facilitates the students' learning.
- 'Just-in-time' learning: resources are made available to learners when required. This facilitates 'on-the-job' learning and the integration of theory and practice.

The two ideas underpinning the above concepts are:

- learners study individually on their own
- learners take charge of the learning process.

Both these features are absent in the lecture but present in independent learning (Fig. 19.1).

In most areas of science, knowledge grows exponentially, and medicine is no exception. With increasing knowledge it is imperative for medical students to develop sound learning habits which will stand them

in good stead throughout their professional life. Such habits include the selection of what is learnt as well as how it is learnt. The latter is one factor which determines whether what is learnt will be remembered long enough to become part of the student's repertoire of knowledge (long-term memory) or will be discarded as soon as it ceases to be of immediate use (short-term memory).

Study skills are those skills which a student should possess in order to undertake independent learning effectively and efficiently. They consist of the following components:

- self-directed learning
- learning with understanding (deep learning), leading to long-term retention, rather than through rote (surface) learning, which is likely to result in short-term retention
- seeking and retrieving information from an increasing variety of resources
- critically reviewing what is read, rather than blindly accepting the written word
- integrating new learning with existing knowledge by seeking links between them, and dealing with dissonance
- assessing oneself on learning that has occurred to ensure that it can be remembered and applied to situations likely to be encountered in professional practice.

Why is independent learning important?

Learning is continuous, with new learning built on what has already been learned. Medical education is a continuum which starts at entry to medical school and ends with cessation of professional practice. Only a

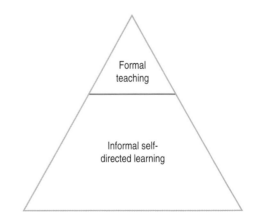

Fig. 19.1 Students make choices in independent learning.

relatively small, though important, part of this continuum takes place in the undergraduate medical school. However, both the content of what is learnt and the process of learning make a significant impact on the remaining phases of the continuum. The future doctor must learn to cope with the ever-expanding body of knowledge in a lifetime of continuing practice.

ACTIVE LEARNING

The independent learner who is properly guided has the opportunity to develop these component skills while in medical school, while adopting a more active approach to learning. Students adopt a deep rather than a superficial approach to learning and search for an understanding of the subject rather than just reproducing what they have learned. They are encouraged to think rather than just recall facts. A learning approach does not describe a particular attribute of the student, but a relationship between the learner and the learning task (Ramsden 1987).

Study skill courses should focus on developing students' awareness of these approaches so that they could select that which is most suited to a given learning task. Superficial reading of text does not guarantee that what is read, and even understood, will be retained in long-term memory. While the most efficient reader may be the 'one who can gather the most amount of information from the printed page in the least amount of time' (Wilcox 1958), he or she may not be the most effective learner, as much of that information may be retained for only a short time. The reflective process involved in the deep approach to learning may, ostensibly, be more time-consuming. However, longer retention of learning makes this approach more effective in the long term. One reason why students complain of the tedious nature of basic science courses may be the lack of time and opportunity for reflection. Students must develop the practice of reflecting on the subject matter, connecting it with what they already know and summarizing new learning in their own words.

 "The best way to learn to appreciate and understand scientific method is to practice until it becomes habitual."

Smith et al 1951

Few would disagree that the attributes and study skills we would desire in a medical student are those embedded in the deep approach to learning. However, many curricula are planned and implemented in ways that promote surface or strategic approaches (Stiernborg & Bandaranayake 1996). The surge of curricula adopting problem-based learning to varying extents favours the deep approach (Newble & Clarke 1987), though the nature of the curriculum does not necessarily dictate the manner in which students undertake self-study in that curriculum. There is no reason, however, for not inculcating a deep approach even in the more conventional curricula. Students accustomed to surface learning may have initial difficulty adopting a deep approach. Effective ways of reflecting on newly learned material are writing essays, discussion with peers, teaching others and entertaining questions.

The traditional curriculum emphasizes the views on a topic of the teacher or lecturer with whom the student is in contact. The student may be seduced into the notion that there is one right answer or one approach to a problem. Independent learning allows him or her to be exposed to the rich environment of many visions and interpretations.

 "Uncertainty should not be hidden away as an embarrassment."

Alderson & Roberts 2000

THE NEEDS OF THE INDIVIDUAL LEARNER

Learners are not a homogeneous group: they have different needs and different aspirations and learn in different ways. For example, in anatomy, learning may best occur for different students through:

- dissection
- prosected specimens
- projected images
- two-dimensional pictures, or
- printed text.

The adoption of an independent learning approach encourages these needs to be recognized and allows for learner choice in terms of content, learning strategy and rates of learning (Fig. 19.2). In 'just-for-you' learning the learning programme is customized to the needs of the individual student or doctor.

 Provide a variety of learning experiences for your students when you help them learn a given topic.

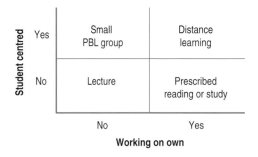

Fig. 19.2 Control of learning by student.

Methods are determined by:

* type of learning objective
* individual preferences and style
* practicalities of a given situation
* priorities in the purpose of learning
* time available for learning.

Students, with the assistance of the teacher, can choose the learning method or approach which suits them best. They can skim material rapidly if they already understand it and spend more time with what is new or challenging to them.

In mastery learning students work with appropriate resource material until they reach the level of mastery required. The key to the development of any skill is practise until perfection is achieved. This applies to both cognitive and psychomotor skills.

STUDENT MOTIVATION

Independent learning gives students more responsibility for their learning and greater participation in the learning process. It allows them to choose the appropriate level for their studies. This in turn gives them a sense of ownership of their learning, which has a positive effect on their motivation. Readiness for learning depends on intrinsic motivation, an inner urge to learn, as well as the acquisition of prerequisite learning on which new learning is built.

Learning occurs as new material is related to previously learned material. If the steps are properly sequenced and studies undertaken accordingly, both horizontal and vertical integration will be facilitated. In other words, the learner will be able to see the links in progressive learning as well as among parallel learning in related areas. Often, lack of synchronization across disciplines hinders horizontal integration between them. The student must learn to develop a study plan (see below) which brings these relationships to the fore, even if it may not correspond to the school's formal timetable.

NEW LEARNING TECHNOLOGIES

 "Web and Internet technologies are transforming our world, presenting opportunities we could only imagine a few years ago."

Horton 2001

Developments in new learning technologies and e-learning are occurring at an astonishingly rapid pace, with profound implications for medical schools (Masters & Ellaway 2008). In addition to the use of the internet, personal digital assistants (PDAs), MP3 players and mobile phones can play podcasts or vodcasts of lectures and tutorials for use by the student

at a time and place convenient to him or her. The potential for the new learning technologies, including their support for the independent learner, is described in Chapters 27 and 28. The development of new social software that allows students to generate their own context and share this with their colleagues supports a more personalized and support-centred view of learning.

 Social networking sites provide several combined features, including instant messaging and logs and could be used to develop personalized learning.

DISTANCE AND BLENDED LEARNING

With the development of e-learning, distance learning has increased in popularity in undergraduate, postgraduate and continuing education. The CRISIS criteria for effective continuing education, developed in the context of distance learning, recognize the potential advantages implicit in independent learning (Harden & Laidlaw 1992):

* Convenience for the student in terms of pace, place and time ('just-in-time' learning)
* Relevance to the needs of the practising doctor
* Individualization to the needs of each learner ('just-for-you' learning)
* Self-assessment by the learner of his or her own competence
* Interest in the programme and motivation of the learner
* Systematic coverage of the topic or theme for the programme.

A blended approach can be adopted where e-learning is combined with face-to-face learning to create an integrated learning experience.

Developing a study plan

 "Systematic methods of learning may require more effort and patience in the beginning, but soon they become habitual and effective."

Smith et al 1951

The medical student, constantly faced with new areas for learning across a spectrum of subjects, must develop a study plan for each significant period of time, such as a week. Often subjects are not organized in a way that enables the student to see the links between them. In some curricula, integration among subjects is achieved through themes, such as organ systems or clinical problems. Yet the student must learn to establish priorities for study, based not on expediency but on importance, difficulty and timeliness. These three characteristics are analysed using 'renal function' as an example.

Importance must be judged in terms of:

- usefulness for professional practice (e.g. understanding how urine is formed is essential for dealing with urinary disorders)
- the degree of understanding required for further learning (e.g. movement of sodium ions for understanding how urine is formed by the nephron)
- the place of new learning in the unfolding of a continuing story (e.g. pathological conditions which affect the nephron and its effects on urine formation).

Difficulty depends on:

- the existence of prerequisite learning (e.g. basic types of epithelia and their functional significance)
- the predilection of the individual for the subject
- the level of abstraction of the subject (e.g. the conceptual nature of the renal countercurrent theory)
- the degree and nature of the initial exposure to the subject.

Each student has to learn to identify areas of individual difficulty and plan study in such a way as to devote more time to such areas.

Timeliness relates to a number of factors, which include:

- readiness for the next phase of study, i.e. what is about to be learnt is considered prerequisite to what is to follow (e.g. histology is prerequisite to histopathology)
- synchronization among different subject areas related to a common integrating theme (e.g. structure and function of the nephron)
- assessment points during the course of study which drive the student to concentrate on certain areas.

This includes the basic skills of language and communication and the ability of the learner to identify discrepancies between what he or she knows and does not know.

In developing a study plan, the student must:

- identify the focus of study
- determine the depth to which study of a particular topic is to be undertaken
- understand the interrelationships of topics by designing a logical sequence of topics for study.

Focus of study is determined by learning objectives. However, a student confronted with a daunting array of objectives must determine priorities among them, based on their relative importance for progressive learning and for future application, and on perceived gaps in knowledge which hinder further learning.

Depth of study is that which is required for understanding and depends on the complexity of the subject matter. As this cannot often be judged prior to actually undertaking study, the student must build into the plan study time in proportion to the relative difficulty of each subject area as experienced previously. The temptation to memorize without understanding should be resisted.

Practice of psychomotor skills is a three-stage process of:

1. observation of a demonstration
2. practise under supervision
3. independent practice until perfect.

In the clinical situation the last step depends on the student's initiative and industry. Recent development of clinical skills laboratories has contributed to expansion of the opportunities available to students to hone their clinical skills. The mere availability of a clinical skills laboratory does not guarantee its adequate use. Students must be encouraged, and time set apart, to use the laboratory under supervision.

 When you have demonstrated a clinical skill to your students, let each in turn practise it under your supervision and then encourage them to practise it by themselves.

Resources for study

 "Learning may be enhanced if a variety of presentation methods is used with students. ... Learning occurs when students use a combination of senses."

Lock 1981

For the individual student, multiple stimuli aid learning as long as there is no dissonance among them. For example, when concepts are presented as descriptive text, graphs and three-dimensional models, students are better able to grasp them. Learning which is reinforced by multiple stimuli is likely to be retained longer.

A skill of paramount importance to the medical student during a lifetime of continuing education is the ability to seek, retrieve and store information. Students must learn to undertake this task efficiently early in their medical education. Many, not having acquired these skills during secondary education, need training in them. While orientation courses at entry to medical school include visits to libraries, relatively few include training in these skills. Locating information from different sources includes the skills of using library filing systems, referring to indices, scanning reading material to determine relevance and importance and referencing for subsequent easy retrieval (Saunders et al 1984).

The tendency to accumulate photocopied material for later use without adequate discrimination should be avoided. Immediate study of the material, highlighting important points and noting them on index cards would save hours of wading through piles of accumulated material subsequently.

With the increasing use of computers in learning, it is now mandatory for the medical student to develop skills in locating and retrieving information from the internet and exercising discrimination by critically evaluating what they are able to retrieve from this valuable source.

 Give your students assignments which require them to study beyond their textbooks and class notes.

There has been a trend towards modularity and flexibility in curriculum planning. Students, individually or in small groups, may rotate through a series of attachments. The advantages of resource material to support the students' learning can help to ensure that different groups receive a similar educational experience and the time-consuming and unnecessary repetition of lectures by staff is avoided. Different groups of students may use the same resource pack and study guide, leaving the teacher free for one-to-one contact with students. In electives or special study modules, where students can choose to study areas in more depth, independent learning has a useful role to play.

The role of the teacher

There is pressure on academic staff to provide coherent and effective teaching and learning programmes despite increasing student numbers and decreasing units of resource. A greater emphasis on independent learning and the sharing of learning resources between institutions can make a contribution. This may be associated with a changing role for the teacher.

The teacher's role as a manager of the students' learning is well accepted and consistent with an independent learning approach (Harden & Crosby 2000). This facilitative role leaves teachers time for more contact with individual students. While many teachers feel most comfortable in the traditional role of lecturing, others have discovered talents in developing resource material, a role which is increasingly being recognized and rewarded.

 In staff development programmes consider the different roles of the teacher in relation to independent learning: the 'guide on the side' and the creator of learning resource material.

Teachers have an important role to play in fostering deep learning among students undertaking self-study. They must devise assignments which compel students to reflect on their learning. Such reflection is encouraged by requiring students to apply their new learning to problems and situations which they have not encountered hitherto. Teachers must also help students relate such learning to their personal goals to enhance motivation.

 In clinical teaching, challenge students with problem-solving exercises based not only on what they know, but also on what they should but do not know.

Review of learning

Review and application of new learning must take place periodically if it is to be built into the student's cognitive framework. Memory is enhanced not only by actively seeking links between new learning and previous learning and experience, but also by deriving logical associations among areas of new learning. For example, the student who is learning about renal function for the first time should seek relationships, on the one hand, with the circulatory system (which may have been learnt earlier) and, on the other, with the microscopic structure of the nephron (which may be introduced at the same time). This helps in acquisition of the new learning as well as review of the old.

 Encourage the student to link the subject you teach with related learning outside your specialty.

In reviewing learning, the student is often confronted with the problem of deciding what topics are important for review. Importance is a matter of perception: to the practitioner, that which is applicable to practice is important; to the teacher, it is that which is essential for understanding the subject; to the student, it is that which is likely to be examined.

In a course which aims to prepare future professionals, rationality dictates that importance be related to practice. However, preparation for practice without understanding the basis of that practice merely results in a technician rather than a professional. Hence emphasis should be placed on understanding the basic sciences rather than memorizing that which is applicable.

Many problem-centred curricula adopt the concept of the spiral problem. The same problem is introduced at increasingly complex levels during successive phases of the curriculum. This helps the student identify content which is considered important for review. When the same content is required for different problems, opportunities are provided for students to review and practise its application in different situations.

"Relevance aids retention of information by increasing motivation to learn as well as by its potential for the learner to make meaningful applications of what is learnt as learning progresses."

Bandaranayake 2011

Constantly encourage students to recall the basic science concepts underlying the clinical knowledge and skills they encounter

A useful technique for review is to organize information that has been learnt into chunks, around certain principles, generalizations or cues. These form pegs on which more detailed information may be hung. Such organization aids easy retrieval of the information, as the pegs are more easily recalled. Thus the student learning about the joints of the body may remember a few principles which govern classification of joints in relation to movement. Even if the details pertaining to a particular joint may be forgotten, recalling the principles would facilitate their retrieval. A student learning about the central connections of the cranial nerves would be aided by categorizing cranial nerve nuclei into functional sets, based on their positions in the developing neural tube. Based on the function of each cranial nerve, then, the student would be able to either recall or work out the positions of its central connections.

Assessment of learning

Assessing oneself is perhaps the most difficult, yet most important, skill that must be undertaken for effective study. Active participation in the process of learning requires insight into one's strengths and weaknesses through self-analysis. Development takes place through capitalizing on strengths and eliminating weaknesses. To identify deficiencies one must not only be a good judge of oneself, but also be aware that a deficiency exists. Students who are coached by a teacher have these deficiencies pointed out to them; those studying in groups are often helped thus by their peers; the individual learner, however, has to depend on certain cues, such as an inability to understand a difficult topic, to identify deficiencies in prior learning. A sound practice is to test oneself on what one has just read using pre-designed questions or

exercises. Frequent reviews help students follow their progress.

Formative assessment is now a regular feature of many medical curricula. Unfortunately, it is often misused in that feedback from such assessment is not provided to students in a way which helps them identify deficiencies. In many instances, formative assessment consists of a series of summative exercises, which contribute to a final grade on which pass–fail decisions are based. While such a practice has the advantage of increased sampling of topics tested, it fails to serve a formative purpose. The problem is compounded by students attempting to hide rather than display their weaknesses, as they are aware of the important decisions that are based on the results.

When you teach, question your students regularly, but react to their responses in such a way that they feel comfortable to display, rather than hide, deficiencies. Only then will they be able to take remedial action.

If student assessment is to play a role in helping students learn, class tests conducted before and during a unit should provide feedback detailed enough to point out areas or skills where deficiencies in learning exist.

It is well known that assessment is the strongest motivator of student learning. While this is unfortunate, teachers should capitalize on this fact and set tests which call upon the students' higher cognitive skills, rather than on the ability to reproduce what is learnt. Assessment should encourage students to search for application of what they learn both in their personal lives and in the context of their future practice, and test their ability to discriminate between fact and opinion, and between assumption and established truth. The critical appraisal of ideas should be an essential ingredient of the total assessment package, as should the ability to gather information pertaining to a given problem.

Unfortunately, most tests in medical education call upon the lower cognitive skills of recall and recognition. We fail to harness the greatest motivator of student learning to bring about desirable learning habits in our medical students. Most study skill courses aim at helping students pass these types of examinations rather than pursue learning which would arm them with the skills and attributes for a lifetime of continuing education.

Trends in independent learning

"The only man who is educated is the man who has learned how to learn."

Rogers 1983

Independent learning is not new. To a greater or lesser extent, students have always worked independently. One can identify, however, a number of changes in current approaches to independent learning, many triggered by developments in e-learning.

It was demonstrated four decades ago in a randomized controlled trial (Harden et al 1969) that medical students learn as or more effectively when they work independently, using learning resources prepared for the purpose, compared with students who attend lectures. Until recently, however, teachers have been slow to move away from an emphasis on lectures. There has been a significant change, however, with independent learning playing an increasingly important role in the curriculum:

- Time previously scheduled for lectures or small-group work is often rescheduled for independent learning.

- Independent learning is now an explicit planned part of the learning activities, and protected time is allocated for it in the timetable.

- The role of the lecture is changing to lend support to independent learning, rather than independent learning being used as an adjunct to support the lecture.

- Students make increasing use of the internet as a learning resource.

Summary

Independent learning has to be carefully planned and not left to chance. The choice is not between a planned programme including lectures and other scheduled activities and students being left to fend for themselves and using any learning resources they can find. Planning by the teacher for independent learning includes:

- Recognizing the role of independent learning in the curriculum, making this explicit to students and scheduling it in the timetable

- Ensuring students have the necessary study skills with which to engage in independent learning in the first instance. Study skills training may include:
  - how to assess needs
  - how to plan learning
  - how to manage study time
  - how to locate and use appropriate resources
  - how to evaluate outcomes of learning
- Identifying the resources to be used by students in their studies, including textbooks, e-learning resources and skills laboratories.

The adoption of independent learning does not imply that the teacher abandons the student to work on his or her own. The role of the teacher as a facilitator in independent learning is important. This can be achieved through interactions between the student and the teacher, face-to-face, by telephone or on the internet. The teacher can also prepare study guides to support the student's learning.

 "A study guide can be seen as a management tool which allows teachers to exercise their responsibilities while at the same time giving students an important part to play in managing their own learning."

Harden et al 1999

A weekly plan of study designed by the student should be based on priorities determined by the importance of the topic for both understanding and application, its relative difficulty and its timeliness. The student should be helped to make decisions with regard to the focus of study as determined by objectives, its depth for understanding and its sequence. While teachers should ensure that students are exposed to a variety of sources for studying a given topic, the individual nature of learning determines which of these is optimal for a given student. Study skills courses should utilize recent findings on the relationship between the learner and the learning task to inform students of the different approaches to learning and help each of them select that which is best suited for a given topic.

Opportunities for repeated independent practice of both cognitive and psychomotor skills should be provided, the former through assignments which call upon the student to apply learning to unfamiliar situations, and the latter through such facilities as skill laboratories. Review of learning should emphasize links between concurrently and progressively learnt topics, thereby promoting horizontal and vertical integration. Formative assessment by teachers, peers and self should be geared to providing feedback on individual strengths and weaknesses. The powerful effect summative assessment has on driving student learning should be capitalized on to promote desirable learning habits by testing higher cognitive skills in examinations.

References

Alderson P, Roberts I: Should journals publish reviews that find no evidence to guide practice? *British Medical Journal* 320:376–377, 2000.

Bandaranayake RC: *The Integrated Medical Curriculum*, London, 2011, Radcliffe Publishing, p 70,

Challis M: AMEE Medical Education Guide no. 18. Personal learning plans, *Medical Teacher* 22(3):225–236, 2000.

Ellington H: Flexible learning – your flexible friend! Keynote address. In Bell C, Bowden M, Trott A, editors: *Implementing Flexible Learning. Aspects of Educational and Training Technology*, vol XXIX, London, 1997, Kogan Page, pp 3–13,

Harden RM, Laidlaw JM: Effective continuing education: the CRISIS criteria. AMEE Medical Education Guide no. 4, *Medical Education* 26:408–422, 1992.

Harden RM, Laidlaw JM, Hesketh EA: AMEE Medical Education Guide no. 16. Study guides – their use and preparation, *Medical Teacher* 21(3):248–265, 1999.

Harden RMcG, Dunn WR, Holroyd C, et al: An experiment involving substitution of tape/slide programmes for lectures, *Lancet* 1:933–935, 1969.

Harden RM, Crosby JR: AMEE Education Guide no. 20. The good teacher is more than a lecturer – the twelve roles of the teacher, *Medical Teacher* 22(4):334–347, 2000.

Horton W: *Leading E-learning*, Alexandria, VA, 2001, American Society for Training and Development (ASTD), pp 130–131.

Lock C: *Study Skills*, 1981, Kappa Delta Pi Northeastern University Publishing Group.

Masters K, Ellaway R: e-Learning in medical education. Guide 32 Part 2: Technology, management and design, *Medical Teacher* 30(5):474–489, 2008.

Newble D, Clarke R: Approaches to learning in a traditional and an innovative medical school. In Richardson JTE, Eysenck MW, Piper DW, editors: *Student Learning: Research in Education and Cognitive Psychology*, Milton Keynes, 1987, Society for Research into Higher Education and Open University.

Ramsden P: Improving teaching and learning in higher education: the case for a relational perspective, *Studies in Higher Education* 12:275–286, 1987.

Rogers C: *Freedom to Learn for the 80s*, Columbus, OH, 1983, Charles E Merrill.

Rowntree D: *Teaching Through Self-Instruction: How to Develop Open Learning Materials*, London, 1990, Kogan Page.

Saunders K, Northup DE, Mennin SP: The library in a problem-based curriculum. In Kaufman A, editor: *Implementing Problem-Based Medical Education*, New York, 1984, Springer.

Smith S, Shores L, Brittain R: *An Outline of Best Methods of Study*, ed 2, New York, 1951, Barnes & Noble.

Stiernborg M, Bandaranayake RC: Medical students' approaches to studying, *Medical Teacher* 18:229–236, 1996.

Wilcox GW: *Basic Study Skills*, Boston, 1958, Allyn & Bacon.

Further reading

Collins R, Hammond M: Self-directed learning to educate medical educators: why do we use self-directed learning? *Medical Teacher* 9(4):425–432, 1987.

Ross MT, Cameron HS: Peer assisted learning: a planning and implementation framework: AMEE Guide no. 30, *Medical Teacher* 29(6):527–545, 2007.

Problem-based learning

A. E. Sefton, M. Frommer

Introduction

Problem-based learning (PBL), now widely adopted in medical programmes internationally, was developed at McMaster University Medical School over 40 years ago. PBL has proved to be effective in promoting active learning, collaboration, communication skills and critical thinking. The principles of PBL have been applied in a variety of other health-related programmes (Dangerfield et al 2009).

What is PBL?

The term 'PBL' means different things in different medical schools, and the diversity of approaches can be represented as a continuum (Harden & Davis 1998). The defining characteristic is that a small group of students is presented with a problem to solve and a structured approach to solving it. The design varies greatly among institutions and with the students' experience or seniority. A problem usually centres on the clinical presentation of one or a few patients (e.g. an individual with Parkinsonism, a child with a metabolic disorder and the child's parents, or a couple presenting with infertility). The problem is usually introduced as an illustrated description of a realistic clinical presentation, but sometimes PBL is conducted in clinical settings with real patients.

The main objectives of PBL are to develop group learning practices; assist students in understanding and learning curriculum content; and support students in gaining skills for problem-solving and reasoning that they will be able to apply in their professional lives. In addition, PBL can enhance the quality of professional communication and collegial interaction.

"A particular goal of this student-centred, problem-based approach is to develop physicians who practice 'science in action' rather than attempting to apply learned formulas to clinical situations."

Tosteson et al 1994

PBL often starts with a vignette summarizing the clinical presentation. At first, students do not have sufficient knowledge to proceed easily: they are deliberately confronted with a problem they cannot solve. By working collectively, they identify key elements and seek out additional information, enabling them to suggest causal hypotheses and identify possible pathophysiological mechanisms. At the start, students are encouraged to think broadly about alternative hypotheses, mechanisms and the sociocultural context. They then refine and test their hypotheses in order to arrive at the most likely explanation. Thus, students are supported as they learn about multiple dimensions of a topic in medicine, greatly enriching and diversifying their learning experiences, especially when they can link PBL to other learning (Dangerfield et al 2009).

In most PBL programmes, a tutor sits in with each group of students for some or all of the problem-solving process. The tutor monitors, facilitates, steers and assists the group learning process and may act as a resource.

Key features and strengths of PBL

PBL is an example of active learning. In contrast to rote learning and memorization, active learning involves interaction, pursuing information, collaborative problem-solving, sharing of ideas, evolving and testing hypotheses. The group collectively gains skills and finds solutions. Thus PBL models effective medical teamwork and communication. Students agree to follow up on specific issues individually or in groups, identifying and sharing information with colleagues. The success of PBL is attributed to the opportunities that it creates to activate and elaborate knowledge in the group situation (Schmidt et al 2011).

PBL processes encourage and support students' learning about multiple dimensions of a medical topic. While the set problem is often precisely defined, it leads students to extend their thinking and examine alternatives.

Some medical topics lend themselves to PBL, while others may not. Obviously, a medical curriculum cannot be covered comprehensively with PBL that is most effective for topics readily 'packaged' into illustrative cases. Even the most circumscribed cases can generate discussion on a broad range of related issues, and a balance must be found between freedom of exploration and allowing the educational messages to become too diffuse.

The PBL problem can be presented in many stimulating ways. The use of an image or video clip of the hypothetical patient can entice students to make careful observations, identify clinical cues, test ideas and note issues for follow-up study. Students particularly enjoy opportunities to develop clinical skills relevant to a PBL case and to engage with real patients who have analogous problems.

Roles, qualifications and training of PBL tutors

The specific roles of tutors vary among medical schools. In general, the tutor's role is to facilitate, encourage active learning and promote collaboration on relevant ideas and concepts. Tutors are trained: they do not impart information or provide ready answers. In a well-functioning group, students themselves actively identify issues, share information and seek clarity on difficult concepts (Woods 1994). Tutors are usually expected to adapt their approach to the level of the students' learning, the quality of the PBL group's interactions and the nature of the current problem.

 To become a confident tutor:
- first observe a class
- access staff training and development (usually mandatory)
- review the sequence of problems
- study tutor guides, websites and relevant literature
- understand requirements for assessment.

Tutors often differ markedly in their backgrounds, qualifications, experience and styles of interaction. The need to select only medically trained tutors is often debated, and recruitment of medical teachers from a range of disciplines is recommended (Norman 2011). Students generally prefer medical graduates as tutors, provided that they respect the need to facilitate group learning, avoiding domination and didacticism. Tutors are not expected to be content experts. Rather, they should have a level of knowledge sufficient to keep the discussion focused and to identify gaps and errors in covering the topic. Tutors need to

ensure that students understand and can summarize key issues.

Tutor training is essential: even experienced medical teachers may be unfamiliar with PBL. They need advice on facilitating and monitoring the group learning process and resolving tensions within a group. Indeed, training is usually mandatory for all new PBL tutors. Training workshops usually provide information on the curriculum context of the PBL sessions, tutors' responsibilities and expectations of students' roles and contributions. Where possible, new tutors observe a few sessions with an established, effective PBL tutor. Tutors are also briefed and/or given written information on the content of each problem.

PBL groups typically meet for about 90 minutes with their tutor in each session. In some programmes, two or three PBL sessions are scheduled each week, but different patterns have emerged. Once the students are inducted into the PBL process, a session can be wholly or partially run by the students, who are supported with some training. Indeed, when students become familiar with the PBL process, the tutor need not be present throughout.

Introduction of PBL problems

The problem or case can be introduced in different ways. If a real patient is the subject of a PBL, the process may begin with a short summary of his or her clinical presentation. If the problem is based on a hypothetical patient, the process begins with a trigger statement that briefly summarizes the characteristics, clinical presentation and circumstances (Box 20.1). The trigger statement may be read out by a student or the tutor, played from a recording or presented as a photograph or computer image to encourage observation. Typically, a recording of the trigger statement

> **Box 20.1 Example of a trigger statement on a hypothetical patient (problem)**
>
> You are an intern on evening duty in the emergency department of a regional hospital when a 65-year-old farmer is brought in by his wife. He has had central chest pain for two hours. The pain radiates to his neck, and he feels nauseated and generally unwell. The pain came on when he was parking his tractor for the night. He looks pale and anxious. He had a similar episode two weeks ago, but it was less severe and of shorter duration, and it resolved spontaneously when he sat down for half of hour.
>
> *Image: A pale, anxious-looking middle-aged man lying on a hospital trolley with his right hand over the centre of his chest. He is wearing nasal prongs (for oxygen). A young woman wearing scrubs marked 'Doctor' is inserting an intravenous cannula in his left arm.*

is played from a computer while a digital image is shown on the screen.

The students examine the trigger statement and image, identifying 'cues' about the case. Students collectively observe and interpret the images that provide the context. They contribute ideas, suggesting and noting relevant information, and then identifying issues to be explored. Group members typically take turns acting as scribe, summarizing ideas on a whiteboard, a computer or paper (Visschers-Pleijers et al 2006). In an effective tutorial, a lively exchange of information and ideas ensues as students identify issues and explore possible mechanisms. The desirable form of the interaction within a PBL group is depicted in Fig. 20.1. Effective tutors avoid taking a traditional didactic teaching role, such as that depicted in Fig. 20.2. The original PBL design assumed that, after a tutorial, students would locate and identify useful information to bring back to the next session, thereby progressing to resolve the problem. However, in recent years, the widespread use of portable computers and handheld devices, with immediate access to published literature and other information sources, has compressed the task of inquiry. Members of PBL groups now find information almost instantaneously during a session, bringing it into the discussion without delay. This is a potentially valuable addition to the learning opportunities of PBL, provided that students' interactions with their computers do not weaken the group interaction. It is important, however, that students do not fall into the habit of uncritically accepting information from electronic sources that are not critically reviewed.

Out of the PBL session, students often work together in informal study groups, sharing understanding and knowledge.

A range of activities and resources relevant to the current problem support students' learning. These may include discussion sessions, seminars, some relevant lectures and practical laboratory classes as well as hospital-based clinical tutorials, communication sessions and demonstrations. Where possible, hospital-based teaching is programmed to coincide with the PBL topics. Staff offer advice on sources of information or facilitate access to learning resources in the medical school or in a community setting. Well-designed online materials can supplement the learning, whether developed 'in house' or acquired commercially.

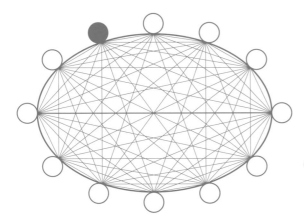

Fig. 20.1 A PBL group: possible interactions.

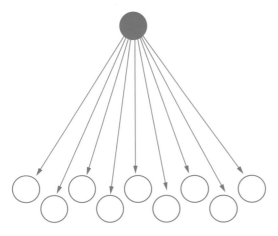

Fig. 20.2 Didactic teaching.

An effective tutor:

- is well-prepared and understands the goals and tutorial processes
- maintains a friendly and open atmosphere
- recognizes characteristics and concerns of individual students
- encourages interactive discussion, avoiding instruction
- knows when to intervene
- handles difficulties with tact and sensitivity.

Development of PBL problems

At the core of an effective problem-based programme is a carefully designed set of relevant 'cases' or problems. The author(s) of the problems ensure(s) that they match the level of students' development and current knowledge. As problems are introduced, tutors and students provide feedback to the author(s) to identify successes or difficulties or to suggest possible improvements.

Preparation of a PBL problem is hard, time-consuming work, requiring planning and concentration. Input is essential from content experts whose knowledge encompasses the basic medical sciences and clinical aspects, as well as input from an individual or team with expertise in educational design and familiarity with PBL. Recent trends in PBL increasingly focus on the process of clinical reasoning, applying and integrating basic medical sciences as the students develop knowledge and skills.

The first step is to define the relevant learning objectives and determine whether PBL is the best way of covering them. Some medical topics are well suited to PBL and others are not. In general, PBL works best with relatively circumscribed topics that can be introduced succinctly. Problems selected for PBL should be realistic and neither too simple nor overly complex. The resources required to run PBL should not be wasted on problems so straightforward that they do not challenge students, or so complex that students cannot get through them in the available time. Complex problems can sometimes be addressed by limiting the scope. For example, a 'case' of alcoholic liver disease might begin where chronic disease has already developed. The PBL time can then be used to focus on the progression to terminal liver failure, rather than covering the entire disease process.

The second step is to identify the main issues represented in the objectives, encompassing basic sciences, pathophysiological mechanism(s), clinical aspects, epidemiology and psychosocial issues. The emphasis inevitably differs depending on the topics and the stage of training. Early in students' training, PBL may be concentrated on basic sciences and how they explain the clinical presentation, with little attention to clinical management. In the latter years of a course, PBL may concentrate on the pathophysiological basis of the management plan.

The third step is to formulate the clinical story. This usually involves creating or selecting a 'patient' who becomes the centrepiece of the problem: this could be a real patient who is actually present, or a real patient drawn from the experience of the content experts, or a hypothetical patient, who could be a composite of two or more known patients. The patient, who must be disguised to prevent any possibility of identification, is the main character in the clinical story. His or her clinical course and personal and social circumstances become the framework for the PBL. The writer must ensure that the patient's problem expresses the agreed learning objectives and encompasses the scope of the topic, structured so that the whole story fits within the duration of the PBL sessions.

The fourth step is an iterative development of both the clinical story and the learning content, listing key issues for the students to consider and major points for the tutor to highlight. When this is complete, radiological images and other illustrative material may be added for the PBL group to access at an appropriate time in the discussion. The temptation to include too many issues needs to be resisted through constant reference to the learning objectives, but with experience, the designer(s) can identify and refine the key issues.

The fifth step is to submit the problem for content and educational experts to review: they need to check the problem comprehensively. Generally, they ensure its currency and face validity. The respective experts should check the basic science, clinical, epidemiological, social, ethical and health law aspects of the problem in more detail as needed. Specialist input may be required, e.g. to ensure that haematological, biochemical and other test results and radiological images correctly match the pathology and reflect current practice.

The sixth step is to trial and evaluate the problem. Useful feedback can be obtained if pilot testing is done by a group of students who are experienced in the PBL process. The evaluation should canvass students' and tutors' views on the coherence of the problem, the quality of documentation, conceptual clarity, how well learning objectives are fulfilled, ease of use, errors of fact, and inconsistencies or other mistakes. Minor errors are often difficult to detect and may persist through several editions of a PBL problem.

Finally, the problem is evaluated on an ongoing basis after it is introduced for regular use. It needs to be updated to accord with new knowledge, changing clinical practice and varying educational needs. Each significant update should be carefully reviewed.

Place of PBL in the medical programme

PBL is generally employed in one or both of two stages of a medical programme. In the first stage, students are learning about basic medical and clinical sciences, the logic of medical thinking and the basic clinical skills of communication, history-taking and physical examination. In a second later stage, students' learning is concentrated on diagnosis and therapeutics: when students are practising their skills in clinical reasoning. Different approaches to PBL can be designed for these two stages to meet students' progressive learning needs. In the first, problems are often based on hypothetical cases constructed to illustrate pathophysiological mechanisms and their clinical manifestations. In the second, the emphasis is on the application of clinical reasoning to medical problems.

The scope of PBL is influenced by the timing of sessions in relation to other aspects of curriculum delivery. Sessions may be timetabled before, during or after the coverage of related curriculum content, or the sessions may be timetabled to span the entire coverage of a topic. These varied situations place different kinds of pressures on students. If the problem is introduced before students encounter the related curriculum content, the PBL group faces the challenge of working through the content from first principles, building on prior knowledge, extrapolating from previous experience, or a combination of these. Undergraduate students are less likely than students in graduate-entry programmes to have prior knowledge and experience. If the problem is introduced after students encounter the related content, the PBL group has the opportunity to reinforce their recently acquired knowledge by applying it or by integrating disparate strands of knowledge to reach a conclusion. This approach, however, may deprive students of working from first principles: a discovery process that many value.

PBL can be applied in multiple ways for different learning objectives: simply placing the PBL activity at different points in the timetable can re-orient the learning process. Timetabling is often complicated by the need to roster small and medium-sized tutorial groups through laboratories and other facilities with limited capacities. Consequently, timetables may be too inflexible to permit varying placement of PBL sessions, and most medical programmes – especially those with large student cohorts – adopt fixed PBL models with constrained objectives. Table 20.1 sets out a typical model with two or three PBL sessions.

The design and pace of PBL can be varied. For students new to PBL, the pace can be slowed, or more time can be allocated. Later, as students acquire knowledge and insight, they may work through problems faster, and indeed may need to be discouraged from cutting corners. Students may then prefer to work in the group without the tutor for some of the PBL session.

Some PBL programmes make only limited use of other modes of learning, while others tend to rely on various additional modes of learning and teaching. Most medical schools use a mixture of PBL and other modes, typically devoting 2.0 to 4.5 hours of timetabled PBL each week.

Table 20.1 The PBL process

Problem introduced: real patient or text and/or image	
Problem analysis and development (one or two tutorial sessions)	Conclusion and resolution (one tutorial session)
Identify cues, explore mechanisms, review learning issues, develop hypotheses.	Diagnostic decision, principles of management, review problem and group process.

Effectiveness of PBL

PBL has proved to be very effective in promoting active learning, the development of communication skills and critical thinking in an environment of mutual support (Schlett et al 2010). Evaluations consistently show that students enjoy PBL and derive great benefit from well-constructed problems and an effective PBL programme (Moust et al 2005). Intending students often give the availability of PBL as a reason for choosing one medical school over another. While acknowledging the time demands of small-group teaching, tutors usually enjoy their contributions and value the enthusiasm of their PBL groups.

"I thought the group I sat in with was doing really well for second year students – their collective knowledge and understanding was impressive. Then I found out that they were actually only a few months into first year!"

Visitor from UK to Medical Program, University of Sydney

PBL may not necessarily be superior to other modes of learning in medical education (Nandi et al 2000). Intuitively, however, comparisons must be affected not only by the theoretical design of each problem but also by many other influences. These include institutional commitment, resources, the quality of programme delivery, the effectiveness of individual tutors, the nature of the learning environment and students' own prior educational experiences and expectations. Whether apparent benefits and the enjoyment of students and staff justify the costs is an issue frequently debated.

Some aspects of a medical curriculum lend themselves well to PBL while others may not. Obviously, a medical curriculum cannot be comprehensively covered solely by means of PBL. PBL works best where topics can be explored through identifiable problems, formulated as illustrative cases. Inevitably, even the most contained cases can generate discussion on a broad or extended range of related issues and questions. A balance must be found between giving each problem a realistic psychosocial and cultural context and loading the story with so many issues that the educational messages become diffuse.

Assessment of student performance in PBL

Formal or semi-formal assessment of students' performance in PBL groups is important in medical programmes that place substantial emphasis on PBL. Both formative assessments (without penalty) and summative assessments (determining progression) are needed. Many PBL tutors observe and grade the performance of individual students in their groups. Criterion-referenced assessment includes the quality of students' preparation and contribution to the group; engagement with the group process; sensitivity to the learning needs and styles of others; general behaviour and organization (e.g. attendance, punctuality and preparedness). On an individual basis, tutors can take account of students' cultural and social attitudes and personal predispositions. They can, for example, make allowance for students who are acculturated to be reticent in the classroom and for students of disparate maturity.

Tensions can arise if competitive grading and ranking discourage students from sharing information or contributing effectively to the group discussions. Peer review has gained some acceptance in PBL programmes. Each student in a PBL group reviews each other student in the same group. The process can be criterion-based but can also allow for comments. Each student's results are compiled from the reviews of all the other students, with the identity of the reviewers kept confidential. Peer review not only provides feedback on PBL performance, but also gives students an opportunity to learn how to give and receive feedback, an important part of all types of professional practice.

Students are also expected to provide formal feedback on the performance of their tutor. This is often done with reference to defined criteria. Students and tutors also provide informal feedback to each other and comment on the group interaction. This is done frequently, sometimes at the end of every PBL session. It should be encouraged, particularly at the end of each block of PBL sessions.

 If difficulties arise in the tutorial, deal with them promptly, don't let them fester:

- Tactfully suggest a new direction to explore.
- Seek support/solutions from the group.
- Offer practical assistance where possible.
- Deal with personal issues in private.
- Identify and recommend local resources and activities for assisting students.
- Don't be tempted to undertake a counselling role; refer to university resources.

What are the challenges of a PBL-based programme?

The main challenges of a PBL programme are that it requires detailed management and maintenance. PBL demands extensive resources of three types.

The first is a sufficient number of suitably qualified tutors to provide for the numbers of small groups. Even if funds are available to pay tutors, it is difficult in almost any educational setting to find enough tutors who have both skills in facilitation and appropriate content knowledge, and who want to tutor. Students regularly comment on the desirability of medically qualified tutors, but finding enough practitioners available to fit in with the timetable is often impossible, even in large institutions. The problem is, of course, compounded by increasing intakes of medical students, a current trend in many countries.

The second is the availability of physical resources. Conventionally, PBL sessions are conducted in small tutorial rooms with one room per group. Ideally, each room is equipped with whiteboards, a computer with internet access, a computer screen large enough to be seen by the group members, access to electronic library materials and comfortable, durable furniture. In some institutions, PBLs are conducted in large rooms with many tables, each group being allocated to one table. With either type of design, PBL requires appropriately equipped, dedicated learning and teaching spaces.

The third comprises the need for resources to sustain the organizational backbone for consistent PBL delivery. An effective PBL programme requires extensive capacity for managing tutor allocations, conducting training and briefing tutors, updating content and pedagogical methods, overseeing student attendance, managing tutors whose approach does not conform with the preferred PBL model and managing students whose performance and behaviours do conform with expectations. In addition, investment must be made in revitalizing pedagogical methods, ensuring that adherence to intended methods does not become eroded over time (Moust et al 2005). All this requires constant work and vigilance. Any slippage soon reveals the frailty of the model.

In addition to these resource requirements, PBL demands a curriculum structure that can be moulded so that PBL sessions are timetabled to coincide with other modes of learning and teaching on related subject matter. Synergy between PBL, clinical tutorials, laboratory sessions and didactic teaching sessions can be very powerful and very rewarding for students and teachers alike. Achieving this synergy requires strong commitment from teaching staff who often have differing and sometimes conflicting priorities. An effort of mediation may be required to ensure that the necessary alignment occurs.

Several solutions to the challenge of sustaining a PBL programme have been tried in different institutions (e.g. University of Sydney: http://sydney.edu.au/medicine/showcase/pbl). Generally, programmes are designed to ensure that students' experiences of PBL are consistently positive while costs are minimized. For example, in programmes that divide PBL sessions into tutored and untutored segments, the latter are structured to encourage students to manage group processes. The untutored time enables a reduction in the number of tutors needed. As students progress, they can both manage and seek increasing independence in their group learning. Different PBL structures can be introduced as students acquire confidence in their problem-solving abilities. Expectations in graduate medical programmes differ from those in undergraduate programmes, with the latter requiring more support and supervision.

Selection of students for a PBL programme

Medical programmes that make extensive use of PBL usually design eligibility and entry criteria to select students who are likely to be orientated towards, and derive benefit from, a PBL programme. Characteristics that can predict fruitful engagement in PBL include an orientation towards teamwork, an aptitude for articulate self-expression, a predisposition to question ideas critically and a sensitivity to the diverse needs and attitudes of others. Many medical programmes utilize multiple-mini interviews (MMIs) for selection. As the cultural and linguistic diversity of students increases, there may be a need to support and assist with language competence: PBL is very highly dependent on language.

The future of PBL

The major factor guaranteeing the place of PBL in medical programmes is its established diversity of purpose and its acknowledged flexibility of design and delivery. Students enjoy PBL, and staff find reward in the close engagement with students during active learning. Tutors value the interactions with a group of students over a period of time and gain great satisfaction from participating in an active group that becomes increasingly cohesive and competent. As a learning method, PBL has the flexibility to absorb new modes of communication and information transfer, such as those that have emerged recently with the increasing availability of low-cost handheld devices.

The major threat is the financial pressure faced by universities almost everywhere. Some other effective modes of learning and teaching are undoubtedly less costly, and the need for PBL is constantly questioned. A possible future is a mixed model in which PBL has a prominent place but not a dominant one, supplementing and reinforcing the other modes of learning as efficiently as possible.

Summary

PBL has formed the educational core of many medical programmes throughout the world in recent decades, promoting an orientation towards active learning in small collaborative groups. Many models of PBL have evolved to fit into different curriculum structures, meet diverse learning needs and accord with available resources. A tutor facilitates the group learning process. The PBL 'problem' may be introduced as a real patient or as a hypothetical case. Students identify the key elements of the case, develop and test hypotheses based on pathophysiological mechanisms, decide on a diagnosis and discuss principles of management. The development of PBL cases is a challenging process, as each case must reflect a defined set of learning objectives, have face validity, suit the students' stage of maturity in medicine and fit with restraints of time and resources. The increasing availability of instant access to information has changed students' approaches and created new opportunities for PBL design.

References

Dangerfield P, Dorman T, Engel C, et al: *A whole system approach to problem-based learning in dental, medical and veterinary sciences – a guide to important variables.* Centre for Excellence in Enquiry-Based Learning. http://www.ceebl.manchester.ac.uk/resources/guides/pblsystemapproach_v1.pdf, 2009.

Harden RM, Davis MH: The continuum of problem-based learning, *Medical Teacher* 20:317–322, 1998.

Moust JHC, van Berkel HJM, Schmidt HG: Signs of erosion: reflections on three decades of problem-based learning at Maastricht University, *Higher Education* 50:665–683, 2005.

Nandi PL, Chan JN, Chan CP, et al: Undergraduate medical education: comparison of problem-based learning and conventional teaching, *Hong Kong Medical Journal* 6:301–306, 2000.

Norman G: Fifty years of medical education research: waves of migration, *Medical Education* 45:785–791, 2011.

Schlett CL, Doll H, Dahmen J, et al: Job requirements compared to medical education: differences between graduates from problem-based learning and conventional curricula, *BMC Medical Education* 40(9):924–931, 2010.

Schmidt HG, Rotgans JI, Yew EHJ: The process of problem-based learning: what works and why? *Medical Education* 48:792–806, 2011.

Tosteson DC, Adelstein SJ, Carver S, editors: *New Pathways to Medical Education: Learning to Learn at Harvard Medical School.* Cambridge, Harvard University Press, 1994.

Visschers-Pleijers AJ, Dolmans D, Degrave WS, et al: Student perceptions about the characteristics of an effective discussion during the reporting phase in problem-based learning, *Medical Education* 40:924–931, 2006.

Woods D: *Problem-Based Learning: How to Gain the Most from PBL*, Hamilton, Ontario, 1994, Donald R Woods.

Team-based learning

D. Parmelee, P. Hudes, L. K. Michaelsen

What is team-based learning?

Team-based learning (TBL) is an active learning instructional strategy that provides students with opportunities to apply conceptual knowledge through a sequence of events that includes individual work, teamwork and immediate feedback. It is very much learner-centred and engages students with the kinds of problems they will encounter in clinical practice. It also promotes the development of professional competencies in interpersonal skills, teamwork and peer feedback (Michaelsen et al 2008a).

"The development of a small group into a learning team is best described as a transformation process."

Michaelsen 2008a

The evidence for its academic effectiveness is beginning to grow, with an emerging track record for improving academic outcomes (Thomas & Bowen 2011, Koles et al 2010, Shellenberger et al 2009). TBL was first developed in the business school domain for large classes. Since 2001, its use in medical and other health professions schools has grown because it enables students to learn a great deal in small groups while still being in a large class setting: there is no need for multiple faculty and separate rooms for each small group.

"Team-based learning (TBL) is an active learning instructional strategy that provides students with opportunities to apply conceptual knowledge through a sequence of events that includes individual work, teamwork and immediate feedback."

How does TBL work?

"...TBL prompts most students to engage in the learning process with a level of energy and enthusiasm that transforms classrooms into places of excitement that are rewarding for both them and the instructor."

Michaelsen 2008b

Team-based learning's sequence of steps are forward thinking, guiding students into thinking progressively, gaining the ability to look beyond the 'now' and constantly asking, 'What's next?' TBL sequences the learning process (Michaelsen et al 2008b) for the students through the following steps (Fig. 21.1).

 Start with a GOOD course design: TBL works best when it complements the other assessments and learning activities.

STUDENTS' PERSPECTIVE

TBL recurring steps

Step 1 – Advance Assignment Out-of-Class/ Individual
Students receive a list of learning activities, accompanied by a set of learning goals. Students study materials in preparation for the TBL session. Learning activities may include readings, videos, labs, tutorials, lectures, etc.

Step 2 – iRAT – Individual Readiness Assurance Test In-Class/Individual
Each student completes a set (10–20) of multiple-choice questions that focus on the concepts they need to master in order to be able to solve the Team Application (tAPP) problems.

TBL Steps
Students' Perspective

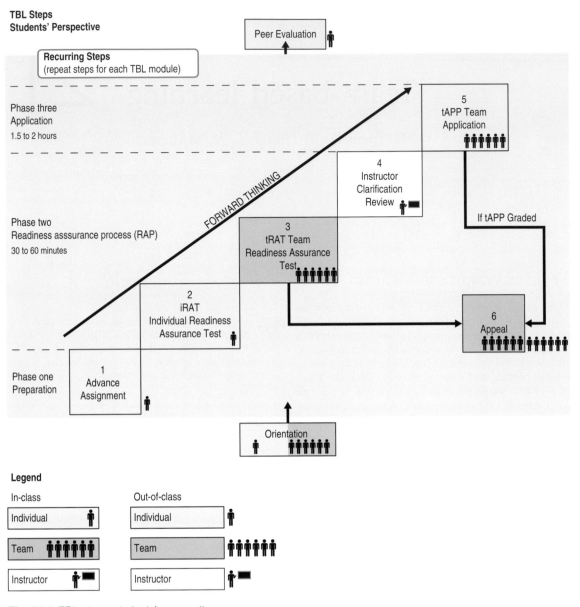

Fig. 21.1 TBL steps: students' perspective.

Step 3 – tRAT – Team Readiness Assurance Test In-Class/Team

This is the same set of questions that each student has answered individually! But now the team must answer them through a consensus-building discussion. There must be a mechanism so that the team knows, as immediately as possible, whether or not they have selected the correct answers because they need this immediate feedback to help them improve their decision-making process.

 Require teams to defend their decisions. This process is the catalyst for deeper learning through discussion, debate and peer instruction.

Step 4 – Instructor Clarification Review In-Class/Instructor

Students get clarification from the instructor on the concepts they have been struggling with during the tRAT. At the end of the Clarification Review, students should feel confident that they are adequately prepared to solve more complex problems for the next TBL step: the Team Application.

Step 5 – tAPP – Team Application In-Class/Team
This is the most important step! Students, in teams, are presented with a scenario/vignette that is similar to the type of problem that they will be grappling with in their careers. They are challenged to make interpretations, calculations, predictions, analyses and syntheses of given information and make a specific choice from a range of options, post their choice when other teams post theirs, and then explain or defend their choice to the class if asked to do so.

The tAPP's structure follows the 4 S's:

- **Significant problem:** Students solve problems that are as realistic as possible. Problems must authentically represent the type of situation that the students are about to face in the workplace or are foundational to the next level of study. The answers must not be able to be found in any source (internet, textbook), but can only be discerned through in-depth discussion, debate, and dialogue within a team.

- **Same problem:** Every team works on the same problem at the same time. Ideally, different teams will select different options for solutions.

- **Specific choice:** Each team must make a specific choice through their intra-team discussion. They should never be asked to produce a lengthy document. Teams should be able to display their choices easily so that all teams can see them.

- **Simultaneous report:** When it is time for teams to display their specific choices to a particular question, they do so at the same time. This way, everyone gets immediate feedback on where they might stand in the posting and they are then accountable to explain and defend their decision.

 For a TBL module, create the team Application Exercise first. Make it authentic: similar to the kind of problem the students are preparing to address in their careers.

Step 3A and/or 6 – Appeal In-Class/Out-of-Class/Team
A team may request that the instructor consider an alternate answer to the one designated as 'best'. The team must provide either a clear and usable re-write of the question if they think it was poorly worded or a rationale with references as to why their choice was as good as the 'best' chosen by the instructor. Only a team that takes the steps to write an Appeal is eligible to receive credit for a particular question.

TBL nonrecurring steps

Orientation Out-of-Class/In-Class/Individual/Team
Students read a brief article about TBL, out-of-class, in preparation for the Orientation session, or the course syllabus as the first Advance Assignment. In-class, students take an iRAT individually, followed by a tRAT in teams and then the tAPP. The instructor clarifies TBL concepts, including how TBL is different from students' previous learning group experiences.

Peer evaluation Out-of-Class/Individual
Each student must evaluate each of his or her teammates on their contributions to the team's success and their own learning. It is best if there is both a quantitative and a qualitative component in which they get practice with framing constructive feedback to one another. It should be done anonymously, but team members are encouraged to speak directly to one another in providing feedback.

What does a TBL session look like?

If you visit a classroom while there is ongoing TBL, you will be impressed by the amount of body movement and talking. No student will be snoozing or reading the news. It is noisy because, for most of the time frame, the students are discussing, debating, even arguing within their teams as they achieve consensus on the instructor's questions. There is a great deal of peer–peer teaching as members of a team ensure that they all 'get on the same page' with what they know and don't know. Those with strong personalities learn to take turns in making their point, listen to those with a different opinion and develop some humility. Reticent students are drawn in to participate because the team needs everyone's brainpower.

If you start class on time with the iRAT, then all students will be in-class early and ready to go. The room will be silent as they answer the set of questions, then when time is called, they will burst into discussion about the questions transitioning into the tRAT.

Students use the Immediate Feedback Assessment Technique (IF-AT) form to answer the tRAT questions. The IF-AT is a multiple-choice answer form with a thin opaque film covering the answer options. Instead of using a pencil to fill in a circle, students scratch off the answer as if scratching a lottery ticket. If the answer is correct, a star appears somewhere within the rectangle indicating the correct answer. Students earn partial credit for a second attempt and learn the correct response for each question while taking the tRAT. One member of a team gets picked by the team to do the scratch off on the IF-AT form, and all are at rapt attention as he or she determines whether or not the team's decision on a question is the preferred one. Generally, teams will give out a small cheer when right and a light groan if wrong. If they do not get it right the first time, they will immediately re-engage on that question and make another selection, but not without careful consideration since the stakes are higher. More information about the IF-AT form is available at the Epstein Educational Enterprises website.

The instructor moves about the classroom, taking a seat with a team to listen in to the discussion to monitor the pulse of their discussions. If many hands go up during the tRAT to ask questions about the questions, then there are problems with the questions, usually regarding how they have been written.

Once all teams have completed the tRAT using the IF-AT form, there should be time for a whole class discussion of one or two of the questions that the class should select (remember, by now, a lot of peer teaching has occurred, as well as immediate feedback). The instructor either makes decisions on the spot about whether or not to accept more than one answer or defers to the Appeal process. The instructor takes the time to assure that all key concepts tested in the RATs are understood by the whole class. If there is a scheduled break between the RAP (Readiness Assurance Process) and the tAPP (Team Application), then the instructor provides guidance to the class on what more they need to master before coming back for the tAPP. Often, the instructor provides a brief, focused presentation (Instructor Clarification Review) that explicates the ambiguities in the key concepts in preparation for the tAPP.

Following the RAP, everyone in the room moves on to the tAPP. The case/problems for this phase can be accessed in envelopes at each team location, displayed on screens in the classroom or posted on a website so that a team can view easily. There is quiet as individual students read through and study the presenting vignettes, which often include CAT scan images, laboratory data or microscopic images that need interpretation. Once members of a team feel that they are ready to discuss, they do so. The noise level rises, students get up and re-position to scrutinize images, and each team discovers its own process to make the best decisions on the options provided in the questions. The instructor calls time and requests the simultaneous response posting of team choices: methods used for posting answers include large colour-coded laminated cards with the options A, B, C, etc., and Audience Response System 'clickers'. When all postings go up, the instructor has to say 'Great choices!' without disclosing the designated 'best' answer.

Next, the instructor must probe for why a team made a specific choice, why not another one, to get all teams engaged in defending their choices. Once there has been sufficient but not excessive presentation of differing positions on a question, the instructor states why he or she likes one or another better. The instructor may concur that two of the choices are equal depending upon how one interprets the data, referring to how a particular team articulated their position. If this component counts for a grade, then Appeals are invited for those teams that disagree with the final in-class answer(s).

What are the ingredients for a successful TBL module?

 Selecting learning activities can be a challenge for those in medical education since the lecture-based pedagogy has been the mainstay for so many years. TBL can eliminate lectures that are primarily 'information transmitting', for the content can be assigned from a text, PowerPoint with notes or even a multimedia online tutorial.

A great deal of thought and planning goes into a successful TBL module. First and foremost, one evaluates the context in which one is teaching (the situational factors) and creates a course design that meets the course goals. We recommend starting with Dee Fink's Integrated Course Design (Fink 2003), which incorporates the backward design paradigm (Wiggins et al 1998): a three-stage design process that delays the planning of teaching and learning activities until clear and meaningful learning goals have been defined and feedback and assessment activities designed (Fig. 21.2).

 "…experience suggests that backward design, that is, designing the feedback and assessment first, greatly clarifies and facilitates answers to the question of what the teaching and learning activities need to be."

Fink 2003

Once course learning goals are established, identifying the feedback and assessment activities that let you know if your students have mastered the goals is

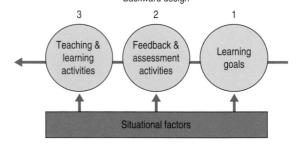

Fig. 21.2 Backward design.

next. Fortunately, TBL is a terrific assessment tool since it provides you and the students with immediate feedback along the way: you and they do not have to wait until the mid-term or final exam for an evaluation of learning.

Selecting learning activities can be a challenge for those in medical education since the lecture-based pedagogy has been the mainstay for so many years. TBL can eliminate lectures that are primarily 'information transmitting', for the content can be assigned from a text, PowerPoint with notes or even a multimedia online tutorial. If you MUST provide a lecture, then either keep it very focused on demonstrating the 'why' and 'how' of key concepts or do it after a TBL session when you know what the students have had the most trouble understanding. Don't waste your or their classroom time by presenting facts they have to learn. Use the classroom to engage them in solving problems!

You should also use the backward design when developing a TBL module. Table 21.1 shows an example of a backward design table for a TBL module on 'the lower extremity'.

Figure 21.3 shows the steps you need to follow to make TBL successful in your course, following the backward design process.

INSTRUCTOR'S PERSPECTIVE

TBL recurring steps

Step 1 – Situational factors and learning goals Identify important situational factors, e.g. students' prior knowledge. Write clear, specific and meaningful learning goals that answer the question 'What do I want the students to be able to DO?' Be specific with exactly how well you want them to master this – use action verbs such as identify, list, explain, calculate, compare and analyse.

 Use 'action-orientated' learning objectives for each TBL module that flow from the course goals.

Step 2 – tAPP – Team Application Create a Team Application exercise that:

- aligns with learning goals: assesses whether students can do what you want them to do
- challenges students: team power is required to solve problems
- is realistic and authentic.

Step 3 – iRAT/tRAT – Individual Readiness Assurance Test/Team Readiness Assurance Test Create Readiness Assurance Test questions that:

- align with the tAPP: focussed on the concepts needed to master for solving the tAPP (not a quiz designed to assess if students did the assignment, i.e. 'picky' questions not related to learning goals)
- are conducive to identifying knowledge gaps
- produce an individual's score that is tightly correlated with performance on any of the course's summative assessments.

Step 4 – Advance Assignment Develop/select appropriate teaching/learning activities (readings, videos,

 Write flawless multiple-choice questions (MCQs) for the Readiness Assurance and have them reflect the key facts and concepts in the Advance Assignment. If they are good questions and are foundational to the team Application Exercise, then you don't have to worry about content coverage: the students will learn it and be able to use it.

Table 21.1 Backward design table for a TBL module on 'the lower extremity'

Situational factors: Anatomy course, Year 1 students, little or no prior knowledge of the lower extremity

1. Learning Goals	2. Feedback and Assessment Activities	3. Teaching and Learning Activities
• Identify and state the significance of all bony landmarks covered in the lab manual related to the lower extremity. • Describe the pattern of cutaneous innervation in terms of dermatomes as well as areas supplied by specific nerves. • Identify and describe the functions of structures associated with the joints of the lower extremity. • Summarize the lymphatic drainage of the lower extremity. • Identify and discuss the relevance of significant surface anatomy features of the lower extremity.	• tAPP (graded) • iRAT, tRAT (graded)	Advance Assignment • Textbook (Chapter 6) • Online tutorials (Lower extremity overview, neuromuscular, joints, imaging) • Dissection labs Instructor Clarification Review session

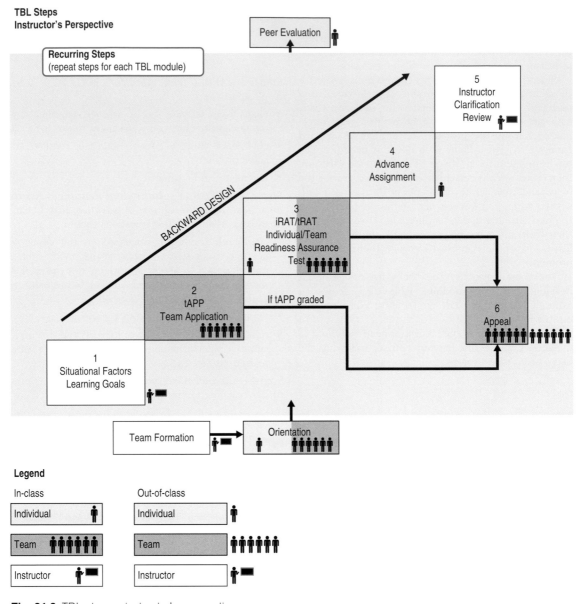

Fig. 21.3 TBL steps – instructor's perspective.

labs, tutorials, lectures) for the Advance Assignment that:

- align with the iRAT/tRAT questions
- are effective and sufficiency for content coverage
- include specific learning goals.

Step 5 – *Instructor Clarification Review* Create an Instructor Clarification Review that:

- predicts/addresses gaps: focused on the concepts students are usually struggling to understand (neither a lecture nor a review of all concepts)

- supports the development of critical thinking skills.

Step 6 – *Appeal* Consider a team's Appeal for an alternate answer to the one you have designated as 'best'. Each team must provide either:

- a clear and usable re-write of the question if they think it was poorly worded, or
- a rationale with references as to why their choice was as good as the 'best' chosen by the instructor.

TBL nonrecurring steps

Team formation Assign students to teams: never let them self-select. Do it by distributing what you consider to be 'wealth factors' across teams, i.e. previous work experience in healthcare, completion of other graduate degrees in science, diversity backgrounds. Make your team selection process transparent so no student is wondering, 'How was I put on this team?' Keep teams working together for the duration of the course or semester.

Orientation Provide an orientation to TBL, using a sample TBL session that explains to students:

- why you are using TBL
- how it is different from previous learning group experiences

Peer evaluation Create a peer evaluation instrument that:

- allows students to evaluate each of his or her teammates on their contributions to the team's success and their own learning
- has both a quantitative and qualitative component
- is accompanied by guidelines on how to provide helpful feedback.

Why does TBL work?

The following sections describe some key characteristics of TBL that make it work.

ACCOUNTABILITY

Students are accountable to come to class having mastered an advanced assignment. Although, at first, they feel accountable because part of their grade depends on the depth of out-of-class mastery of course content, they come to feel accountable to their teammates because they want to contribute all they can to their team's productivity.

IMMEDIATE FEEDBACK

The main driver of TBL is frequent and immediate feedback on everything students decide: whether as individuals or in teams. This enhances their development of deliberate practice.

SOLVING AUTHENTIC PROBLEMS

Once students have mastered course content and key concepts, evaluated in the Readiness Assurance Process, they must tackle complex problems that are similar to the ones they will encounter in their professional activities.

ENGAGEMENT WITH COURSE CONTENT

Students become fully engaged with course content both outside of class, with the Advance Assignment, and in the classroom, with the set of activities that involve and embroil them in discussions on the course content that must lead to decisions. The tighter the fit of the instructor's components for the TBL module with the course learning goals and the greater the authenticity of the Team Application questions, the greater the student engagement.

LEARNING TO WORK COLLABORATIVELY

Teams stay together for as long as possible, and since there are clear incentives to collaborate for the good of the team, students learn how to communicate effectively with peers, resolve conflicts and stay focused on the tasks at hand.

What can go wrong with TBL?

The most common stories of TBL going awry are the following.

1. **'The students hated it because they do not like to prepare for class.'**

   Solution: Prepare students for TBL.

   You must prepare your students for the shift to TBL in which they learn the content outside of class and apply it in the classroom. One of the quickest ways is to provide an orientation session for your students as a sample TBL session. You can create the sample session by using TBL content (based on a brief TBL article) or using the course syllabus as the first Advance Assignment (imagine students reading what the course is about before the first class!). The TBL Collaborative website has a link called 'Orienting Students' with more tips on how to introduce TBL to your students.

2. **'The students hated the RAT questions and argued so much with me that we had no time for the Team Application.'**

   Solution: Write good questions and use the Appeal process.

   You need to write better MCQs and make sure that they are tightly linked to the learning goals, Team Application and Advanced Assignment. The questions should also be well-constructed: a great source for writing effective MCQs is the National Board of Medical Examiners (NBME) Item Writing Manual, downloadable at their website.

   Use an Appeal process that enables students to challenge either the wording or content of a question.

3. **'The students hated it because they did so poorly on the RAT as individuals and the team scores weren't so good either; the mood was grim and angry before we got to the Team Application.'**

Solution: Adjust questions' level of difficulty.

The mean iRAT score for the class should be close to their performance on any of the course's summative assessments; the tRAT mean score should be in the high 80s–90s. If the mean iRAT score is low, then your questions were poorly written and/or there is not a good fit between the questions and what you provided them for the Advanced Assignment. Craft your Advanced Assignment such that they know to what depth they must master it to be successful in the TBL module; adding a few sample questions can guide them. The difficulty level of the RATs should not be a surprise, like 'I gotcha' quizzes. Make the questions match your goals and be meaningful for their learning.

4. **'Everything went well until it was clear we would not get through the Team Application because of time; then everyone was frustrated.'**

Solution: Use fewer questions.

Ensuring that there is enough time for the Team Application is essential, and the most common mistake is to include too many questions. It is far better to have just two to four really probing, thought- and debate-provoking questions that explore the 'why' and 'how' of the problem than trying to cover more content: the most common driver of medical education pedagogy. Sometimes, it is best to separate the RAP from the tAPP by a few hours or even a day or two; consider having two sessions for the tAPP, the second one more challenging than the first.

5. **'It was chaos because the lecture hall has fixed seating, the acoustics were terrible and there was no room for any team clustering.'**

Solution: Use efficient strategies to better organize the TBL session.

Few institutions will have ideal space for TBL since either they have a lecture-based curriculum that uses the sage-on-the-stage design or PBL is well-established and there are many small group rooms and few larger ones to contain the whole class or a good portion of it. We have several suggestions about how to better organize your TBL classroom experience.

Divide the TBL session into two groups: There does need to be space in the classroom for clustering, so if the classroom is completely full with the class, then consider doing the TBL session twice after dividing the class in half.

Require students to stand up when asking/answering questions: Require that a student stand up when he or she speaks and face the class as much as possible. Almost always, when this happens the others will be quiet. If they are allowed to remain sitting when they speak, few can hear, and few will really pay attention. Restate what is asked and what is said so that you are sure everyone in the class has heard. Using roving microphones can also work, but still require students to stand when they speak.

Develop systems for identifying teams and for simultaneous reporting: Find some marker system so that you and everyone in the class knows where the teams are (e.g. poles or tents displaying team number), and when it is time for simultaneous reporting, have a way to display the choices. Methods used for posting answers include large colour-coded laminated cards with the options A, B, C, etc., and Audience Response System 'clickers'.

Package materials in advance: Keep the chaos factor down by having all TBL materials carefully prepared, packaged and ready to use at the team site, including IF-AT forms and clear instructions on how to record individual and team answers for grading. Ideally, you will keep all materials secure, meaning none of the materials leave the classroom.

6. **'The students got a lot out the Readiness Assurance but seemed unengaged in the Team Application because they felt the questions were too much like the Readiness Assurance ones.'**

Solution: Design an effective Team Application.

Your case/problem for the tAPP must closely resemble what students will be encountering soon in their careers (authentic), and it must require them to apply all the content and concepts they have learned to come up with the best answers to your questions. Make it challenging: don't underestimate the power of a small group of students who are working collaboratively to make really good choices. Be creative: use a video clip of a patient describing his or her symptoms; post laboratory or diagnostic information that is real but appears contradictory to the rest of the patient's presentation. This is not something that can be thrown together the week before a module! It takes much planning and peer review.

Is TBL worth the effort?

Designing an effective and successful TBL module can be labour intensive; however, there are many reasons that make it worthwhile, depending upon your context, how much time you have to plan ahead and your commitment to using classroom time for solving problems. Is it more work than putting together a set of scintillating lectures? Yes, it is. But do you ever really know that your students were engaged with the course material in a lecture? At the end of your lectures, do you ever know if they could apply what you taught? When composing a lecture, do you ever consider *how* your students think?

Transforming your course or instructional unit to TBL will require that you shift from an emphasis on covering content to determining how students can apply content to answer meaningful questions. It also requires students to give up the expectation that 'spoon-feeding' lectures will provide them with what they need to know to pass the exams and to understand that learning how to work collaboratively with others is a key goal in education.

Some additional points to consider are the following.

ONE INSTRUCTOR; SAME MESSAGE

Only one instructor is needed without losing any of the benefits of 'small-group' learning, and the instructor need not be trained or talented in group process: he or she need only be a content expert and adhere to the structure and principles of the process. This provides the additional dividend of all students getting the same message, which is hard to achieve with multiple small group instructors.

 Make your 'teaching moments' brief and in direct response to where you see gaps in student knowledge. The TBL process will provide you with continuous information about what your students know and don't know: if you pay attention!

ONE CLASSROOM; NO SPREADING AROUND OR FINDING MORE FACULTY

An entire session is done in one classroom; no need for the small groups to be divided up and spread around the building or set of buildings. The classroom may become noisy, but the students are sharing, learning and very actively engaged in the process. There is no need to beg colleagues to leave their labs/clinics to come teach a small group or worry about what they say in their small group!

IN-CLASS MEETINGS; ALL HAPPENS IN THE CLASSROOM

Students do not have to meet outside of class to either prepare or complete any project. Except for the individual study as part of the Advanced Assignment, everything happens in the classroom.

INDIVIDUAL ACCOUNTABILITY; NO SOCIAL LOAFING

Social loafing is extinguished by the accountability components: (1) the iRAT counts as part of the course grade: 'If I want to do well in this course, I have to prepare for each class'; (2) the tRAT and tAPP count as part of the course grade: 'What I contribute to my team will mean a lot for my course grade'; (3) peer evaluation: 'How I behave towards my peers and help them learn more counts!'

SIMULTANEOUS REPORTING; NO PRESENTATIONS

Simultaneous reporting on specific choices and decisions eliminates having students take turns presenting findings, which students uniformly find boring and a waste of time.

INSTRUCTOR CLARIFICATION; IMMEDIATE FEEDBACK

There is a content expert, the instructor, who, at the appropriate times, does share his or her expertise to elucidate, clarify and amplify when the class gets stumped or needs new direction. Students master the course content (facts) and concepts because they have to apply both to solve the problems in the Team Application. Therefore, they complete a module feeling confident in what they know and how to apply it and are clear about what they don't know so that they might learn it before any next assessment.

NATURALLY FUNCTIONAL TEAMS; NO TEAMWORK INSTRUCTION

There is no need to instruct students in teamwork. They learn by doing, and the immediate feedback on their thinking both as individuals and as team members shapes collaborative behaviours. They become committed to the team's performance and make behavioural changes that lead to improved performance. It is extremely rare for there to be a dysfunctional team that persists, and if it occurs, it is because there may be a severely disturbed member or the team selection process was flawed, e.g. teams were allowed to select their own members.

Summary

TBL can be an exhilarating learner-centred instructional strategy for both the instructor and students, providing students with regular opportunities to learn how to collaborate with peers. For an individual module or a whole course using TBL to be successful, one must adhere to the steps and principles emphasized in this chapter. Based on our many years of experience with TBL, we are convinced that it is ideal for medical education because of its emphasis on accountability, decision making, and collaboration with peers: all essential competencies for healthcare professionals.

References

Fink LD: *Creating Significant Learning Experiences: An Integrated Approach to Designing College Courses.* 2003, Jossey-Bass Higher and Adult Education.

Koles PG, Stolfi A, Borges NJ, et al: The impact of team-based learning on medical students' academic performance, *Academic Medicine* 85(11):1739–1745, 2010.

Michaelsen LK, Parmelee DX, McMahon KK, Levine RE: *Team-Based Learning for Health Professions Education: A Guide to Using Small Groups for Improving Learning.* 2008a, Stylus.

Michaelsen LK, Sweet M, Parmelee DX: *Team-Based Learning: Small Group Learning's Next Big Step. New Directions for Teaching and Learning.* 2008b, Jossey Bass.

Shellenberger S, Seale JP, Harris D, et al: Applying team-based learning in primary care residency programs to increase patient alcohol screenings and brief interventions, *Academic Medicine* 84(3): 340–346, 2009.

Thomas PA, Bowen CW: A controlled trial of team-based learning in an ambulatory medicine clerkship for medical students, *Teaching & Learning in Medicine* 23:31–36, 2011.

Wiggins G, McTighe J: *Understanding by Design.* 1998, Merrill Education/ASCD College Textbook Series.

Online resources

Epstein Educational Enterprises, Immediate Feedback Assessment Technique (IF-AT) form: http://www.epsteineducation.com

National Board of Medical Examiners (NBME) Item Writing Manual: http://www.nbme.org/publications/item-writing-manual-download.html

Team-Based Learning Collaborative website: http://www.teambasedlearning.org

Integrated learning

D. Prideaux, J. K. Ash

Introduction

Medical education courses draw on disciplines from the physical, human and biological sciences, humanities and the social and behavioural sciences and clinical sciences. Traditionally, in a Flexnerian manner, the disciplines were taught separately with an emphasis on the basic sciences in the early years and clinical experiences in the later years. Students, however, were expected to combine all the knowledge and skills from the disciplines and apply them to their clinical work.

In the later part of the 20th century medical education reformers advocated the combination of the disciplines and the organization of integrated learning experiences for students where they called upon knowledge and skills from across the disciplines in addressing patient cases, problems and issues. Integration was promoted in teaching and learning approaches rather than assuming that students would somehow integrate their disciplinary knowledge on their own. While integration was once regarded as a mark of innovation in medical education, it is now more widely accepted as a feature of all programmes. The degree of integration varies. Harden (2000) conceptualized a 'ladder' of integration with 11 steps or stages ranging from treating the disciplines in 'isolation' from each other to 'interdisciplinary' and 'transdisciplinary' designs (Fig. 22.1).

Types of integration in medical education

There are two main types of integration in medical education: integration through dedicated approaches and integration through specific contexts. In the first of these the programme is deliberately structured to organize or facilitate learning across the disciplines around key concepts, themes or problems. There are two common approaches in medical education:

- horizontal integration
- vertical integration.

In horizontal integration there is integration among the various disciplines within any one or each year of the course such as in courses organized on a body systems basis. In vertical integration there is integration of disciplines taught in the different phases or years of the course. The early introduction of clinical skills and their development alongside basic and clinical sciences is a good example of vertical integration.

Integrated learning through context is more common in the clinical components of medical

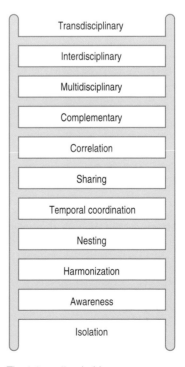

Fig. 22.1 The integration ladder.

courses. As clinical services become more integrated so too do the learning experiences available for students. The increased emphasis on clinical experience in community, ambulatory, primary care and general practice settings has brought additional opportunities for integrated learning in current medical school curricula.

The rationale for integrated learning

The rationale for integrated learning is frequently unstated or not argued strongly. It is assumed that integrated learning will result in a more relevant, meaningful and student-centred curriculum, but the assumption often remains untested.

A rationale for integrated learning can be found, however, in some of the writings in cognitive psychology. Regehr and Norman (1996) have summarized these writings. It is easier to retrieve and use information when it is combined in meaningful schemata.

 "Information in isolation is inert and unhelpful."
Regehr & Norman 1996

Regehr and Norman (1996) also refer to the concept of 'context specificity'. The ability to retrieve an item from memory depends on the similarity between the condition or context in which it was originally learned and the context in which it is retrieved.

 Context specificity: what is learned in one context is more readily retrieved in another similar context.

There are at least three ways to address context specificity for curriculum integration. One is to promote students' elaboration of knowledge in 'richer' and 'wider' contexts. Horizontally integrated system or case-based curricula can provide opportunities for such elaboration. Repeated opportunities to use information in different system or case contexts can also reduce the effects of context specificity. Such opportunities can be found in vertically integrated courses where there is revisiting of knowledge in different situations and in different combinations of disciplines.

A third way of reducing the effect of context is to make the learning contexts as close as possible to the context in which the information is to be retrieved. This provides an argument for integrated learning within integrated clinical contexts such as in community settings, primary care, family medicine or general practice and for providing a clinical context for learning of basic knowledge prior to clinical placements.

Approaches to integration

HORIZONTAL INTEGRATION

In horizontally integrated courses the disciplines are combined, organised around concepts or ideas in each year or level of the course. Commonly this is done using a body system approach. The early years of medical courses are frequently organized into blocks or units corresponding to body systems such as:

- cardiovascular
- respiratory
- renal
- gastrointestinal
- endocrine/reproductive
- musculoskeletal.

Within these blocks students learn the basic sciences of anatomy, physiology and biochemistry together with social and behavioural sciences and clinical sciences as applied to normal and abnormal structures and functions within the systems (Fig. 22.2). More recently, some schools have adopted the concept of life cycle as a means of integrating content. The blocks or units which provide the basis for integration are organized according to stages in the life cycle.

Horizontally integrated courses are becoming more popular as increasing numbers of medical schools around the world adopt problem-based or case-based learning approaches. In these approaches, specifically constructed cases become the focus for a week or 2 weeks of study. The cases may be organized by system or life cycle blocks, but each case in itself is also integrated. They are designed so that students must draw on knowledge, ideas and concepts from across the disciplines in order to generate and pursue learning goals. Problem-based learning, in particular, emphasizes elaboration of learning as students generate learning goals and discuss them in small groups, calling on all relevant knowledge across the disciplines.

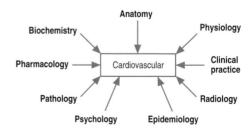

Fig. 22.2 Horizontal integration.

VERTICAL INTEGRATION

In vertically integrated courses the disciplines are organized into themes or domains which run throughout all years of the course. Many medical courses are now organized around four main themes which, while given different names, generally deal with the following:

- clinical and communication skills
- basic and clinical sciences
- social, community and population health
- law, ethics and professionalism.

A common way of organizing a vertically integrated curriculum through the themes is to use a spiral approach. Within each of the themes there may be sub-themes or blocks which provide the basis for integration across the years of the medical course. For example, there may be a sub-theme such as growth, development and ageing which is present in each year of the course in one or more themes. The studies in each year revisit those from the previous year or years, build upon the sub-theme and extend the learning to higher levels and greater complexity. Each turn of the spiral represents an extension of the studies from the previous turn (Fig. 22.3).

There are few medical courses which now rigidly maintain a preclinical/clinical divide, with the former presented in the earlier years of the course and the latter towards the end. Students now have early clinical learning experiences which increase in emphasis as they proceed through the course. There is a corresponding decrease in emphasis on the basic sciences,

but they still have an important part to play in the clinical years in providing an explanation of the mechanisms of disease and disease processes. This increases the potential for integration of clinical and science disciplines. For example, anatomy and imaging are being presented in an integrated approach throughout medical courses. The establishment of clinical skills units, where students have opportunities to learn and practise skills in an intensive way, has also fostered integration, including the immediate application of concurrently learned anatomy and physiology. Dent et al (2001) have reported on an Ambulatory Care Teaching Centre (ACTC) in which students' early experiences in the clinical skills centre integrate with patient-based experiences in the ACTC during subsequent system blocks.

Contexts for integrated learning

In the rationale for integrated learning set out here it is argued that one way to achieve such learning is to ensure that the learning context is itself integrated. With medical practice becoming more specialized, particularly in large teaching hospitals, this is becoming increasingly difficult to achieve. This is one of the reasons underlying the calls for more clinical experiences for students in community settings, ambulatory services, general practice, family medicine and primary care. It is claimed that these contexts will provide opportunities for students to experience a patient-centred approach rather than a disease-oriented one and will enable them to experience a broad spectrum of illness to which they can apply the integrated knowledge from the studies in their medical courses.

 "When students learn complex tasks in an integrated manner, it will be easier for them to transfer what they have learned to the reality of day-to-day work settings."

Janssen-Noordman et al 2006

The Parallel Rural Community Curriculum (PRCC) model pioneered in the School of Medicine at Flinders University enables students to take a whole year of clinical studies in rural general practices and associated small rural hospitals. They learn the same content from the major clinical disciplines as those students who take the year in a teaching hospital, but do it in an integrated patient-based approach. Students in the integrated approach perform better in end-of-year examinations than their teaching hospital-based peers, thus providing evidence for the importance of matching integrated learning programmes with integrated learning contexts (Worley et al 2004) (see Chapter 13, In the community). This programme and the increasing interest in enabling students to undertake

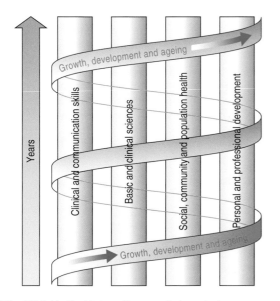

Fig. 22.3 Vertical integration: a spiral curriculum.

clinical studies in rural, ambulatory, community health centres and district general hospitals has led to the implementation of further integrated longitudinal learning experiences in many parts of the world. The Consortium of Longitudinal Integrated Clerkships (CLIC) is a group dedicated to the organization of longitudinal integrated clinical experiences across the range of hospital and non-hospital settings.

One of the additional features of the PRCC and other longitudinal programmes is that students make a contribution to the clinical and other services of the general practices, health services and hospitals in which they work. This idea is encapsulated in the 'symbiotic' approach to clinical education, which emphasizes that medical schools should enter a mutually reinforcing relationship with their health services (Prideaux et al 2007). In such a relationship, student learning should be enhanced by the health services, and, in turn, the students and their programme should make a contribution to the enhancement of the clinical services in which they are placed.

 In a symbiotic curriculum, education and clinical service are mutually enhanced.

A symbiotic relationship can be achieved by enabling students to have longer placements in clinical services and by providing guidelines and support for students to direct their own learning from patients rather than expecting them to be constantly directly 'taught' by busy clinical staff. Bleakley and Bligh (2006) have advocated a shift from the 'primacy' of the doctor–student relationship to the relationship between student and patient. In patient-centred approaches students can have extended placements across clinical services with opportunities for integrated learning facilitated by study guides or learning logs. 'Parallel consulting' systems in general practice enable students to see and learn from patients on their own without reducing the number of consultations by the general practitioners. It also provides opportunities for general practitioners to focus on the students' history taking and clinical reasoning when they interact with patients and students together (Walters et al 2009).

Achieving integration in medical education programmes

It is regarded as paradoxical by some medical educators that integrated curricula require a greater degree of structuring than those based on traditional disciplines. In a course based on separate disciplines, concepts and key ideas can be defined by the well-structured approaches existing in the disciplines. In an integrated curriculum, concepts and key ideas from several disciplines must be combined in some logical way. Hence there has been increasing interest in medical education in approaches to the organization and articulation of curriculum and curriculum content.

Outcomes-based approaches to curriculum design and development are advocated for medical courses (Harden et al 1999). In an outcomes approach those responsible for the course define broad and significant outcomes that students must attain on graduation. There is then a process of 'designing down' so that learning and assessment systems match the outcomes. The course can be defined by outcomes, not by disciplines. Competency-based approaches can also foster integration, as competencies cross disciplinary boundaries and do not require discipline-based blocks or units. As with an outcomes approach, care must be taken to ensure that the medical course is not reduced to those attributes that are readily translated into competencies and that complexity is not lost.

 Integrated curriculum designs can be achieved through use of outcomes or competencies that transcend disciplines, but complexity must not be lost.

Integrated curricula can also be defined by key concepts or key ideas that transcend disciplines. For example, 'homeostasis' can be used as a key concept to integrate content from biochemistry and physiology. Clinical studies can be integrated by examining the effects and outcomes of disordered homeostasis. The key is to define a set of concepts that will effectively integrate all the content required in the course (Fig. 22.4).

Curriculum maps can be employed effectively in this process. One way of designing maps is to place the key concept or idea in the middle of a diagram and then draw the content from across the disciplines that will contribute to the understanding of the concept. There then can be a selection of the linked content to provide the material for study in the medical course. Maps can also be used as a double-check on the curriculum. Those responsible for the disciplines can draw up their own maps of essential concepts and content to be covered. These can be

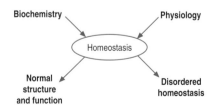

Fig. 22.4 Homeostasis is an example of a key learning concept.

matched against the material covered in the integrated approach to identify omissions or overlapping content.

Searchable computer databases provide an effective way of determining the coverage of content in integrated courses and are increasingly employed in medical schools across the world. Course content can be logged onto the computer and can be subject to searches according to a number of criteria, including discipline, key concepts, common presentations or illnesses and system complexes. Students can have access to the databases as a guide for their own learning and preparation for assessment. They can match what they learn in their integrated programmes to what is expected in the course as a whole, by careful examination and searching of the database. This gives them responsibility for their own learning. Databases can be linked to electronic resources to support student learning. In this way students can access learning resources which may be shared by different medical schools. Many medical schools now have a distributed approach to clinical education across rural, urban, community and hospital sites with integrated experiences in the distributed sites. This has been made possible by the ability of students to access databases of course content.

These approaches require a greater degree of central rather than departmental control of the curriculum. Indeed, they require the breaking down of so-called departmental 'silos'. In most medical schools the responsibility for curriculum content and organization now lies with a central committee or decision-making body representative of the disciplines and groups in the course. It is this body which oversees curriculum content and the contribution of the disciplines.

Learner integration

An important distinction made by curriculum writers is that between the 'intended' curriculum and the 'real' curriculum as it is experienced by students. There may well be a difference between the curriculum as it is intended and written down by its designers and how it is actually received by the students who experience it. Thus the real measure of the degree of integration of a curriculum is not what is written down in plans, statements and booklets but rather how much integration takes place in student learning.

 "A number of empirical studies have shown, however, that effective competence-based learning is not achieved by offering students separate building blocks because this does not facilitate transfer of what students have learned."

Janssen-Noordman et al 2006

Contemporary medical education curricula emphasize self-direction in learning, and there is much interest in the concept of 'constructivism'. In constructivist approaches students actively construct or develop their own learning from the range of experiences available to them. Again, this makes the question of achieving integration more problematic. In a didactic approach the integration can be presented to students in a prepackaged way, although, of course, the question still remains as to whether it will necessarily be received in that way. In more self-directed and constructivist approaches, learning plans and goals, study guides and learning pathways should be designed to facilitate integrated learning, but in the final analysis it will be up to the students to construct their learning in an integrated or nonintegrated way.

 "The point of education is to improve the quality of meanings we construct."

Newman et al 1996

Newman and colleagues (1996) have provided a critique of constructivist approaches where student engagement has become an 'end in itself' rather than the pursuit of quality learning and 'intellectual' outcomes for students. They use the term 'authentic learning', which they argue has three central components:

- the construction of knowledge
- disciplined inquiry
- 'value beyond' the school or educational context in which the learning takes place.

These three components bring together some of the preceding discussions. As indicated above, a major task for curriculum designers will be to design learning tasks that enable students to construct their learning in integrated ways. This can be facilitated through the use of:

- study guides
- learning logs and portfolios
- online materials
- independent projects.

This construction of knowledge should be underpinned by a process of rigorous inquiry. The central elements of the process of inquiry as set out by Newman and colleagues are the following:

- building on a prior knowledge base
- providing for in-depth learning
- providing for elaborated learning.

These match the central elements of problem-based learning. Thus problem- or case-based approaches will provide a strong foundation for authentic integrated learning.

Problem- or case-based learning provides a strong foundation for authentic integrated learning.

Providing integrated clinical contexts for learning will demonstrate the value of what is being learned beyond the medical school environment and indicate its relevance to clinical practice. This potentially is the most important area of all. If student learning is to be meaningfully integrated, it must be anchored in the realities of clinical practice. There must be a high degree of involvement of students in the actual tasks and activities of integrated clinical services so that they can clearly see that integrated learning is not just something important for success in medical school, but will be an important part of their continued development as medical professionals. The interprofessional learning experiences offered at Linköping University in Sweden are an example of this. Students from different health disciplines work together in the authentic tasks of actually running an interprofessional patient care service.

The frequently quoted adage in medical education that 'assessment drives learning' must not be ignored. If integrated learning is to be achieved it must be driven by integrated assessment. As in the process of structuring the curriculum, integration must be deliberately incorporated into the assessment process. The most important step is to ensure that integrated learning is represented in assessment blueprints. This requires a central process of test and examination construction, with responsibility for assessment residing with the medical school overall rather than with individual departments, similar to the design of the curriculum as indicated earlier.

There are now established methods for assessing integrated clinical learning once it has been represented in the blueprints. The objective structured clinical examination (OSCE) format is ideal for assessing integrated clinical learning. Similarly, portfolio-based assessment and the Mini-CEX can promote this form of learning. There is renewed interest in work-based assessment, where students can be assessed in holistic ways as they interact with patients. Written assessments, too, can be focused on integrated learning. Many medical schools using problem-based formats have adopted case-based assessment methods which attempt to evaluate the processes of problem-based learning as well as the integration of student knowledge. Multiple-choice and short-answer questions which are focused on the assessment of application, analysis, synthesis and evaluation rather than recall do provide opportunities for students to demonstrate that they can integrate and apply their learning and knowledge base. There is growing interest in progress testing, where students are regularly assessed

through integrated exit level items with student achievement documented and recorded.

 Assessment items that test higher-order cognitive skills allow students to demonstrate integrated learning.

Conclusion: Building an evidence base about integrated learning

Despite the advocacy of integrated learning, many of the claims made for it remain largely untested. As yet, there is not clear evidence about the impact of integrated learning nor about the best ways to achieve it. Certainly Newman and colleagues found some support for their concept of authentic pedagogy and the interrelationship between pedagogy, assessment and performance in the school population. However, there have been few studies of integrated learning in the medical education context.

There is a need for some programmatic research on the concept of integrated learning. It is important to ask and to seek responses to questions such as those below:

- What factors promote integrated learning?
- What factors limit it?
- What curriculum designs promote integrated learning?
- What is the perceived relevance of integrated learning for students?
- What is the effect of integrated assessment on integrated learning?
- Does integrated learning provide value beyond medical school?
- Is integrated learning promoted by student participation in authentic integrated clinical contexts?

Is integrated learning promoted by student participation in authentic integrated learning contexts? This is an important question for future research.

There will be a need to pay careful attention to questions of research design. Simple comparison of student performance in integrated and nonintegrated programmes may not prove to be productive because of the interrelationships of variables and the very real difficulty in classifying programmes as wholly integrated or nonintegrated. Nevertheless, answers to the questions above and others like them will assist in establishing both the nature and place of integrated learning in medical education and, ultimately, in assessing the effect of student engagement in integrated learning on subsequent practice as a medical professional.

Summary

Contemporary medical educators have increasingly called for the integration of student learning across the disciplines contributing to medical courses. A rationale for this kind of learning can be drawn from cognitive psychology through the concept of 'context specificity'. Retrieval of learning is enhanced where there is similarity between the context of initial learning and the context of retrieval. Horizontal integration addresses context specificity by enabling elaboration of learning in richer and wider contexts such as those provided in case-based or systems-based curriculum designs. Vertical integration provides repeated opportunities for use of information in different contexts in theme-based or spiral curricula. Integrated learning is also promoted where the learning context itself is integrated, as in community, general practice or family medicine clinical services.

Integrated curriculum designs require structure around outcomes, concepts or maps. Nevertheless, irrespective of what is intended, it is the reality of integration for the learner that is important. Constructivism and authentic learning can promote integration, and integrated assessment will drive integrated learning.

However, despite widespread advocacy of this approach, there is little evidence about integrated learning. There is a need for research evidence about its nature and place in medical education so that its contribution to the ongoing medical practice of medical graduates can be assessed.

References

Bleakley A, Bligh J: Students learning from patients: let's get real in medical education, *Advances in Health Sciences Education* 13(1):89–107, 2006.

Dent JA, Angell-Preece HM, Ball HM-L, Ker JS: Using the Ambulatory Teaching Centre to develop opportunities for integrated learning, *Medical Teacher* 23(2):171–175, 2001.

Harden RM, Crosby JR, Davis MH: An introduction to outcome-based education. Part 1 AMEE no. 14 Outcome-based education, *Medical Teacher* 21(1): 7–16, 1999.

Harden RM: The integration ladder: a tool for curriculum planning and evaluation, *Medical Education* 34:551–557, 2000.

Janssen-Noordman AMB, Merrinboer JJG, van der Vleuten CPM, Scherpbier AJA: Design of integrated practice for professional learning competences, *Medical Teacher* 28(5):447–452, 2006.

Newman FM, Marks HM, Gamorgan A: Authentic pedagogy and student performance, *American Journal of Education* 104:280–312, 1996.

Prideaux D, Worley P, Bligh J: Symbiosis: a new model for clinical education, *The Clinical Teacher* 4(4):209–212, 2007.

Regehr G, Norman GR: Issues in cognitive psychology; implications for professional education, *Academic Medicine* 71(9):988–1001, 1996.

Walters L, Prideaux D, Worley P, et al: What do general practitioners do differently when consulting with a medical student? *Medical Education* 43(3):268–273, 2009.

Worley P, Esterman A, Prideaux D: Cohort analysis of examination performance of undergraduate medical learning in community settings, *BMJ* 328:207–209, 2004.

Interprofessional education

J. E. Thistlethwaite

Introduction

The adjective interprofessional describes a strategy in which practitioners learn and work together for a common goal. It implies dialogue and negotiation, consensus and compromise, as well as mutual understanding and respect. The most widely used definition for interprofessional education (IPE) is that of the UK-based Centre for the Advancement of Interprofessional Education (CAIPE), which was updated in 2002: 'occasions when two or more professions learn from, with and about each other to improve collaboration and the quality of care' (CAIPE 2002). Here 'professions' refers to health and social care and to both prequalification students and qualified practitioners. The prepositions 'from', 'with' and 'about' are important as they imply that learning is interactive and equitable. Collaboration, and therefore collaborative practice, as a goal of IPE is now becoming a commonly used term, along with teamwork.

 Interprofessional collaboration is "the process of developing and maintaining effective interprofessional working relationships with learners, practitioners, patients/clients/families and communities to enable optimal health outcomes."

The Canadian Interprofessional Health Collaborative 2010

A number of educational, psychological and sociological theories underpin the development and delivery of IPE. These include, but are not limited to, professional socialization, communities of practice, adult learning theory and transformative learning.

 Aspiring interprofessional educators should become familiar with the theories linked to IPE and venture outside the medical education literature into other disciplines.

The rationale for IPE

For many programme planners the impetus for introducing interprofessional outcomes into a course is that they are now mandated or recommended by increasing numbers of professional accreditation bodies, for example, the General Medical Council (GMC) in the UK and the Interprofessional Education Collaborative of the United States. The underlying rationale is the changing international health and illness profile, with an increase in chronic and complex disease as the population ages, as well as the patient safety agenda and the importance of health promotion. Health and social care is now predominantly a team-based enterprise as practitioners specialize and patients move between primary, secondary and, potentially, tertiary care sectors. Beyond the core team, collaboration also occurs on a wider scale and may include interactions with schools, the police and the judiciary as well as diverse health and social care providers.

 "Learn effectively within a multi-professional team:

- Understand and respect the roles and expertise of health and social care professionals in the context of working and learning as a multi-professional team;

- Understand the contribution that effective interdisciplinary team working makes to the delivery of safe and high-quality care."

GMC 2009

Planning for IPE

Successful delivery of IPE is not easy, but too often the difficulties are highlighted and used as an excuse for stifling development and innovation. The first requirement in any institution or postgraduate programme is an interprofessional champion: a highly committed health or social care professional with experience in the area who is able to lead by example, motivate others, challenge stereotypes and role model 'being interprofessional'. Such a person needs to be able to engage with all the professional education leads whose students or practitioners will be joining the programme(s) and have options for solutions to the common difficulties that will arise while enabling people to suggest their own strategies for successful implementation. The interprofessional educator often straddles departments in universities and clinical settings and will need a colleague within each profession or faculty with whom to liaise and plan. The profession of the IP lead should not be important, but the planning team should be inclusive of all the professions who will be learning together.

 "Being interprofessional means that we:

1. Know what to do: think through what action is needed in a particular setting and how to do what is needed

2. Have the skills to do what needs to be done: being competent

3. Conduct ourselves in the right way when carrying out a particular action: appropriate attitudes, suitable values and beliefs about what we are doing."

Hammick et al 2009

Once the planning team is in position, consideration needs to be given to the following: the number of students/learners and what professions will be involved; whether all activities are mandatory or if there will be a choice; the timing of the activities (early, late or throughout the course); the number of hours and over what time frame; where learning will take place (classroom, clinic, ward, etc.); the type and timing of assessments; and how many rooms and facilitators will be required. In addition, the people responsible for coordinating the timetables and for overseeing the budget need to be identified.

 When planning new interprofessional activities, remember to build in an evaluation and/or research plan and consider whether ethical approval is required if there is an intention to disseminate the results.

 The reason for evaluation is to "provide accountability for health and social care resources to those who provide or control them – regional/national authorities, research and service funders, consumers and foundations."

Reeves et al 2010

Learning outcomes for IPE

The logistical and capacity barriers to effective prequalification IPE are of course immense: large numbers of students, with profession-specific timetables, often learning in academic and clinical environments with limited space. The work required to negotiate these hurdles is only rewarded if there is an added value to students' learning through bringing them together (face-to-face and/or online). Therefore, it is extremely important that careful consideration is given to explicit learning outcomes for interprofessional activities. These will derive in part from any professional accreditation standards set for prequalification or postqualification continuing professional development (CPD) programmes. The published learning outcomes should be such that they would be unlikely to be achieved without interprofessional interaction. The aim is, thus, shared learning rather than common learning, i.e. 'from', 'with' and 'about'.

For example, for students learning how to measure blood pressure (a common skill for many healthcare professions), there should be outcomes over and above profession-specific and generic skills such as patient communication and clinical skills. Moreover, students and facilitators should know what the outcomes are, how they can be met and how they will be assessed.

The most frequently defined outcomes fall into six main areas: teamwork, communication, understanding of roles and responsibilities, ethical issues, the patient and learning/reflection (Thistlethwaite & Moran 2010). There are a number of frameworks for IPE in which outcomes are also referred to as competencies, capabilities and objectives. As demonstrated by the GMC quote above, the terminology in these documents varies, and often multiprofessional, multidisciplinary and interdisciplinary are used interchangeably.

 "Seven objectives of interprofessional education

1. Modify reciprocal attitudes

2. Establish common values, knowledge and skills

3. Build teams

4. Solve problems

5. Respond to community needs

6. Change practice

7. Change the professions."

Barr in Bluteau & Jackson 2009

Learning activities

As IPE has been undertaken in various formats, locations and learning environments since the 1960s, there is a rich menu of learning activities that can be scrutinized when planning new initiatives. The decision about activities should be based on the need to align the defined learning outcomes with learning opportunities, but programmes are also constructed pragmatically, taking into account student numbers and available resources such as space and trained facilitators.

PREQUALIFICATION

In higher education, not everyone will have the luxury of starting new programmes with completely blank curricula through which interprofessional activities can be woven. More commonly, interprofessional learning is added into already crowded curricula, or it may take the form of student-selected options or electives.

The common curriculum model involves students from different health and social care professional training spending 1 or more weeks learning together full-time. This may be a full first year of study. For example, at the Auckland University of Technology (AUT) in New Zealand, students undergo a common first year before differentiating into professional groups and undertaking profession-specific modules. The New Generation project of Southampton University in the UK has students undertaking interprofessional units over 2 weeks for a number of times during their first year (O'Halloran et al 2006). Implementing this sort of activity requires curriculum renewal across health and social care professional programmes in order to integrate fully the interprofessional learning into each profession's timetable.

Interprofessional modules may involve classroom activities based on teamwork and professionalism. There may be early patient/client contact in community or clinic settings with mixed groups of students interviewing patients/clients.

In Canada, the model proposed by Curran and Sharpe (2007) adopts a curricular approach, which exposes students to interprofessional education at an early stage in their training with subsequent regular reinforcement. Early evaluation has shown satisfaction amongst students and faculty as well as significant effects on attitudes toward interprofessional teamwork and education. At Leicester University (UK), interprofessional student groups visit patients in their homes, adopting a biopsychosocial approach to eliciting their stories and planning management.

 All health professional students undergo clinical attachments at various points in their training; by mapping such attachments, it should be possible to bring the professions together at some point to provide team-based experiences that are as authentic as possible.

Rural rotations, where students are able to live together as well as work together, offer rich interprofessional experiences. Such placements have been described in Australia and Canada, whose rural and remote locations are ideal for interprofessional activities. Learning here becomes informal as well as formal, as students interact both professionally and socially.

The interprofessional student training ward, first implemented at Linköping University, Sweden, in 1996, requires a high commitment from both the higher education institution and the national health system for its development and delivery. The training ward model is now running in modified forms at the Karolinska Institutet, Stockholm, since 1998 and at St George's Medical School at the University of London, while a further ward is in the planning stages at Curtin University in Western Australia. On the ward, which is a functioning patient care delivery unit, between five and seven students work in teams to plan and deliver care to in-patients, under supervision. They learn about teamwork, handover and communication.

POSTQUALIFICATION

Interprofessional learning activities should be easier to implement for qualified health professionals as they can be undertaken by existing healthcare teams. However, much of CPD is profession specific and accredited for re-licensure or revalidation by uniprofessional colleges or boards. Moreover, if professions do come together for education focused on specific illnesses or conditions, the activity may be learning in common (multiprofessional) rather than an interactive session with the added value of interprofessional learning outcomes. Mixed professional groups attending a lecture on diabetes management are likely to be passive learners. Education should therefore be developed at the level of the healthcare team, and facilitated by trained educators who use the experience of the participants to ensure learning from and about each other.

ONLINE LEARNING

E-learning is a method applicable to both pre- and postqualification learners which may stand alone or complement face-to-face activities. Online modules are common in masters programmes and for CPD. They can help overcome many of the logistical problems associated with large numbers of participants.

The universities of Coventry and Warwick in England have partnered to provide an interprofessional learning pathway (IPLP) for 1000 students across 15 professions and at three levels (Year 1, Year 2 and the final year of study). Students interact online in mixed groups of 15 with a facilitator trained in both IPE and e-learning. Students work through cases and tasks that provide material for interprofessional discussion and comparison of roles and responsibilities. While feedback has demonstrated that many students would prefer a face-to-face component, this has proved difficult to implement. Evaluation is ongoing, and student satisfaction is highly dependent on the skill of the facilitator (Bluteau & Jackson 2009).

 To help ensure high levels of student and facilitator satisfaction with e-learning, there needs to be prompt and accessible technical support.

Evidence and theory-based education

It is imperative that IPE is interactive and learner-centred, with an emphasis on adult learning techniques. Small-group and experiential learning with time for reflection and authentic clinical experiences is important.

INTERACTIVE SMALL-GROUP LEARNING

Obviously, such groups contain a mix of professions: the size of the group and the mix are often determined pragmatically by the overall number of learners, facilitators, clinical placements and/or rooms. The optimum group size in a classroom is six to eight, but this is rarely possible with cohorts of students in an institution often numbering several hundred. Having more than eight learners interacting in a clinic or at the bedside is difficult for everyone concerned, including the patients.

AUTHENTIC EXPERIENCES

An assumption of adult learning theory is that learning experiences should be relevant to the student. For IPL this means engaging students in authentic clinical and team-based environments, which should motivate them to engage in IPE activities. This could range from interviewing patients about their healthcare needs in their homes or in clinical settings to participating in organized interprofessional clinical placements, such as the training ward or rural health centres. A major issue, however, is that of the hidden curriculum: what students learn from observation and role models. Students may not observe interprofessional teamwork in action during their clinical placements, because such teamwork is not explicit, does not look like the models they have learnt about, or does not exist. This lack of experience undermines any classroom learning and leads students to question the very nature of interprofessionalism and IPE. Educators need to ensure that students are exposed to interprofessional practice at some time within their programmes; they may attend multidisciplinary team meetings in hospital or primary care, work within operating theatres, or be placed in well-functioning diabetes clinics. After any interprofessional activity students need to be debriefed about what they have seen and learnt, be given time to discuss the type or lack of teamwork they have observed and be encouraged to consider how teamwork and collaborative practice may be fostered in the environments in which they have been placed.

REFLECTION AND TRANSFORMATION

Learning activities should include a time for reflection. Reflection and discussion led by a skilled facilitator enable the transfer of new learning into practice. We can adapt Mezirow's 1991 theory of transformative learning by stating that transformative IPL reveals distorted assumptions and stereotypes.

TIMING OF ACTIVITIES

There is still considerable discussion regarding the stage at which prequalification health and social care students should be introduced to interprofessional learning. The rationale for early immersion is that it will prevent the formation of misconceptions about other health professionals and stereotyping. However, it is argued that students should gain knowledge and confidence within their chosen profession before they are able to interact effectively with others. Ideally, students will have interprofessional experiences integrated throughout their courses and beyond, into their working lives.

Impact and effectiveness of IPE

There have been a number of systematic reviews of the effectiveness of IPE in the last decade. There is also an extensive body of descriptive evaluative literature, which has its place in demonstrating participant satisfaction with interprofessional activities. As educational researchers know, the gold standard for biomedical research – the randomized controlled trial – is difficult to apply in educational settings due to confounding and ethical factors. Taken together, publications informing the body of knowledge do point to positive impact and learning. It is also difficult to argue convincingly that teamwork is not enhanced by learning about teamwork, and that interprofessional collaboration should only be learnt when doing the job, rather than there being preparation beforehand. However, there is certainly need for further research into what works and how it works.

To highlight the problem, the most recent Cochrane Collaboration review (Reeves et al 2008) identified only six studies (all postqualification), through a systematic search process, that met its inclusion criteria of randomized controlled trials, before-and-after studies and interrupted time series studies, which reported objectively measured or self-reported outcomes related to patient care or healthcare processes. Four of these reported positive outcomes; two studies reported mixed results; and two studies reported no impact. Moreover, all six focused on postqualification interventions. The BEME (Best Evidence Medical Education) Guide (2007) included 21 papers, the majority of which (15) evaluated prequalification IPE (Hammick et al 2007). Most studies looked at learner reaction while indicating minimal impact of interprofessional activities on learner attitudes towards other professional groups. However, a few prequalification studies demonstrated a positive effect of IPE interventions on student behaviour.

Assessment

To stress the importance of interprofessional education to students, assessment of learning outcomes is necessary. As IPE is an interactive, collaborative learning process, formative assessment is ideally team-based. Students can be assessed on team-based activities such as projects and presentations, simulations involving multiple professionals, team-based OSCE stations and the preparation of patient care plans. Educators need to decide whether the responsibility for the 'end product' is a collective responsibility, with all students in a team receiving the same mark, or whether individuals are assessed on individual team performance, with students marking each other. After all, overall team functioning is dependent on all team members, including the leader.

Summative assessment is more problematic, as professional accreditation bodies have different requirements in terms of grading and types of examinations and may insist that students are assessed by members of the same profession. Portfolios, with reflective components and with students' collected evidence of achieving outcomes, are a good vehicle, but there are issues relating to reliability and feasibility. Multisource feedback (MSF) forms may also be included, with students asking for feedback on performance from a number of different health professionals with whom they come into contact. MSF is also a valuable method for assessment of postqualification clinicians.

Faculty development for IPE

For the successful implementation of IPE at any time and at any level, facilitators and educators who have experience of working with one profession will not have all the necessary attributes. Therefore, there must be a commitment to staff or faculty development. As interprofessional learning activities may be deployed within a diverse range of settings from the classroom to the clinical environment, from the community to the hospital, and in postgraduate education centres and within the workplace, faculty development is a complex process. Educators in these settings have varying levels of teaching expertise and clinical experience; their time commitment and motivation will also vary, and they will have different employers, e.g. the university, the health service or private practices. Some potential facilitators have multiple roles; research and clinical practice may take precedence over education. One size of faculty development will therefore not fit all, but it may be difficult to offer tailor-made courses to fit in with other commitments and experiences.

 An interprofessional educator is "attuned to the dynamics of interprofessional learning, skilled in optimizing learning opportunities" and should value "the distinctive experience and expertise which each of the participating professions brings."

Barr 1996

THE ATTRIBUTES OF AN EFFECTIVE INTERPROFESSIONAL FACILITATOR

There are a number of lists of attributes in the literature which include some or most of the following:

- Competencies relating to teamwork theory and team building
- Experience of working in a healthcare team – ideally interprofessional rather than multiprofessional
- Experience of collaborative practice and the ability to promote this within the workplace
- Knowledge of others' professional roles and responsibilities
- Awareness of boundary issues and the issues regarding blurring of professional roles
- An understanding of the process of professional socialization and how this might impact on interprofessional interactions
- Skills in negotiation and conflict resolution
- Knowledge of the evidence for IPE.

In addition, the generic attribute for all facilitators in higher education is an up-to-date knowledge of educational theory, including adult learning theories.

DEVELOPING INTERPROFESSIONAL FACILITATORS

One question for discussion is whether it is mandatory that interprofessional facilitators are still practising clinicians. On the one hand, being in clinical practice ensures that the facilitator's knowledge is up to date and that he or she has credibility. On the other hand, we might argue that the facilitation process is more important than content knowledge and clinical experience and that having only one health professional lead a group is a disadvantage for learners from other professions; the nonclinical educator is seen as neutral.

 Cofacilitation or team teaching involving one expert facilitator and one clinical expert helps achieve balance; if clinical experts also have facilitation experience, then the facilitators can be from two different professions.

Interprofessional facilitation involves observation of learner interaction and collaboration and includes giving feedback on team processes and facilitating reflection on roles, responsibilities and language. The facilitator may need to challenge stereotyping, if the group members do not challenge this themselves, and draw parallels between group work in learning and teamwork in clinical settings.

A 'train the trainer' approach to IPL facilitator development is an effective way of preparing facilitators and should mirror the type of interprofessional interaction that learners will subsequently undergo. Therefore, faculty development sessions should be organized, developed and facilitated by two or more professional educators who role model the process while discussing content. Applying social constructivism theory is helpful, as within IPE there is an emphasis on learning with and from others, experientially and in the environment in which we work. In their development sessions, novice IPL facilitators should not only participate in sessions but also observe the interprofessional interactions taking place around them. The expert faculty development facilitator should reflect how one's own profession or background impinges on the interactions and language within the group and must be open to alternative points of view, being empathic to other professionals' values, work practices and feelings. There should be the potential for equal participation by all students in discussion, bearing in mind the similarities and differences between them. Students may be at different stages of training, maturity and life experience.

Overcoming potential challenges

Within the IPE literature barriers to successful implementation of professional development programmes tend to focus on logistics. But there are also factors such as lack of support from teachers/tutors for IPL generally; some faculty certainly do not consider that the effort required to put the students in the same space at the same time is merited. Institutional and organizational buy-in is so important; the trickle-down effect of motivated champions who enthuse others with their passion and belief in IPL as a means to enhanced interprofessional teamwork and practice is paramount to engage educators in a new way of working. Many of these educators will remain to be convinced of the evidence for IPL and will become disaffected if 'forced' to teach in this way. A concise, well-written summary of the evidence should be part of the development package, highlighting the move of health service delivery to a patient-centred/client-centred team approach.

Another potential problem is the perceived academic elitism and stereotyping of professions, found not only in students but also in their teachers. In both undergraduate and postgraduate education, there may be a prevailing culture of deferring to medical doctors, which is resented by some health professionals. If such attitudes and behaviour emerge during group (or even faculty development) sessions, the facilitator should draw attention to the process and ask the participants why they think this is happening and how it should be tackled.

There may be a fear that IPE and interprofessional practice will lead to a loss of status, a loss of professional identity and a dilution of the role of individual professions in patient care, with blurring of role boundaries. This worry needs to be anticipated and dealt with by careful handling and acknowledgement of all concerned.

 "It was an encouraging feeling to have the support, camaraderie and cooperation of the other students and preceptors in the community, and it gave us the opportunity to experience both learning and teaching roles with each other. It made me aware of some of the misconceptions existing between professions and the limitations of our own profession."

Medical student, WHO 2010

Summary

The changing nature of modern health and social care delivery, with an increasing emphasis on collaboration between practitioners, is the stimulus for greater awareness and development of IPE. There is growing evidence for the effectiveness of learning together. It is important that interprofessional learning outcomes are explicit and align with activities and assessment. Postqualification learning is best carried out in established teams for relevance. Faculty development is crucial for success. As further research is needed in this field, rigorous evaluation should be planned for and research questions considered. Successful IPE is challenging but also rewarding and helps us share values and experience with other colleagues.

References

Barr H: Ends and means in interprofessional education: towards a typology, *Education for Health* 9:341–352, 1996.

Bluteau P, Jackson A, editors: *Interprofessional Education. Making It Happen*, Basingstoke, 2009, Palgrave Macmillan.

CAIPE: *Interprofessional education: a definition*, London, 2002, Centre for the Advancement of Interprofessional Education.

Canadian Interprofessional Health Collaborative (CIHC): A national interprofessional competency framework. Available at: http://www.cihc.ca/files/CIHC_IPCompetencies_Feb1210.pdf, 2010.

Curran VR, Sharpe D: A framework for integrating interprofessional education curriculum in the health sciences, *Education for Health* 20(3). Available at: http://www.educationforhealth.net/publishedarticles/article_print_93.pdf, 2007.

General Medical Council: *Tomorrow's Doctors*. London, 2009, GMC.

Hammick M, Freeth D, Koppel I, et al: A best evidence systematic review of interprofessional education. BEME guide no. 9, *Medical Teacher* 29:735–751, 2007.

Hammick M, Freeth D, Copperman J, Goodsman D: *Being Interprofessional*, West Sussex, 2009, Polity Press.

Mezirow J: *Transformative Dimensions of Adult Learning*, San Francisco, 1991, Jossey-Bass.

O'Halloran C, Hean S, Humphris D, et al: Developing common learning: The New Generation Project undergraduate medical curriculum, *Journal of Interprofessional Care* 20:12–28, 2006.

Reeves S, Zwarenstein M, Goldman J, et al: Interprofessional education: Effects on professional practice and health care outcomes, *Cochrane Database of Systematic Reviews* 1, 2008.

Reeves S, Lewin S, Espin S, Zwarenstein M: *Interprofessional Teamwork for Health and Social Care*, Oxford, 2010, Blackwell Publishing.

Thistlethwaite JE, Moran M: Learning outcomes for interprofessional education (IPE): literature review and synthesis, *Journal of Interprofessional Care* 24:503–513, 2010.

World Health Organisation: *Framework for Action on Interprofessional Education and Collaborative Practice*, Geneva, 2010, WHO.

Section 4

Tools and aids

Instructional design

J. J. G. van Merriënboer

Introduction

People learn in many different ways. They learn by studying examples, by doing and practicing, by being told, by reading books, by exploring, by making and testing predictions, by being questioned, by teaching others, by making notes, by solving problems, by finding analogies, by rehearsing information and by many, many other activities. Learning is basic to all goal-directed human activity; people cannot deliberately do something without learning from it. This is not to say that learning is always optimal: there are many factors that may either hamper or facilitate learning. Instructional design is that branch of knowledge concerned with, on the one hand, research and theory about instructional strategies that help people learn and, on the other hand, the process of developing and implementing those strategies. Sometimes, the term instructional design (ID) is reserved for the *science* of doing research and developing theories on instructional strategies, and the term instructional systems design (ISD) is reserved for the *practical field* of developing, implementing and evaluating those strategies. The main aim of this chapter is to briefly introduce the reader to the field of ISD and ID.

 Instructional design is both a *science* and a *practical field.*

The ADDIE model

ISD models typically divide the instructional design process into five phases: (1) analysis, (2) design, (3) development, (4) implementation, and (5) evaluation. In this so-called ADDIE model (see Fig. 24.1), the evaluation phase is mainly summative, while formative evaluation may be conducted during all phases. Though the model appears to be linear, it does not have to be followed rigidly. Often, the model is repeatedly used to develop related units of instruction (iteration), phases are skipped because particular

information is already available (layers of necessity) or later phases provide inputs that make it necessary to reconsider earlier phases (zigzag design). It is thus best seen as a project management tool that helps designers think about the different steps that must be taken. Moreover, the ADDIE model does not suggest or follow specific learning theories: it can be used for all instructional design projects irrespective of the preferred learning paradigm.

In the first phase of the ADDIE model (Fig. 24.1), the focus is on the analysis of the desired learning outcomes and on the analysis of fixed conditions. With regard to fixed conditions, analyses pertain to the analysis of the *context* (availability of equipment, time and money, culture, setting such as school, military or

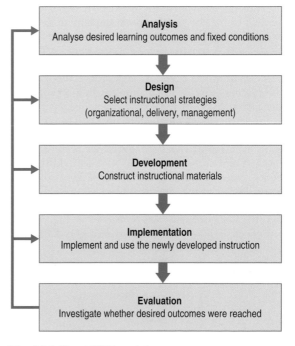

Fig. 24.1 The ADDIE model.

work organization, etc.), the analysis of the *target group* (prior knowledge, general schooling, age, learning styles, handicaps, etc.), and the analysis of *tasks and subject matter* (tools and objects required, conditions for performance, risks, etc.).

 Optimal instructional strategies are determined by both desired outcomes and fixed conditions.

In the second phase of the ADDIE model, instructional strategies are selected that best help to reach the desired outcomes given the fixed conditions. A distinction may be made among organizational strategies (How is the instruction organized?), delivery strategies (Which media are used to deliver the instruction?) and management strategies (How and by whom is the instruction managed?). The basic idea is that both desired outcomes and fixed conditions determine the optimal strategies to select. For example, if the desired outcome is memorizing the names of skeleton bones, rehearsal with the use of mnemonics is a suitable organizational strategy, but if the desired outcome is performing a complex surgical skill, guided practice with feedback on a wide variety of scenarios is a more suitable organizational strategy. In addition, if there is sufficient equipment or money available, the use of high-fidelity simulation might be a suitable delivery strategy for teaching a complex surgical skill, but if there is no equipment or money available, guided on-the-job learning is more suitable.

The remaining phases of the ADDIE model provide guidelines for the development, implementation and evaluation of selected strategies. Development refers to the actual construction of instructional materials, such as learning tasks and assignments, instructional texts, multimedia materials, slides for lectures, guides for teachers and so forth. Implementation refers to the introduction of the newly developed instruction in the setting in which it will be used and to the actual use of the instructional materials. Evaluation investigates whether the desired outcomes were actually reached and answers questions such as: Did the students achieve the expected outcomes? What did they learn? How can the instruction be improved? Each of these phases represents a whole field of research and development in itself. The remainder of this chapter will focus on ID models rather than ISD models, thus on the former two phases.

The universe of ID models

Close to 100 ID models have been described in the literature (for overviews, see Reigeluth 1983, 1999, Reigeluth & Carr-Chellman 2009) and on the internet (see, e.g. www.instructionaldesign.org,

http://carbon.ucdenver.edu/~mryder/itc/idmodels). ID models differ from each other in several dimensions. One dimension pertains to the learning paradigm they adhere to, which may reflect, for example, a behaviorist, cognitive or social-constructivist perspective. A second dimension, discussed in the next section, is between models directed at the level of message design, lesson design and course and curriculum design. A third dimension pertains to outcomes-based models and whole-task models.

OUTCOMES-BASED MODELS

Outcomes-based models typically focus on one particular domain of learning, such as the cognitive domain, psychomotor domain or affective domain (Bloom 1956), which roughly corresponds with the triplet knowledge, skills and attitudes. In one particular domain of learning, desired outcomes are analyzed in terms of distinct objectives or learning goals, after which instructional strategies are selected for reaching each of the separate objectives. Gagné (1985) introduced a widely used taxonomy in the cognitive domain. His taxonomy makes a distinction between verbal information, intellectual skills, cognitive strategies, attitudes and psychomotor skills. The intellectual skills are at the heart of the taxonomy and include five subcategories:

1. Discriminations
2. Concrete concepts
3. Defined concepts
4. Rules
5. Higher-order rules.

This taxonomy reflects the fact that some intellectual skills enable the performance of other, higher-level skills. For instance, the ability to apply rules or procedures is prerequisite to the use of higher-order rules (i.e. problem solving). If you teach an intellectual skill, it is important to identify, in a so-called *learning hierarchy*, the lower-level skills that enable this skill. In teaching, one starts with the objectives for the skills lower in the hierarchy and successively works towards the objectives for the skills higher in the hierarchy.

Many researchers introduced alternative classifications of objectives. But a common premise of all outcomes-based models is that different objectives can best be reached by the application of particular instructional strategies (the *conditions of learning*; Gagné 1985). The optimal strategy is chosen for each objective; the objectives are usually taught one by one and the overall educational goal is believed to be met after all separate objectives have been taught. For instance, if complex skills or professional competences are taught, each objective corresponds with one enabling or constituent skill, and sequencing the objectives naturally results in a part-task sequence. Thus, the learner is taught only one or a very limited number of constituent skills at the same time. New constituent skills are gradually added to practice, and it is not until the end of the instruction – if at all – that the learner has the opportunity to practise the whole complex skill.

Outcomes-based instructional design models are very effective for teaching objectives that have little to do with each other, that is, require little coordination. But in the early 1990s, authors in the field of instructional design started to question the value of outcomes-based models for reaching 'integrative' goals or objectives (e.g. Gagné & Merrill 1990). For complex skills or professional competencies, which are dominant in the medical domain, there are many interactions between the different aspects of task performance and their related objectives: with high demands on coordination. Then, an outcomes-based approach yields instruction that is fragmented and piecemeal and thus does not work. Whole-task models provide an alternative because they pay explicit attention to the coordination of all task aspects.

 Outcomes-based instructional models are very effective for teaching isolated objectives.

WHOLE-TASK MODELS

Whole-task models explicitly aim at integrative goals, or *complex learning*. They take a holistic rather than atomistic perspective on instructional design (van Merriënboer 1997). First, complex contents and tasks are not split over different domains of learning (e.g. knowledge is taught in lectures, skills are taught in a skills lab and attitudes are taught in role plays), but knowledge, skills and attitudes are developed simultaneously by having the learners work on whole, integrative tasks. Second, complex contents and tasks are not reduced into simpler elements up to a level where the single elements (i.e. isolated objectives) can be transferred to learners through presentation and/or practice, but they are taught from simple-to-complex *wholes* in such a way that relationships between the elements are retained. Thus, whole-task models basically try to deal with complexity without losing sight of the relationships between elements.

Rather than starting from a specification of objectives, instructional design starts with the identification of a representative set of real-life tasks and an analysis of the cognitive schemas that people need in order to perform those tasks (also called *cognitive task analysis* or CTA; Clark et al 2008). Cognitive schemas can be seen as the building blocks of cognition and integrate knowledge, skills and attitudes. The process of competence development can be described as the construction and automation of increasingly more complex cognitive schemas. Subprocesses of schema construction are inductive learning and elaboration. Learners *induce* new cognitive schemas and modify existing ones as a result of their concrete experiences with a varied set of tasks. They *elaborate* their cognitive schemas by connecting newly presented information to the things they already know.

 Whole-task models start with the identification and analysis of a set of representative real-life tasks.

Subprocesses of schema automation are knowledge compilation and strengthening. Learners *compile* new knowledge when they construct cognitive rules that always yield the same reaction under particular conditions. Repetition helps learners to *strengthen* these rules; each time the rule is used and yields desired effects, the chance it will be used again under similar conditions is increasing. Whereas schema construction helps learners to develop non-routine behaviors (problem solving, reasoning, decision making), schema automation helps them to develop routine behaviors. Typically, a mix of non-routine and routine behaviors is necessary to efficiently perform real-life tasks. From a design point of view, the specification of increasingly more complex schemas helps to define a series of simple to complex learning tasks. It also helps to identify the non-routine and routine aspects of performance, so that learners can be provided with the necessary information, feedback and assessments on all the different aspects of whole-task performance.

 Complex learning is driven by rich, meaningful learning tasks such as problems, projects or cases.

Whole-task models thus assume that complex learning takes place in situations where student learning is driven by rich, meaningful tasks which are based on real-life or professional tasks. Such tasks are called *problems* (in problem-based learning), *cases* (in the case method), *projects* (in project-based learning), and so forth. Van Merriënboer and Kirschner (2007) use the generic term 'learning tasks' to refer to all whole tasks that help learners reach integrative goals. Merrill (2002) compared a large set of whole-task models and found that they all shared five 'first principles of instruction', stating that meaningful learning is promoted when:

1. Learners are engaged in solving real-world problems
2. Existing knowledge is activated as a foundation for new knowledge
3. New knowledge is demonstrated to the learner

4. New knowledge needs to be applied by the learner

5. New knowledge is integrated into the learner's world.

Examples of ID models

This section will discuss three examples of ID models, at the level of instructional message design, lesson design, and curriculum and course design. All three models can be seen as whole-task models.

COGNITIVE LOAD THEORY

Nowadays, the most popular theories for instructional message design are Sweller's cognitive load theory (CLT) (Sweller 1988; van Merriënboer & Sweller 2010) and Mayer's cognitive theory of multimedia learning (Mayer 2010). Both theories have much in common; we will focus our discussion on CLT. The central notion of CLT is that human cognitive architecture should be a major consideration when designing instructional messages. This cognitive architecture consists of a severely limited working memory with partly independent processing units for visual/spatial and auditory/verbal information, which interacts with a comparatively unlimited long-term memory. The theory distinguishes between three types of cognitive load, dependent on the type of processing causing it, namely:

- *Intrinsic load.* This is a direct function of performing the task, in particular, of the number of elements that must be simultaneously processed in working memory. For instance, a task with many constituent skills that must be coordinated (e.g. dealing with an emergency) yields a higher intrinsic load than a task with less constituent skills that need to be coordinated (e.g. stitching a wound).

- *Extraneous load.* This is the extra load beyond the intrinsic cognitive load mainly resulting from poorly designed instruction. For instance, if learners must search in their instructional materials for information needed to perform a learning task (e.g. searching for the checklist of how to operate a piece of machinery), this search process itself does not directly contribute to learning and thus causes extraneous cognitive load.

- *Germane load.* This is related to processes that directly contribute to learning, in particular to schema construction and schema automation. For instance, consciously connecting new information with what is already known and self-explaining new information are processes yielding germane cognitive load.

Intrinsic, extraneous and germane cognitive load are additive in that, if learning is to occur, the total load of the three together cannot exceed the available working memory capacity. Consequently, well-designed instructional messages should decrease extraneous cognitive load and optimize germane cognitive load in such a way that available cognitive capacity is not exceeded, because otherwise cognitive overload with negative effects on learning will occur. A first set of principles generated by CLT aims to decrease extraneous cognitive load. The *goal-free principle* suggests replacing conventional learning tasks with goal-free tasks that provide learners with a nonspecific goal (e.g. ask students 'Please come up with as many illnesses as possible that could be related to the observed symptoms' rather than asking them 'Which illness is indicated by the symptoms of this patient?'). Whereas conventional tasks force learners to identify the means to reach a specific goal, which causes a high cognitive load, goal-free tasks allow learners to reason from the givens to the goal, which causes a much lower cognitive load. Similar principles are the *worked example principle*, which suggests replacing conventional tasks with worked examples that provide a full solution learners must carefully study (e.g. let students criticize a ready-made treatment plan, rather than having them independently generate such a plan), and the *completion principle*, which suggests replacing conventional tasks with completion tasks that provide a partial solution learners must finish (e.g. let medical interns closely observe a surgical operation and only perform part of it, rather than having them perform the whole operation independently).

 Within the limits of available cognitive capacity, well-designed instructional messages should decrease *extraneous* cognitive load and increase *germane* cognitive load.

Other principles to decrease extraneous cognitive load are particularly important for the design of multimedia materials. The *split attention principle* suggests replacing multiple sources of information, distributed either in space (spatial split attention) or in time (temporal split attention), with one integrated source of information (e.g. provide students instructions for operating a piece of medical equipment just in time, precisely when they need it, rather than providing them the information beforehand). The *modality principle* suggests replacing a written explanatory text and another source of visual information (unimodal) with a spoken explanatory text and the visual source of information (multimodal, e.g. give students spoken explanations when they study a computer animation of the working of the digestive tract, rather than giving them written explanations on screen). The *redundancy principle* suggests replacing multiple sources of information that are self-contained (i.e. they can be understood on their own) with one source of information (e.g. when providing learners with a diagram of the flow of blood in the heart, lungs and body, eliminate a description verbally describing the flow).

Another set of principles aims to optimize germane cognitive load. The *variability principle* suggests replacing a series of tasks with similar features with a series of tasks that differ from each other on all dimensions on which tasks differ in the real world (e.g. when describing a particular clinical symptom, illustrate it using patients with different sex, ages, physiques, medical histories, etc.). The *contextual interference principle* suggests replacing a series of task variants with low contextual interference with a series with high contextual interference (e.g. if students practise different variants of a particular surgical task, order these variants in a random rather than a blocked order). The *self-explanation principle* suggests replacing separate worked examples or completion tasks with enriched ones containing prompts, asking learners to self-explain the given information (e.g. for students learning to diagnose malfunctions in the human cardiovascular system, present an animation of how the heart works and provide prompts that ask them to self-explain the underlying mechanisms).

NINE EVENTS OF INSTRUCTION

At the level of lesson design, Gagné's nine events of instruction (1985) provide general guidelines for the organization of lessons, which can be applied to a wide range of objectives or integrative objectives in the case of complex learning. Table 24.1

Table 24.1 Gagné's nine events of instruction

Event	Illustration
Gain attention	Did you hear about?
Inform learner of objectives	Today we are going to …
Stimulate recall of prior information	Two days ago we learned how to …
Present information	This is a demonstration of how to …
Provide guidance	Now this is a guide for performing …
Elicit performance	Now you try it yourself …
Provide feedback	Alright, but you need to …
Assess performance	We will now have a performance test
Enhance retention and transfer	Alright, now suppose you have to do it on the job …

summarizes the nine events and illustrative remarks made by a teacher; they are roughly sequenced in the order in which they will typically occur in a lesson.

The first three events prepare the students for learning. First, their attention should be gained by presenting an interesting problem or a topical subject or asking them questions on a topic of their interest. This will help to ground the lesson and motivate the learners. Second, the goals of the instruction should be made explicit, so that learners know what they will be able to accomplish after the lesson. A demonstration might be given so that the students can see how they can apply the new knowledge. Third, the relevant prior knowledge of the learners needs to be activated, by making explicit how the new knowledge is connected to the things they already know, providing them with a framework that helps learning and remembering or having them brainstorm on the topic of the lesson.

The next four events steer the actual learning process. First, the new knowledge is presented and examples or demonstrations are provided. Texts, graphics, simulations, figures, pictures and verbal explanations may all help to present the new knowledge. Second, the learners need to practise with the newly presented knowledge. Performance is elicited so that the learners do something with the newly acquired knowledge; for example, they apply new knowledge or practise new skills. Third, learners should receive guidance that helps them to be successful in the application of the new knowledge and skills. Guidance is different from the presentation of content because it primarily helps students to learn (e.g. help them to process new information). Fourth, the learners receive informative feedback, which helps them to identify weaknesses in their behavior and provides hints for improvement.

 The presentation of new information should *always* be accompanied by guided practice and feedback.

The final two events mark the end of a lesson. First, learners' performance should be assessed to check whether the lesson has been successful and the learners have acquired the new knowledge and/or skills. Often, it is worthwhile to give the learners information on their progress over lessons. Second, explicit attention should be paid to enhancing retention and transfer of what has been learned. One might inform the learners about more or less similar problem situations in which the acquired knowledge and skills can be applied, let them review the lesson and come up with new situations in which the acquired knowledge and/or skills can be applied or actually let them perform in such transfer situations.

FOUR-COMPONENT INSTRUCTIONAL DESIGN (4C/ID)

At the level of course and curriculum design, four-component instructional design (van Merriënboer & Kirschner 2007) is a popular whole-task model aimed at the training of complex skills and professional competencies. It provides guidelines for the analysis of real-life tasks and the transition into a blueprint for an educational programme. It is typically used for designing and developing substantial educational programmes ranging in length from several weeks to several years.

The basic assumption of 4C/ID is that blueprints for complex learning can always be described by four basic components, namely: (1) learning tasks, (2) supportive information, (3) procedural information and (4) part-task practice. The four components are based on the four learning processes discussed previously: inductive learning, elaboration, compilation of rules, and strengthening. Learning tasks provide the backbone of the training programme; they provide learning from varied experiences and explicitly aim at transfer of learning. The three other components are connected to this backbone (Fig. 24.2).

Learning tasks include problems, case studies, projects, scenarios and so forth (indicated by the large circles in the figure). They are authentic whole-task experiences based on real-life tasks and aim at the integration of skills, knowledge and attitudes. The whole set of learning tasks exhibits a high variability of practice, because learning from varied experiences facilitates transfer of learning. The learning tasks are organized in easy-to-difficult task classes (indicated by dotted boxes around sets of circles) and have diminishing learner support and guidance within each task class (indicated by diminishing filling of the circles). The basic underlying process for learning from learning tasks is induction, that is, learning from concrete experiences.

Supportive information helps students learn to perform non-routine aspects of learning tasks, which often involve problem solving, diagnostic reasoning and decision making (indicated by L-shaped forms connected to equally difficult learning tasks or task classes). It explains how a domain is organized (e.g. knowledge of the human body) and how problems in that domain are best approached (e.g. a systematic approach to differential diagnosis). It is specified per task class and is always available to learners. It provides a bridge between what learners already know and what they need to know to work on the learning tasks. The basic underlying process for learning from supportive information is elaboration, that is, learning by connecting the new information to what is already known.

> Supportive information is what teachers typically call 'the theory'.

Procedural information allows students to perform routine aspects of learning tasks that are always

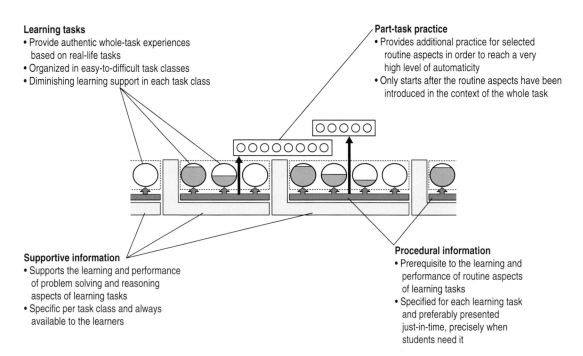

Learning tasks
- Provide authentic whole-task experiences based on real-life tasks
- Organized in easy-to-difficult task classes
- Diminishing learning support in each task class

Part-task practice
- Provides additional practice for selected routine aspects in order to reach a very high level of automaticity
- Only starts after the routine aspects have been introduced in the context of the whole task

Supportive information
- Supports the learning and performance of problem solving and reasoning aspects of learning tasks
- Specific per task class and always available to the learners

Procedural information
- Prerequisite to the learning and performance of routine aspects of learning tasks
- Specified for each learning task and preferably presented just-in-time, precisely when students need it

Fig. 24.2 Schematic overview of the four components in 4C/ID.

performed in the same way (indicated by the dark beam with upward pointing arrows to the learning tasks). It specifies exactly how to perform the routine aspects of the task (i.e. *how-to* information) and is best presented just in time, precisely when learners need it. This can be done by an instructor, but also by a quick reference guide, job aid or mobile application. It is quickly faded as learners gain more expertise. The basic underlying process for learning from procedural information is knowledge compilation, that is, learning by transforming new information into cognitive rules.

Finally, part-task practice pertains to additional practice of routine aspects so that learners can develop a very high level of automaticity for selected aspects for which this is necessary (indicated by the series of small circles). It is mostly used for critical task aspects (e.g. CPR, auscultation, stitching). Part-task practice typically provides huge amounts of repetition and only starts after the routine aspect has been introduced in the context of a whole, meaningful learning task. The basic underlying process for learning from part-task practice is strengthening, that is, automating routine skills through repetitive practice.

Van Merriënboer and Kirscher (2007) describe 10 steps which specify the whole design process typically employed by a designer to produce effective, efficient and appealing programmes for complex learning (see Table 24.2). The four blueprint components directly correspond with four design steps: The design of learning tasks (step 1), the design of supportive information (step 4), the design of procedural information (Step 7), and the design of part-task practice (step 10). The other six steps are auxiliary and are only performed when necessary. Step 2, in which task classes are sequenced: organizes learning tasks in simple to complex categories. They ensure that students work on tasks that begin simply and smoothly increase in complexity. Step 3, where objectives for the different task aspects are set: specifies the standards for acceptable performance. They are needed to assess student performance and to provide learners with useful feedback on all different aspects of whole-task performance. Steps 5, 6, 8 and 9, finally, pertain to in-depth cognitive task analysis. It should be noted that real-life design projects are never a straightforward progression from step 1 to Step 10. As in the ADDIE model, new findings and decisions will often require the designer to reconsider previous steps, yielding zigzag design approaches.

Summary

Instructional design pertains, on the one hand, to the science of doing research and developing theories on instructional strategies, and, on the other hand, to the practical field of developing, implementing and evaluating those strategies. The latter is also called instructional systems design and is characterized by the ADDIE model, which describes the process as a progression through the phases of analysis, design, development, implementation and evaluation.

Close to 100 instructional design models have been described in the literature. Outcomes-based models describe desired learning outcomes in instructional objectives and then select the best instructional strategy for each objective. Whole-task models aim at the development of complex skills or professional competencies; they describe desired learning outcomes as one integrative objective and then select instructional strategies that help students develop professional competencies in a process of complex learning by working on whole, meaningful learning tasks. Three representative examples of ID models on the level of instructional message design, lesson design, and course and curriculum design are, in order, Sweller's cognitive load theory, Gagné's nine events of instruction, and van Merriënboer's 4C/ID model.

In the field of medical education, we see an increased interest in integrative objectives and the development of competence-based curricula in order to facilitate transition from the school to the clinic. In addition, there is a diversification of delivery strategies with increased use of media such as medical simulation, animation and other e-learning applications. As a result, instructional design models are becoming more and more important to the field of medical education.

Table 24.2 Ten steps to complex learning

Blueprint components	Ten steps to complex learning
Learning tasks	1. Design learning tasks 2. Sequence task classes 3. Set performance objectives
Supportive information	4. Design supportive information 5. Analyze cognitive strategies 6. Analyze mental models
Procedural information	7. Design procedural information 8. Analyze cognitive rules 9. Analyze prerequisite knowledge
Part-task practice	10. Design part-task practice

 ID models are becoming increasingly important in medical education due to the popularity of complex learning approaches and e-learning.

References

Bloom BS: *Taxonomy of Educational Objectives, the Classification of Educational Goals – Handbook I: Cognitive Domain*, New York, 1956, McKay.

Clark RE, Feldon DF, van Merriënboer JJG, et al: Cognitive task analysis. In Spector JM, Merrill MD, van Merriënboer JJG, Driscoll MP, editors: *Handbook of Research on Educational Communications and Technology*, ed 3, Mahwah, NJ, 2008, Erlbaum/Routledge, pp 577–594.

Gagné RM: *The Conditions of Learning*, ed 4, New York, 1985, Holt, Rinehart & Winston.

Gagné RM, Merril MD: Integrative goals for instructional design, *Educational Technology Research and Development* 38:23–30, 1990.

Mayer RE: Applying the science of learning to medical education, *Medical Education* 44:543–549, 2010.

Merrill MD: First principles of instruction, *Educational Technology Research and Development* 50(3):43–59, 2002.

Reigeluth CM, editor: *Instructional-Design Theories and Models: An Overview of Their Current Status, vol 1*. Hillsdale, NJ, 1983, Erlbaum.

Reigeluth CM, editor: *Instructional-Design Theories and Models: A New Paradigm of Instructional Theory, vol 2*. Mahwah, NJ, 1999, Erlbaum.

Reigeluth CM, Carr-Chellman AA, editor: *Instructional-Design Theories and Models: Building a Common Knowledge base, vol 3*. New York, 2009, Routledge.

Sweller J: Cognitive load during problem solving: Effects on learning, *Cognitive Science* 12:275–285, 1988.

Van Merriënboer JJG: *Training Complex Cognitive Skills*, Englewood Cliffs, NJ, 1997, Educational Technology Publications.

Van Merriënboer JJG, Kirschner PA: *Ten Steps to Complex Learning*, Mahwah, NJ, 2007, Erlbaum.

Van Merriënboer JJG, Sweller J: Cognitive load theory in health professions education: Design principles and strategies, *Medical Education* 44:85–93, 2010.

Simulation-based medical education

D. Østergaard, P. Dieckmann

Introduction

Simulation-based medical education (SBME) in its widest sense should be defined as any educational activity that utilizes simulative tools and methods in order to create learning opportunities for participants.

 "Simulation is a technique – not a technology."
Gaba 2004

The rapid technological evolution has made it possible to develop tools to be used across all stages of professional development. Training approaches range from basic skill training to training of complex medical situations, like interprofessional critical care and complex scenarios addressing patient safety issues and human factors. In this chapter we focus on how to *do* simulation to create learning opportunities in the different settings. We interpret the term 'medical' in a wide sense, including all healthcare settings and professions. The principles of doing simulation will not vary much between settings and target groups, while the content of scenarios and debriefings will. Here, we focus on the principles.

Rationale for using simulation

Traditionally, medical education has been rooted in clinical practice and based on apprenticeship learning. Organizational and economic challenges in healthcare make it important to change the way we train healthcare professionals and to find ways to optimize learning in the clinical setting:

- The number of people in training in hospitals has increased significantly, and at the same time, the training opportunities are fewer due to a reduction in working hours.

- Today's patients do not want to be trained on.

- New guidelines, methods, drugs and tools are introduced frequently, but their full adaptation in practice takes up to 15 years. Simulation can help shorten this implementation phase. One of the many reasons for slow adaptation is resistance from the senior staff. Simulation can provide a safe yet convincing learning environment, also for senior staff, to stimulate the learners' reflection of current practice. Such changes of attitude and introduction of new ways of working are often difficult for the adult learner. SBME seems to be a promising tool, as it is based on concrete experiences and reflections (Issenberg et al 2005).

- Patients are harmed as a result of incidents, and patient safety data indicate a need for improvement of skills; not only medical expertise skills, but also skills such as interdisciplinary communication and teamwork. The principles of crisis resource management (CRM) were derived from aviation and other high-risk industries and contribute to addressing these challenges. CRM is intended to help prevent and manage difficulties during healthcare, reflecting both the social-team-oriented and cognitive-individual-oriented aspects of human factors (Rall et al 2010a). Learning about CRM is a means to learning new skills and unlearning others, as well as changing attitudes. Anaesthesiology was one of the first specialties to adapt CRM training, and it is believed that this early adoption has contributed considerably to improvements in patient safety. Later, the term non-technical skill was introduced to describe the skills needed to supplement medical expertise or technical skills.

- Healthcare professionals are educated in silos of care, and this makes it difficult to function as a team. We need to change the way health professions are trained: a paradigm shift from mono-professional training to multi- and interprofessional training in order to improve patient safety. Crisis situations are especially challenging, as diagnosing and treatment might be difficult and time constraints might make the challenge greater. Such a complex situation requires a well-functioning team of experts from different specialties and different professions. Simulation provides the opportunity for the team to train together, exchange experiences and learn about mutual expectations and differences in the norms, values and beliefs of professionals from different backgrounds. This will help bridge the silos, especially when introduced in pre-graduate curricula.

- From a pedagogical view, we need to help adult learners to learn by introducing interactive methods. Adult learners are experimental learners, and they learn by going through certain steps in the learning cycle and doing so in different styles (Kolb 1984). SBME provides these types of opportunities. According to Knowles (1990), adult learners are problem centred, and they value learning that can be applied to actual problems that they meet in their clinical life. SBME provides the link between knowing and doing. Simulation scenarios combined with debriefings support reflection and improvement of own competences.

SBME and the simulation technology have the potential to improve training conditions by systematically training on the prevention and management of critical situations, by repeating training scenarios and by continuing the training until a specified level of competence is obtained.

 Why use simulation-based training?
- To improve patient safety
- To provide training opportunities for novices and experts
- To facilitate learning at the individual level
- To facilitate learning in teams of health professions.

ADVANTAGES AND DRAWBACKS OF SIMULATION

The advantages of SBME are numerous. It is possible to train in a safe environment without endangering the patient. The design and implementation of scenarios can be adjusted according to the learner's need. If, for instance, the learner needs more time for decision making, the deterioration of the patient can be slowed down. This is in contrast to the clinical situation, where physiology follows natural laws and the senior person will have to take over the treatment of the patient. In the simulated setting, education can be the primary priority, whereas in the clinical setting, patient safety always comes first. It is also possible to repeat the situation if the objectives are not met or the learner needs more training.

The major drawbacks of SBME are the high costs of the technology and the need for qualified instructors. The costs of taking the participants and the facilitators away from their clinical work are also substantial. On the other hand, the cost of harming the patients or delaying treatment is certainly higher, apart from the human suffering by all involved. One of the challenges is that it is difficult to prove that training has an impact on patient outcome.

Evidence in favour of using simulation

There is overwhelming evidence that participants and facilitators are in favour of SBME.

 "Simulation has been found to be educational effective and to complement clinical training."

Issenberg et al 2005

There is, however, only a limited number of studies demonstrating a positive effect on learning and transfer to the clinical setting using patient simulators.

 "Residents trained in a laparoscopic simulator performed better in the clinical setting than residents trained without exposure to simulation."

Larsen et al 2009

An improvement in perinatal outcome has been demonstrated after simulation-based team training (Draycott et al 2006). Most of the studies evaluating the effect of SBME do not have the sufficient power or proper design to be able to demonstrate an effect. Multicentre studies with a sufficient number of participants are needed, but so are studies focusing on how to use SBME best, as our understanding of how to use SBME to optimize learning is limited (Issenberg et al 2011).

SIMULATION MODALITIES

Simulators used in medical education are educational tools that fall into the broad context of simulation-based medical education. A wide variety of different trainers and methods are available:

1. Skill trainers, animal or human models, can be used for learning practical procedures such as invasive procedures, examinations and procedures where time issues makes it difficult to train in clinical practice (e.g. airway management and basic resuscitation skills).

2. Simulated patients are volunteers (actors, health professionals) or trained patients. They are often used for communication training or for examining purposes, as for instance with rheumatological conditions/patients.

3. Screen-based simulators range from simple programs to advanced programs that allow interaction

with the participant and with the ability to provide automated feedback. Programs are developed for basic science, medical expertise skills and non-technical skills. The advantages of these programs are the ability to use them when it suits the participants and the low cost of running them, once they are ready. The drawbacks are high development costs, the time needed to learn how to use the program and the absence of a teacher.

4. Virtual reality (VR) simulators are advanced screen-based simulators based on 3-D and other immersive technologies. They seem in many ways to be a promising technology both for education of novices and for clinical procedures done by experts. Based on individualised data (for example, from MRI scans) it might be possible to simulate a given procedure with actual patient data before it is performed on that patient.

5. Surgical or procedural simulators are computer-driven devices combined with audio-visual and advanced tactile feedback systems. The advanced simulators provide feedback to the participant based on performance assessment. Endoscopic and minimally invasive surgery simulators are available with a selection of cases/diseases representative for both novices and experts within a given specialty. Advanced simulators are also available for invasive procedures such as catheterization or pacemaker insertion and noninvasive procedures such as ultrasound.

6. With patient simulators (or manikin-based simulators) learners engage in a scenario: a patient case developing according to a set of learning objectives. A patient simulator consists of a computer program (software), a control interface and a realistic full-size manikin placed in a realistic clinical environment, such as the OR, the emergency room or a ward room. The physiological parameters are generated by the computer and displayed on a monitor. The manikin can be a neonate, child or adult with different features. The manikin can be diagnosed (e.g. heart and breath sounds, pupil reaction), procedures can be performed (e.g. handling the airway, insertion of IV) and treatment can be applied (e.g. drugs and fluid administration). A loudspeaker placed in the manikin (the patient's voice) makes is possible to communicate with the patient. The computer program can be pre-programmed to mimic a certain case/scenario and the program will respond to the actions taken by the participant.

Different combinations of these modalities are frequently used, like a part task trainer and a simulated patient or a surgical simulator and a simulated patient or a patient simulator. Screen-based simulators are often used as pre-course preparation or post-course follow-up to maintain capabilities. Often a given learning objective is obtained by combining modalities on a course, for instance, training practical skills on a part task trainer and later in a procedural/surgical or patient simulator. At times the distinction between the modalities is not clear-cut and related to their use. Both manikin-based simulators and surgical simulators can be used and seen as task trainers as well as advanced simulators. Basing the distinction on the feature list of a simulator alone might not be adequate.

Improved simulation technology and concepts have resulted in greater acceptance by health professionals and an increased use of SBME (Khan et al 2011). Over the last two decades, the use of SBME has significantly increased, especially the use of advanced simulators. Contents of training vary with the tools available and between disciplines. For example, surgical simulators are primarily used for procedural skills training (medical expertise skills) and training is done by the individual doctor, at times immediately before this type of procedure is to be applied in an actual clinical case (Kneebone et al 2007). This is in contrast to SBME using patient simulators, which is often conducted for a group of learners or a real clinical team. Manikin-based simulations are frequently used to improve knowledge, attitude and behaviour towards patient safety. In any case, the role of a tutor and the responsibility for this type of training are very different from the role of a lecturer and tutor in a skills centre. Therefore, there is an increased interest in train-the-trainer concepts (see below). In the following sections, we discuss in more detail how and when to use SBME. We will focus on manikin-based simulators, but the principles are similar for other simulation modalities as well.

How to start using patient simulators?

In the following sections, we focus on patient simulation training. The different simulation applications are diverse and can be categorized by 11 dimensions related to, for example, purpose and learning objectives, participant level of experience and domain, the technology and site of training and feedback method (Gaba 2004).

 How to start using patient simulators:
- Identify the learning objectives
- Select the right tool
- Consider context and setting
- Develop the scenario script including patient data, room set
- Include sufficient time for debriefing.

SBME can aim at the 'knows', 'knows how', 'shows' and 'does' levels. Learning objectives can address medical expertise skills, non-technical skills or combinations of these. Enthusiasts have a tendency to use patient simulators for everything. We recommend, due to the high costs, that the technology is chosen according to the learning objectives and that a combination of different methods is used, as described in the previous section. Some content is still best acquired by reading a book and thinking about what the author wanted to say. Several publications have described a set of principles and provided guidelines for how to use SBME most efficiently (Burke et al 2006, Rall et al 2010b).

For all the use of simulation, it is essential that the instructors know how to best use the tools in a given context.

Surgical simulators are primarily used for procedural skills training.
Manikin-based simulations are frequently used to improve knowledge, attitude and behaviour towards patient safety.

TRAIN THE TRAINERS

In the simulation literature, the trainer is called (and functions as) either a facilitator or an instructor. The learning objectives and the context are implying which role to take. In patient simulation it is advocated that the primary role is the facilitator role. A facilitator is described as a person who facilitates learning, who guides and stimulates reflection in the group of learners.

The facilitator should be able to shift to the role of instructor. This can be necessary if the learners, for instance, do not fully understand the situation or the recommended treatment. The trainer should shift back to the facilitator role when possible to stimulate the group of learners to self-reflection and learning.

"The facilitator should be enthusiastic and trained in guiding the participants through all 8 phases of a simulation course."

Dieckmann et al 2009

Selection and training of the facilitators are of paramount importance. The facilitator should be able to reflect on the activities and be ready for continuous development based on critical reflection of the participants' learning and own competence. Professionally, the person should be humble, be respectful and yet be able to take the lead. He or she should be able to adjust on the fly, if necessary. This could be adapting the scenario to make it a good learning experience or the debriefing to dig deeper into a certain learning point. Facilitation is the keyword.

Collaborating with the simulator operator is important. It can be difficult during the scenario to take notes; the use of a marker system can make it easier to identify relevant recordings that illustrate good and bad performances and other interesting points. Where SBME addresses interprofessional teamwork, the role-modelling function of an interprofessional team conducting the course is especially important. An important first step for any course and scenario development is the conduction of a thorough needs analysis.

NEEDS ANALYSIS

The three-circle model of competence presented by Harden et al (1999) describes the core circle as the ability to perform the task, the second circle as the ability to approach the task and the outer circle as professionalism. This nicely describes the skills needed for health professionals. Often a combination of skills needs to be trained. The importance of non-technical skills for applying the medical expertise skills has to be addressed.

In specialist training programmes the learning objectives are clearly stated, but other sources of information are needed such as patient safety data and the learner's confidence/experience with a given objective. In some institutions simulation is used as a method to analyse the working environment and the system's weaknesses. This method can also demonstrate the necessary competences at the individual and team level and hence the need for training. The areas which are difficult to train/learn or should be trained as a team should be addressed in SBME. Also, procedures that are dangerous for the patient or where time (urgency) is of importance for survival should be the first to address using SBME.

Complex skills or tasks can be trained using a combination of technologies. Advanced cardiac life support training for the team could, for instance, consist of a combination of mini lectures (knowledge of algorithms and of the importance of team skills), skills training (compression, ventilation and the use of a defibrillator) and patient simulation (decision making and teamwork).

SELECTING THE RIGHT TOOL

In earlier years, the level of fidelity and realism of the simulator were highlighted, whereas now, the focus is on how to establish a valuable learning experience for the participants. Realism of simulation should be distinguished from the relevance of simulation and whether simulation is necessary to reach the goals. A good and relevant simulation in medical education is the simulation that allows the creation of the learning opportunities required by the curriculum. Whether the simulation is realistic or not is then a secondary question. However, for some learning goals realism to the right degree is needed. Realism concerns the comparison between two entities: the simulator and the patient who is simulated. As opposed to aircraft simulators, the patient simulations cannot be compared so easily to the 'simulated system', as patients account for much larger variability than airplanes do.

To determine what level of realism is needed for which learning goals requires further differentiations. Realism is not a mono-dimensional concept, as many different works have shown. We suggest the three dimensions of physical, semantical and phenomenal realism (Dieckmann et al 2007, Dieckmann et al 2009). Physical realism concerns all and only what can be measured in centimetres, grams and seconds (e.g. weight of a simulator in pounds, wavelengths of the light that is reflected by the pupils of the manikin). Semantical realism concerns the cognitive meaning that can be assigned to the situation (e.g. interpreting the clinical and vital signs of the patient as a case of asthma). Phenomenal realism concerns the experience that participants have during the actual simulation case and how well it corresponds to the experience they would have with an actual clinical case of an asthma patient (e.g. feeling tense because of difficulties in finding the right treatment and, simulation-specific, the tension of being observed and debriefed).

For some learning goals physical realism of simulation is needed (e.g. when learning the psychomotor skills of placing an IV line). If the physical force patterns are wrong, participants might have difficulties in actually placing an IV line on the patient. For many other learning goals, however, it can be very beneficial to depart from physical realism while still preserving semantical and phenomenal realism (e.g. many simulative exercises work with abstract situations that are still relevant for clinical treatment). When designing and implementing courses and scenarios, it is important to optimize (not maximize!) the realism in the right form for the specific learning goals. One might very well reflect on one's performance in highly unrealistic simulations in the physical sense.

CONTEXT/SETTING

The scenario takes place in realistic surroundings. The number of participants will vary depending on the scope of scenario or the size of the team. Often, a few of the participants are chosen to be the main participants in the scenario, while other team members can be assigned a role later in the scenario. Some of the participants will have the role of an observer, who is taking notes and preparing questions to the team to be used in the debriefing session after the scenario (see later). The scenario is recorded, and sequences from the recording are used in the debriefing session.

SBME is used both in universities for medical students and for teams of students from the same or differing professions such as nursing or respiratory therapy. This implies that training takes place in the university in a realistic environment. SBME is implemented in postgraduate training programmes in many countries. Often training is mono-disciplinary, but there is a clear need for multi-professional training programmes to promote a culture of safety and knowledge of collaborators' competence. Many hospitals have implemented training programmes for multidisciplinary and interprofessional teams in handling emergency situations. At first training was introduced for emergency teams such as cardiac arrest, medical emergency and trauma teams. Later, training of ward staff was introduced to improve teams' ability to identify the deteriorating patient and initiate initial treatment. It is important that training is conducted for the real team and for team members to play their own role in the scenario. Changing roles might be beneficial in order to get an understanding of other team members' tasks and conditions, but is usually difficult to do.

Often, training of staff takes place in simulation units in the hospital or in regional simulation centres. Training can also be conducted locally, in the ward room or in the ambulance. This is called in situ training. Instead of bringing the learner to the simulation centre, the simulator is brought to the learner. The advantage is that training can take place in the real setting, using local manuals and having people find the necessary equipment and drugs; the local procedures are then tested. Shorter scenarios are often run during the day, making it possible for more people to attend the training and to some extent reduce the time away from the department. One should, however, be realistic about how much to include in the training and balance the number of learning objectives with the length of the scenario. This type of training is ideal for creating attention or re-training purposes. The drawback is the time and effort spent on preparing the scenario locally and moving the simulator and other equipment. Also finding space in a busy department (ward) locally might be difficult.

THE EIGHT PHASES OF SBME

An eight-phased model has been used to describe the elements of a SBME course (Dieckmann et al 2009):

1. Setting introduction: establish a safe learning environment and a confidentiality agreement
2. Simulator briefing: familiarization with the simulator and the environment
3. Theory input: presentation of concepts related to the course
4. Scenario briefings: participants are given details about the scenario

5. Simulation scenario: conduction of the patient case

6. Debriefing: facilitated group discussion, often combined with the use of clips from recordings

7. Breaks: refreshments and possibility to communicate with team

8. Course ending: evaluation of the course, preparation of learning plans.

TYPES OF SCENARIOS/PRINCIPLES OF SCENARIO DESIGN

The scenario should have well-defined and clear learning objectives, describing what we expect the learners to learn. The facilitators' task is to transform the clinical tasks into meaningful scenarios that help this process. Real cases (after de-identification) can be used as an inspiration for developing a scenario that can illustrate the necessary learning objectives and provide many of the clinical data (BP, HR, etc.); laboratory data, ECG and X-rays are also very useful to develop the scenario and the patient record. After the development of the scenario, it can be scripted. It is recommended to pilot test the scenario to find out whether the learning objectives can be met and to adjust the lists used for preparation. A pilot test will hopefully also make it obvious whether the level of difficulty for this type of learner is appropriate or should be adjusted. Often a given scenario can easily be used or slightly modified for other types of learners. Ideally, instructors are able to adjust the scenario to learners for whom it would be 'too easy' as well as for those for whom it would be 'too hard' by using 'scenario life savers' (Dieckmann et al 2009).

A scenario script includes learning objectives, patient demographics, patient data background, baseline and development of parameters during scenario, manikin and room set-up description, list of needed drugs and equipment, and information for 'hot seat' participants, role players and observers. If possible, evidence-based guidelines to support the medical treatment should be included. Supplementary information for the facilitator and simulation operator is included to make it easier for them to run the scenario. This part includes a plan B (and C) if the learners deviate from the case. A structured, centre-standardized approach to scenario scripts is recommended.

One of the burning issues in the simulation community is the question: Will you allow the patient to die? The answer is yes, if part of the learning objectives is to be able to stop treatment if needed or to train communication with relatives (providing the bad news). On the contrary, the answer is no, if only due to insufficient treatment of the simulated patient.

KEY ELEMENTS OF DEBRIEFING

The debriefing element in SBME is the cornerstone of the course, but also the most difficult part for the simulation instructor. Here the participants can reflect on actions taken in the scenario and discuss them with the team. Adult learners are capable of evaluating their own skills, so the learners are asked to reflect and explore. For the participants to grow professionally, they must develop meta-cognitive skills, including the ability to critically analyse one's own performance.

The many terms used to describe the simulation instructor using SBME indicate the differences in the underlying philosophies and tasks that the person has to perform. The most important role in the debriefing phase is to steer the discussion and, by the use of questions, to give insight into frames (mental models) behind the participants' reaction and action (Rudolph et al 2008). The role here is more a facilitating role than an instructor role. Small clips from the recording can be used to illustrate learning objectives.

 The debriefing is where the learning takes place. The role is more a facilitating role than an instructor role.

Debriefing is a complex task and can be conducted in different ways. A structured approach is advocated. In the literature several methods are described (Fanning & Gaba 2007). Most methods involve a setting-the-scene phase, where the rules and timeline are presented. Often the emotions created by the simulation are taken care of first. A three-phased structure is often used: description, analysis and application (Steinwachs 1992). Most facilitators find it natural to begin with a positive round or comment: reinforcement of good behaviour, building up competence and establishing a constructive atmosphere in the room. The learner who made a wrong decision in the scenario but who is aware that this is the case should be given the opportunity to express his or her awareness and how he or she should have acted. The instructor should be a role model for how to communicate to the team during the debriefing session. Constructive feedback is recommended, but it is also necessary to address undesirable behaviour.

Facilitators might be in a situation where a learner is complaining about the realism of the simulation, finding it difficult to participate in the scenario. Often this is due to the participant feeling unprepared for the simulation. This might imply that the facilitator could have interacted differently during or before the scenario.

ESSENTIAL FACTORS FOR SUCCESS

 The most essential factors for success of simulation-based training is providing feedback and integrating the training into the curriculum.

According to Issenberg et al (2005), some of the most essential factors for the success of SBME include providing feedback and integrating SBME into the curriculum, whereas the fidelity of the simulator is less important.

According to Knowles it is important for adult learners to feel safe in the professional image of who they are, which is related to their roles and job responsibilities (Knowles 1990). One should remember that SBME is a strong learning tool and that participants can feel very exposed. Creating a safe and engaging learning environment is a challenge. This can be achieved by sending out material in advance to make learners comfortable and to prepare the facilitators and by helping the learners to identify their own learning needs.

In the preparation of the learning experience, the most important factors are:

- Establishing a safe learning environment
- Preparation of the participants for simulation
- Designing scenarios with well-described learning objectives
- Designing scenarios with different levels of difficulty
- Describing the roles of the participants in the scenario
- Training the facilitators in providing feedback
- Stimulating reflection on own competences and assisting in preparing learning plans.

Integration of SBME in the curriculum can be a challenge if not all stakeholders are interested in a change, as introducing SBME means taking out something else. Establishment of national or regional workgroups that include all stakeholders might be a way forward. This has been done successfully in some specialties in European countries.

If a positive effect of team training in a hospital is seen, leaders and decision makers should take advantage of this and discuss how to implement this type of training in the organization.

Summary

SBME combines educational methodologies, concepts and frameworks which can be used to help participants improve their capabilities: no matter on which level they start. Many aspects are of importance for optimizing the learning. SBME should be used following a needs analysis and should address relevant learning objectives for the participants. The most cost-effective (SBME) modality should be used to obtain the given objectives. The human resources and conceptual frameworks are at least as important as the technology used.

SBME challenges instructors, and training programmes should be implemented to prepare them for the different roles they need to play using SBME. SBME is a powerful tool and thus needs to be used by capable instructors. However, the literature on how best to use this tool in order to facilitate learning is still limited. Further development should include adaptive training addressing the individual needs of the learners.

Combining different types of SBME in a goal-oriented fashion will probably (and hopefully) be used more often in the future, making it possible for specialists to train together using realistic tools: for instance, combination of a surgical and an anaesthesia simulator. To spread this powerful tool, it will need to be integrated more strongly into the curriculum.

References

Burke CS, Salas E, Wilson-Donelly K, Priest H: How to turn a team of experts into an expert medical team, *Quality and Safety in Health Care* 13 (Suppl 1):96i–104i, 2006.

Dieckmann P, Gaba D, Rall M: Deepening the theoretical foundations of patient simulation as social practice, *Simulation in Healthcare* 2:183–193, 2007.

Dieckmann P, Manser T, Wehner T, Rall, M: Simulation settings for learning in acute medical care. In Dieckmann P, editor: *Using Simulations for Education, Training and Research*, Lengerch, 2009, Pabst.

Draycott T, Sibanda T, Owen L, et al: Does training in obstetric emergencies improve neonatal outcome? *BJOG* 113:177–182, 2006.

Fanning RM, Gaba DM: The role of debriefing in simulation-based learning, *Simulation in Healthcare* 2:115–125, 2007.

Gaba DM: The future vision of simulation in health care, *Quality and Safety in Health Care* 13:2–10, 2004.

Harden RM, Crosby JR, Davis MH: AMEE Guide No. 14: Outcome-based education: Part 1 – An introduction to outcome-based education: a model for the specification of learning outcomes, *Medical Teacher* 21:7–14, 1999.

Issenberg SB, McGaghie WC, Petrusa ER, et al: Features and uses of high-fidelity medical simulations that lead to effective learning: a BEME systematic review, *Medical Teacher* 27:10–28, 2005.

Issenberg B, Ringsted C, Østergaard D, Dieckmann P: Setting a research agenda for simulation-based healthcare education. A synthesis of the outcome from an Utstein style meeting, *Simulated Healthcare* 6:155–167, 2011.

Khan K, Pattison T, Sherwood M: Simulation in medical education, *Medical Teacher* 33:1–3, 2011.

Kneebone R, Nestel D, Vincent C, Darzi A: Complexity, risk and simulation in learning procedural skills, *Medical Education* 41:808–814, 2007.

Knowles M: *The Adult Learner: A Neglected Species*, ed 4. Houston, TX, 1990, Gulf Publishing Company.

Kolb DA: *Experiential Learning: Experience as the Source of Learning and Development*, Englewood Cliffs, NJ, 1984, Prentice Hall.

Larsen CR, Sørensen JL, Grantcharov T, et al: Impact of virtual reality training in laparoscopic surgery. A randomised controlled trial, *British Medical Journal* 338:b1802, 2009.

Rall M, Gaba DM, Howard SK, Dieckmann P: Human performance and patient safety. In Miller RD, editor: *Miller's Anaesthesia*, Philadelphia, 2010a, Elsevier Churchill Livingston.

Rall M, Gaba DM, Dieckmann P, Eick C: Patient simulation. In Miller RD, editor: *Miller's Anaesthesia*, Philadelphia, 2010b, Elsevier Churchill Livingston.

Rudolph JW, Simon R, Raemer DB, et al: Debriefing as formative assessment: Closing the performance gaps in medical education, *Academic Emergency Medicine* 15:1010–1016, 2008.

Steinwachs B: How to facilitate a debriefing, *Simulation and Gaming* 23:186–195, 1992.

Simulated/standardized patients

M. Cantrell, E. A. Gephardt

Introduction

Lay people who have been trained to portray patients have come under many names since the 1960s. Initially they were called *programmed patients*, followed by *simulated patients* in the 1970s. When used for assessment of medical students, they came to be known as *standardized patients* and then, in good medical acronym fashion, came the term SP. The term 'standardized' eventually replaced the original term 'simulated' to reinforce the fact that the patient's situation can be made fundamentally the same for every student encounter. This terminology is attributed to Canadian psychometrician Geoffrey Norman (Wallace 1997). People who are portraying parents or relatives of a patient, or other healthcare members in a clinical situation who are not the patient, are termed standardized participants (Monaghan et al 1997).

 A standardized patient is always simulating, but a simulated patient is not always standardized.

In this chapter, SP will be used interchangeably to mean standardized patient, simulated patient or standardized participant.

SPs are particularly useful for teaching beginning students who are developing their interviewing and examination skills in preparation for interactions with real patients. Medical students often lack clinical experience with real patients. By learning through realistic SP scenarios, they increase their experience, and faculty are able to see how students practically use their new knowledge. With SPs, students can learn to take a patient history and perform a physical exam in a structured and efficient manner. Students learn to ask questions about medical, surgical and social histories in a systematic way. SPs are also helpful with upper-level students, assuring that what has been taught in the curriculum has been integrated by students ready to go out into practice.

 In what areas of your curriculum would SPs enhance a student's understanding and proficiency?

What can an SP do?

 "An SP is defined as a person who has been carefully coached to simulate an actual patient so accurately that the simulation cannot be detected by a skilled clinician."

Barrows 1993

The SP can replay a case over and over again in a consistent and believable way. An SP can be trained to give information on a patient case, display physical findings in an examination and give feedback to the student in the form of verbal feedback or by filling out a checklist.

The best way to see if a medical student can perform a medical interview or physical exam in a correct way is to observe them as they interview or examine a patient. Any student who works with patients will behave in the same way with an SP as they do in the actual clinic setting. This accurate reflection of their actions, decisions and behaviours has been thoroughly researched and validated by many professionals (Barrows 1993). Since it can be difficult to find real patients with the diseases and findings necessary for students to see, using SPs guarantees that students study the preferred patient cases. An added benefit of using SP cases is the ability to schedule them as needed.

SPs can give information and also be scripted to ask for any information that is needed in the case. They can have examinations performed on them including breast, pelvic and male genitourinary examinations. There is special training for those exams, and special attention should be given to how many exams are performed daily. An SP can be trained to successfully record an encounter on a written checklist, recalling what happens and stating what they have experienced. In their written feedback, they may not address the medicine behind any procedure performed during the encounter. For example, for a heart exam, the SP can record on a checklist where the student placed the stethoscope during the exam, but cannot make a judgment about what the student heard or diagnosed in regard to heart disease.

The SP can also score a communication checklist based on his or her experience during the encounter with the student. For example, the SP can comment on a student's degree of caring or lack of eye contact, based on the SP's experience during the encounter.

In general, the use of SPs allows faculty control of clinical content and assurance that patients are available on schedule. In addition, using SP cases is:

- Convenient: available anytime, any place
- Reliable: cases are standardized and reproducible
- Valid: comparable to real patients
- Controllable: faculty can adjust the learning objectives
- Realistic: faculty can integrate psychosocial issues into a case
- Corrective: learner can receive feedback immediately
- Practical: learners can practise invasive exams (pelvic or breast exams)
- Repeatable: learners can rehearse clinical situations they are not ready to manage alone
- Measurable: learners' performances can be compared
- Safe: inconvenience, discomfort or potential harm to real patients are limited
- Efficient: may provide a longitudinal experience in a compressed time frame and reduce time demands on physician teaching faculty.

SPs are used in many medical schools around the world as well as other healthcare educational programmes including pharmacy, nursing and dentistry. Any healthcare team members who interact with patients can benefit from working with an SP in order to evaluate how they actually work with patients in their field.

If an institution has an SP programme, then a valuable resource is already available. Contacting the institution's SP educator can save time and make case and curriculum development a much easier process.

If the institution does not have an SP programme, it is still worth the time and effort to use an SP to teach medical students how to conduct an interview, communicate with a patient or family member and examine a patient. It is also helpful to teach clinical reasoning and can take a student through an entire disease state from diagnosis to treatment and follow-up. This can all be completed in 2 hours instead of 2 weeks, 2 months or longer.

 What kind of patient cases would translate to SP methodology?

How to use an SP

SP RECRUITMENT

Finding a person who becomes a successful SP is not always easy. Recruitment requires imagination! Most programmes start small and gradually build a pool of well-trained and dependable SPs. It is necessary to find people who are intelligent and can understand that this work is educational. The use of people from outside the institution creates a better outcome of a realistic encounter for the learner. When students know the SP, whether a colleague or the staff secretary, they are less likely to take the simulation seriously. People outside of the medical profession can easily be trained to portray cases without having an understanding of medical knowledge. Friends, neighbours and family members who are interested in the programme's success are often a good initial source for recruitment.

Retired teachers and educators make excellent SPs because they understand educational objectives. Other reliable SPs have been homemakers, students in undergraduate non-medical programmes, health club members, part-time teachers, waiting staff and actors. Use caution when using actors as SPs. This work is not about their ego or applause, but is strictly about education. Actors working as SPs must clearly understand that their role is in the field of education, not theatre.

 A good SP is intelligent and can understand that SP work is about education, not entertainment.

Once there is a core group of SPs, they will spread the word about the programme and recruit individuals with whom they would like to work. When a more formal approach is needed, place small posters near elevators in hospitals and clinics. When special populations are needed, like adolescents or elderly persons, approach schools or assisted living facilities. Advertising in local papers can produce an adverse response to recruitment. People who respond to advertising for 'fake' or 'pretend' patients are often not the most mentally stable or reliable employees. This seems to be especially true for cases involving psychiatric issues, as when the applicant responding to the advert requests psychiatric cases.

When recruiting SPs, these characteristics are of primary importance:

- appropriate for role (age/gender/physical characteristics)
- accurate (on time, every time)
- accessible (by telephone, e-mail)
- able to accept/use constructive feedback/criticism
- able to maintain confidentiality.

SP TRAINING

Schedule the first training session for approximately 2 weeks before the event. It is suggested that the SP have multiple training sessions, with the first session covering an introduction of the case being portrayed and the SP's educational role in that portrayal. At the first session, give the SP a brief orientation to the activity and describe the role. During training, an SP should be given information in small bites. Ask the SP to write down everything said about who the character is and what he or she knows about the patient: this is a good way to reinforce the knowledge of the case. After the first training, allow the SP a few days to study the material independently.

The next training session will consist of answering any questions about the case and introducing the SP to other educational components of the case such as checklists and feedback processes. Next, walk the SP through the physical encounter if there is one associated with the case. Let the SP feel where he or she will be in the room and where to enter and exit. Allow the SP to experience each item on the checklist. When confident, the SP should practise the encounter under the observation of the author or trainer. During this second training, the SP should practise a sufficient number of times to ensure accuracy.

A third and fourth training session will be used for running the case repeatedly until the SP is portraying the case in a consistent and reliable way. A final run-through, or dry run, of the case allows the medical faculty to experience the encounter from the student's perspective and to make small adjustments to the case as needed. Allow the case author to see the dry run using an upper level student with no prior knowledge of the case to see how it will flow during teaching or testing. This dry run also allows the checklist to be clarified and, if necessary, adjusted by the faculty prior to the student encounters. Showing an audio-visual (A/V) recording to the SP will validate his or her progress in portraying the encounter. The ability to capture an A/V recording of the SP/ student encounters makes this methodology very efficient. Faculty can review the recordings based on their own schedules. Students can review their encounters privately to reflect on and self-assess their performance.

Remember that the overarching goal of SP training is that the SP will be so carefully coached that the simulation cannot be detected by a skilled clinician. General training tips for SPs include:

- Dress the part: make sure you are dressed just like the patient might be, with the same props, such as bags, purse, shoes
- Don't answer before a question is finished (telegraph information)
- Speak slowly
- Use conversational style when appropriate: don't sound like a robot, spitting out checklist items as if reading
- Only answer the questions that you have been asked (don't volunteer information unless directed to do so)
- Answer questions by using the checklist item as your statement, not just yes or no; this will help with recall ('No, I am not on any medications')
- Make sure your body language supports the personality of the patient you're portraying (open and welcoming, slumped over and tired, closed and angry).

TEACHING WITH AN SP

Teaching students to work with SPs

The key to interacting with SPs is to relate to them exactly as a real person who has either a professional or a personal relationship to the simulation. SPs will not interrupt a learner during an encounter, nor will they volunteer any information unless directed to do so. Learners should not attempt to communicate with an SP out of role. This is unprofessional and will embarrass both the SP and the learner.

When SPs are used in small-group teaching sessions, the 'time-in/time-out' format is used. The guidelines are very simple:

- Imagine that the SP is sitting in a clinic room, waiting to be seen. The SP will not acknowledge the group until addressed as a real patient.
- One student begins the interview by introducing him- or herself and eliciting the reason for the visit (or the chief complaint).
- If the student in the encounter becomes uncomfortable or does not know what to say, he or she can signal by saying 'time-out'. The SP will go into suspended animation and act as if waiting for the doctor. When the student is ready to resume, he or she will call 'time-in'.
- The student can ask for help in 'time-out', but this is not the time for a lecture or lengthy discussion.

- If a preceptor needs to correct a student or to emphasize something the student has done, he or she may also call 'time-out'.

- Only the facilitator or student in the encounter can call 'time-out'.

- Once all the students who wish to interview the patient have done so, the preceptor will ask the SP to step out of role and give feedback to each student who participated in the encounter.

Teaching associates (TAs)

TAs are professional patients who have been trained to teach physical examination manoeuvers on their own bodies. SPs facilitate 'hands-on' teaching of clinical skills while avoiding inconvenience, discomfort or potential harm to real patients. TAs provide specific guidance about examination techniques, such as appropriate palpation pressures and sequencing for patient comfort, and this immediate feedback enhances the learning process. TAs can make awkward first-time exams more comfortable. They can also serve as expert recorders in testing situations. TAs need to have careful training and coaching by physicians in order to teach exactly how these exams should be done. Coaching is also very important for how they will communicate with the student. They will need to be reminded that what they are teaching is a technique and not medicine. It is helpful to have a physician on hand during these exams to answer any medical questions that might arise.

Feedback and debriefing

Students should receive immediate and constructive feedback at all levels of training. Well-trained SPs can give constructive feedback based on how they feel during the encounter. Using the model, 'When you did this, I felt this' keeps the feedback on a communication level and not about the student's medical knowledge. An example of this might be, 'When you walked in the exam room and forgot my name, I felt angry.'

 Using the patient's unique perspective, the SP can tell the student what the physical exam actually felt like and how well the student communicated.

Practising this with the SP during the training will help the SP develop feedback skills that can work with almost any student encounter. A debriefing process with the faculty helps students learn by reflecting, analysing and talking about the SP experience. A faculty member or trained facilitator should guide the process by asking questions, giving feedback or clarifying information. For most teaching

simulations, we recommend debriefing participants immediately after the simulation, while the experience is fresh and it is easy to demonstrate a key point or repeat part of the simulation (Schwid et al 2001).

Testing with an SP

INSURING ACCURACY

When SPs are used for testing, consistency and accuracy are much more important than for a teaching session. SPs must portray each encounter in a consistent way so that each student would describe the exact same person in their encounter. Important to each case is the checklist and what responses are elicited for each checklist item. Writing a simple checklist guide for the SP will help with accuracy. For example, if the checklist item is 'I only take a baby aspirin and a multivitamin each day, nothing else', you might list the questions a student would ask to get that checklist item correctly, such as 'Are you on medications?', 'Do you take any kind of pills regularly?', 'What kind of drugs do you take?' or 'Are you on medication right now?'. The case writer should be the one to give the guidelines to the SP in order for the SP to consistently and accurately be able to answer questions in a standardized way.

 We can standardize the patients, but not always the student.

CONSIDERATIONS

Testing also requires more SP training than teaching encounters. When using SPs for testing, make sure the checklist is introduced in the first or second training session and make sure complete checklist items are spoken while portraying the patient. Simply answering yes and no to questions does not make for easy scoring or recall of the checklist item. For testing, there may be more than one dry run session needed. To ensure checklist accuracy, have the SP portraying the case fill out a checklist whenever he or she watches an encounter or watches a replay of the encounter. The case author and anyone helping with the case should complete a checklist as well: so that comparisons can be made and inconsistent scores of checklist items can be discussed and agreed upon. If an SP cannot consistently score, consider using a replacement or having the SP do more training.

Hybrid or multimodality simulation

SPs represent the wide variety of roles that are represented in healthcare encounters. These SPs may portray nurses, physicians, allied health professionals and/or the patient's friends and family (Monaghan et al 1997). Many patients are not alone when they come into a hospital setting. This is especially true in paediatric hospitals. With a movement towards patient- and family-centred care, there can be many players in the exam room and hospital setting.

According to the Bristol Medical Simulation Centre's database, there are currently over 1550 simulation centres around the world, confirming that many healthcare education programmes are establishing simulation centres (Jones 2011). An SP educator is a beneficial member of that simulation team. When SP methodology is integrated into high-fidelity simulation using manikins, the realism of a scenario increases and standardization of the simulation makes it reproducible for multiple learners. Some things to consider when adding an SP to a simulation encounter with a manikin are the level of emotion the encounter will have and what kind of feedback the SP will give to students. Manikin simulation often relates to crisis situations and how a medical team reacts in a crisis. Adding the SP to the crisis provides a richer, more complex encounter for the team. For example, the team may need to deliver bad news to the family about what happened during the crisis situation. The learning objectives now include not only team communication but also the family-centred care communication that make the encounter more holistic.

Another use of hybrid simulation is to incorporate partial task trainers with SPs so that students can practise both clinical procedures and patient communication skills (Kneebone et al 2002). This technique is done by putting the SP and task trainer together so that the task trainer becomes an extension of the SP's body. Examples of this include seating an SP behind a pelvic trainer or catheterization model and then draping the SP to the model. The student must then perform the procedure and talk the patient through the procedure as it is being done. Other possible hybrid simulations can include using simulated skin tissue strapped to an SP's arm or leg for wound care or injections. The risk of the SP being stuck or harmed can be avoided by careful training. The use of dry runs is particularly important to ensure the SP's thorough understanding of any possible harm that might occur during the simulation. This training then allows the SP to pay special attention during the encounters.

Summary

While SPs do not replace real patients in the curriculum, they provide a dynamic educational resource for a safe and supportive medical learning environment. They are a useful tool for clinical demonstrations, interactive small-group sessions, physical examinations, high-fidelity simulation using manikins or partial task trainers and video portrayals. Students generally respond well to experiences with SPs, and a well-trained SP can provide valuable feedback that is more authentically given from the patient's perspective. Imaginative and creative minds can always find new ways to incorporate standardized patients into any kind of simulation education. An institution with a strong SP programme allows its faculty to expand curriculum and enhance teaching.

References

Barrows HS: An overview of the uses of standardised patients for teaching and evaluating clinical skills, *Academic Medicine* 68(6):443–451; discussion 451–453, 1993.

Jones A: World Simulation Centre Database, 2011. Available at: http://www.bmsc.co.uk/sim_database/centres_europe.htm.

Kneebone R, Kidd J, Nestel D, et al: An innovative model for teaching and learning clinical procedures, *Medical Education* 36:628–634, 2002.

Monaghan M, Gardner S, Hastings J, et al: Student attitudes toward the use of standardised patients in a communication course, *American Journal of Pharmaceutical Education* 61:131–136, 1997.

Schwid HA, Rooke GA, Michalowski P, Ross BK: Screen-based anesthesia simulation with debriefing improves performance in a manikin-based anesthesia simulator, *Teaching and Learning in Medicine* 13(2):92–96, 2001.

Wallace P: Following the threads of an innovation: the history of standardised patients in medical education, *Caduceus (Springfield, IL)* 13(2):5–28, 1997.

Resources

The Association of Standardised Patient Educators (ASPE), http://www.aspeducators.org/

ASPE is the international organization for professionals in the field of standardized patient methodology. ASPE is dedicated to professional growth and development of its members, advancement of SP research and related scholarly activities, setting standards of practice and fostering patient-centred care. They have over 600 members and are often a good resource for the nearest SP programme to many medical institutions. Peggy Wallace's article entitled 'Following the threads of an innovation: the history of standardized patients in medical education' can be found at this site.

Wallace P 2006 Coaching Standardised Patients for use in the Assessment of Clinical Competence. Springer. http://springerpub.com/prod.aspx?prod_id=02247

Working with SPs has become so important in medical education that it is now a component of the USMLE clinical skills assessment exam. To ensure best practice, the coaches who prepare SPs now need general guidelines. This book is a thorough guide and a support for those who are involved in training SPs, encouraging each coach to develop a system that will deliver the best results and, in the end, help train the most competent doctors. Included are tips to help develop coaching skills and be a director to SPs, cast standardized patients, get the best performance from actors, perfect SPs' timing of fact delivery during examinations, improve the SPs' written feedback to students and streamline training regimens.

Digital medical education

R. H. Ellaway

Introduction

There has been a long history of educational technologies that have both defined and enabled the development of medical education. Pre-digital technologies such as books, buildings, photography and chalkboards have all played a critical role. However, we tend to only see recent innovations as 'technologies' while overlooking more familiar forms. Technology today has become synonymous with our interconnected and interdependent computing devices, software and network infrastructures. It would be inappropriate to discuss digital technologies without considering the ways in which they are used. This chapter will therefore consider the tools, applications and social and cultural organizations associated with digital media as a single phenomenon: 'the digital'.

We are currently training the last generation of doctors who can remember a time before the internet, the first who will learn in an environment dominated by digital technologies and the first who will practise in a predominantly e-health environment. At the same time, medical teachers who trained in a pre-digital environment (and therefore have little or no experience of e-learning or e-health as learners) are those who are defining and running contemporary medical education. This time of transition therefore requires teachers and their students to be attentive, reflective and considered in how they shape the future of healthcare in a digital age.

 "We are training the last generation of doctors who can remember a time before the internet."

The breadth of interactions between medical education and the digital makes a discrete review of its use in medical education particularly challenging. Lecturing involves using PowerPoint, video recording and audience response systems ('clickers'); curriculum preparation now involves configuring and populating virtual learning environments (VLE); and running exams now means using online question banks and e-assessment delivery systems. We track clinical encounters through electronic logbooks, our libraries' collections are predominantly online and our learners make significant use of the web and other electronic resources above and beyond that required by their tutors. The two essential challenges facing us are how to make the best use of the digital in medical education, and how to best configure medical education in a digital age.

Why use digital?

Educational technologies may be used for many reasons, only some of which directly relate to instruction. Institutions, as well as teachers, are often more interested in other benefits, such as tracking learners, improving administrative efficiency or expanding the reach of their programmes (Ellaway 2011). The shift to more explicitly accountable forms of medical education is supported by digital technologies providing detailed logs of what participants in a programme are actually doing (at least through online institutional systems). Whether this is based on the frequency of learners' postings to a discussion board or the numbers and mix of their logged patient encounters, knowing who is doing what and when they are doing it may be as important to an institution as the quality of their learners' educational experiences. This is not to endorse such perspectives, but the medical teacher should be clear as to the drivers in and around the tools they use. See Box 27.1 for some of the key ways the digital can drive and shape education.

Increased reach is another reason for adopting the digital in medical education. Online tools and information can be made available at any time of day and anywhere a network connection can be found. Similarly, teachers and learners are now regularly online and accessible well outside regular working hours. The digital also allows for more rapid and assured publishing of information. While printed copies of anything (including this book) can rapidly lose their currency, online information can be provided as a single 'golden' copy that can be kept up to date more easily than print. Other noninstructional reasons for using technology in medical education include meeting learner expectations, seeking cost savings in programme administration and delivery, connecting with other online service providers, and meeting accreditation requirements for communication and curriculum management.

The use of digital media for instructional purposes may be limited by the greater value associated with face-to-face rather than virtual encounters, particularly by learners. Indeed, where educational multimedia is used in an educational setting, it is often to accommodate logistical rather than educational ends. For instance, the number of lectures in a course may be reduced and their content reallocated to

multimedia applications, or a distributed student population (particularly in community teaching sites) may be provided with asynchronous access to the same teaching resources to allow for local variations in scheduling.

PRESENCE

One defining aspect in designing and using digital media for instructional purposes is to what extent and in what way the teacher is, or is not, co-present with their learners. Teachers often consider classroom and independent study as binary opposites, but new media technologies have blurred this distinction. Table 27.1 sets out a continuum between presence and absence and the different kinds of activities and tools that apply to these different settings.

Mitchell (2000) presents the concept of 'economies of presence' as the cost–benefit ratio for different kinds of presence, both physical and digital. Despite faculty concerns over poor attendance at lectures, most medical learners continue to seek the most authentic, hands-on, face-to-face encounters they can find. The use of digital media typically does not provide the same experiential richness as embodied experiences and can therefore be perceived as less valuable. Despite this, there are situations where economies of presence lead learners to favour the use of digitally mediated activities. For example, digital media can establish or enhance educational presence when learners and teachers are working at a distance from each other, when learners need to access resources out of hours or when shared activities persist over time and involve many participants. Similarly, groups of learners may work as a collective, using digital tools to pool lecture and research notes and other resources, for instance, in small-group learning activities.

By allowing medical teachers to extend their teaching presence to work with learners and colleagues beyond the limitations of the classroom or clinical workplace, different kinds of digital media can alter the way that the participants in medical education interact with each other and their learning environment. Medical teachers should understand and make the most of the extended forms of presence afforded them and are encouraged to explore what it means to be an educator when not co-present with their learners.

ACTIVITIES

Another key construct regarding the use of digital technologies in medical education is 'activity'. Learning doesn't happen spontaneously; learners and teachers participate in different educational activities (lectures, PBL, exams, bedside teaching and so on). Table 27.1 shows how different forms of presence

---

Box 27.1 Internet dimensions

Because the internet has many influences on the things with which it interacts, it can be difficult to anticipate what effects it will have (for good or ill) in fields such as medical education. Nevertheless, the following five dimensions describe the kinds of impacts that any internet-related activity may have in an educational setting:

- **Acceleration:** the internet can make communication, processing and access much faster. This means that tasks can be undertaken more quickly but with less and less time to reflect on the consequences of one's actions.

- **Reach:** the internet can significantly extend the reach of one's actions. For instance, geographically remote learners can study together and patients and physicians at different locations can be connected via telehealth networks. One reaction to this extended reach has been a tendency to value face-to-face encounters more than online ones.

- **Integration:** the internet can integrate a variety of services and information, reflected for instance in the proliferation of virtual learning environments (aka learning management systems) such as Blackboard and Moodle. Integration also means more interdependence, which can in turn make otherwise resilient education systems more and more vulnerable to errors and failures.

- **Observation:** the internet can track and record almost any action. While this provides the ability to provide rich feedback and modelling of learner behaviours, it can also reduce learners' autonomy to explore and their freedom to express themselves.

Table 27.1 A continuum of teacher presence and associated technology enhanced learning methods.

	Face-to-face teacher presence	Synchronous teacher telepresence	Asynchronous teacher telepresence	Teacher represented in software
Location	Teacher and learners are in the same place at the same time using technology in a 'blended learning' mode.	Teacher is online at the same time as their learners.	Teacher interacts episodically and at different times to their learners.	Software is designed to take on the role of the teacher
Activity	Learning activities are constructed between the participants with little activity encoded in the artefacts and resources used.	Learning activities are constructed between the participants. Activities partly depend on the capabilities and functionality of the medium being used.	Learning activities are very much defined by the capabilities and functionality of the medium being used.	Learning activities and the range of variability within them are largely predefined and encoded in the software.
Examples	Learning makes use of digital resources as part of a classroom activity or lecture.	Learning is undertaken through webconferencing, videoconferencing or virtual worlds.	Learning is undertaken through discussion boards, wikis or blogs.	Learning is undertaken using self-study multimedia teaching packages and virtual patients.

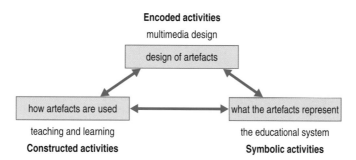

Fig. 27.1 Three activity levels associated with educational technologies (after Ellaway R, Davies D: Design for learning: deconstructing virtual patient activities, *Medical Teacher* 33(4):303–310, 2011).

work with different forms of educational activity, with face-to-face teaching being typically the most improvised, and 'computer-as-teacher' designs the most predefined. We can expand on this to consider three levels of activity: encoded, constructed and symbolic (Ellaway & Davies 2011; see Fig. 27.1).

Encoded activities are what learners and teachers need to do to allow them to interact with, operate or otherwise control a technical artefact. At the most basic level this involves watching or listening to what the computer is doing and then clicking, typing or touching items on the screen in response. Other input devices include joysticks (such as game handsets), the motion or orientation of a handset (such as for a Wii) or whole device (such as tablets and smartphones) or physical gestures (using sensors such as the Kinect). Medical education-specific devices such as manikins

and laparoscopic simulators support more clinically focused encoded activities through observing, touching and manipulating a simulated human body. It should be noted that while each of these activities involves a mixture of cognitive and hand–eye components, the latter are often overlooked. The physicality of computing can assist or impede learning just as much as its cognitive aspects; indeed, it is an unavoidable hidden curriculum issue associated with using educational technologies.

More complicated encoded activities are built up from these basic forms, such as multiple-choice questions, 3-D anatomical models or a series of management decisions within a virtual patient. All of the things that a software artefact can do are encoded as part of its build; even the ability to be adaptable needs to be explicitly designed and built (such as in a VLE or a virtual world). There are three organizing principles for encoded activities: the way they are sequenced, the way they are presented, and their convergence with the objectives of the activities in which they are used.

- The presentation principle involves visuals, audio and video. For instance, a series of multimedia design principles have been identified to guide how encoded activities are presented (Mayer 2009). These are essentially about reducing the 'cognitive load' on the learner and are summarized in Box 27.2. Multimedia principles should be applicable to any kind of encoded activity involving onscreen or paper-based materials, including lecture slides, handouts and study guides.

- Sequencing is concerned with the order in which different encoded activities are presented (this before that, this after that) and the logic that refines the ordering (this if that, that if not this). Although sequencing has been identified as important to learning (Ritter et al 2007) the role and

---

Box 27.2 Mayer's multimedia principles

1. Coherence: remove any material not relevant to the task in hand.

2. Signalling: add cues regarding the organization of the material.

3. Redundancy: images and narration are better than images, narration and text.

4. Spatial: corresponding words and images should be adjacent to each other.

5. Temporal: corresponding words and images should be presented at the same time.

6. Segmenting: user-paced segments are better than a single presentation.

7. Pre-training: learn key concepts before applying them.

8. Modality: image and narration are better than image and text.

9. Multimedia: words and images are better than words alone.

10. Personalization: using a conversational narrative style is better than using a formal one.

11. Voice: a real human voice is better than a machine-generated one.

12. Image: seeing the speaker's image, such as a 'talking head', does not improve learning.

After Mayer R: Multimedia Learning, 2nd edn, Cambridge New York, NY, 2009, University Press.

---

impact of sequencing are still being explored. Both presentation and sequencing are important, not just to instructional use of digital technologies but to all systems and tools used in medical education.

- The alignment between different encoded activities and their ability to support different learning objectives is also important. For instance, if the task in hand is to work through a virtual patient diagnostic pathway, how well does that prepare a learner to make similar decisions in practice? From this perspective we can ask similar questions to those raised with regard to simulation and simulators, such as the validity and the extent to which knowledge and experience transfers to medical practice. While the relationships between a simulator and its real-world equivalent are usually apparent, the same cannot always be said about instructional multimedia. Dormans (2008) identifies three aspects of simulation in digital games that can also be applied to educational technologies in medical education:

  ○ *Iconic simulation* is concerned with how much a technical artefact mirrors key aspects of the real world. For instance, an online lecture about a particular clinical presentation would arguably be less iconic than a virtual patient, where the learner can make practice decisions and deal with the simulated consequences.

  ○ *Indexical simulation* is concerned with simplification of or abstraction from the real world. For instance, PBL cases or virtual patients are written to exclude what the authors would consider irrelevant details. Only certain choices and outcomes are allowed, typically reflecting the intended learning objectives.

  ○ *Symbolic simulation* is concerned with the arbitrary or non-real representation of the real world. For instance, requiring a learner to interact with a virtual patient using mouse clicks and key presses is more symbolic than physically interacting with a mannequin.

Collectively, these three dimensions can be used to guide the design of a learning resource or they can be used to evaluate an existing one. It should be noted that simplification (indexical) and abstraction (symbolic) are neither good nor bad in and of themselves; they may be desirable, even essential, in certain circumstances and less desirable in others. They should therefore be seen as tools to help medical teachers understand the options available to them. For instance, the use of virtual worlds (such as Second Life) is superficially quite iconic (as physical objects are recreated as 3-D models) but in use they are quite indexical (the detail of action and the range of available actions are quite limited) and symbolic (interaction with objects and other 'players' is through clicks translated to vague onscreen gestures).

While encoded activities are expressed in the different ways that an educational technological artefact can be used or manipulated, constructed activities focus on what the artefact is used for and how it is used. For instance, a website on joint pain may be used in a tutorial, for independent study, for patient education or even as an example of good (or bad) communication. It is axiomatic that any given digital resource may be used for multiple constructed activities, and any given constructed activity may use multiple digital resources. Although the encoded activities within a digital resource are typically designed with one or more constructed activities in mind, a constructed activity may not use all of a given resource's available encoded activities. For instance, a tutor may focus on just one part of a virtual patient such as history taking, or an online lecture may be used to critique teaching methods rather than its content.

Medical education technologies

A full exploration of constructed activities is outside the scope of this chapter; indeed, it is arguable that the rest of this book (and much of the rest of medical education) is primarily concerned with constructed activities. There are many good generic texts on using educational technologies, and the reader should refer to them to understand the basic principles of technology-enhanced education and its application to a range of different circumstances (Clark & Mayer 2008, Ellis & Goodyear 2009, Horton 2006). Although there is much that is generic to higher education (such as VLEs, repositories, wikis, blogs and e-portfolios), there are a number of essential forms and practices that are critical to medical education (Ellaway 2007). This section will consider a few key examples.

The first form focuses on computer-mediated simulators. Although they have been given many names (e-cases, electronic patients, computer-based cases and so on), the most common term at present is 'virtual patients'. Whatever label is used, this is a broad category of educational technologies that simulate different kinds of patient or other professional encounters. By combining aspects of case narrative, simulation and computer games, virtual patients can offer all sorts of different activities including history taking, decision making and dealing with complexity and psychosocial issues. Activity structures may be linear (with a preset path) or branching (where decisions change the direction of the activity) or make use of some kind of artificial intelligence, although the latter is relatively rare because of the effort required to develop it. At an encoded level activities may be presented either as pages (of text, images and video)

or within simulated physical environments (such as Second Life); again, the relative ease of development and portability of the former make this the more common format. Virtual patients can be used for independent or group study, for PBL or for formative or summative assessment, or the act of creating them can be used for educational purposes. See Box 27.3 for more information on virtual patients. Other onscreen educational simulators include tools for practising prescribing, running simulated biomedical experiments and using virtual microscopes.

A second form of health profession-focused constructed activity is based on using educational technologies at the bedside. There are a number of ways in which this can be realized including using decision support tools (such as educationally focused pharmacopoeia or clinical pathway databases), just-in-time refresher materials (such as clinical skills videos) or patient encounter logging. The latter type has become a key part of many clerkships and residencies, both as a way of collecting evidence that individual learners have had the core experiences they require and as a way of supporting reflective practice. A critical factor in ensuring the success of encounter logging is the quality and quantity of the feedback given on a

---

Box 27.3 Getting started with virtual patients

There are many benefits to using virtual patients including on-demand access, educationally focused activity designs and the ability to rehearse practice patterns such as ABC (airway, breathing, circulation) or HEIDR (history, examination, investigation, diagnosis and therapy). The activity design should be aligned both to the learning objectives and to the level of the intended learner. For instance, more advanced learners tend to need fewer graphics and multimedia and more sophistication in the choices available to them than their junior colleagues.

Despite a common name, there are many different designs of virtual patients and many ways in which medical teachers can get started with this medium. For instance, there are many examples in the MedEdPortal repository (www.mededportal.org), while others are available through subscription services such as MedU (www.med-u.org) or project websites such as eViP (www.virtualpatients.eu) or PINE (http://pine.nosm.ca/pine). Alternatively, teachers may wish to build their own cases or adapt existing ones, in which case they could use a dedicated authoring tool (for a list of interoperable tools see www.medbiq.org/virtual_patient/implementers) or more generic tools such as Adobe Captivate.

learner's logged encounters, whether it be from tutors or from their peers. This reinforces the point that it is the activity (rather than the tools or content that support it) what should be the focus for medical teachers.

The use of short videos for teaching or rehearsing clinical skills, whether from respected journals like the *New England Journal of Medicine* or from more generic repositories such as YouTube, is also growing, not least because a procedure can be reviewed immediately before performing the procedure. The rapid adoption of smartphones such as the iPhone or various Android devices has been a significant enabler for the use of technology-enhanced point of care learning. Chapter 28 on mobile learning goes into more detail on this. A third form involving the use of e-health technologies is discussed later in this chapter.

While some activity designs have been translated from non-digital forms (such as e-books and MCQs), others have been developed within a digital environment (such as Web 2.0 tools like blogs and wikis). Either way, new forms are almost always developed from existing forms. This is because in order to make technologies understandable to their users, they need to be presented in ways that are familiar as well as efficient. Larger gaps in familiarity can create adoption problems, such as learning to use a multi-button mouse or game controller for the first time. Making tasks simpler can also make their adoption less challenging: for example, multitouch interfaces for tablets and smartphones. When considering the adoption of an educational technology, the medical teacher should consider both its utility and its familiarity to those that will be using it.

Appraising and selecting educational interventions are central to teaching. In doing so, teachers need to be able to appreciate the efficacy, efficiency and alignment to programme and learner needs for technological as well as more traditional methods. The modern medical teacher should therefore be able to appreciate the many forms and roles of digital and nondigital technologies in medical education and the reasons why they are, or at least might be, used.

Preparing for e-health: medium as message

As a discipline, medical informatics is concerned with the effective organization, analysis, management and use of information in support of healthcare. Although its scope is broader than the use of computers, to paraphrase Marshall McLuhan, the computing medium is very much the message in terms of developing medical informatics competencies. Although there is a clear need for tomorrow's doctors to be prepared to practise in an electronic practice environment, e-health investment has tended to focus on developing and deploying new technologies rather than on preparing people to use them.

Key e-health technologies and systems include electronic health records (EHRs) and electronic medical records (EMRs), imaging (picture archiving and communication systems [PACS]), order entry and prescribing, point of care information, decision support and guidelines, logistics (scheduling, organization management), communication with patients and colleagues and patient access to information and support resources (such as public health websites, hotlines and personal health records). All of these forms can be taught by using them for educational as well as practice purposes. For instance, an EMR can be populated with the cases learners will encounter in their PBL or clinical skills sessions. Clerking and managing their patients through the EMR therefore becomes a part of the broader course experience rather than a thing set apart. Digital competencies for clinicians involve much more than operator skills for a particular system; physicians need to know how to work in e-health ecologies. This includes developing a practical knowledge of the following:

- *Coding:* this involves understanding how patients and their health are represented in electronic systems. Examples include the specificity and directing nature of coding systems such as DSM or LOINC as well as billing and other practice management models.

- *Workflow:* teaching and learning can consider how different players contribute to patient journeys through different electronic systems. This can include topics such as interprofessional teamworking and an exploration of the different ways in which different professions see and represent their patients through the creation and management of health information.

- *Quality improvement:* electronic health systems are primarily intended to improve the efficiency and efficacy of the healthcare system, often with a focus on reducing the number of errors associated with handling information. Teaching and learning can be designed to explore how systems can improve safety as well as introducing problems.

- *Confidentiality:* while aspects of patient confidentiality inform much of medical education, they should include the challenges of maintaining confidentiality in distributed health information systems. For instance, email communication with a patient can be used to explore questions such as who gets access to the messages and whether they are entered in to the patient record.

Some consideration should also be given to the impact of the digital on the healthcare system as a whole and on the profession of medicine. Rothman and Blumenthal observe that 'IT may exert its greatest impact on medical professionalism not directly, by changing what practitioners do, but indirectly, by changing with whom they collaborate in doing it' (2010, p. 133) and that 'physicians should be – and will have to be – much more capable of using the internet for health care purposes than their patients' (ibid, p. 20).

At present it would seem that relatively few institutions have engaged with these issues. If the disconnect between professional training and the development of e-health is not addressed, then medical learners may well enter practice with no appreciation of the strategic role of informatics or a clear or consistent idea of their responsibilities in an e-health environment. As long as we invest in e-health but fail to connect this to the training of those who will use it (beyond that of operator training), then it is arguable that we are eroding the role of physicians and their ability to be effective leaders within the healthcare system as a whole.

Educational ecologies

Up to this point this chapter has considered relatively distinct components of technology-enhanced learning. However, any such application should be understood as a component, a species perhaps, within broader educational ecologies, not just technical but encompassing all aspects of an educational system or culture. As an illustration, integrated software systems, such as VLEs, have become a key part of many medical education programmes. However, most off-the-shelf VLEs are organized around the generic modular format of most higher education programmes and are somewhat limited in their ability to support the complexity and integration found in much contemporary medical education. Issues of fit and alignment are clearly ecological in nature, but this metaphor goes further; an ecological perspective makes the information flows between different players easier to perceive.

 Technology-enhanced learning should be understood as a component of broader educational ecologies.

Considering a medical programme as an educational ecology also suggests that it is not self-contained; it interacts with the other ecologies around it. For instance, the use of online social networking has allowed learners (and sometimes faculty) to say or do things in public forums that impact their own reputations as well as those of their institution and professions. While there have always been indiscretions, the difference with social media is that it

---

Box 27.4 Principles of digital professionalism for medical learners, teachers and health professionals

1. Establish and sustain an on online professional presence that befits your responsibilities while representing your interests ... but be selective where you establish a profile.

2. Use privacy controls to manage more personal parts of your online profile and do not make public anything that you would not be comfortable defending as professionally appropriate in a court of law or in front of a disciplinary panel.

3. Think carefully and critically about how what you say or do will be perceived by others and how what you say or do online reflects on others, both individuals and organizations: act with appropriate restraint.

4. Almost everything online can be monitored, recorded or data mined by multiple groups. Think carefully and critically about how what you say or do online will be perceived in years to come and consider every action online as permanent.

5. Be aware of the potential for online attack or impersonation, know how to protect your online reputation and what steps to take when it is under attack.

6. Your professional identity extends into all online communities you join, and you are still a professional there.

7. Pretence and deceit are inappropriate behaviours for health professionals – do not impersonate or seek to hide your identity for malicious or unprofessional purposes.

8. Theft and piracy are not acceptable for any professionals – work within the law.

9. Curation of information is a serious responsibility. Do not expose information to unnecessary risk and consider wisely the potential impact of any use or exchange of information you make.

10. Behave professionally and respectfully in all venues and using all media and take responsibility for modeling positive digital professionalism for others.

Reproduced from Ellaway R, Tworek J: The net generation illusion: Challenging conformance to social expectations. In Ferris SP, editor: Teaching and Learning with the Net Generation: Concepts and Tools for Reaching Digital Learners. Information Science Reference, 2012.

makes indiscretions far more public far more rapidly. While some institutions have responded by punishing or proscribing the use of social media around medicine or medical education, others have tried to take a more positive approach. Box 27.4 sets out a 'digital professionalism' framework to guide learners, teachers and health professionals in working in an ambiently digital environment.

Medical school ecologies also interact with those of other schools, for instance, through the exchange of digital resources, sometimes on a one-to-one basis but more often through shared online repositories. While some of these resources are provided on a commercial basis, others are provided for free or even as open source (allowing them to be edited and adapted). There have been many approaches to exchange over the years including conceiving of digital content as reusable learning objects (RLOs), as open educational resources (OERs) or as Open Courseware (www.ocwconsortium.org). More generic systems, such as iTunes, YouTube or Flickr, are being used more and more frequently as ways of publishing and exchanging digital materials. Box 27.5 describes the use of repositories for the exchange of digital materials. These ecologies of exchange depend on technical standards that allow materials to be moved from one system to another. The role of standards as a critical part of establishing broader educational ecologies is demonstrated by groups such as MedBiquitous (www.medbiq.org).

e-Teachers

The use of web technologies for education has been popularly dubbed 'e-learning' even though it is usually defined and led by teachers rather than learners. It therefore helps to separate out two distinct kinds of practice: e-teaching (what the teacher does) and e-learning (what the learner does). E-teaching tasks include selecting the appropriate tools (both digital and non-digital), operating, and, to an extent, troubleshooting the technologies used, facilitating learners' activities through and around digital media, and evaluating and appraising their performance. In the early years of educational technology teachers were often also the designers of the tools they used, and, despite the widespread availability of online educational resources, it is arguable that design remains a critical skill for contemporary medical teachers. Even if they don't build things from scratch, they still need to be able to configure and structure their teaching within and around digital technologies.

"There are two distinct kinds of practice: e-teaching (what the teacher does) and e-learning (what the learner does)."

> **Box 27.5 Repositories**
>
> Digital repositories are systems for storing digital content of different kinds, supporting their users in managing and tagging these resources, and allowing them to search for resources based on different search criteria. A particularly notable example for medical education is the Association of American Medical College's (AAMC) MedEdPORTAL (www.mededportal.org), a collection of 2000+ peer-reviewed resources for medical educators. At the time of writing MedEdPORTAL support 1000 downloads a week by users from around the world. Other repositories of note include HeAL (www.healcentral.org), eViP (www.virtualpatients.eu), and MedPedia (www.medpedia.com).

E-teachers also need to decide where their educational technology efforts are going to be targeted. The more efficient an educational artefact is, the more it tends to catalyse or otherwise support learning for the greatest number of learners. However, it is an ongoing challenge that the best learners tend to make use of every opportunity afforded them and that those with most need use such supports least. If the goal is to help less able learners, then the resource needs to align with their needs and the ways that they approach their learning; simply making a resource available may increase the gap between the most and least able rather than closing it. Quizzes with targeted feedback can often help less able learners or those struggling with certain core concepts much more than multimedia rich resources can.

It is also important for medical teachers to ensure that their technology-enabled activities are integrated into the curriculum; if they are not, then they are unlikely to be used, particularly by those who need them most. Managing the alignment between e-teaching and programme objectives and outcomes is critical. Biggs (1999) states that: 'in aligned teaching there is maximum consistency throughout the system'. This alignment should extend to the online as well as the offline aspects. If e-teaching is not in alignment with the rest of the curriculum, then it can introduce dissonance and confusion for the learner as well as confuse what is and is not important. Furthermore, e-teaching does not sit in isolation from other methods and techniques; it interacts with, borrows from and ultimately better prepares teachers for more traditional face-to-face practice. The idea of blended learning (combining the best of traditional and new media and techniques) is now well established, but the parallel concept of blended e-teaching is less so, although much blended e-learning clearly involves teaching.

Negotiating alignment and the blend between e-teaching and other methods are skills that are best learnt from practical experience.

It is highly recommended that those wishing to take on an e-teaching role seek out opportunities to learn first-hand what is like to be an e-learner, perhaps as faculty development or continuing medical education activities. There are also opportunities to learn and develop through connecting with the many online e-teaching communities. One last issue, and one that experience as an e-learner will help to highlight, is that all technologies change. Some change quite rapidly, while others change more slowly. Either way, focusing on operator skills alone will not suffice; developing an understanding of the broader issues of e-teaching is no longer an esoteric specialty but a core part of being a medical teacher.

e-Learners

Medical teachers also need to appreciate the roles and identities of their e-learners. There has been a tendency over the last decade, particularly in the media, to assume youth have greater computing skills and abilities than their seniors. Labels such as 'digital natives' or 'net generation' have become a powerful meme that has persuaded many learners and faculty (Ellaway & Tworek 2012). This is problematic for a number of reasons. While some learners have certainly embraced a digital lifestyle, others have not. Every class will typically have a few students with strong IT skills, while there will be others with relatively little practical ability or interest. This can be exacerbated by learners' generally poor assessment of their ability to use digital technologies; typically they have greater confidence than competence. Faculty, on the other hand, often have less confidence than competence, perceive greater risks in using technologies and may as a result cede control of the digital to their learners with the belief that they are more able (Beetham et al 2009). Learners need their teachers to guide them in becoming digital professionals. Box 27.6 describes a range of key issues to guide curriculum development around health informatics but covering a broader range of issues associated with the digital.

Despite the ability of educational technologies to track learners' activities, much of what learners do remains invisible to their teachers. For example, in the last few years the use of online social networking sites has become a staple online social activity for students worldwide, largely displacing such activity from university systems. Similarly, instant messaging allows discrete groups of learners to interact without the scrutiny or knowledge of their teachers. There is also an apparently significant level of online exchange and discussion between learners at different institutions.

Box 27.6 Key curricula themes in healthcare informatics for medical students

Healthcare informatics is a growing discipline that has yet to have a profile in medical education proportionate to its place in contemporary healthcare. The following themes can serve to create a structured and integrated informatics curriculum within student training and assessment:

A. Evidence-based medicine, critical appraisal and knowledge translation

B. The role and use of information systems such as health records and imaging

C. Legal, ethical and professional dimensions of informatics

D. Informatics in communication and education: with other professionals and with patients

E. Technical skills in using different technologies

F. The semantic dimensions of information use: coding, tagging and structuring information

G. Information management, governance, reporting and audit skills

H. Telehealth for individual patients and whole populations as well as connecting health professionals.

Teaching materials from one school can easily end up being used (and valued) by learners at another with no faculty involvement. With learners seeking venues where they will not be observed and assessed by their faculty and their extended social network and their participation in professional networks, many of today's students have become digital nomads even if they are not digital natives.

Summary

This chapter is not intended to be a generic text on e-learning, not least because there are many excellent texts on this area already. The goal has rather been to provide a briefing on the wider themes and issues that accompany the use of digital technologies in medical education.

From a practical point of view medical teachers need to be able to function in a range of different digitally enhanced environments, both as learners and as teachers. They need to be able to appreciate the dynamics of such environments, critiquing the options and selecting those tools and processes that best meet their needs. They also need to appreciate how e-health and other profession-focused digital developments intersect with the education of those who will use them. Although there is likely to be an ongoing role for educational technology specialists to cover the more strategic and involved aspects of digital medical education, all medical teachers are now to some extent medical e-teachers.

 "All medical teachers are now medical e-teachers."

The balance between digital and non-digital forms is still in flux with issues such as long time storage and curation still creating major challenges. As a medium, the digital remains quite ephemeral, particularly when compared with the resilience of books and other printed matter. It may be that the use of digital content may prove to be less important than its use as a medium for educational activities. This chapter has set out a series of concepts around educational activities that allow both learners and their teachers to make better use of their time both together and apart. The greatest promise of the digital therefore may and probably should be to enhance and improve traditional models of medical teaching and learning, rather than to simply sweep them away. Future editions of this book will have the benefit of hindsight to validate or challenge this perspective.

References

Beetham H, McGill L, Littlejohn A: *Thriving in the 21st Century: Learning Literacies for the Digital Age*, Glasgow, 2009, Glasgow Caledonian University/JISC.

Biggs J: *Teaching for Quality Learning*, UK, 1999, OU Press.

Clark RC, Mayer RE: *e-Learning and the Science of Instruction*, San Francisco, 2008, Pfeiffer.

Dormans J: Beyond iconic simulation. IADIS Gaming Conference proceedings, 2008. Online at http://www.jorisdormans.nl/article.php?ref=beyondiconicsimulation.

Ellaway R: Discipline based designs for learning: the example of professional and vocational education.

In Beetham H, Sharpe R, editors: *Design for Learning: Rethinking Pedagogy for the Digital Age*, 2007, Routledge, pp 153–165.

Ellaway R: E-learning: Is the revolution over? *Medical Teacher* 33(4):297–302, 2011.

Ellaway R, Davies D: Design for learning: deconstructing virtual patient activities, *Medical Teacher* 33(4):303–310, 2011.

Ellaway R, Tworek J: The net generation illusion: challenging conformance to social expectations. In Ferris SP, editor: *Teaching and Learning with the Net Generation: Concepts and Tools for Reaching Digital Learners*. Information Science Reference, 2012.

Ellis R, Goodyear P: *Students' Experiences of e-Learning in Higher Education: The Ecology of Sustainable Innovation*, Abingdon, UK, 2009, Routledge.

Horton W: *E-Learning by Design*, San Francisco, 2006, Pfeiffer.

Mayer R: *Multimedia Learning*, ed 2, New York, 2009, Cambridge University Press.

Mitchell WJ: *E-topia: "Urban Life, Jim—But Not As We Know It"*, Cambridge, 2000, MIT Press.

Ritter FE, Nerb J, Lehtinen E, O'Shea TM, editors: *In Order to Learn: How the Sequence of Topics Influences Learning*, New York, 2007, Oxford University Press.

Rothman D, Blumenthal D, editors: *Medical Professionalism in the New Information Age*, Piscataway, NJ, 2010, Rutgers University Press.

Further reading

Ellaway R, Masters K: AMEE Guide 32: e-Learning in medical education Part 1: Learning, teaching and assessment, *Medical Teacher* 30(5):455–473, 2008.

Masters K, Ellaway R: AMEE Guide 32: e-Learning in medical education Part 2: Technology, management and design, *Medical Teacher* 30(5):474–489, 2008.

Mobile learning (m-learning)

J. E. Sandars, G. S. Frith

Introduction

Over the last few years, an increasing range of devices with computing capability have become available for use whilst on the move. These mobile devices have become smaller in size but have continued to offer most of the computing power and functions that are provided by personal computers. Originally there were distinct differences between the various types of device, such as the PDA (personal digital assistant) or the web-enabled mobile phone, but their functions have now started to merge. The result has been the smartphone, with its wide range of functions, and this convergence of technology has created exciting new possibilities for teaching and learning on the move. This is the world of m-learning.

 M-learning: Learning with mobile devices.

 Mobile devices offer flexible learning opportunities created by high portability (any time and any place).

The types of mobile device

There are a wide variety of mobile devices. Their use was originally determined by the group using the device and the particular function of the device. Laptop computers and PDAs (personal digital assistants) were mainly used in a professional environment for various administrative functions, such as e-mail, and the provision of information, such as access to clinical guidelines. In contrast, digital media players (iPods and MP3 players) were mainly used by a younger generation for entertainment, such as listening to music. Mobile phones were originally used for communication, by either speech or text messages. However, over the last few years these boundaries have started to become less distinct and increasingly there is *convergence*, where one device has the same functions as those provided by another device.

 Convergence: Multiple functions provided by one mobile device.

Most mobile phones are now 'smartphones' and have the additional functions of a PDA, an MP3 player and a digital camera. These smartphones have connectivity not only to cellular telephone networks but also to wireless networks that provide easy access to the internet. The mobile phone now has similar functions to a laptop computer. The latest innovation is the tablet device (such as the iPad), which combines a range of different functions that previously could only be obtained from a single device, yet it is lightweight, is relatively inexpensive and has a convenient screen size. The introduction of high-quality touch-screen technology has significantly increased the usability of both smartphones and tablet devices.

The choice of device for teaching and learning will significantly depend on the rapidly changing global marketplace that is dictated by both the preference of the users and the functionality of the devices supplied by the manufacturers (Box 28.1). The degree of connectivity (availability of wireless or mobile phone networks) in the various situations where the devices are expected to be used is usually also an important consideration.

 The choice of a mobile device for teaching and learning is determined by the preference of users, the functionality of the devices and usually the connectivity to networks.

Currently, Apple has a significant share of the market with their operating system for the iPhone, iPod Touch and iPad (iOS), but there is increasingly strong competition from other manufacturers who are offering similar functionality with their own operating systems, such as Android OS and Blackberry OS (Box 28.1). Unfortunately, there is little compatibility

---

Box 28.1 Types of mobile device

- Laptop computers
- Tablet computers (including iPads)
- PDAs (personal digital assistants)
- Smartphones
- e-book reader
- Digital media players (iPods and MP3 players)
- Mobile phones

---

between these operating systems at the device level. The focus for compatibility has, however, now moved to the availability of the various applications and the capability of the device to connect to wireless and/or mobile telephone networks.

The functions of mobile devices that can enhance teaching and learning

The great value of any mobile device is that a range of functions can be easily provided in a busy workplace or remote community setting. The immediacy of obtaining information also often engages a reluctant learner.

A wide range of learning resources can be downloaded directly onto the device from a desktop computer or by a connection to a wireless or mobile phone network. These resources can be text (such as standard textbooks and revision aids) or audio and/or video (podcasts). The two latest trends are the use of 'apps' (which are small software programs that can be downloaded onto smartphones and tablet devices) and e-readers that are designed primarily for the purpose of reading digital books and periodicals. All of these resources that are loaded onto the device can be viewed at any time, and most importantly, at any place.

Data can be uploaded from the device. Assessment templates can be completed and sent to computerized data banks. The learner can make audio or video recordings, either as self-reflection or from encounters with patients, which can be sent to an e-portfolio.

An internet connection can provide access to the same vast number of web-based resources that are available to static computers. Institution based e-learning systems, such as a VLE (virtual learning environment), can usually be accessed.

A wireless or mobile phone connection allows communication between users, by voice, text e-mail messages or electronic alerts. Tutors can mentor their

students but also revision notes can be sent to students.

Managing the process of learning is essential, and an administrative function can be provided with calendars, reminders and log books.

 Mobile devices can connect learners to content, learners to learners and tutors to learners.

The impact of mobile devices on teaching and learning

The use of mobile devices to enhance teaching and learning has been increasingly evaluated over the last few years, and there are some important themes that can inform their further widespread use. It is sometimes stated that only undergraduate medical students prefer to use m-learning and other new technologies for teaching and learning, but a recent survey has highlighted that both established doctors and doctors in training also are highly aware of and use these new approaches, albeit less than medical students.

 M-learning offers high acceptability and usefulness to learners.

PDAs (PERSONAL DIGITAL ASSISTANTS)

Most of the documented experience of mobile devices has been with PDAs since these devices have been widely used by both doctors and students over the last few years. Many medical schools, especially in the United States, have either provided PDAs or insisted that students provide their own devices. A large variety of clinical support resources have become available from numerous commercial providers and academic institutions. Many standard textbooks and clinical guides have PDA versions, often called e-books. There are also quick reference cards for basic sciences and clinical management, videos to demonstrate clinical skills and drug reference resources. A vast range of web-based resources, including the PubMed database, can also be instantly accessed through an internet connection. These resources can also be used to enhance teaching and learning since they provide 'learning on the go' in busy clinical workplaces.

An important use of PDAs has been in the administration of student placements, especially when these are based in the community. The profile of cases seen can be easily noted and tracked to ensure that a variety of appropriate learning experiences have been encountered.

Numerous evaluations have noted the high user acceptability of PDAs. These devices are also perceived to be very useful by learners and they have been shown to increase learning outcomes, especially for evidence-based medicine skills. Immediate access to resources motivates learners and makes the tasks more relevant. The functionality of the PDA has now been absorbed in to the smartphone, but much of this experience is relevant to today's devices.

PODCASTS AND PODCASTING

Most undergraduate medical students and many post-graduates will be very familiar with the use of podcasts, often delivered through iTunes, for personal entertainment. Worldwide sales and ownership of media players, such as iPods, are extremely high and their cost has dramatically fallen over the last few years. The latest mobile phones from a wide range of manufacturers also commonly have an integrated media player.

The regular broadcasting of an audio or video file by an RSS (Really Simple Syndication) feed is called podcasting, and the downloaded media file is called a podcast. These terms are often more loosely applied to any use of an audio or video file, especially in the context of teaching and learning. The main problem with any sound or video recording is that it creates a large file size, but these files can be compressed into an MP3 file to provide ease of uploading and downloading. Some podcasts only contain audio, others have a sequence of visible bullet points (often called an enhanced podcast) and some may be video (often called a vodcast). A digital media player is needed to open the MP3 file and listen to or view it. An example is iTunes, which can be played on many Apple devices.

The main use of podcasts in medical education has been to provide recordings of lectures. There are often called 'profcasts' in recognition of the expert providing content about a topic. Sometimes these are edited to offer a shorter version; occasionally the editing is done by students. A variant of this approach has been 'potcasts', which provide an audio guided tour of a pathology museum. Evaluation of the use of podcasts by medical students has shown that they particularly value podcasts for revision since they are able to repeatedly review the content after face-to-face lectures and prior to examinations. There is no evidence that students avoid attending lectures.

There are a large number of available podcasts that can be easily downloaded when required from a variety of providers, including medical and general publishers, professional societies and academic institutions. Many are 'mini' lectures or presentations, but there are also interviews with a wide range of experts. Most educators will not want to produce their own podcasts, but they can use these resources for blended learning by providing a link to the resource so that students can download the relevant podcast to enhance their learning.

APPS

Increasing the capability of smartphones and tablet computers by downloadable software, called apps, has become a rapidly expanding emergent trend in the use of mobile devices. There are thousands of apps on an incredible range of topics for devices using the Apple, Android or Blackberry operating systems. For practical purposes, these apps are equivalent to the various resources that were provided for PDAs, and the same suppliers have now started to shift their focus to the development of apps. The increased capability of the smartphone has, however, led to an explosion in the number of people writing apps (especially for Apple devices) both paid for and free. There are now a large number of apps for clinical care (such as drug dose calculation) and administrative support (such as electronic medical records and billing), as well as some apps which can be used as learning resources, including basic sciences and clinical topics.

There has been little evaluation of the use of apps and iPhones/iPads for teaching and learning, but high levels of perceived usefulness and usability are expected since these resources and devices are widely used for various purposes outside education: such as games, news and travel information.

Recent advances have seen the development and use of interactive e-books as a way of delivering content. An interactive e-book is a category of apps designed specifically to create an experience beyond the printed format, enabling users to actively interact with multimedia content.

M-learning provides new opportunities for teaching and learning

The success of any teaching and learning that uses technology, including mobile devices, depends less on the technology than on how it will be used to enhance the learning journey. However, the constant and easy access of mobile devices in the daily social and work life of the learner provides an exciting opportunity to enhance teaching and learning. This ubiquitous nature of mobile devices offers the possibility of learning that is also ubiquitous.

 M-learning should focus how the devices are used to enhance learning and not what is the latest technology.

An essential aspect of learning that is ubiquitous is that the learner can engage in authentic and personalized learning that is situated in the classroom or clinical workspace. This approach is more than simply consulting a textbook or guideline that has been

Table 28.1 Key digital competences for teaching and learning

Enquiry
Formulate questions as online enquiries
Find, gather and collate information
Evaluate online content and services

Production
Create digital artefacts (diagrams, designs)
Capture digital media (visual, audio)
Edit digital media (visual, audio)
Publish digital content (web, PDF, e-book)

Participation
Communicate and share information and media
Contribute appropriately to networked community activities
Work collaboratively online towards a goal
Moderate and manage the activities of an online group

Digital literacy
Understand online security and privacy
Understand and respect digital property rights
Compose communications to suit target recipients

(After Next Generation User Skills, A Report for Digital 2010 & the SQA, www.sqa.org.uk/sqa/files_ccc/ HNComputing_NGUSReport_NextGenerationUserSkills.pdf)

downloaded on the mobile device. Learners are frequently faced with a learning challenge: something that they need to quickly explore and investigate. For example, a learner may need to understand why the patient's blood pressure is not being controlled by a prescribed medication. The learner can immediately look at one or two previously downloaded favourite information resources on their mobile device, search the internet for a relevant article and contact a colleague for information and opinion by e-mail or via a chat room. The various options can be considered and a plan of action implemented. After the event, the learner can reflect on his or her experience and perhaps complete an online knowledge quiz related to the topic and share the experience with a wider online community of learners. What has been described in this hypothetical sequence is an illustration of how a unique and personalized learning experience can be constructed by assembling a range of different learning resources. The uniqueness of this approach is that it is directly related to the learning challenge and each challenge can be responded to by assembling a different variety of learning resources that are highly relevant to the challenge. This approach is in contrast to the learner who mainly uses a limited range of resources, such as a textbook or website, to respond to educational challenges.

 M-learning should focus on how the devices are used to enhance learning and not the technology.

A new approach to learning with mobile devices requires new competences by both the tutor and the learner. The development of digital competence covers four main areas, including the identification and appraisal of online resources (Table 28.1). Other competences include producing content to share with others, effectively communicating with others in a digital environment, and being fully aware of the ethical issues, such as copyright of shared materials and maintaining patient confidentiality.

Future directions in m-learning

Technology will continue to rapidly develop, and there are some emergent trends that are likely to impact on teaching and learning. This will create exciting new potential uses of m-learning in medical education.

Many mobile phones have GPS (Global Positioning System) capabilities, which can also be a function of a mobile device used for teaching and learning. This system identifies the geographical position of the user and can be used to authenticate reports from community placements, ensuring that the student is where they say they are, and to provide text message reminders of tasks that need to be performed in particular situations. More exciting is the opportunity to provide specific learning resources depending on where the learner is within a designated learning space. For example, in museums and art galleries, resources can be instantaneously downloaded as the learner faces a particular exhibit. Techniques such as augmented reality allow the use of the smartphone's camera and GPS to layer information on the particular view that the user is looking at through the camera. This has an exciting potential use in clinical learning environments.

The use of multimedia in teaching and learning leads to creative possibilities, such as video diaries and digital storytelling for reflective learning, but previously it has been slow to progress because of the complex technology that was required. However, most mobile devices now have integrated cameras and many have editing software. Many of these capabilities are embryonic and will only be fully realized when mobile networks and public wireless networks improve both their availability and capacity. Time, however, moves very rapidly in the mobile communications world, and providers are investing heavily in new technology to increase coverage and capacity.

A more futuristic concept is wearable mobile devices that are 'always on'. The rapid development of seamless wireless networks and mobile devices that can be worn like clothing offers exciting opportunities for teaching and learning but also raises new challenges that will have to be considered.

Cloud computing may be an unfamiliar term at the moment but it is likely to significantly develop in the near future. The concept is that through the web browser, services such as storage and applications can be provided to a range of smaller devices. The cloud servers augment the capabilities of the device by running applications and providing file space away from the device. The computing power resides in the master server, and this can be accessed when 'under the cloud' (that is, any place and anywhere). Mobile devices are 'thin' with minimal memory and software, allowing them to be smaller and there to be fewer security concerns if they are lost.

Use of m-learning in developing countries

Wireless and mobile phone networks have been extensively introduced into most developing countries since there is a poor, or nonexistent, fixed-line telephone and broadband infrastructure. This creates an ideal opportunity to use m-learning for medical education in these countries.

Most mobile devices are relatively inexpensive to buy and to maintain. Their power consumption is low and the battery can be recharged using solar energy. The high mobility and low technology of these devices are ideal for rural health workers.

Low-cost text messages using mobile devices can be used to provide regular clinical updates, and these can be combined with the many initiatives that routinely use mobile devices to collect epidemiological data. Podcasts can be sent to mobile phones or downloaded at base stations onto portable media players that can then be taken to remote areas.

It is an exciting thought that media globalization could be applied to medical education. High-quality learning resources that have been developed for mobile devices could be made instantly available in a remote area of the developing world, and a two-way conversation, via either voice or text, could occur with a world expert who is thousands of miles away. This potential remains to be explored.

Constraints on the use of m-learning

The implementation of m-learning, both in the curriculum and in healthcare organizations, requires careful planning. It is essential that the use of mobile devices is embedded within existing curriculum design, instead of something that is simply bolted on and optional. This lack of embedding is often associated with the use of the devices as a simple course administrative tool or as a mobile textbook that only provides content. A blended approach allows the full potential of mobile devices to be realized, but this requires integration of the devices into daily teaching and learning, such as at the end of patient encounters or for projects. The experience of large-scale implementation within healthcare organizations can lead to mistrust by both patients and staff who may regard the use of mobile devices, in a busy clinical environment, as a social communication device (such as uploading to social network sites) instead of a useful teaching and learning resource.

 Effective m-learning requires consideration of how it is embedded in the curriculum and in healthcare organizations.

The main technical problems noted with the use of mobile devices in medical education have been related to the small size of the screen and the method of data entry (keyboard, touchscreen or stylus). Battery life can also be short, leading to sudden loss of data, and there may be interoperability problems between the various types of device and institutional IT systems and VLEs. However, manufacturers are aware of these issues, and recent advances in technology are helping to rapidly resolve these problems.

Concerns have been raised about the safety and inappropriate use of mobile devices. The main response has been to ban mobile devices in clinical areas where they could be most useful. It has been suggested that the use of mobile phones is associated with harm to users and interference with electronic equipment, but there is no real evidence to support these concerns. Ethical issues have been raised about the use of camera phones in clinical areas and patient consent, but these concerns are part of a wider debate and sensible guidelines need to be developed. Tutors and students may also find mobile devices difficult to use, especially if they have certain disabilities. Concerns about equity of learning opportunities should also be part of a wider debate.

Summary

The use of mobile devices to enhance teaching and learning is here to stay. The relatively low cost of devices, the multiple functions of individual devices, the high portability and the possibility of constant connectivity have been the main factors for the increasing popularity of mobile devices in social, leisure and educational contexts. Exciting new potential learning opportunities can be created by mobile devices. However, this is dependent on applying key educational principles as to how technology can be used to enhance teaching and learning instead of concentrating on what is the latest technology.

Further reading

Iacono A, Frith G: Mobile media – from content to user. In Earnshaw RA, Vince J, Carr R, editors: *Digital Convergence – Libraries of the Future*, London, 2008, Springer, pp 273–294.

Lindquist AM, Johansson PE, Petersson GI, et al: The use of the Personal Digital Assistant (PDA) among personnel and students in health care: a review, *Journal Medical Internet Research28* 10(4):e31, 2008.

Luckin R: The learner centric ecology of resources: A framework for using technology to scaffold learning, *Computers and Education* 50(2):449–462, 2008.

Sandars J, Murray C, Pellow A: Twelve tips for using digital storytelling to promote reflective learning, *Medical Teacher* 30:774–777, 2008.

Sandars J, Dearnley C: Twelve tips for the use of mobile technologies for work based assessment, *Medical Teacher* 31:18–21, 2009.

Sandars J: Twelve tips for using podcasts in medical education, *Medical Teacher* 31:38–389, 2009.

Sandars J: Developing competences for learning in the age of the internet, *Education for Primary Care* 20:337–422, 2009.

Sandars J, Murray C: Digital storytelling for reflection in undergraduate medical education: a pilot study, *Education for Primary Care* 20:441–444, 2009.

Free downloadable books

Ally M (ed) 2009 Mobile Learning: Transforming the Delivery of Education and Training. Athabasca University Press, Edmonton, Canada. http://www.aupress.ca/index.php/books/120155

The whole book or separate chapters can be viewed.

Pachler N (ed) 2007 Mobile Learning: Towards a Research Agenda. Work-Based Learning for Education Professionals (WLE Centre), Institute of Education, University of London, UK. http://www.wlecentre.ac.uk/cms/files/occasionalpapers/mobilelearning_pachler2007.pdf

This book has an interesting chapter on the theoretical pedagogical aspects of mobile learning.

Websites

Assessment and Learning in Practice Settings (ALPS): www.alps-cetl.ac.uk

ALPS is a collaboration between five higher education institutions in the UK and spans 16 health and social care professions across the partnership, from audiology to social work. The ALPS research and development work with over 900 students has produced a range of resources (teaching and learning tools as well as publications and reports) which are freely available from the website. The areas in which the ALPS partnership has significant experience and expertise include mobile learning, competency mapping, interprofessional assessment, reflective tools development, ePortfolios, accessibility, service user and carer engagement and collaborative working.

The main relevant downloadable reports are the following:

- Embedding mobile enabling technologies (EMET)
- Implementing a large-scale mobile learning programme
- Exploring and reducing the barriers to service user engagement with the ALPS assessment suite: a multi-disciplinary approach
- ALPS Research Capacity Report – Mobile enabled disabled students (MEDS). An investigation into the benefits, barriers and essential specifications of mobile devices used for learning and assessment purposes with disabled students
- ALPS cost benefit analysis.

The International Association for Mobile Learning (IAmLearn): www.iamlearn.org
IAmLearn is a membership organization to promote excellence in research, development and application of mobile and contextual learning. It organizes the annual mLearn international conference series and manages the website to collate and disseminate information about new projects and emerging technologies.

Resources

Lists of medical apps for mobile devices:

iPhone/iPad/android: www.imedicalapps.com
Android: www.pepid.com/android

Review of latest smartphones: www.telegraph.co.uk/technology/mobile-phone-reviews

Lists of medical podcasts: http://lib.georgiahealth.edu/resources/podcasts.php

Section 5

Curriculum themes

Basic sciences and curriculum outcomes

W. Pawlina, N. Lachman

Introduction

The role of the basic sciences and, consequently, the role of the basic science educators in the medical curriculum have undergone significant change in the context of even more dramatic change in both healthcare delivery systems and medical education. Over the last two decades, a debate has ensued challenging the very existence of medical basic science departments. From this argument, it has been shown that a traditional delivery of the basic sciences no longer has a place within the medical curriculum. As medical curriculum evolves, conventional courses need to adopt a new system of basic science instruction. As our understanding of the science of learning progresses, new knowledge transforms educational strategies in basic science.

 Three tips for faculty teaching basic sciences in medical school:

- You are NOT teaching basic sciences to future basic scientists (… but to future physicians)
- When teaching basic sciences you are NOT only teaching basic science content (… but other discipline-independent subjects)
- Teaching basic sciences should NOT be for 'breakfast' only (… but distributed as a regular 'meal' throughout the entire length of medical curriculum).

The changing medical curriculum

With the dissolution of input-based curricula that nurtured the traditional format of basic science teaching, the challenge now lies in teaching an 'old subject in a new world' (Haase 2000). Regarding undergraduate programmes, a multiplicity of forces have changed the roles and responsibilities of medical educators. These forces include:

- Revision of medical curricula that progressively decreases the time alloted for basic sciences
- Adoption of student-centred, flexible curriculum design that promotes the well-being of students
- Increased presence of innovations and electronic technologies
- Attention to the science of healthcare delivery systems with an emphasis on systems engineering
- Emphasis on clinical translational (bench-to-bedside) research
- Emphasis on value, safety, quality and other measurable outcomes in patient care
- Inclusion of discipline-independent subjects such as professionalism, ethics, leadership and interprofessional teamwork.

Therefore, educators must now produce scientifically competent graduates able to function as professionals in the climate change of healthcare reform. This means that they must practise evidence-based medicine, adhere to outcomes-based standards of care, translate scientific discoveries into clinical applications, utilize electronic information technology, comply with safety and quality measures and provide accessible, affordable, accountable and affable medical care (Srinivasan et al 2006).

 "Understanding the scientific foundation of medical practice and using this knowledge to inform decisions for patient care is an essential competency of a physician."

Fincher et al 2009

The overarching objective of a basic medical science course is to provide fundamental scientific theories and concepts for clinical application. Traditionally, basic science subjects have included anatomy, histology, physiology, biochemistry and pathology. The current teaching model includes genetics, cell and molecular biology, epidemiology, nutrition and energy metabolism and the science of healthcare delivery and bioinformatics. The medical curriculum has shifted from the Flexner model to an integrated model in which basic science courses are either paired with related clinical disciplines (e.g. anatomy/radiology, immunology/pathology, neuroscience/psychiatry) or taught in blocks by organ system. Blocks are coordinated by faculty from both basic science and clinical departments, ensuring that students are given early exposure to patients in a clinical setting (Gregory et al 2009).

 Elements of an effective basic science course with distribution of faculty efforts:

- Specific course objectives (10%)
- Didactic component designed on the active learning platform supported by modern instructional technologies with critical thinking activities (60%)
- Formative feedback on students' performance (5%)
- Discipline-independent subjects (10%)
- Assessment of knowledge and skills (5%)
- Summative feedback on course performance and directions for professional development (10%).

Basic science courses that used to focus on content knowledge are morphing to incorporate the longitudinal objectives of the medical arts. Often termed 'holistic education', this movement encourages intellectual, social, creative and emotional development alongside knowledge acquisition. Technology offers new platforms upon which to build integrative innovations, but its use comes with many challenges. In e-learning, entire curricula are accessible via electronic content management systems on websites. This non-classroom didactic setting creates a challenge for the teacher when presented with the imperative to incorporate basic science into lessons in clinical medicine and professionalism through holistic learning. Teachers and learners alike must be flexible and adapt to this rapidly changing educational environment.

The active learning environment

Another didactic shift in this movement is the transition away from passive learning towards a more active learning environment. In active learning, students learn to restructure the new information and their prior knowledge into new knowledge (McManus 2001). Among the most utilized formats for active learning are discussions in small groups (problem-based learning [PBL]), learning through clinical scenarios (case-based learning [CBL]), team-based

learning (TBL) and learning through reflection (Lachman & Pawlina 2006).

 "The basic science lesson can, through the implementation of creative exercises, present an ideal opportunity for initiating independent, self-directed learning that allows for integration and validation of key learning areas, both theoretically and practically."

Lachman & Pawlina 2006

One of these approaches has become a commonly applied strategy in basic sciences: PBL (Bowman & Hughes 2005, Kinkade 2005). PBL shifts the emphasis from didactic instruction to self-directed learning. So for teachers with more experience in traditional education, the implementation of PBL requires not only a change in mindset, but also major adjustments in preparation to teach in this programme. The PBL approach is labour intensive, demanding more time for preliminary work to integrate appropriate skills and knowledge within the programme.

To facilitate student-centred learning, the TBL approach supports small-group activities where students teach one another. TBL was designed for use in large classrooms, and so TBL is often used in undergraduate courses such as anatomy, histology and microbiology during medical training. There is evidence that TBL has the ability to balance cognitive skills through group interaction of factual assimilation and application (Michaelsen et al 2008, Vasan et al 2008). Since this type of strategy requires a small-group set-up and is highly collaborative in nature, teachers must master group facilitator skills while serving as content experts. Rather than lecturing, teachers debrief on the problems presented during TBL sessions (Michaelsen et al 2008). While this level of interaction usually requires more in-depth understanding of the subject material by the facilitator, it also promotes more critical thinking and reflection.

 "As medical schools are creating integrated and interdisciplinary courses during the preclinical years, TBL is particularly useful because of its emphasis on teamwork, mastery of content, and problem solving for clinical application."

Vasan et al 2009

CBL is learning stimulated by active discussion on clinical cases specifically constructed to emphasize basic science principles. Cases should portray authentic, often complex, problems resolved by applying basic science knowledge and critical analysis. Independently or in extracurricular study groups, students review the case ahead of the CBL session to identify and research the critical concept. During the CBL session, a facilitator advances learning objectives by asking a sequence of trigger questions that stimulate students to articulate their perspective: proposing problem-solving strategies, actively listening to group discussion and promoting reflection (Bowe et al 2009). The multidisciplinary basic and clinical science faculty collaboration may enhance the outcomes of CBL sessions.

As coaches and facilitators instead of lecturers, teachers still manage the overall instructional process in which students have the opportunity to master course objectives and solve problems. As teachers continue to learn alongside their students, they serve as role models of lifelong learning. Additionally, mentorship may develop among teachers and students that self-select to serve as teaching assistants. In these apprenticeships, students find themselves on the way to becoming colleagues of their teachers, capable of working in effective, self-managed interprofessional teams and moving education forward.

Use of reflective practice, critical thinking and clinical reasoning

The use of reflection as a practical tool has become an important component of curriculum design for basic science. Reflective exercises support the practice of critical thinking for problem solving and the development of humanistic qualities desired in healthcare practitioners.

Within the learning environment, students may reflect individually through writing, or they may engage a team to explore or share experiences that lead to better comprehension and understanding. Reflection involves the synthesis of fragmented lessons, integration into one's personal experience, and application to the larger narrative in which students find themselves in the world. In this process students cease to be educational automatons and develop personal epistemological initiative based on their values, which usually champion knowledge as a form of progress. From a theoretical standpoint, a student reflects by making an association with the learning objective, integrating the new concept with prior knowledge, validating the knowledge and, finally, applying the material (Lachman & Pawlina 2006).

In designing a curriculum to include critical thinking through reflective exercises, it is important to leave the course methods open to challenge and review. Explicit training in clinical reasoning naturally begins with the basic science courses, as it is important for the development of a systematic and efficient approach to clinical cases. This foundation serves medical trainees well indeed in all subsequent educational endeavors to come (Elizondo-Omaña et al 2010). It entails bridging the gap between theory and practice, a chasm that can be crossed through reflection.

The implementation of reflective exercises may be achieved through the application of various techniques and learning activities. An effective way of teaching critical thinking and reflection in basic sciences is to encourage self-directed learning. Again, in this setting, the educator takes on the role of a facilitator rather than a director of knowledge. When assigned tasks that require investigation outside of the classroom, the student must reflect on the information given and decide upon a relevant interpretation of core objectives for the subject to be mastered. Critical thinking skills are further enhanced through collaboration and team interaction. The use of teamwork to facilitate conceptual understanding has proved to be effective in stimulating collective thinking. In many cases, this can be accomplished by utilizing e-learning technologies.

Reflection and clinical reasoning should also be incorporated into assessment strategies. Questions may be designed for critical thinking by including clinical cases that demonstrate core basic science concepts. Providing formative assessment allows students to monitor their own learning process. In many institutions, audience response systems (ARSs) are used to provide immediate feedback on individual student performance in relation to overall performance within the group. The use of a combination of questioning styles such as multiple-choice questions (MCQs) and short answer questions (SAQs) promotes both discernment and writing skills. Additionally, peer and self-evaluation are effective assessments of critical analysis of teamwork dynamics.

Conceptual knowledge:
- Understanding the process and concept rather than memorizing details
- Providing knowledge of resources for obtaining detailed information (e.g. finding gene structure and location on variety of genetic databases).

Applied knowledge:
- Applying content to situations that are clinically relevant
- Teaching reasoning skills through virtual patients/clinical cases
- Bridging the gap between basic science and clinical thinking.

Innovations in teaching basic sciences

Dramatic changes in basic science teaching are paralleled with advances in electronic media. The development of more powerful computers (tablet and notebook computers), 3-D gaming and simulation, smartphones and mobile technologies, and high-speed wireless internet connections has allowed medical educators to incorporate high-quality imaging, animations, virtual reality interactive training modules and learning management systems into the classroom. What were once considered advanced and sophisticated teaching methods and technologies are now commonplace or outdated (Pawlina & Lachman 2004). The benefit of computer-assisted learning (CAL) is that it has great potential for enhancing knowledge acquisition as it appeals to the 21st century learner (McNulty et al 2009). However, educators must be aware that CAL has different characteristics when compared with conventional scenarios, especially as it impacts social communication, message exchange, cognitive load and participation of the learner.

However daunting, basic science teachers should take advantage of innovative technology (Philip et al 2008). For example, the ARS serves as an interactive solution for teachers trying to engage their students in active learning. Employing ARS in the classroom allows students to continuously monitor their progress in the class (Alexander et al 2009). Simulation laboratories are increasingly utilized in teaching basic sciences. Animal physiology laboratories have been replaced by simulation centres that utilize high-fidelity manikins that can demonstrate the basic physiological concepts, respond to pharmacological compounds, and encourage diagnostic reasoning skills in medical students (Rosen et al 2009).

In addition to high-fidelity simulators, educators often use simple techniques and low-fidelity physical models in teaching the basic sciences. For instance, body painting in gross anatomy improves student knowledge of surface anatomy needed for palpation and auscultation in clinical practice (McMenamin 2008). The active and kinesthetic nature of body painting, coupled with the strong and highly memorable visual images of underlying anatomy, contribute to the success of body painting as a learning tool (Finn & McLachlan 2010). The use of simple physical models to demonstrate the spatial relationship of the represented structures within the human body aids understanding of its more complex function. These simple techniques and models serve as memory aids, reduce cognitive overload, facilitate problem solving, and arouse students' enthusiasm and participation (Chan and Cheng 2011).

The use of new techniques and tools in basic science education is essential for the training of a medical student. Innovations must bear relevance to clinical practice and incorporate principles of functional science within integrated and practically digitized environments.

Basic science integration throughout the curriculum

In addition to preserving prior knowledge, undergraduate students must also incorporate recent advances that occur in clinical practice and correlate their understanding through the interpretation and integration of basic science concepts. Frequently, areas well known to the basic scientist but rarely explored by the clinical specialist become crucial to the success of new clinical procedures. For example, the use of surgical robots and interventional procedures with minimal access surgery, as in radiofrequency ablation of cardiac arrhythmias, necessitates a solid understanding not only of detailed anatomical relationships within the heart but also of the heart's electrophysiology. Detail once considered extraneous has renewed significance and is often critical to the success of a clinical procedure. Therefore, integration of basic sciences into the later years of the medical curriculum and, more so, in postgraduate specialization is growing in popularity. A return to the basic sciences during the latter years of medical curriculum, when students' clinical reasoning and analytical skills are more refined, enables learners to better integrate basic science concepts into their clinical experience (Spencer et al 2008).

However, this also means that while modern medical education may not favour the retention of the classical basic scientist, the success of modern medical education is thoroughly dependent on the classical details of foundational medical sciences. Basic scientists can no longer exist in isolation from clinical disciplines and need to contribute to clinical outcomes. Whereas in the past their expertise was limited to the first few years of medical training, the new era of medicine requires the basic scientist to be engaged throughout the medical curriculum.

 "The most effective leaders are those who can communicate effectively, generate trust, and motivate others to work together."

Jensen et al 2008

Nontraditional discipline-independent basic science skills

Moving forward, basic science will more likely extend throughout the curriculum (Spencer et al 2008). Therefore, basic science courses must incorporate longitudinal objectives that will be revisited in clinical courses (Hamilton et al 2008). These may include discipline-independent subjects such as leadership, teamwork, professionalism, effective communication and promoting students' well-being:

- Leadership
  - Skills fostered through team-based activities
  - Demonstrated by the success with which a group is able to achieve set objectives under the direction of the designated team leader (Pawlina et al 2006)
- Teamwork
  - Essential part of successful patient care
  - Fosters collaboration in obtaining, sharing and presenting knowledge (O'Connell & Pascoe 2004)
  - Involves learning teams as an instructional strategy (Michaelsen et al 2008)
- Professionalism
  - Entails acts of dutifulness and showing respect for others
  - Based on traditional duties and responsibilities of the profession
  - Anchored in clinical practice of medicine; also should apply to basic sciences (Bryan et al 2005, Lachman & Pawlina 2006)
- Communication skills
  - Early emphasis equips students with the ability to effectively transfer information between the members of the team and later in the patient setting
  - Early introduction of peer and self-evaluations to enhance assessment skills (Bryan et al 2005)
- Student well-being
  - Protection of nonscheduled curricular time for self-learning, reflection and activities that promote well-being of learners
  - Didactic review sessions and practice practical examinations utilizing format of final examinations
  - Incorporation of flexible 'consolidation days' into the course curriculum with students' self-directed activities.

Learning basic science outside curricular structure

Advances in healthcare delivery are taking place at a staggering pace. There are many examples of lessons once strictly within the domain of basic science that are now a part of everyday clinical practice. Starting early in medical school, teaching faculty should advocate for, mentor and provide opportunities for students to be engaged in research projects that enrich their appreciation for translational research. Many schools have protected research time within the curriculum for medical students, usually dispersed among clinical clerkships. Others offer summer programmes for students who are interested in further research. In curricula without designated time for research activities, the basic science faculty should provide opportunities for students to participate in research activities during unstructured time in the medical curriculum. Under the guidance and direction of their mentors, students may elect to conduct research within a spectrum of possible projects including basic science bench research, medical education research and clinical research. Extracurricular research fosters closer relationships between students and their faculty mentors, gives students the opportunity to meet distinguished visiting physicians and scientists and allows them to gain experience in diverse laboratory and patient care settings.

These opportunities are likely to create a culture of scientific research as the students come to be clinicians (Fincher et al 2009). If this approach generates an abundance of clinician-scientists, it will likely increase the translation of knowledge from the bench to the bedside and improve patient outcomes.

Summary

Basic sciences should no longer be taught in the traditional manner in the medical curriculum. The design of the contemporary medical curriculum incorporates clinical and translational research, an increased presence of electronic technology, the implementation of student-centred learning, and the increased emphasis on professionalism, ethics and interprofessional teamwork. Teachers should assume the roles of coaches and facilitators rather than directors. They need to mentor students into becoming lifelong learners – apprentices on the way to becoming colleagues – capable of working within interprofessional communities. Students also need concrete knowledge of fundamental basic science alongside its application to clinical practice, and they must appreciate the process of scientific inquiry and translation (Fincher et al 2009) within the digitized environment of electronic medical records and resources. Furthermore, basic scientists cannot exist in isolation from the clinical disciplines and must contribute to clinical outcomes. For the basic scientist, in framing a more modern concept of medical education, it will be necessary to shift the paradigm of tradition passed down over the centuries and integrate the foundations into clinical practice. Basic scientists must remain learners in this new age of medical education, and must strive so that all efforts benefit students: the future generation of healthcare providers.

References

Alexander CJ, Crescini WM, Juskewitch JE, et al: Assessing the integration of audience response system technology in teaching of anatomical sciences, *Anatomical Sciences Education* 2(4):160–166, 2009.

Bowe CM, Voss J, Aretz TH: Case method teaching: an effective approach to integrate the basic and clinical sciences in the preclinical medical curriculum, *Medical Teacher* 31(9):834–841, 2009.

Bowman D, Hughes P: Emotional responses of tutors and students in problem-based learning: lessons for staff development, *Medical Education* 39(2):145–153, 2005.

Bryan RE, Krych AJ, Carmichael SW, et al: Assessing professionalism in early medical education: experience with peer evaluation and self-evaluation in the gross anatomy course, *Annals of the Academy of Medicine, Singapore* 34(8):486–491, 2005.

Chan LK, Cheng MM: An analysis of the educational value of low-fidelity anatomy models as external representations, *Anatomical Sciences Education*, 4(5):256–263, 2011.

Elizondo-Omaña RE, Morales-Gómez JA, Morquecho-Espinoza O, et al: Teaching skills to promote clinical reasoning in early basic science courses, *Anatomical Sciences Education* 3(5):267–271, 2010.

Fincher RM, Wallach PM, Richardson WS: Basic science right, not basic science lite: medical education at a crossroad, *Journal of General Internal Medicine* 24(11):1255–1258, 2009.

Finn GM, McLachlan JC: A qualitative study of student responses to body painting, *Anatomical Sciences Education* 3(1):33–38, 2010.

Gregory JK, Lachman N, Camp CL, et al: Restructuring a basic science course for core competencies: an example from anatomy teaching, *Medical Teacher* 31(9):855–861, 2009.

Haase P: The challenges of teaching an old subject in a new world – a personal perspective, *Clinical Investigations in Medicine* 23(1):81–83, 2000.

Hamilton SS, Yuan BJ, Lachman N, et al: Interprofessional education in gross anatomy: experience with first year medical and physical therapy students at Mayo Clinic, *Anatomical Sciences Education* 1(6):258–263, 2008.

Jensen AR, Wright AS, Lance AR, et al: The emotional intelligence of surgical residents: a descriptive study, *American Journal of Surgery* 195(1):5–10, 2008.

Kinkade S: A snapshot of the status of problem-based learning in US medical schools, 2003–04, *Academic Medicine* 80(3):300–301, 2005.

Lachman N, Pawlina W: Integrating professionalism in early medical education: the theory and application of reflective practice in the anatomy curriculum, *Clinical Anatomy* 19(5):456–460, 2006.

McManus DA: The two paradigms of education and the peer review of teaching, *Journal of Geoscience Education* 49(5):423–434, 2001.

McMenamin PG: Body painting as a tool in clinical anatomy teaching, *Anatomical Sciences Education* 1(4):139–144, 2008.

McNulty JA, Sonntag B, Sinacore JM: Evaluation of computer-aided instruction in a gross anatomy course: a six-year study, *Anatomical Sciences Education* 2(1):2–8, 2009.

Michaelsen LK, Parmelee DX, McMahon KK, Levine RE: *Team-Based Learning for Health Professions Education: A Guide to Using Small Groups for Improving Learning*, 229, Sterling, VA, 2008, Stylus Publishing LLC.

O'Connell MT, Pascoe JM: Undergraduate medical education for the 21st century: leadership and teamwork, *Family Medicine* 36(Suppl):S51–S56, 2004.

Pawlina W, Hromanik MJ, Milanese TR, et al: Leadership and professionalism curriculum in the gross anatomy course, *Annals of the Academy of Medicine, Singapore* 35(9):609–614, 2006.

Pawlina W, Lachman N: Dissection in learning and teaching gross anatomy: rebuttal to McLachlan, *Anatomical Record. Part B, New Anatomist* 281(1):9–11, 2004.

Philip CT, Unruh KP, Lachman N, et al: An explorative learning approach to teaching clinical anatomy using student generated content, *Anatomical Sciences Education* 1(3):106–110, 2008.

Rosen KR, McBride JM, Drake RL: The use of simulation in medical education to enhance students' understanding of basic sciences, *Medical Teacher* 31(9):842–846, 2009.

Spencer AL, Brosenitsch T, Levine AS, Kanter SL: Back to the basic sciences: an innovative approach to teaching senior medical students how best to integrate basic science and clinical medicine, *Academic Medicine* 83(7):662–669, 2008.

Srinivasan M, Keenan CR, Yager J: Visualizing the future: technology competency development in clinical medicine and implication for medical education, *Academic Psychiatry* 30(6):480–490, 2006.

Vasan NS, DeFouw DO, Compton S: A survey of student perceptions of team-based learning in anatomy curriculum: favorable views unrelated to grades, *Anatomical Sciences Education* 2(4):150–155, 2009.

Vasan NS, DeFouw DO, Holland BK: Modified use of team-based learning for effective delivery of medical gross anatomy and embryology, *Anatomical Sciences Education* 1(1):3–9, 2008.

Further reading

Davis MH, Harden RM: Planning and implementing an undergraduate medical curriculum: the lessons learned, *Medical Teacher* 25(6):596–608, 2003.

Norman G: Teaching basic science to optimize transfer, *Medical Teacher* 31(9):807–811, 2009.

Clinical communication

J. R. Skelton

Introduction

The importance of clinical communication is now taken for granted. It is routinely taught and tested at the undergraduate and postgraduate level, often with a set of 'communication skills' in mind which are perceived as the conduit for patient-centred medicine. A key document which drew attention to the literature and placed the issue centre stage was the so-called Toronto Consensus Statement (Simpson et al 1991): the most fully developed list of skills derives from Silverman et al (2005) and is available online. Maguire and Pitceathly (2002) give a brief summary of 'key communication skills', and von Fragstein et al (2008) outline a consensus on the undergraduate curriculum for the UK.

Mainstream research links skills such as 'eye contact' or 'listening' with desirable outcomes such as patient satisfaction and better health (but for a detailed critique, see Skelton 2008). The communication skills movement has been of exceptional importance in reworking a timeless theme for a contemporary audience: the good doctor needs more than clinical knowledge. However, scrutiny of what constitutes 'good skills' has tended to divert attention from the wider context in which communication is practised.

Firstly, there is at present considerable attention on aspects of (nonclinical) professional competence. In the UK, this has been closely linked to the heart searching following the Shipman tragedy and the events at Bristol which led to the Kennedy Report (2001). The latter asks for a broader definition of 'clinical competence', and the range of issues with which communication is bracketed is instructive (see Box 30.1). Secondly, teaching has centred on a particular kind of professional interaction: spoken, doctor–patient, with a broadly counselling approach. Other communication types are mentioned below.

However, the centrepiece of most clinical communication teaching remains doctor–patient interaction through role play.

Box 30.1 Broadening the notion of clinical competence

Greater priority than at present should be given to nonclinical aspects of care in six key areas in the education, training and continuing professional development of healthcare professionals:

- Skills in communicating with patients and with colleagues
- Education about the principles and organization of the NHS, and about how care is managed, and the skills required for management
- The development of teamwork
- Shared learning across professional boundaries
- Clinical audit and reflective practice
- Leadership.

From Kennedy I: The report of the public enquiry into children's heart surgery at the Bristol Royal Infirmary 1984–1995 ('The Kennedy report'), paragraph 57, London, 2001, HSMO, (www.bristol-inquiry.org.uk/final_report/rpt_print.htm), with permission.

Using role play

RATIONALE

'Role play' is an unfortunate label: even in the UK, it has overtones of amateur dramatics, and in the United States it has perhaps even less credibility. But alternative labels for similar activities (e.g. 'simulated patients') are unfortunately used in different ways, so I have retained the term 'role play' to mean a serious, challenging educational activity.

The fundamental rationale for role play is that you cannot become a better communicator except by practising communication any more than you can become a good driver except by driving. Role play provides a safe environment for mistakes and experimentation and can offer the same, educationally useful, performance repeatedly.

Behind this rationale are other important characteristics. Education through role play is essentially inductive in nature; it moves from a focus on a particular case to a discussion which seeks to induce general principles. For example, 'Mr Smith responded in this way – is this typical of how people might respond in these circumstances?' It therefore fits well with contemporary educational practice in starting with individual cases rather than lecture-based generalities. It also fits neatly into the common pattern of clinical life: contact with patients, one by one.

 Role play is a serious, challenging, and above all *educational* activity. It isn't a piece of drama.

FORMATS FOR ROLE PLAY

There are unlimited variations of the role play formats outlined below, which are indicative rather than prescriptive.

1. *Forum theatre:* One role player, one or two facilitators. Audience of any size up to several hundred. In lecture theatre or similar large venue. One hour in length.

   Role player and facilitator act out a scenario in a less-than-perfect way. Facilitator subsequently invites comments from audience (or second facilitator does, with roving microphone). Repeat scenario, building in changes suggested. Draw conclusions.

2. *Large group:* Role player and facilitator, audience of 8–20. This can be done as a version of forum theatre, but the smaller group size makes it more flexible. Two hours in length. 'Time outs' can be introduced, so that everyone (including role player and facilitator) can stop, review, ask questions or make suggestions.

   With a group of this size, it becomes reasonable to ask participants to play the part of the doctor. Depending on levels of confidence, other participants can offer detailed advice beforehand (this shares the burden of responsibility if things go badly) or none at all.

   With a group of up to 20, it isn't usually realistic to offer everyone a chance to role play. Notoriously, those most in need are least likely to volunteer, but it may be reasonable to allow some to take a back seat, participating in targeted observation. This means asking individuals to look for certain key elements – 'How is the doctor achieving empathy?' or, at a lower level, 'How many open questions is the doctor asking?' (A variant of this, particularly with students on attachment, is to make explicit use of the clinical tutor as a model, with students looking at the tutor's clinical communication in

practice). This kind of activity can form part of the feedback offered. Discussion often lasts at least as long as the role play itself, and is at least as interesting. This is particularly so with qualified health professionals who have more experience to draw on and often more confidence to discuss.

The best role players are essentially educators, and contribute detailed feedback.

 When you set up role play, be confident, matter-of-fact and serious. If you're not relaxed about it, the learners won't be.

3. *Small group:* Role player and facilitator, or facilitator only, group of up to 8. With this number of participants it becomes realistic to offer everyone a chance to role play, either seeing a consultation through from beginning to end or undertaking part and then handing over to someone else during a time out.

   Educators often suggest asking health professionals to take the part of patients, on the grounds that this will help them to understand what it's like to be on the receiving end of bad news, a peremptory doctor, etc. Where the budget doesn't run to a professional role player, this is inevitable. Most people can at least play a version of themselves tolerably well ('Just imagine that you personally are in this situation').

   A standard (but costly) variant is to subdivide a larger group into smaller groups of four to six, each with a facilitator, and with a number of role players rotating round the groups.

4. *Single participant role play:* Role player-facilitator, or role player plus facilitator, one participant.

   It's clear that this is an expensive resource but, particularly in cases where the aim is remedial support, the intensity of the contact and the possibility of very detailed discussion make it cost-effective. A 2-hour session can make a real difference. And it is very likely to reveal a great deal about other areas such as attitude.

CONDUCTING A ROLE PLAY SESSION

Of central importance prior to the interaction is that the atmosphere is right. If participants have never undertaken role play before, they may be nervous and, often for this reason, sceptical. It's therefore vital that the facilitator and role players are confident, matter-of-fact and serious. (If you Google the phrase 'the dreaded role play' you'll find plenty of examples of trainers anxiously saying, 'It's not that bad, really': exactly the line *not* to take). There needs to be a shared understanding that all participants are there to support each other and engage together in learning.

This brings us to the question of feedback. At an elementary level (for example, with junior undergraduates, or for remedial support), there is a need for feedback centred on the basic skills: the use of questioning styles, appropriate body language, checking of understanding and so on. This is vital partly because it may be done poorly, but mostly so that participants are made aware of these skills and have a vocabulary with which to discuss them.

This is, however, basic stuff: a course in 'advanced eye contact' is hardly plausible. One of the real values of role play is the opportunity it gives for discussion at a higher level, for reflection about oneself and others and about the profession. There is a basic hierarchy of questions, in fact (see Box 30.2), which perhaps most people employ, but which is seldom made explicit. At the heart of the issue here is that good communication is not a matter of the mechanical application of skills, but judicious, insightful choices about when and how to deploy them.

Level 1, clearly, deals with behavioural skills. We know very little about *how much* of these skills is the right amount for particular circumstances, nor about *why* the amount might vary from one occasion to the next. The facilitator's role at this level, then, is to ensure that the participant and observers can describe accurately what they have seen, and evidence it. Thus, not 'You were very empathic' but 'When you leaned forward and murmured, 'Take your time' that made you appear very empathic'. And – moving as quickly as possible on to the next level in the hierarchy – ensure that they can justify what was done. The third level in the hierarchy represents the classic movement of inductive teaching: it compares the particular instance against general patterns. A common way of linking the two is through the facilitator or one of the participants, saying 'This happens a lot – I had a patient once …'.

The higher-order questions are invitations to reflect. 'What do you make of this patient?', 'What kind of person are they?' or, 'What does this role play tell you about being a doctor?'

 Move as quickly as you can up the 'hierarchy of questions': the higher the level of the questions, the more interesting the session.

The wider context

CLINICAL SKILLS AND CLINICAL COMMUNICATION COMBINED

Role play has tended to invoke a quasi-counselling setting and approach. However, clinical communication typically happens alongside clinical skills. For

---

> **Box 30.2 Hierarchy of question types after role play**
>
> 1. *Describing skills:* Did you maintain eye contact? The right amount? How do you know?
> 2. *Justifying skills:* Why did you do it that way? What if you'd done it differently?
> 3. *Generalizing skills:* Are there general principles here, e.g. about how to defuse aggression? ('I had a patient who …')
>
> **Higher-order questions**
>
> 4. *Assessing people:* What was the patient like? Is this typical or unusual for patients of this type, or with this problem?
> 5. *Assessing self:* What kind of person are you? What did the experience tell you about, e.g. your response to stress, breaking bad news … how did it make you feel?
> 6. *Assessing the profession:* In the light of this scenario, what does it mean to be a doctor? What kind of things do doctors do?

---

many students, early in their clinical career, the requirement to perform a clinical skill while sounding professional is difficult, as is the language which surrounds clinical examination: a request for a patient to undress is an obvious example. In addition, good communication with a patient in a clinical setting such as the ward may often be a matter of seconds rather than minutes, which makes the counselling model less relevant. Yet the doctor who spends 10 seconds with a patient is creating a foundation of trust which might be of considerable importance.

 The competencies that doctors need to communicate well involve much, much more than quasi-counselling skills.

The most detailed form of clinical communication teaching is what happens on simulated wards. Here, typically, a group of participants is faced with a patient or patients and required to undertake a series of tasks. The patients may be role players who are happy to have a range of clinical skills practised on them. Alternatively, manikins may be used, with the 'communication' element being between the various participants rather than the plastic model. The comparison is often made between this kind of activity and the training which airline pilots have on flight simulators, where the trainee has to deal with unexpected and potentially catastrophic situations. The training in consequence often focuses on the risk which arises from such 'human factors' as the clumsiness, forgetfulness and general confusion that arise from working under pressure.

COMMUNICATION BETWEEN COLLEAGUES

As the previous example makes clear, clinical communication does not occur merely between a doctor and a patient. A great deal of it happens between colleagues. A method often taught is known as 'SBAR' (NHS Institute 2011): situation, background, assessment, recommendation. (SBAR too was first developed in an aviation and military context). The idea is that, 'at any stage of the patient's journey', the template can be used to 'shape' communication between colleagues. This works well for referral letters, aspects of handover, asking the consultant to come to the ward and many other things. As regards teaching, it lends itself to a wide variety of different approaches. A paper case can be offered to a group, for example, and they can be invited to agree what elements matter: that is, how to fill the SBAR template. This is obviously a good prioritization task in itself. One of the participants can then actually report the case, perhaps under psychological pressure (it's the middle of the night, you're on the phone, the consultant is horrible …).

Other common issues which surface in colleague interaction centre on aspects of teamwork, leadership, negotiation and the like (see Box 30.1). It's probably reasonable to say that most medical students and young doctors find this kind of communication difficult. In particular, there are issues of what is known as *register*, i.e. how to express the correct level of formality and, by extension, appear appropriately polite without being obsequious (with seniors) or patronizing (with juniors). This evidently also lends itself to role play, but there are simple consciousness-raising activities which are possible as well. Most TV dramas with a hospital setting represent atrocious professional interaction: usually people shouting at each other for dramatic purposes.

ACADEMIC READING AND WRITING

Much of professional communication is academic in nature, or written, or both. Unfortunately, a great deal of the advice floating around consists of vacuous exhortations to 'be clear' and 'remember your audience'. In the absence of useful generalities, a lot of formal presentation skills teaching, for instance, happens through a kind of forum theatre. The presenter gives a presentation which is deliberately poor, and the audience advises on improvements.

Academic reading is important for all doctors, not just for those seeking to pursue an academic career. The more approachable doctors find an article in *The Lancet*, the more likely they are to develop and maintain the faculties of careful scrutiny and reflective practice which medicine demands. Generally, critical reading courses (see also Greenhalgh 2006) incorporate some aspects of 'reading skills', as the phrase is normally used. What is often missing is the kind of standard reading exercise done in other disciplines: exercises in skimming, reading for gist and so on. This type of exercise is often undertaken against the clock, e.g. 'Here's a *JAMA* article without its abstract. In 20 seconds, tell me what the authors acknowledge as the main shortcomings of their paper'. This confirms for participants that 'good reading' can consist of things other than reading a piece intensively from beginning to end: professional life involves quick, sensible choices about what to read and at what level of detail. It also requires readers to know where they are likely to find shortcomings stated (by convention, usually early in the discussion section), and this in turn gives them an understanding of the structure of academic papers (see also Chapter 47, Publishing).

The core of successful teaching of academic writing, in all disciplines, is an understanding of its conventional structure. A personal favourite activity to sensitize participants to aspects of structure is to invite them, in a group of up to six, to write up an imaginary randomized controlled trial (RCT) to test the hypothesis contained in a well-known proverb such as 'a stitch in time saves nine'.

 Examples of 'communication' can be spoken or written, brief or extended, with colleagues or patients. Think creatively about what will benefit your learners.

Shorter pieces of writing are best handled not in the 'writing class' but in the context of professionalism. The doctor who doesn't fill in handover notes or makes poor records on the ward of tasks to do and tasks done is also a risk to patient safety. Of the tasks which are slightly longer, a key one is reading and writing referral letters. These can partly be taught as part of SBAR, as indicated above, but there is the further issue of reading between the lines ('I am referring this anxious patient …'), which doctors need to be able to do, and of making requests, offering criticisms and the like in language which is clear yet courteous and professional. Rewriting tasks work well in these areas: improving a letter too vague or discourteous to be effective. Or the instruction to the class might be: 'Write back to the GP telling him politely not to be such a blithering idiot …'.

LANGUAGE, CULTURE AND THE INTERNATIONAL MEDICAL GRADUATE (IMG)

IMGs, and for that matter international medical students, are likely to encounter substantial difficulties (Whelan 2005), even when they are fluent speakers of the main local language. The UK, for example, has many doctors who speak vigorous, confident South Asian, West African or other well-established (and equally good) varieties of English. Often, however, these doctors struggle with UK 'communicative competence': that is, they *know* the language, but cannot *use* it: they know the phrase 'That's wrong' and the phrase 'I wonder if I could possibly disagree?' but are at risk of using them to the wrong people. Such issues become serious everyday hurdles: 'Who should I be on first name terms with? How should I talk to a junior nurse?'

The best advice for the IMG is usually exposure to the target culture, e.g. through local friends, TV and radio. In addition, they should listen for, make a note of and practise the words and phrases they hear others using to make requests, offer a suggestion, ask a difficult question, etc.

Of course, the multicultural nature of many parts of the modern world is such that many doctors encounter dozens of different cultural groups in the course of a year. Learning the rules of communicative competence for all these groups would be impossible: here, what matters is a more general sensitivity to the possibility of cultural difficulty.

Professionalism

'Communication' is a term which, exasperatingly, can mean more or less anything. The clothes we wear 'communicate', as does our accent, or the architectural style of the local town hall, which perhaps 'communicates' the bourgeois values if its builders. It's impossible to set precise boundaries. For example, the relationship between written communication and the intellectual ability to construct an academic argument has been hinted at above, as has the relationship between communicating well and taking due professional care.

 Think carefully about how to use 'communication' sessions to develop the wider issue of professionalization.

The boundaries set on 'clinical communication' will vary in place and time. At the moment, broadening the notion of clinical competence to include communication and areas related to it, as suggested by some of what is expressed in Box 30.1, offers a more interesting agenda for the future than we have seen over the last generation and suggests ways in which clinical communication can be situated within the wider framework of developing professionalism, which is now regarded as a key area.

This seems to be particularly well-illustrated in the area of remedial support. 'Poor communication' is often given as a frequent cause of patient or colleague complaint, but it is often the symptom rather than the disease. Common sense suggests that the doctor who communicates bad news in a manner perceived as uncaring may actually *be* uncaring rather than merely poorly skilled.

'Communication' is a label that gets slapped on many of the nonclinical, professional problems that doctors encounter and is often the entry point for remediation. Thus particular doctors may be perceived as bullying (with the 'poor communication' being that they shout at people, for example), and this may in turn be because they are anxious, or set impossible standards, and so on. Or perhaps they 'lack leadership qualities', meaning that they don't talk much: which in turn may mean that they need to find a leadership style which allows them to be their true, quiet selves, yet carry authority, and so on (Skelton 2008). (For remedial support in communication in general, see Dowell et al 2006.)

 Tomorrow's Doctors (2009) talks of the requirement for graduates in the UK to communicate 'sensitively', as you would expect. But it also says they should (italics added):

- Communicate effectively with patients *and colleagues*
- Communicate by spoken *written and electronic methods (including medical records)*
- Communicate effectively in various roles, for example, as patient advocate, teacher, manager or improvement leader.

Assessment

Assessment of clinical communication, at least for doctor–patient interaction, is well-accepted. Typically, summative assessment happens through OSCEs with role players. The only major difficulty here is instructive. The more one tries to break down the 'good consultation' into its constituent skills, the more it turns communication into a mechanistic exercise, but the more holistic one is, the more subjective the judgment.

This is a specific example of a generic problem in testing, of course, and the solution, such as it is, is this: be as holistic as you can, and as reductive as you have to be.

Other types of assessment include simple observation and feedback, 360-degree appraisal, and the like. It is difficult to be sure, however, what the level of expertise is of the raters under these circumstances, or whether they all understand 'communication' the same way. This perhaps makes them more appropriate for formative assessment.

Conclusion

Clinical communication has found its niche in medical education over the last 30 years. There are still some who labour the obvious point that a clinically competent but tongue-tied doctor is better than a silver-tongued ignoramus, but for most, the case has been made: communication matters. What the discipline has been less good at, however, is integrating itself fully within a clinical curriculum, rather than being handled separately as a kind of counselling. Nor is it yet well understood as a gateway to the wider professional competencies doctors need. The power of communication teaching to develop these last two areas is considerable.

Summary

Teaching and assessing clinical communication, particularly of doctor–patient interaction, is taken for granted these days. The skills involved in good communication are much discussed and widely available, and there is general agreement that they can be taught, particularly through role play activity. The wider context of communication in medicine is less well-understood, however. Much less is understood about how communication relates to other professional areas such as teamwork and leadership, or the exercise of clinical skills, or about written communication.

References

Dowell J, Dent J, Duffy R: What to do about medical students with unsatisfactory consultation skills? *Medical Teacher* 28(5):443–446, 2006.

Greenhalgh T: *How to Read a Paper*, ed 3, Oxford, 2006, Blackwell.

Kennedy I: *The report of the public enquiry into children's heart surgery at the Bristol Royal Infirmary 1984–1995 ('The Kennedy report')*, London, 2001, HSMO. http://www.bristol-inquiry.org.uk/final_report/rpt_print.htm.

Maguire P, Pitceathly C: Key communication skills and how to acquire them, *British Medical Journal* 325(7366):697–700, 2002.

NHS Institute for Innovation and Improvement: Situation, background, assessment, recommendation: SBAR. http://www.institute.nhs.uk/safer_care/safer_care/Situation_Background_Assessment_Recommendation.html, 2011.

Silverman J, Kurtz S, Draper J: *Skills for Communicating with Patients*, Oxford, 2005, Radcliffe.

Simpson M, Buckman R, Stewart M, et al: Doctor-patient communication: the Toronto consensus statement, *British Medical Journal* 303:1385–1387, 1991.

Skelton J: *Language and Clinical Communication: This Bright Babylon*, Oxford, 2008, Radcliffe.

von Fragstein M, Silverman J, Cushing A, et al: UK consensus statement on the content of communication curricula in undergraduate medical education, *Medical Education* 42:1100–1107, 2008.

Whelan G: Commentary: Coming to America: the integration of international medical graduates into the American medical culture, *Academic Medicine* 81(2):176–178, 2005.

Teaching resources available online

The amount of interesting, easily accessible material for use with students or doctors learning about – or simply reflecting on – clinical communication is considerable. This is a sample only.

1. For those with access to the UK RCGP website, the e-learning package includes much on communication (module 2): http://e-lfh.org.uk/projects/general-practitioners/

2. Examples of role play in a clinical setting are available at the following website, which emanates from St. George's: www.virtualpatients.eu/resources/other-resources-2/communication-skills-online

3. Tokyo Medical University has an extensive website (in English) to support medical students and doctors. It is designed to support non-native speakers of English, but is of considerable value for anyone, and includes both reading support and videos of consultations: www.emp-tmu.net

4. On the issue of giving feedback, see this, from the London Deanery (in general, an excellent educational website): www.faculty.londondeanery.ac.uk/e-learning/feedback/models-of-giving-feedback

5. This website (also of value for many educational areas) looks in detail at the approach associated with Silverman, Kurtz and Draper: www.skillscascade.com/models.htm#Calgary-Cambridge

6. The Picker Institute, which promotes patient-centred care, has interesting information on clinical communication: www.pickereurope.org

7. Finally, although this is more properly 'patient narrative' rather than communication in itself, there is a great deal of potential value for

teaching and learning communication in this extensive website: www.healthtalkonline.org.

Other teaching resources

1. Wiskin C, Skelton JR, Morrison K, Smith P: *Dialogues in Dying*. Oxford, 2009, Radcliffe Medical Press,

    This follows the (fictional) narrative of a young man with motor neurone disease.

2. Hull M, Skelton JR, Wiskin CM: *Consulting: Communication Skills for GPs in Training*, London, 2006, RCGP

    Designed, as the title indicates, for primary care, but there are obviously a great many generic issues. A series of simulated consultations.

3. For cross-cultural issues, see the following:

    Kai J, editor: *Proceed: Professionals Responding to Ethnic Diversity and Cancer*, London, 2006, Nottingham University/CRUK.

    Kai J, editor: *Valuing Diversity*, ed 2, London, 2006, RCGP.

4. Medilectures in partnership with the UK Council of Clinical Communication in Undergraduate Medical Education offers a series of simulated consultations for medical students: www.ukccc.org.uk/consultations-e-learning

Support for the international doctor

For better or (usually) worse, there are any number of websites directed at doctors seeking to pass the UK PLAB exams and their equivalents in other countries. Some of this, of course, involves support for communication.

1. By far the best-known language textbook for those at an intermediate level of English is the following. Glendinning has worked in this area for many years:

    Glendinning EH, Holmström BAS: *English in Medicine*, Cambridge, 2005, Cambridge University Press.

2. There is a huge tradition in applied linguistics of support for reading and (especially) writing skills for international students and professionals. In fact, most of what is known and taught is of value to doctors in their first language as well. A key text is the following.

    Swales JM, Feak CB: *Academic Writing for Graduate Students: Essential Tasks and Skills*, ed 2, Ann Arbor, MI, 2004, University of Michigan Press,

3. The concept of 'communicative competence' dates back to the following (quite technical) paper:

    Hymes D: On communicative competence. In Pride JB, Holmes J, editors: *Sociolinguistics: Selected Readings*, Harmondsworth, 1972, Penguin Books, pp. 269–293.

Reviews of the literature

Aspegren K: Teaching and learning communication skills in medicine: a review with quality grading of articles, *Medical Teacher* 21(6):563–570, 1999.

Fallowfield L, Jenkins V: Communicating sad, bad and difficult news in medicine, *Lancet* 363:312–319, 2004.

Lane C, Rollnick S: The use of simulated patients and role play in communication skills training: A review of the literature to August 2005, *Patient Education and Counseling* 67:13–20, 2007.

Ong LM, de Haes JC, Hoos AM, Lammes FB: Doctor-patient communication: a review of the literature, *Social Science and Medicine* 40:903–918, 1995.

Ethics and attitudes

A. V. Campbell, J. Chin, T. C. Voo

Introduction

 Current accepted standards of medical ethics education:

- Multidisciplinary and multiprofessional
- Academically rigorous and related to research
- Fully integrated horizontally and vertically
- Focused on clearly defined outcomes
- Sound teaching methods and valid assessment.

Medical ethics has seen a remarkable development in the last three decades everywhere in the world, mostly in the UK, Europe and the United States, but also more widely. There is international consensus that it should be an important part of any medical curriculum (WHO 1995, WMA 2005)

As the field 'comes of age' (Goldie et al 2000, Miles et al 1989), there is now wide acceptance, firstly, that medical ethics is no longer the concern of a single profession or academic discipline but has to be multidisciplinary and multiprofessional; secondly, that it should be academically rigorous and, like other academic subjects that are taught in the medical curriculum, related to current research and ongoing debates in its field; and thirdly, that ethics education must be fully integrated into the medical curriculum, both horizontally and vertically, so that there is seamlessness between what is being taught at any given time and pertinent ethical issues, along with continuous reinforcement for professional growth.

However, medical ethics education today faces pressing questions about the effectiveness of what is currently offered in medical schools. Although the vast majority of medical schools teach medical ethics to some extent, there is a broad range in terms of how it is taught, who teaches it and how frequently. These findings were reported by Mattick and Bligh (2006) in a survey of medical schools in the UK where, in spite of having a well-accepted core curriculum in medical ethics, there is wide diversity in teaching, assessment methods and staffing levels (GMC 1993, Consensus Statement 1998 [updated in Stirrat et al 2010]). There is no clear and consistent picture in the current literature of the efficacy of existing forms of ethics education (Campbell et al 2007). Systematic approaches to teaching and assessing legal literacy in relation to ethical thinking should also be developed for the formation of professional identities inclined and confident to engage with the law as a means to guide, protect and empower patients (Preston-Shoot & McKimm 2011, Preston-Shoot et al 2011).

This chapter illustrates the practical implementation of the current standards of medical ethics teaching, using the innovation of an integrated ethics curriculum as a case study. It also highlights the ethical values, skills and attitudes that the future practitioner must acquire through a discussion of the critical challenges facing the medical profession. To nurture the ethical doctor, ethics education must be based on clearly defined outcomes and matching assessment methods in the key areas of students' ethical development, viz. knowledge, habituation and action. The success of this endeavour lies in addressing some theoretical and practical issues with the assessment of ethics and professional attitudes.

Critical challenges

 Challenges for medical ethics education:
- Profound social change and the meaning of professionalism
- Global standards and cultural diversity
- Countering the hidden curriculum.

CHALLENGE 1: THE CHANGING DOCTOR–PATIENT RELATIONSHIP

In the last 20 years, international trends to privatize medicine have nurtured a 'healthcare industry' aimed primarily at profit. This has created role conflicts for medical practitioners, who are caught between their responsibilities to patients, on the one hand and, on the other, the notion of 'entrepreneurship' that encourages personal business success combined with loyalty to corporate employers (Breen 2001).

Thus, the search for new standards by the medical profession has to focus on those values that distinguish medicine from business, that define fiduciary responsibilities to the vulnerable sick and that bind doctors together as a committed body of persons with judgement and stewardship of knowledge and skill (Pellegrino 2002, Working Party of the Royal College of Physicians 2005). To meet this challenge, medical ethics education must put an emphasis on qualities that all patients look for in a practitioner: they seek a trustworthy advocate, committed first and foremost to patient welfare, empathetic, reflective and able to face up to the complexity of the rapidly changing world of medical practice. But today's doctors also have to be stewards of scarce resources. They have to seek just uses of finite healthcare budgets that provide the best available healthcare for patients, balancing fee-for-service care to meet growing (and at times unrealistic) consumer demands with publicly provided healthcare (Michels 1999); and to do this, they have to create effective relationships with corporate administrators that preserve rather than absolve or diminish professional responsibility (Breen 2001). This stewardship will also involve assessing the effectiveness of new healthcare delivery channels, including 'disruptive' technologies such as telemedicine and internet medicine.

The changing doctor–patient relationship

"Until recently, physicians generally considered themselves accountable only to themselves, to their colleagues in the medical profession and, for religious believers, to God. Nowadays they have additional accountabilities – to their patients, to third parties such as hospitals and managed healthcare organizations, to medical licensing and regulatory authorities, and often to courts of law."

WMA 2005

The growth of the pharmaceutical and biomedical research industries has exerted additional pressures on doctors' professionalism. As they are increasingly encouraged to participate in the recruitment of patients in clinical trials and to occupy the often uneasy role of 'clinician researchers', a whole new range of ethical skills must be learned: medically responsible participant enrolment in approved randomized controlled trials, checking evidence of a participant's suitability for enrolment against peer judgements, swift withdrawal or change of treatment when adverse events occur regardless of clinical equipoise protocols and research integrity, which includes intellectual honesty (accuracy, due credit, proper disclosure) and accountability (vigilant supervision of people and funds, and safety for whistle-blowers).

CHALLENGE 2: CULTURAL PLURALISM

Globalized societies must deal with bewildering questions about the translation of standards and ethical paradigms across diverse cultural contexts. No wholesale application of global standards is possible. The importance of culture has been illuminated by Canadian philosopher Charles Taylor. Taylor emphasized the truth that people are self-creating and culture-bearing individuals whose unique identities are formed through integration, reflection and modification of their heritage in response to, and in dialogue with, others (Taylor 1994).

Multiculturalism

"The process of bridging the cultural divide does not imply uncritical acceptance of all cultural norms as being intrinsically equal, as there may not always be room for compromise. It does imply, however, that discussion about values should be open and transparent and that questions of cultural conflict arising from the inevitable collision of different paradigms of health, illness, society, law and morality should be debated in a critical and reflective manner."

Irvine et al 2002

One implication of this for medical ethics is that patients will differ in their beliefs concerning matters such as the meaning of life, human suffering and illness, obligations to others in decision making or the extent of interventions upon nature. Today's doctors must be prepared to test their own ethical beliefs and cultural assumptions against other cultural frameworks. But how will 'ethical contours' be discerned in a world that is increasingly flattened by late capitalist imperatives of individualism, universalism, commodification and unrelenting conquest of, and dissociation from, the natural world? Some considerations that are emerging include greater attention to deep and long-standing cultural values that put limits upon medical intervention for ethically and ecologically important reasons; the relationships of family and community in the lives of individuals and their impact on decisions; the avoidance of cultural stereotypes and genuine embrace of an ethics of virtue that commands trust and values true autonomy or 'self-rule', as contrasted with a mere ethics of obligation that emphasizes only procedural requirements in dealing with disagreement or outright conflict of values (Irvine et al 2002).

Today's doctors and doctors-in-training are presented with opportunities for deep reflection about human values as advancement of medical science raises unprecedented and perplexing issues. Medicine can enrich the world if it will face these issues squarely. In a climate of global medical tourism and urgent need for transnational dialogue, it will be important for students to recognize and uphold medicine's social obligation to maintain equitable healthcare and professionally worthy conduct wherever they may practise as doctors. Good doctors are not just dutiful doctors. In an age that is unremittingly self-conscious about difference, identity and the burdens of choice, medical practitioners, and especially medical students who have the luxury of academic shelter, would do well to recognize, respect and use their own cultural heritage as starting points of reflection and learn to listen to, and integrate, different points of view.

CHALLENGE 3: THE POWER OF THE HIDDEN CURRICULUM

It has been clearly established that extracurricular factors can have harmful effects on the ethical development of medical students and junior doctors (Hafferty & Franks 1994). However, there continues to be a mismatch between the pedagogical efforts of medical schools and the challenge of reforming environments that impair ethical development (Hafferty 2000). It has been observed that while medical education professes explicit commitment to traditional values such as compassion, empathy and altruism, the reality is that its underbelly is a tacit, nonreflective acceptance of detachment and professional self-interest (Coulehan & Williams 2001). This easily leads to a narrowing of professional identity to that of the competent technician, devaluing relationship-centred approaches to medicine. Patients are seen as objects of technical services and medical students as apprentice technicians or trainee medical scientists. It is commonplace that medical graduates' spirits can be broken by the tough discipline of hospital managers and senior clinicians, and fair to say that the educational model of most hospital internship programmes may often be likened to a hierarchical 'militaristic' command structure (Leeder 2007). The 'soft' influence of pharmaceutical companies in undergraduate medical education is also an area of concern, particularly its effects on the practice of evidence-based medicine. Students' interaction with industry is found to be associated with positive attitudes towards industry marketing, including the reception of gifts, and scepticism about

possible negative influence on their prescribing patterns (Austad et al 2011).

 Hidden curriculum – teaching teachers

"Character formation cannot be evaded by medical educators. Students enter medical school with their characters partly formed. Yet, they are still malleable as they assume roles and models on the way to their formation as physicians."

Pellegrino 2002

How can this 'hidden curriculum' be countered? Part of the answer may lie in the teacher–student relationship which prefigures the student–patient relationship (Reiser 2000). As Reiser puts it, 'Students first learn about the use of authority in medicine from the faculty: how those with power and knowledge treat those who lack it.' But beyond this, as he points out, there is enormous educational potential for good or ill in the policies and pronouncements of the medical school, its traditions and ceremonies, and the atmosphere of scientific, technical and ethical commitment that its entire staff in unison with administrative personnel creates. Formal ethics training has its part to play in this cultural reformation through its encouragement of critical and independent thinking and its rejection of the false idea that seniority alone is a guarantee of ethical perceptiveness and considered judgment. That is why 'teaching the teachers' must be an integral part of medical ethics education.

 "As we expect greater professionalism from our students, we need to expect the same from teachers and organizational leaders. Anything else is disingenuous. For example, students have every right to expect that mistreatment by residents and faculty is taken just as seriously as unprofessional behaviour on the part of students."

Stern & Papadakis 2006

Undergraduate education

ORGANIZING UNDERGRADUATE ETHICS EDUCATION

The nuts and bolts of setting up an ethics curriculum are best explained with reference to a specific example, and we shall focus here on a new integrated medical curriculum that is currently being planned at the National University of Singapore's Yong Loo Lin School of Medicine. The revised structure of the curriculum is aimed at early patient contact; strengthening areas of growing importance such as ambulatory and community care experience, geriatrics and rehabilitative medicine; quantitative and evidence-based research skills and information literacy; healthcare financing and patient safety; horizontal and vertical integration of content with emphasis on the applications of biomedical sciences to clinical practice; developing professionalism; facilitating self-directed and lifelong learning habits; and broadening student choices for training in clinical specialties, research, scholarship or administration.

The medical school recently established a Centre for Biomedical Ethics (CBmE) whose main responsibility is to implement health ethics, law and professionalism components as a longitudinal track in the new medical curriculum. A core collaborative group of clinicians trained in medical ethics and law, and nonclinician specialists in philosophy, bioethics, law and pedagogy was set up to do the detailed planning.

ETHICS IN AN INTEGRATED MEDICAL CURRICULUM

The health ethics, law and professionalism (HeLP) track aims to develop ethical sensitivity, theoretical understanding, reflective and critical skills and professional attitudes in medical undergraduates. The principles that are applied to its design are that it has to be student- and patient-centred; research-based and fully integrated into the curriculum; case-related, multidisciplinary and interprofessional; fully assessed, formatively and summatively; and dialogue-enabling within the profession, between professions and with the general public.

In line with the educational aims of a global university, the selection of topics has been aligned to core medical ethics curricula around the world including those of the UK and Australasia (Consensus Statement by Teachers of Medical Education and Law in UK Medical Education 1998, Stirrat et al 2010, Australasian Core Curriculum 2001), but adapted to the medicolegal and cultural context of Singapore.

The HELP track follows the five phases of the revised curriculum (which remains under a process of review and improvement at time of writing):

- Normal structure and function (Phase I)
- Abnormal structure and function (Phase II)
- Core clinical practice (Phase III)
- Advanced and specialty clinical practice (Phase IV)
- Student internship programme (Phase V).

Phase I teaching begins with a 3-week introductory module on health and disease, which is taught alongside foundational aspects of medical ethics, medical law and professionalism. Ethical issues within topics such as blood and stem cell donations and health promotion will then be covered following lessons on body systems. Continuing from Phase I, Phase II of the HeLP track will complete students' basic knowledge of ethics, law and professionalism by integrating pertinent topics in ethics and law with the teaching of pathology and patterns of disease in the medical curriculum (Fig. 31.1).

In Phase III, the core clinical phase, students can embark on special study modules or research projects in bioethics supervised or assisted by the multidisciplinary staff of CBmE. All students are required to write a reflective report on the ethics, professional and communication aspects of a patient encounter as part of their learning portfolio. In the clinical practice stage of Phase IV and the student internship programme, lectures and workshops focused on the social aspects of medical practice such as the fostering of trust and cultural sensitivity will be conducted in relation to issues or practices such as iatrogenic injuries, resource allocation (including healthcare services and organs) and consumerism. 'Ethics OSCEs' may be introduced (i.e. the Objective Structured Clinical Examinations will include an ethics station in addition to the traditional medical OSCE stations).

Assessment of ethical and professional attitudes

FITTING OUTCOMES AND INNOVATIVE METHODS

A strategy of ethics education in a medical school should aim to create a valid programme for educating and certifying graduates who are knowledgeable, ethically sensitive and reflective and able to act with clinical ethical competence. These are key areas of a medical ethics education, the development of which can be illustrated with an ascending pyramid with specific learning outcomes and matching methods of assessment (adapted from Miller 1990; see Fig. 31.2).

ASSESSMENT: SOME DIFFICULTIES

Much current research is now focused on measuring medical professionalism and ethical attitudes, after a sustained period of scepticism about the possibility of making such assessments. But efforts in this field have led to better understanding of the limits of measurement (Parker 2006) and a growing realization of the conceptual and practical issues involved in assessment (Self et al 1992, 2003, Self & Olivarez 1996).

Firstly, an interesting study by Hodges identified four models of competence found in competency assessments around the world: competence as knowledge, competence as performance, competence as reliable test score and competence as reflection. It was discovered that overemphasis on an aspect of

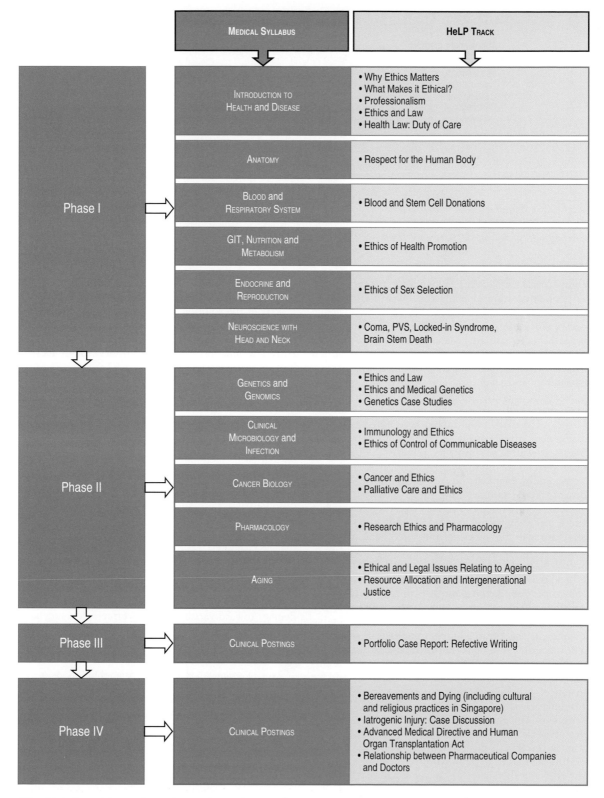

Fig. 31.1 Organizing undergraduate ethics education (schematic © Syahirah A Karim, 2011).

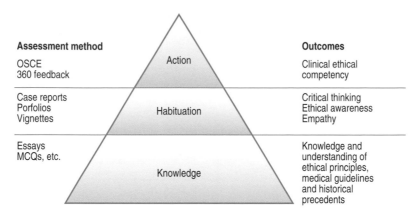

Fig. 31.2 Outcomes and assessment methods (adapted from Miller GE: The assessment of clinical skills/ competence/performance, *Academic Medicine* 65(9 Suppl):S63–67, 1990).

competency may lead to 'hidden incompetence', such as poor integration of knowledge with performance. For example, a student who had acquired knowledge competency but clearly displayed a kind of incompetence asked a patient, 'Madam, do you have higher conjugated or unconjugated bilirubin?' Other hidden incompetencies included a performance 'checklist' mentality and lack of appropriate interpersonal behaviour, merely producing portfolios without appropriate self-awareness and remedial self-learning. Critics of the reflection model have noted that self-assessment often correlates poorly with peer assessments, as well as performance (Hodges 2006, Kaslow et al 2007).

Secondly, there are also problems in assessment design. For example, the much beloved clinical vignette is often used to assess ethical sensitivity, but there are unanswered questions about how such an attribute can be properly measured, and whether ability to analyse cases correlates to it (Herbert et al 1992). Vignette tests are also frequently used to assess ethical reasoning, but no obvious connection has been shown between helping students to reason things out and defend their point of view, on the one hand, and on the other hand, acting in an ethically acceptable manner in the future. Indeed, increase in reasoning ability seems a minimal criterion for measuring success in ethics education: necessary, no doubt, but is it sufficient? Innovative ideas continue to be tested, for instance, Goldie's attempt to assess the effect of teaching in ethics using an instrument he calls 'consensus professional judgement'. This was a set of vignettes in which there was a consensus on the best way of resolving a given dilemma, both from the literature and from experts who were consulted about the issues in the vignette. They were administered to measure how far ethics teaching improved the student's ability to make judgements that were

consistent with what would be the judgement of the experts (Goldie et al 2000, 2001).

Part of the solution in addressing these difficulties is helping students to integrate knowledge, skills, dispositions, self-perceptions, motives and belief-attitudes and fostering the capacity for reflective lifelong learning (Kaslow et al 2007).

ASSESSMENT: SOME GUIDELINES

Integrating formative and summative assessments

Formative assessments should be ongoing, developmentally informed and focused on giving students feedback for achieving higher levels of competence. Summative or end-point assessments can be effective and optimally enhance competence, if well-aligned with formative training (Weber 2000). Curriculum managers should take account of the curriculum's effects on students' attitudes and progress and be prepared to intervene when deficiencies are identified. Where supervisors perform both formative and summative evaluations, they should be alerted to tendencies toward variability, 'halo' effects, leniency and supervisor defensiveness.

 Assessment guidelines:

- Formative assessments should be ongoing, should be developmentally informed and should give students feedback for achieving higher levels of competence.

- Summative assessments optimally enhance competence if well-aligned with formative training.

- Assessment of attitudes should cease to require demonstration of competence across a slew of summative hurdles, but should be assessed 'negatively' by a consensus on whether a student falls below an acceptable standard.

- Educators and assessors should receive training in interpretation and management of assessment results, correction of examiner biases and how to give specific and accurate feedback.

The special nature of attitudes

While the possibility of objective measurement of competence is highly defensible so that no excuse can be made for failure to implement such assessments (Cruess & Cruess 2006, Stern & Papadakis 2006), it is equally important to note the special nature of attitudes and their evaluation. Parker points out that we can reasonably assume that students have basic attitudinal competence upon entry to medical school, but a requirement of positive demonstration of such competence across a slew of 'summative hurdles' assumes precisely the opposite! Assessment of attitudes, he argues, is rather like evaluating a person's decisional capacity, where it is up to the doctor to rebut the presumption of decision-making competence. It is easier to come to a consensus that a person lacks (falls below a certain threshold of) a capacity than to agree that he or she has it, and at what precise level. In practice, this type of assessment can be done by setting clear expectations of behaviour, training teachers to deal with issues of misconduct and providing a remedial mentoring programme (Whiting 2007, Field 2008). Repeated misdemeanours such as absenteeism, dishonesty, unreliability, disrespect or recalcitrance should then trigger a need to decide whether a student fails the ethics and professionalism course. Consensus is usually not difficult at this point, as Parker observes (Parker 2006).

Training educators and assessors

Educators and assessors should be trained in the areas of inter-rater objectivity and awareness of common and personal biases, giving direct, specific and accurate feedback to students regarding their strengths and deficits and means of improving in a collegial setting. Training should also be provided in the interpretation and management of assessment results. Finally, guidelines for writing competency-based letters of recommendation and appropriate forms should be made available for use in selection of postings and the internship year (Kaslow et al 2007).

Consistent expectations

The medical school's programme of certifying students professionally competent should be consistent with expectations of professionalism later in their careers. Standards should therefore be congruent with those of licensing boards, but levels of competency must be adjusted suitably in line with student experience.

Summary: Effecting culture shift

Medical ethics education is in a progressive, exciting phase, and ideas about implementation are burgeoning. The best approach to teaching and assessing ethics and professionalism, however, remains an unresolved debate. Despite this, there is wide acceptance that ethics education should be fully integrated both horizontally and vertically with the clinical curriculum so that students can experience and appreciate the centrality of ethics to clinical practice. With profound changes to healthcare landscapes worldwide, ethics education must seek to foster contemporary professional qualities in doctors in training while inculcating in them the time-honoured virtues of trustworthiness, empathy and commitment to patient welfare; expose them to the vibrant pluralism of viewpoints on the human body, relationships, life and death; and actively counter any negative influence of the hidden curriculum. While the methods remain contentious, assessment is recognized as necessary to foster learning, enable curricular evaluation and change and facilitate accountability for the profession and the public (Kaslow et al 2007). For proper assessment to take place, outcomes in key ethics competencies must be specified and pursued with matching, rigorous instruments. Success in medical ethics education is measured in terms of producing reflective, responsive and self-regulating doctors. To this end, a culture shift towards concerted teaching and assessment of professional attitudes and ethical behaviour must be affected.

References

Austad KE, Avorn J, Kesselheim AS: Medical students' exposure to and attitudes about the pharmaceutical industry: A systematic review, *PLos Medicine* 8(5):e1001037, 2011.

Australasian Core Curriculum: An ethics core curriculum for Australasian medical schools. A Working Group, on behalf of the Association of Teachers of Ethics and Law in Australian and New Zealand Medical Schools (ATEAM), *Medical Journal of Australia* 175:205–210, 2001.

Breen KJ: The patient–doctor relationship in the new millennium: Adjusting positively to commercialism and consumerism, *Clinics in Dermatology* 19:19–22, 2001.

Campbell AV, Chin J, Voo TC: How can we know that ethics education produces ethical doctors? *Medical Teacher* 29(5):431–436, 2007.

Consensus Statement by Teachers of Medical Ethics and Law in UK Medical Education: Teaching medical ethics and law within medical schools: a model for the UK core curriculum, *Journal of Medical Ethics* 24:188–192, 1998.

Coulehan J, Williams PC: Vanquishing virtue: The impact of medical education, *Academic Medicine* 76(6):598–605, 2001.

Cruess RL, Cruess SR: Teaching professionalism: general principles, *Medical Teacher* 28(3):205–208, 2006.

Field L: Deciding when students are not fit to practice, *Student BMJ* 16:64–65, 2008.

General Medical Council: *Tomorrow's doctors: recommendations on undergraduate medical education*, London, 1993, GMC.

Goldie J, Schwartz L, Morrison J: A process evaluation of medical ethics education in the first year of a new curriculum, *Medical Education* 34:468–473, 2000.

Goldie J, Schwartz L, McConnachie A, Morrison J: Impact of a new course on students' potential behaviour on encountering ethical dilemmas, *Medical Education* 36:489–497, 2001.

Hafferty FW, Franks R: The hidden curriculum, ethics teaching, and the structure of medical education, *Academic Medicine* 69:861–871, 1994.

Hafferty FW: In search of a lost cord. In Wear D, Bickel J, editors: *Educating for Professionalism: Creating a Culture of Humanism in Medical Education*, Iowa, 2000, University of Iowa Press, pp 11–34.

Herbert PC, Meslin EM, Dunn EV: Measuring the ethical sensitivity of medical students: A study at the University of Toronto, *Journal of Medical Ethics* 18:142–147, 1992.

Hodges B: Medical education and the maintenance of incompetence, *Medical Teacher* 28 (8):690–696, 2006.

Irvine R, McPhee J, Kerridge IH: The challenge of cultural and ethical pluralism to medical practice, *MJA* 176:175–176, 2002.

Kaslow NJ, Rubin NJ, Bebeau MJ, et al: Guiding principles and recommendations for the assessment of competence, *Professional Psychology: Research and Practice* 38(5):441–451, 2007.

Leeder SR: Preparing interns for practice in the 21st century, *Medical Journal of Australia* 186(7) Supplement: S7–S8, 2007.

Mattick K, Bligh J: Teaching and assessing medical ethics: Where are we now? *Journal of Medical Ethics* 32:181–185, 2006.

Michels R: Medical education and managed care, *New England Journal of Medicine* 340:959–961, 1999.

Miles SH, Lane LW, Bickel J, et al: Medical ethics education: Coming of age, *Academic Medicine* 64:705–714, 1989.

Miller GE: The assessment of clinical skills/ competence/performance, *Academic Medicine* 65(9 Suppl):S63–S67, 1990.

Parker M: Assessing professionalism: theory and practice, *Medical Teacher* 28(5):399–403, 2006.

Pellegrino ED: Professionalism, profession and the virtues of the good physician, *Mount Sinai Journal of Medicine* 69:378–384, 2002.

Preston-Shoot M, McKimm J: Towards effective outcomes in teaching, learning and assessment of law in medical education, *Medical Education* 45(4):339–346, 2011.

Preston-Shoot M, McKimm J, Kong WM, Smith S: Readiness for legally literate medical practice? Student perceptions of their undergraduate medico-legal education, *Journal of Medical Ethics* doi:10.1136/jme.2010.041566, 2011.

Reiser SJ. In Wear D, Bickel J, editors: *Educating for Professionalism: Creating a Culture of Humanism in Medical Education*. Iowa, 2000, University of Iowa Press.

Self DJ, Baldwin DC Jr, Wolinsky FD: Evaluation of teaching medical ethics by an assessment of moral reasoning, *Medical Education* 26:178–184, 1992.

Self DJ, Jecker NS, Baldwin DC: The moral orientations of justice and care among young physicians, *Cambridge Quarterly of Healthcare Ethics* 12:S54–S60, 2003.

Self DJ, Olivarez M: Retention of moral reasoning skills over the four years of medical education, *Teaching and Learning in Medicine* 8(4):195–199, 1996.

Stern DT, Papadakis M: The developing physician health ethics, law and professionalism becoming a professional, *New England Journal of Medicine* 355:1794–1799, 2006.

Stirrat GM, et al: Medical ethics and law for doctors of tomorrow: The 1998 Consensus Statement updated, *Journal of Medical Ethics* 36(1):55–60, 2010.

Taylor C: The politics of recognition. In Gutmann A, editor: *Multiculturalism*, 25–73, Princeton, 1994, Princeton University Press, pp 25–73.

Weber ML: Evaluation and learning: An impossible task? *Royal College of Physicians and Surgeons of Canada* 33:339–344, 2000.

Whiting D: Inappropriate attitudes, fitness to practise and the challenges facing medical educators, *Journal of Medical Ethics* 33:667–670, 2007.

WHO. *The Teaching of Medical Ethics: Fourth Consultation with Leading Medical Practitioners*, Geneva, 1995, World Health Organization.

World Medical Association: Medical Ethics Manual. Ferney, Voltaire, France/Online. Available at: http://www.wma.net, 2005.

Working Party of the Royal College of Physicians: *Doctors in Society: Medical Professionalism in a Changing World*, London, 2005.

Further reading

Beauchamp T, Childress JF: *Principles of Biomedical Ethics*, ed 5, New York, 2001, Oxford University Press.

British Medical Association: *Medical Ethics Today*, ed 2, London, 2005, BMJ Publishing Group.

Campbell AV, Gillet G, Jones G: *Medical Ethics*, ed 4, Oxford, 2005, Oxford University Press.

Hope T, Savulescu J, Hendrick J: *Medical Ethics and Law: The Core Curriculum*, ed 2, Edinburgh, 2008, Churchill Livingstone.

Mason K, Laurie GT: *Mason and McCall Smith's Law and Medical Ethics*, ed 7, Oxford, 2006, Oxford University Press.

Stern DT: *Measuring Medical Professionalism*, New York, 2005, Oxford University Press.

Wear D, Bickel J: *Educating for Professionalism: Creating a Culture of Humanism in Medical Education*, Iowa, 2000, University of Iowa Press.

Chapter

32

Professionalism

P. M. Gliatto, D. T. Stern

Introduction

Consider the following scenarios:

- A professor strongly urges his preclinical students to attend a session on the doctor–patient relationship because one of his patients is going to participate. 'You will learn more from her story than from any textbook,' he states. The session is one day before a pharmacology examination, and he is disappointed when only a third of the class attends.

- A resident physician feels uncomfortable when she laughs at a joke her senior colleague makes regarding the appearance of one of the patients.

- An attending physician sees a student speak rudely to a nurse because she had failed to draw a set of blood cultures prior to the patient's first dose of antibiotics. The student snaps, 'Now we'll never know what this poor patient has, and it's because of your incompetence!' The physician wonders how to handle the student's outburst.

- A junior faculty member is embarrassed when he learns that a friend posted photos of him on a social networking page. In the photo he is clearly inebriated and the picture is labelled 'Dr Phillips – at it again!'

All of these scenarios represent issues of medical professionalism. While professionalism has become a buzzword in the medical education literature, training in professionalism still largely occurs through subtle mechanisms like role modelling and socialization and is influenced profoundly by institutional, cultural and socioeconomic forces. The goals of this chapter are to provide a working definition of professionalism and examples of how to teach and evaluate it. How to remediate unprofessional behaviours is an evolving area that is beyond the scope of this chapter.

Helping future and current doctors to meet professional standards should be one of the central missions of any medical education endeavour. Concerns about physicians' conflicts of interest (Campbell et al 2007) and evidence that certain behaviours in training are correlated with future loss of licensure for issues of professionalism (Papadakis et al 2005) demonstrate the need to teach and evaluate professionalism formally. Moreover, disruptive behaviours by physicians may be linked to poor team performance, patient dissatisfaction, increased litigation and medical errors (Joint Commission 2008). Medical schools, graduate medical education programmes and professional organizations have advocated formalizing the education and evaluation of professionalism (General Medical Council 2006, Accreditation Council for Graduate Medical Education 2008).

Defining professionalism

Educators and regulatory bodies have attempted to define professionalism to facilitate discussion and scholarship, as well as for teaching and evaluating trainees and physicians. From the day that a student enters medical school, he or she begins the process of becoming a professional. Being a professional means many things, including internalizing and adhering to a set of values, behaving according to standards that define acceptable medical practice and being ultimately accountable to the patients he or she serves. These attributes of the 'professional' create an identity distinct from personal identity (Mostaghimi & Crotty 2011). With this identity is a set of expectations for behaviours and appearance, as well as entitlements. A recent review formulated three ways of thinking about professionalism: as an individual trait, as the result of an interpersonal process and as a social phenomenon. Each of these approaches has advantages and drawbacks and can inform how professionalism is taught and assessed (Hodges et al 2011).

 "The central act of profession . . . is an active, conscious declaration, voluntarily entered into and signifying willingness to assume the obligations necessary to make the declaration authentic."

Pellegrino 2001

Edmund Pellegrino (2001) defines the medical professional as one who:

> *'declares aloud' that he (or she) has special knowledge and skills, that he (or she) can heal, or help, and that he (or she) will do so in the patient's interests, not his (or her) own.*

Herbert Swick has noted that these two dimensions of professionalism, expertise and a commitment to apply that expertise for the good of others, may be out of balance in today's environment, with serious consequences to the legitimacy of the profession in the eyes of the public. The rapid advances in medical knowledge and technology have caused the medical profession to become 'more closely linked to the application of expert knowledge and less closely linked to the functions central to the good of the public they serve' (Swick 2000). He argues that without its public and social purpose, medicine as a profession risks losing its 'distinctive voice' that inspires society to trust in the profession and allow it considerable latitude to regulate itself. Swick states that to try and restore the balance, one must begin by defining professionalism by what physicians actually do: 'how they meet their responsibilities to individual patients and communities.'

Behaviours that are common to several proposed definitions and discussions of professionalism (ABIM Foundation 2013, Epstein 1999, Stern 2006, Swick 2000) include the following:

- Fiduciary obligation: in offering their skills and expertise, physicians are expected to subordinate their own interests to the interests of their patients.
- Responsiveness to societal needs: physicians are expected to understand and address society's pressing health needs, including access to care.
- Empathy: physicians are expected to demonstrate that they understand their patients as persons who are often in a state of vulnerability.
- Respect for others: physicians are expected to demonstrate a deep respect for a patient's culture, autonomy and confidentiality. Physicians should also respect the contributions of other professionals in the care of patients.
- Accountability: physicians are expected to adhere to standards of practice and commit to measures that ensure that all members of the profession meet these standards. As a corollary, the profession has an obligation to regulate itself in terms of setting up standards for licensure and certification.
- Commitment to quality and excellence: physicians are expected to maintain their knowledge and skills and analyse their practices to be able to deliver state-of-the-art care.

- Ability to deal with ambiguity and complexity: physicians are expected to be able to engage in medically and morally complex situations and be willing to make judgements even in the face of limited data.
- Reflection: physicians must be open to critically examining their own practices, skills, and limits.

 Delineating the behaviours and contexts that define professionalism can facilitate a staged, level-appropriate curriculum.

The above elements are often combined and re-sorted under a variety of different headings. For example, humanism, which can encompass altruism, empathy, respect for others and reflection, has been identified by some as a core element of professionalism (Stern 2006). Additionally, ethical and legal principles can inform professionalism, and communication skills can be a manifestation of it (Stern 2006).

Professionalism: How to teach it

Professionalism is multifaceted and dependent on context. How one might respond to a nurse's phone call for a minor concern when well-rested on a small inpatient service, might differ strikingly from how one might respond when covering a large complex service in the middle of the night. So teaching professionalism cannot be easily compared to teaching the knowledge of medicine: it is not as simple as identifying the principles of antibiotic treatment and expecting students to apply them rationally. In addition, the professional issues to be taught change depending on the level of the trainee: from cheating on tests by a medical student, to copying notes in an electronic chart by a physician in postgraduate training, to misrepresenting patient findings in order to justify procedures limited by insurance by a practising physician. As such, while the principles of professionalism should be clearly articulated at a programmatic or institutional level, the 'teaching' of professionalism occurs best in real-life contexts or high-fidelity simulations. Some suggestions for teaching professionalism are detailed in the following paragraphs.

COURSES

Most medical schools offer courses on doctoring or clinical skills that cover ethics, the rules that govern doctor–patient relationships and moral reasoning (Self et al 1992, Stern & Papadakis 2006) (see Chapter 31, Ethics and attitudes). There are underlying principles, historical precedents and decision-making models that can be learned, even in the most noninteractive style of formal lectures. Some courses use team-based learning techniques that require students to be collaborative and accountable to fellow students in order to foster the professional attitudes and behaviours requisite for the multidisciplinary care of complex patients (Stern & Papadakis 2006). Whether the principles learned in this way lead to changes in practice settings has yet to be shown.

Some educators have used literature, art and film to teach elements of professionalism. The development of empathy and respect requires an ability to imagine the viewpoints of others. Reading patient narratives or watching films depicting patient–doctor interactions, combined with guided reflection, is intended to lead to a better understanding of the patients' perspective and, in turn, greater empathy (Charon 2001). Hafferty (2000) has called for even more explicit coursework in professionalism that draws on sociology, history, economics and cultural studies.

ROLE MODELLING AND MENTORING

Role modelling and mentoring are powerful forces in the development of trainees' professional identities. Mentoring is a more formal relationship in which a senior and established member of a community takes a special interest in the personal and professional growth of a specific trainee (Grady-Weliky et al 2000) (see Chapter 17, Mentoring). Role modelling happens in more day-to-day situations and does not necessarily have the length or intensity of a mentoring relationship. Trainees model their behaviours and actions on those who they see around them through a process of emulation or socialization (Hafferty 2000). Role models can be positive or negative. Negative role models serve a purpose to inspire students to 'never act like Dr X when I graduate' (Branch et al 1993). Role modelling may be enhanced with explanation or by making actions explicit. A faculty member can behave in a fashion he or she expects to be modelled, but the modelling may go unnoticed or misinterpreted. For example, a physician may model a behaviour, like washing hands, to teach the importance of preventing nosocomial infection and demonstrating respect to the patient, yet a student may interpret the behaviour as the physician's concern about contracting disease. Therefore, learning through role modelling is haphazard and the lessons learned may not be those the teacher intends. Following the lead of other professions, the principle of reflective practice (Schön 1983) encourages the demonstration of a behaviour, then the explicit discussion of the behaviour as a more certain method for transmitting professional behaviours. This pattern of 'explicated' role modelling has potential for increasing the positive impact of the best teachers (Stern & Papadakis 2006).

REFLECTION

 "In a world where the past often comes to reach back no further than the last exam, one should not be surprised to find medical trainees residing (often unwittingly) in an ever expanding (and nonreflective) here and now."

Hafferty, in Wear & Bickel 2000

 Any effort to foster professionalism in trainees must take into account the effects of the hidden and informal curricula.

Trainees should have a chance to reflect upon their experiences and their growing skills in order to develop a sense of perspective and solidify experiences into more durable learning. Reflection provides opportunities for trainees to generate insight into how they perceive themselves and their roles. It also allows for them to explore the rationale behind their behaviours and attitudes (Ginsburg & Lingard 2006). Such mental processes are essential in the acts of complex decision making that physicians engage in every day. In what he terms 'mindful practice', which characterizes a reflective practitioner, Epstein (1999) writes that the goals are

… to become more aware of one's own mental processes, listen more attentively, become more flexible, and recognise bias and judgments, and thereby act with principles and compassion.

Because trainees may have limited practise in self-assessment, it is best if reflection is structured and involves assistance of faculty. Faculty must keep in mind when facilitating reflection that reasoning and many components of professionalism are developmental processes, and therefore teaching exercises should be designed that are level-appropriate (Ginsburg & Lingard 2006).

Reflection can take the form of small-group discussions, essays, journals or portfolios (see below). Trainees can draw upon their own experiences or can reflect on different scenarios provided to them, like examples from art or literature, as mentioned previously.

SERVICE LEARNING

Medicine at its core is a service endeavour (Pellegrino 2001). The physician has a fiduciary commitment to the patient and a duty to try to heal disease, palliate symptoms and/or preserve function. Junior trainees may or may not get to participate in this singular activity of medicine, as key decisions about patient care may be made outside of their circle of influence. There are concerns that the way medicine is currently modelled is too focused on the technical aspects of biomedical knowledge and procedural skills and therefore may not promote a sense of duty in trainees. Emphasis on efficiency and expediency may devalue compassion (Eckenfels 2000). It is important that trainees have opportunities to recharge their idealism and get a sense of the deep commitment to patient welfare that drew them into medicine in the first place. Service endeavours, especially those that are spearheaded by trainees, can help fill this large gap in professional education. Likewise, global health initiatives can be highly instructive and enriching experiences that emphasize accountability, dealing with uncertainty and altruism and acknowledging and addressing the healthcare needs of a community or population (Stern & Papadakis 2006). These topics may be difficult to truly teach in a formal curriculum but are essential in helping a trainee develop as a professional (Eckenfels 2000). Controversy exists over whether explicit service should be mandated of trainees (Eckenfels 2000).

Professionalism: How to evaluate it

"Our failure to measure professionalism sends a conflicting message to both students and practicing physicians. While we profess and encourage professionalism, we do little to ensure its presence."

Stern 2006

Regulatory and educational bodies internationally and across the continuum of medical education have called for increased attention to the measurement of medical professionalism. Evaluating professionalism can be done formatively or summatively, be targeted at educational ends or accreditation, be used to measure the effects of educational programmes, or be used to reward individuals or promote practises in an institution (Stern 2006). Like the teaching of professionalism, its evaluation is best done in a longitudinal fashion, by different methods, and across different contexts, since professionalism is context-specific (Hafferty 2006) and its manifestations are in actions and behaviours as well as attitudes and motivations. Because of its complexity, professionalism cannot be accurately assessed in a single action at a single point in time.

Choosing appropriate evaluation methods is essential to reinforcing educational goals and trainee expectations regarding professionalism. Deciding on the stakes of the evaluation process is also important, as a system that does not adequately reward trainees or physicians for exemplary professionalism or have consequences for those who fail to meet expectations will be unlikely to promote professionalism in individuals, teams or institutions. Conversely, using exclusively high-stakes methods may stifle the input of evaluators and thereby render the evaluation less useful as an educational method to foster professionalism (Norcini 2006).

Means of assessing professionalism, and methods of determining outcomes of an individual's professionalism, are still largely in development. This section details some established ways of evaluating the professionalism of trainees. Some of these methods may also apply to the evaluation of practising physicians.

EVALUATIONS BY SUPERVISING FACULTY

Faculty is able to observe interactions of trainees with patients, peers and staff. Evaluations based on these observations have the advantages that they are easy to collect, can be made transparent to the evaluator and trainee and reflect the context of real scenarios (Norcini 2006). Disadvantages include the fact that evaluators differ in their opinions on what constitutes acceptable performance and therefore several evaluations are required to achieve reliability, especially in regards to the observable behaviours that pertain to professionalism. The evaluator may have many other competing responsibilities (like patient care or documentation requirements) that leave only limited, fragmented and unstructured time to observe, assess and provide feedback to trainees.

The context of the evaluation is also important, because an observed behaviour in one particular context may not be generalizable to other contexts. Lastly, as mentioned above, the stakes of the evaluation can influence the comfort of the evaluator and the accuracy and quality of the evaluations. For example, a faculty member might feel easier offering formative feedback on directly observed behaviours or skills rather than making summative evaluations that are more judgmental in nature, like those that may be used for grading or promotion (Norcini 2006).

INCIDENT REPORTS

Incident reports, in which faculty document notable professional or unprofessional incidents ('sentinel events') that they observe in trainees, have the advantage of occurring over longer periods of time and across more contexts than in a single course, clerkship or rotation. While each incident may only represent a 'snapshot' of performance, several reports, over time and in aggregate, may detect trainee traits, attitudes and/or behaviours that are sustained and generalizable. Alternatively, a single event that may be concerning in isolation may not in fact define a trainee as unprofessional if the remainder of the record is not consistent with that conclusion. Having more than one documented event for a trainee should trigger a careful review of the trainee's performance. Such incident report programmes need to be developed, implemented and monitored at an institutional level (Papadakis & Loeser 2006).

PEER ASSESSMENT AND 360° EVALUATIONS

Peer evaluations offer special insights into a trainee or practitioner that can be used to assess elements of professionalism. Peers, since they are at the same level of training or experience, and because they may have longer and more intimate exposure to each other, may offer unique perspectives on humanistic attributes and collaborative behaviours. Because such interactions tend to be less formal, they may represent authentic traits and practices that are less prone to gaming. Peer evaluations can take the form of rating forms, nominations, rankings or qualitative assessments, and can be required or voluntary and anonymous or signed. These ratings require the honest participation of peers, so developing evaluations with the peers themselves is highly recommended. Because of the implications of 'whistle-blowing', the most acceptable form of peer assessment is anonymous and formative. Non-anonymous and summative evaluations may result in a lack of reliable reporting. Formative peer assessment (particularly for rewards) is highly recommended as an effective and important component of any system of assessing professionalism (Arnold & Stern 2006).

In addition to the above assessments from faculty and peers, 360° evaluations also add assessments from patients, nursing and ancillary staff. These perspectives can augment the evaluation process and offer unique perspectives on qualities like compassion, respect for others, cultural awareness and ability to work as part of a multidisciplinary team.

PORTFOLIOS

Assessments of observed behaviours tend to best isolate individuals at the extremes of performance but may not promote reflection. Trainees may quickly learn how to modulate their behaviours to meet the expectations of the observer, and evaluations may serve more to promote adaptive behaviours than motivate a self-regulatory, thoughtful, respectful and altruistic practitioner (Hafferty 2006).

Portfolios have been used to document outcomes across a variety of educational objectives. They may be used as teaching tools and evaluation methods, based on how they are constructed and scrutinized, and lend themselves well to the multifaceted and experiential nature of clinical education, including professional development. The portfolio operationalizes the theory that reflection on experience can result in deeper, more permanent learning. Reflecting on

experience, and documenting the reflection, may be a particularly useful way to promote the kind of 'mindful practice' detailed earlier.

 Reflection is an essential component in teaching and evaluating professionalism.

Essential to the effectiveness of portfolios in learning is access to experienced faculty members who can serve as mentors and reviewers of portfolio content (Fryer-Edwards et al 2006). Please see Chapter 39 on portfolios and their use in medical education for more details on how these can be constructed and assessed.

SIMULATION

Simulated scenarios using standardized patients, role play or other modalities can evaluate certain elements of professionalism or related skills like communication, response to stress and ability to work as part of a team.

Promoting a culture of professionalism

 "Students need to see that professionalism is articulated throughout the system in which they work and learn. In our academic medical centers, this means providing an environment that is consistently and clearly professional not only in medical school but throughout the entire system of care."

Stern & Papadakis 2006

Any efforts to teach and evaluate professionalism will have little efficacy if they occur within an institutional culture that does not reinforce the fundamental messages of the educational endeavour. The contextual and experiential nature of medical education can very easily undermine any curricular goals aimed at teaching professionalism. Some aspects of the culture or setting may be difficult or impossible to change. The 'informal' or 'hidden' curriculum, which is partly determined by the institutional culture, strongly influences the learning environment. Educational efforts that take these contextual factors into account will be more effective. What factors align with educational goals? What factors will potentially undermine them? For the latter, are there ways to modify these factors, and if not, are there ways to highlight them so that the individual learner can be conscious of them? Getting the input of trainees will provide a grounds-eye view that is essential to understanding these influences.

Potential threats to the teaching and learning of professionalism that can occur at an institutional level may include the following:

- lack of a shared standards of professionalism among teachers and trainees
- lack of, or notable differences in, consequences for trainees and faculty who engage in unprofessional behaviours
- lack of meaningful recognition for those whose professionalism may be exemplary
- the fast pace and intensive nature of clinical medicine that encourages reflexive as opposed to reflective thought and action
- the brief, episodic nature of interactions between faculty and trainees, such that faculty lacks opportunities to sufficiently observe trainees, and conversely, to model professional behaviours
- processes for selecting candidates for medical school and higher medical training, as well as for promoting faculty, that may not include explicit considerations of professionalism, or the potential for it (Wagoner 2006)
- the pervasiveness of conflicts of interest in academic medical centres and community practices (Campbell et al 2007).

There are a number of ways to begin to address these issues. First, institutional or programmatic recognition of the importance of professionalism is essential. Awards that recognize students and faculty for exemplary professionalism or humanism exist at many schools. Making such recognition count in more concrete ways, as in criteria for promotion for faculty appointments, may make it even more meaningful. Likewise, unprofessional conduct by faculty and trainees should have consequences that are applied to both groups.

Opportunities for reflection must be built into the curriculum so trainees can convert their experiences into more durable learning. Reflection is one way the informal and hidden curricula can be used for explicit teaching rather than tacit socialization.

Many institutions have policies about conflicts of interests that faculty must understand and adhere to. Trainees should also understand potential conflicts of interests, and how to identify, acknowledge and address them.

Fundamental to the development of professionalism is learning in environments that promote it. Healthcare systems may find the most powerful method for instilling professionalism is to operationalize and implement innovations at the institutional level that promote empathy, respect and accountability.

Return to the scenarios

Please refer to the scenarios that started the chapter. A discussion of these scenarios will be used to demonstrate some practical aspects to teaching and evaluating professionalism.

In the first scenario the professor aimed to expose his students to a patient's perspective on illness, a thoughtful strategy to encourage empathy. However, his timing is off and he may be trying to teach something that is not yet meaningful to such students early in their training. Likely they are principally concerned about the immediate consequences of not performing well on the pharmacology exam. This scenario demonstrates that teaching professionalism must be relevant to the learner's needs. Perhaps a student in his or her first year is not yet ready to learn the value of empathy in a clinical context because his or her direct contact with patients is limited, and therefore learning about empathy at this stage is not something that will have enduring benefit. This does not mean that professionalism cannot be taught to junior students, or that students do not have obligations that one could consider professional in nature. However, the learning should be meaningful and level-appropriate. One option for junior students would be to focus more on professional attributes like accountability or respect for others. For example, some basic science courses now require faculty to evaluate students on things like ability to work with others and self-directed learning, skills and attitudes that fit nicely with other educational designs like small group learning. Such evaluations may contribute to grades, which reinforce their importance. Also, the evaluation of preclinical professional behaviours may have predictive validity. Student behaviours such as being accountable for routine administrative matters like completing course evaluations or health requirements correlate with faculty evaluations of professionalism in clinical situations (Stern et al 2005).

In the second scenario the resident physician feels uncomfortable for laughing at the joke her senior colleague made about a patient. If given the opportunity to reflect upon this experience, the physician may actually learn something, rather than just feeling bad about her actions or, worse, rationalizing her feelings away. A forum free of punitive consequences, like an essay assignment or a discussion group with peers, would be an excellent way for the physician to think about the consequences of the behaviour for herself (is it a mark of eroding values?), her juniors (if students see her laughing, will they think it is okay?) and her patients (would the patient trust her if he overheard?). She could also explore her feelings and values. Was this a symptom of burnout, or just a needed release? Lastly, the incident could prompt her to think about professional norms and their importance. Is laughing about a patient ever acceptable? Is there humour even beneath the surface of the pain and suffering of illness? Reflective learning requires that programmes and institutions provide a time and space for reflection and encourage trainees to recognize 'sentinel events' within their own professional development. The power, and the liability, of experiential learning is its episodic nature. Without some effort to 'capture' these events and allow learners to process them into something more durable, the teaching power of the experiences will be lost. Faculty need to help trainees to recognize these teaching moments.

In the third example the faculty member may be inclined to avoid giving the student feedback about how he spoke to the nurse. The physician may fear the consequences of such feedback, upon himself (will the student view him as an adversary?), or for the student (could the feedback teach him not to advocate for his patients?). The physician may need to consider submitting an incident report, since he is unsure whether this is a lapse for a student who usually behaves professionally, or whether the incident is a marker of a deeper character flaw. Regardless, giving the student feedback is important for two reasons. First, it may encourage reflection in the student. A simple labelling of the incident as 'professional' or 'unprofessional' will be unlikely to lead to durable learning. The faculty member can maximize the teaching if he approaches it in a nonpunitive way and encourages the student to perform a kind of 'root cause analysis' for his behaviour, as well as to consider the potential consequences of the behaviour. Second, monitoring the student's response to feedback may be very instructive about the student. If he reacts defensively, it may signal that the student may require more intense scrutiny or remediation. Poor capacity for self-improvement (Papadakis et al 2005) has been linked to future loss of licensure.

The final example demonstrates what can happen when professional and personal identities become blurred. This is a real liability in the era of various online activities and social networking. While social media can be a useful tool to communicate with colleagues, and in some cases, patients, trainees and faculty must be very conscious of how they use such media (Mostaghimi & Crotty 2011). There are obvious pitfalls in regard to patient confidentiality, personal information and how posted material may be interpreted, altered or disseminated. Misuse of these technologies can damage reputations, undermine relationships and breach trust. While there are times that such misuse is out of the individual's control (as in this case), trainees and faculty must be conscious about their professional and personal online activities and make every effort to separate them. Additionally, trainees and faculty should adhere to any policies on the use of social media that their institutions have created. In this case, the physician should request that his friend remove the photograph.

Summary

The pedagogy of professionalism has become more formalized at all levels of the medical education continuum. Concerns about eroding values of practitioners and trainees, expressions of public dissatisfaction with medical care, and threats to the profession's primacy and autonomy have all contributed to the renewed attention to professionalism. Professionalism is transforming from 'something that has (too long) been considered a natural by-product' (Hafferty 2006) to an essential facet of medical training that requires careful planning and implementation. Such efforts are challenging because they require not only innovative curricula and measurement tools but also attention to educational institutions and their cultures. Much progress has been made in delineating the dimensions of professionalism that are essential to medical practice and developing valid and feasible evaluations of professionalism, like faculty and peer assessments. While education naturally focuses on observable, measurable behaviours and outcomes, developing a professional identity is a complex matter that involves attitudes, feelings and beliefs. While reflection can start to make some of these processes more explicit and perhaps more teachable, a major challenge to educators is how to ensure that trainees internalize these lessons, so that their claims to expertise and service are authentic ones (Hafferty 2006).

References

ABIM Foundation: Advancing Medical Professionalism to Improve Health Care, 2013. Available at: http://www.abimfoundation.org/Professionalism/Physician-Charter/Commitments-of-the-Charter.aspx.

Arnold L, Stern DT: Content and context of peer assessment. In Stern DT, editor: *Measuring Medical Professionalism*, New York, 2006, Oxford University Press, pp 175–194.

Accreditation Council for Graduate Medical Education: Program Director Guide to the Common Program Requirements, 2008. Available at: http://www.acgme.org/acgmeweb/Portals/0/PDFs/commonguide/IVA5_EducationalProgram_ACGMECompetencies_Introduction_Explanation.pdf.

Branch W, Pels RJ, Lawrence RS, Arky R: Becoming a doctor: critical-incident reports from third-year medical students, *New England Journal of Medicine* 329:1130–1132, 1993.

Campbell EG, Gruen RL, Mountford MD, et al: A national survey of physician-industry relationships, *New England Journal of Medicine* 356:1742–1750, 2007.

Charon R: Narrative medicine: a model for empathy, reflection, profession, and trust, *Journal of the American Medical Association* 286:1897–1902, 2001.

Eckenfels EJ: The case for keeping community service voluntary: narrative from the Rush Community Service Initiatives Program. In Wear D, Bickel J, editors: *Educating for Professionalism: Creating a Culture of Humanism in Medical Education*, Iowa City, 2000, University of Iowa Press, pp 165–173.

Epstein RM: Mindful practise, *Journal of the American Medical Association* 282:833–839, 1999.

Fryer-Edwards K, Pinsky LE, Robins L: The use of portfolios to assess professionalism. In Stern DT, editor: *Measuring Medical Professionalism*, New York, 2006, Oxford University Press, pp 213–234.

General Medical Council: Good Medical Practise, 2006. Available at: http://www.gmc-uk.org/guidance/good_medical_practice.asp.

Ginsburg S, Lingard L: Using reflection and rhetoric to understand professional behaviours. In Stern DT, editor: *Measuring Medical Professionalism*, New York, 2006, Oxford University Press, pp 195–212.

Grady-Weliky TA, Kettyle CN, Hundert EM: The mentor–mentee relationship in medical education. In Wear D, Bickel J, editors: *Educating for Professionalism: Creating a Culture of Humanism in Medical Education*, Iowa City, 2000, University of Iowa Press, pp 105–119.

Hafferty F: Professionalism and medical education's hidden curriculum. In Wear D, Bickel J, editors: *Educating for Professionalism: Creating a Culture of Humanism in Medical Education*, Iowa City, 2000, University of Iowa Press, pp 11–34.

Hafferty F: Measuring professionalism: a commentary. In Stern DT, editor: *Measuring Medical Professionalism*, New York, 2006, Oxford University Press, pp 281–306.

Hodges BD, Ginsburg S, Cruess R, et al: Assessment of professionalism: recommendations for the Ottawa 2010 Conference, *Medical Teacher* 33(5):354–363, 2011.

Joint Commission: Behaviors that undermine a culture of safety, 2008. Available at: http://www.jointcommission.org/assets/1/18/SEA_40.PDF.

Mostaghimi A, Crotty BH: Professionalism in the digital age, *Annals of Internal Medicine* 154:560–562, 2011.

Norcini J: Faculty observations of student professional behaviour. In Stern DT, editor: *Measuring Medical Professionalism*, New York, 2006, Oxford University Press, pp 147–158.

Pellegrino E: Toward a reconstruction of medical morality: the primacy of the act of profession and the fact of illness. In Bulger RJ, McGovern JP, editors: *Physician and Philosopher, the Philosophical Foundation of Medicine: Essays by Dr Edmund Pellegrino*, Charlottesville, VA, 2001, Carden Jennings Publishing, pp 18–36.

Papadakis MA, Loeser H: Using critical incident reports and longitudinal observations to assess professionalism. In Stern DT, editor: *Measuring Medical Professionalism*, New York, 2006, Oxford University Press, pp 159–174.

Papadakis MA, Teherani A, Banach M, et al: Disciplinary action by medical boards and prior behaviour in medical school, *New England Journal of Medicine* 353:2673–2682, 2005.

Schön DA: *The Reflective Practitioner: How Professionals Think in Action*, London, 1983, Temple Smith.

Self DJ, Baldwin DC, Wolinsky FD: Evaluation of teaching medical ethics by an assessment of moral reasoning, *Medical Education* 26:178–184, 1992.

Stern DT: A framework for measuring professionalism. In Stern DT, editor: *Measuring Medical Professionalism*, New York, 2006, Oxford University Press, pp 3–13.

Stern DT, Frohna AZ, Gruppen LD: The predication of professional behaviour, *Medical Education* 39:75–82, 2005.

Stern DT, Papadakis MA: The developing professional – becoming a physician, *New England Journal of Medicine* 355:1794–1799, 2006.

Swick HM: Toward a normative definition of medical professionalism, *Academic Medicine* 75:612–616, 2000.

Wagoner NE: Admission to medical school: selecting applicants with the potential for professionalism. In Stern DT, editor: *Measuring Medical Professionalism*, New York, 2006, Oxford University Press, pp 235–264.

Evidence-based medicine

C. Heneghan, P. Glasziou

Introduction

The process of lifelong, self-directed learning includes recognition of clinically important questions about diagnosis, therapy, prognosis and other aspects of healthcare when caring for our patients. The methods of evidence-based medicine (EBM) aim to provide skills that help clinicians to rapidly answer these questions and assimilate new evidence and ideas and put them into practice.

We can summarize the EBM approach as a four-step process (Straus et al 2005):

- asking answerable clinical questions
- searching for the best research evidence
- critically appraising the evidence for its validity and relevance
- applying the evidence to groups and individuals.

To remind us to evaluate and improve our skills at these steps, a fifth step is often suggested: evaluating your own self education performance.

In this chapter we outline a possible curriculum plan for teaching EBM, moving from awareness and principles to skills and practice.

Introductory lecture: an hour on raising awareness

 "Evidence Based Medicine is the conscientious, explicit and judicious use of the best current evidence in making decisions about the care of individual patients."

Sackett et al 2000

Initial concepts in an introductory lecture should include what EBM (sometimes called 'evidence-based practice') is and isn't, the problem of our information overload, our need to discriminate between good-and-poor quality evidence and how EBM skills can help.

Important themes to develop are trying to keep up to date and the problem of overcoming the increasing world literature: over 1500 new medical research articles are published daily (Fig. 33.1). You might stop and ask your learners to reflect on how they currently learn and keep up to date. You might also ask them how much time is being spent on each process. Activities usually identified include attending lectures and conferences, reading articles in journals, tutorials, textbooks, clinical guidelines, clinical practice, small-group learning, study groups, using electronic resources and speaking to colleagues and specialists. There is no right or wrong way to learn; a mixture of all of these methods will be beneficial in the overall process of gathering information.

It is helpful to think of learning needs as a process of gathering information in two different ways: 'push' and 'pull'. The 'push' is learning from the deluge of information that arrives in our post or email, on a variety of topics. This type of learning can be thought of as 'just-in-case learning'. When the information is filtered to provide only what is important to clinical practice and has already been appraised for certain validity criteria, it can be very useful. But most of our learning should focus on information 'pull': answering the questions that arise in practice (also called 'just-in-time' learning).

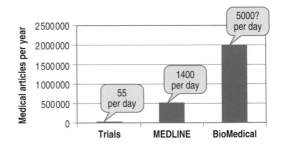

Fig. 33.1 The amount of medical research.

EVALUATE YOUR OWN LEARNING STRATEGIES AND YOUR LEARNERS

- Write down one recent patient problem.
- What was the critical question?
- Did you answer it? If so, how?

Samples of an introductory presentation are available free from the Centre for Evidence Based Medicine website (Oxford Centre for Evidence-Based Medicine downloads, www.cebm.net).

Asking answerable questions

You should consider following or combining this session (1–2 hours) with a searching skills laboratory (1–2 hours). Your librarians may have skills unbeknown to you that might help in this area. Use the PICO principle to formulate the clinical questions:

Population/patient: what is the disease problem?

Intervention/indicator: what main treatment is being considered?

Comparator/control: is this in relation to an alternative?

Outcome: what are the main outcomes of interest to the patient?

(And sometimes we add a **T** for the **T**ime to the outcome, e.g. 5-year survival).

Learners should practise dissecting the question into its component parts and then restructuring it so that the components can be used to direct the search. Prior to clinical work, scenarios are useful for teaching question building. For the less experienced, you might begin with short scenarios that lend themselves to dissecting the question(s) easily.

One way to begin is by giving an initial patient presentation and asking students what medical knowledge they need to 'solve' the clinical problem. List all the questions, and then classify them using the typology below (the type will affect where you look for the answer, and what type of research you can expect to provide it):

Clinical findings: how to interpret findings from the history and examination

Aetiology: the causes of diseases

Diagnosis: what tests are going to aid you in the diagnosis?

Prognosis: the probable course of the disease over time and the possible outcomes

Therapy: which treatment are you going to choose based on beneficial outcomes, harms, cost and your patient's values?

Prevention: primary and secondary risk factors which may or may not lead to an intervention

Cost-effectiveness: is one intervention more cost effective than another?

Quality of life: what effect does the intervention have on the quality of your patient's life?

Phenomena: the qualitative or narrative aspects of the problem

HOW YOU ARE GOING TO INTEGRATE ASKING QUESTIONS INTO YOUR OWN PRACTICE?

The challenge to the teacher is to identify questions that are both problem based and orientated to the learners' needs; at the same time you will also be identifying gaps in your own knowledge which may need to be addressed. Think of how you and your students are going to keep track of the questions and come to a clinically useful answer.

Remember to recognize potential questions which are clinically useful to you and your learners, decide which of the questions to focus on, guide your learners into developing useful questions and assess their performance in building and asking answerable questions.

Searching for the evidence

Resources which you will need are the following:

- if available, a computer laboratory with internet access
- one terminal for every two students
- if available, data projection linked up to a computer with database access for students to view searches in action
- internet access or access to medical research databases.

We recommend starting with MEDLINE for searching for the evidence.

PUBMED

Using PubMed (www.ncbi.nlm.nih.gov/PubMed) allows all the concepts of proficient searching to be taught. The most useful is the 'Clinical Queries' section, a question-focused interface with filters for identifying the more appropriate studies for questions of therapy, prognosis, diagnosis and aetiology. Ask students to do a search with and without the filters, and contrast the number of 'hits' found. Warn students that the first searches will take 15–30 minutes, but with regular practice they should get key information in a few minutes.

The session will take 1–2 hours, and there are several good guided tutorials on the web.

THE SUCCESS OF PROBLEM-BASED LEARNING DEPENDS ON THE ABILITY TO FIND THE CURRENT BEST EVIDENCE EFFECTIVELY

Finding answers to questions, when done well and quickly, can be highly rewarding or, when done poorly, can be frustrating and time consuming. A study of 103 GPs showed that they generated about 10 questions over a 2.5-day period. They tried to find the answers for about half of them. The most critical factor influencing which questions they followed up was how long they thought it would take to obtain an answer. If they thought the answer would be available in less than a couple of minutes, they were prepared to look for it. If they thought it would take longer, they would not bother. Only two questions in the whole study (0.2%) were followed up using a proper electronic literature search (Ely et al 1999).

HOW ARE YOU GOING TO MAINTAIN SEARCHING SKILLS?

In teaching searching skills think of the resources you have available to you. Librarians often have knowledge in this area far beyond the skills of a busy clinician. They often run courses and workshops; if they aren't currently, then consider approaching them to begin setting them up. On a personal level you should be proficient in searching. Often you will be asked questions about searching strategies: Which database to use? Why do I seem to get so many articles?

It is often best to have a prepared scenario which generates a four-part question and demonstrates some of the key components of an effective search strategy.

- In a five-year-old with a fever and a red bulging tympanic membrane, should I prescribe antibiotics or watch and wait?

    (See the clinically useful systematic review in Glasziou et al 2004.)

- A 35-year-old woman came to the clinic with a fresh dog bite and wanted to know whether she should have some prophylactic antibiotics.

    (See the clinically useful answer in PubMed/Medline, in Cummings 1994.)

There are two main strategies for searching bibliographic databases: thesaurus searching (all articles are indexed under subject headings) and text-word searching (where you search for specific words or phrases in the title or abstract). Once the question has been broken down into its components, it can be combined using the Boolean operators 'AND' and 'OR' (Fig. 33.2, Table 33.1).

In combining terms into a search strategy, it can be useful to represent them as a Venn diagram (Fig. 33.3). Complex combinations can then be structured.

Critically appraising the evidence for its validity and relevance

Initially it is worth communicating to your audience in a lecture format some of the key concepts of critical appraisal and why it is important as well as some of the potential pitfalls. Flecainide use in the treatment of ventricular arrhythmias (Anderson et al 1981, Echt et al 1991) is one illustration of potential pitfalls.

If you are about to embark on teaching appraisal, consider how proficient you are in appraisal in the following study types:

- therapy
- diagnosis
- systematic reviews
- harm/aetiology
- prognosis
- optional: economic analysis.

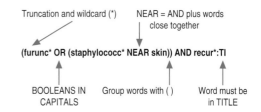

Fig. 33.2 Tips and tactics for searching.

Table 33.1 Convert your question into a search strategy

Question: In a 65-year-old man with heart failure, does the addition of a β-blocker compared with usual care improve survival?

Question part	Question term	Synonyms
Patient/problem	Adult, heart failure	Left ventricular failure, congestive heart failure, NYHA classification
Intervention	β-blocker	Metoprolol, carvedilol
Comparison	Usual care, standard therapy	
Outcome	Mortality	Death, survival

If you are not feeling confident, then refer to the EBM book by Straus et al (2005) or consider attending a workshop on teaching and practising EBM (Oxford Centre for Evidence-Based medicine; www.cebm.net).

CRITICAL APPRAISAL

Teaching the details of critical appraisal is best done as small-group work, with a specific article and flip-chart or whiteboard. Small-group work allows generation of free discussion of these new concepts between the group leader and the participants, enabling them to gain knowledge from their peers. As with many intellectual skills, practice, discussion and feedback are helpful for faster and deeper learning. Each of the six topics above will take a session of 60–90 minutes, so the full set may take 6–9 hours of small-group work.

WORKING THROUGH CRITICAL APPRAISAL

To help you in the process, we suggest that you have some prepared critical appraisal worksheets available to guide the process. You can design your own, but there are many available which will help you, for example:

- Oxford Centre for Evidence-Based Medicine free downloads of critical appraisal worksheets (www.cebm.net)

OR

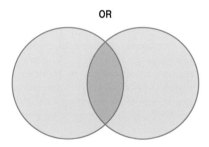

Retrieve all articles with either word

AND

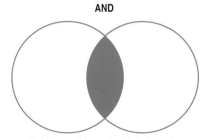

Retrieves articles only with both words

Fig. 33.3 A search strategy represented as a Venn diagram.

- Centre for Health Evidence University of Alberta (www.cche.net/che/home.asp)
- Centre for Evidence-Based Medicine, Mount Sinai, Toronto (www.cebm.utoronto.ca).

CRUNCHING THE NUMBERS

Learners should become proficient with most common outcome measures used in trials. Results can be expressed in many ways and you should feel comfortable in demonstrating the calculations involved:

- relative risk (RR)
- relative risk reduction (RRR)
- absolute risk reduction (ARR)
- number needed to treat (NNT)
- odds ratios (OR)
- sensitivity and specificity of diagnostic tests
- pre-test probabilities, likelihood ratios and post-test probabilities.

Do not expect your learners to calculate all of these every time, but they should be able to calculate NNTs and RRs; however, the more complex calculations may put them off. Introduce the use of a nomogram (Fig. 33.4) to aid diagnostic decision making.

CONFIDENCE INTERVALS AND *P* VALUES

Statistics will often bring fear to some of your students. Remember that most people will only need to be *users* of statistics, not *doers*. So emphasize interpretation, not calculation. You might explain that all studies are subject to some random error, and that the best we can do is estimate the true risk based on the sample of subjects in a trial (called the 'point estimate'). Statistics provide two ways of assessing chance:

- *P* values (hypothesis testing)
- Confidence intervals (estimation).

Do not go into the statistical methods of calculating the answers. Provide discussion about the relevant methods and why an intervention can only be considered useful if the 95% confidence interval (CI) includes a clinically important treatment effect. A useful exercise is a 'forest plot' from a meta-analysis. Ask students to read off which are the largest and smallest studies, which are statistically significant, which are clinically significant, etc.

Make clear the distinction between statistical significance and clinical importance:

- Statistical significance relates to the size of the effect and the 95% CIs in relation to the null hypothesis.

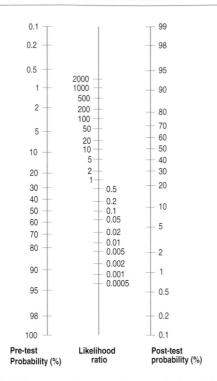

Pre-test Probability (%)   **Likelihood ratio**   **Post-test probability (%)**

Fig. 33.4 Nomogram for converting pre-test probabilities into post-test probablilties for a diagnostic test result with a given likelihood ratio (reproduced with permission from the Oxford Centre for Evidence-Based Medicine from www.cebm.net/index.aspx?o=1161).

- Clinical importance relates to the size of the effect and to a minimum effect that would be considered to be sufficiently important to change practice.

Applying the evidence

The questions you should think of before you decide to apply the results of the study to your patient are the following:

- Is the treatment feasible in my setting?
- Are your patients similar to those of the study?
- What alternatives are available?
- Will the potential benefits outweigh the harms?
- What does the patient value?

Evaluating your own performance

The most important evaluations are the ones you and your learners design and carry out yourselves. The questions you might want to ask include the following:

- How many questions are you recording?
- Are you using different databases in your search strategies?
- Are you challenging your colleagues about everyday decisions?
- Are you answering your questions?
- Has your practice changed?

Think of how you might want to be evaluated. Small presentations such as in a journal club can be a valuable way of appraising students, whilst increasing everyone's knowledge. Are you creating critically appraised topics (CATs)? These are structured appraisals incorporating all of the relevant points you would want to know from a study. There is a free downloadable version of a CATmaker available at the CEBM website (Oxford Centre for Evidence-Based Medicine, www.cebm.net).

Are you setting clearly defined objectives in your small groups, and is this meeting the needs of your students? If your learners are creating important information, think of how you might want to store this resource. You could create a database that could be accessed by others in your related fields.

Integrating EBM into your curriculum

Think of finding a like-minded individual who will help you to design and carry out the introduction and maintenance of an EBM course. You can have a rapid introduction to EBM in one-day courses: there are several good workbooks available to guide you in this process (Glasziou et al 2007). A one-day course would comprise an introductory lecture, searching skills and critical appraisal (of just one study type) in small groups. It is possible to integrate EBM throughout the course of a year, making your scenarios relevant to the different disciplines that a student will face. It is essential to demonstrate that you are practising EBM in your own clinical duties; leading by example is an excellent way to illustrate how evidence can be incorporated into your patient care. Be adventurous and try different strategies; mix and match lectures and small-group work; think about introducing a journal club for all those questions that still need answering. Join up with practitioners from different areas, and consider refreshing your skills at one of the many courses available.

Summary

The traditional continuing medical education flow is for research to be formulated into guidelines or reviews (evidence-based, we hope!), packaged into

CME, and presented in written form (in journals) or at educational sessions, to be later retrieved and applied at the appropriate clinical moment. Instead, we suggest that the traditional flow be reversed, and the choice of topics on which to gather information should come directly from caring for our patients (Del Mar & Glasziou 2001). Use a variety of strategies to incorporate the five steps of EBM into your course. Essential to this process is the teacher's role as an effective practitioner of EBM.

References

Anderson JL, Stewart JR, Perry BA, et al: Oral flecanide acetate for the treatment of ventricular arrhythmias, *New England Journal of Medicine* 305:473–477, 1981.

Cummings P: Antibiotics to prevent infection in patients with dog bite wounds: a meta-analysis of randomized trials, *Annals of Emergency Medicine* 23:535–540, 1994.

Del Mar CB, Glasziou PP: Ways of using evidence-based medicine in general practice, *Medical Journal of Australia* 174:374–450, 2001.

Echt DS, Liebson PR, Mitchell LB, et al: Mortality and morbidity in patients receiving ecainide, flecainide, or placebo. The Cardiac Arrhythmia Suppression Trial, *NEJM* 324:781–788, 1991.

Ely JW, Osheroff JA, Ebell MH, et al: Analysis of questions asked by family doctors regarding patient care, *British Medical Journal* 319:358–361, 1999.

Glasziou PP, Del Mar CB, Sanders SL, Hayem M: Antibiotics for acute otitis media in children (Cochrane Review). In *The Cochrane Library, Issue 1*, Chichester, 2004, John Wiley.

Glasziou P, Del Mar C, Salibusry J: *Evidence-Based Practice Workbook*, Oxford, 2007, BMJ Books.

Straus SE, Glasziou P, Richardson WS, Haynes RB: *Evidence-Based Medicine: How to Practice and Teach EBM*, ed 3, New York, 2005, Churchill Livingstone.

Further reading

Clinical Evidence. http://www.clinicalevidence.com.

Green ML, Ciampi MA, Ellis PJ: Residents' medical information needs in clinic: are they being met? *American Journal of Medicine* 109:218–233, 2000.

Oxford Centre for Evidence-Based Medicine.http://www.cebm.net/.

Patient safety

I. Dror

Introduction

Patient safety is obviously not only paramount, but stands at the very crux of medical care. Why then, despite huge investments and efforts, does patient harm resulting from medical care remain a problem (Landrigan et al 2010)? What is the role of medical teachers in achieving patient safety? And how can they contribute to patient safety?

When thinking of teaching patient safety we need to realize that it mostly relates to dealing with avoidance of unintentional error and patient harm by those who are there to actually provide patient care. Understanding the obstacles and difficulties in achieving patient safety will lead the way to teaching this elusive topic. Many of the failures to combat patient harm stem from misconceptions as to the root of the problems and how to deal with them most effectively.

To begin with, where is patient safety within the teaching curriculum? Is patient safety a topic that requires its own dedicated specialized educational module, or a designated lecture added within each topic taught? Or is patient safety a theme that cuts across modules and lectures and is 'everywhere'? And if so, how is it accomplished?

In addition, achieving patient safety is a challenge because most often patient safety is compromised unintentionally, within a highly qualified, motivated and caring environment. If (when) patient harm is a result of intentional behaviour or incompetence, then the problem is relatively simple and easy to deal with. However, when patient harm results from attentive and professional medical care, then it is harder to see how education can contribute to patient safety (Dror 2011a).

Even when considering one's own personal self-regarding life behaviours, people often compromise their own safety, for example, crossing a road in a red light or having unprotected sex. The point is that if one's self-regarding behaviours are lacking in safety, then it is no surprise that there are also deficiencies in other-regarding behaviours.

Finally, actions and efforts to reduce unsafe behaviours (such as TV commercials) are not very effective. The multi-million advertisements and campaigns aimed at increasing awareness and changing behaviours – even those that use disturbing emotional images – have for the most part failed (e.g. people continue to drink and drive, have unprotected sex, etc.).

 Patient safety should be continuously integrated into teaching by letting students make errors and 'burn' themselves, so as to create the more effective, salient and long-lasting mental representations necessary for actually achieving patient safety.

These are some of the reasons that patient safety is an elusive objective, and teaching it in a way that makes a difference is no small headache. I say this not to discourage medical teachers, but to lay out the challenges and difficulties, so that innovative and effective ways to teach and increase patient safety are utilized. It is not straightforward, but it is possible, and I will suggest some very practical ways to go about it.

Causes of problems with patient safety

Any effective teaching aimed at increasing patient safety must be underpinned by an understanding of the issues and causes that result in patient harm/ safety. However, these must be in depth, looking at and understanding the environment in which they occur, as well as the underlying cognitive processes that lead to patient safety/harm. One must get into the practical and effective ways of actually creating awareness and a culture of safety, and get beyond directive approaches of avoiding errors, such as instructing health professionals to 'wash their hands' or to 'make sure they give the correct medication, to the correct patient, at the correct time, and in the correct dosage'. Understanding cognition of errors, and why and how they occur in the medical environment, will lead to new and better teaching of patient safety. Current approaches have not been very effective (Landrigan et al 2010). Even with extensive teaching and comprehensive programmes (that include visible posters and reinforcing a supportive culture) the effectiveness – for example, of simple checklists – still encompassed 30% noncompliance with following all the steps in a checklist (Pape et al 2005).

Human cognition

Cognition involves perception of information, judgement, interpretation and decision making that determines if and what actions should be taken. The human cognitive system has limited resources and therefore cannot process all the information provided by the environment. Therefore, it has developed a variety of mechanisms that enable it to operate effectively, despite the lack of sufficient computational resources. In a nutshell, the human mind is not a camera. For example, it actively interacts with information and is conceptually driven, uses selective attention and specialized cognitive modules (e.g. distinct decision-making modules: one for rational/analytic choices and another for intuitive/experiential ones) (Payne & Bettman 2004).

The organization of the brain and the cognitive mechanisms that allow intelligence also mean that errors occur. In fact, expertise entails greater use and reliance on these mechanisms, allowing greater and superior performance, but at the same time it introduces vulnerabilities and more opportunities to make mistakes (Dror 2011b). This is an important point in medical teaching, a highly skilled domain that requires expertise.

The medical environment

 By understanding the cognitive weaknesses, and how they are manifested in the medical profession, one can develop proper and effective teaching of patient safety.

We also need to remember that medical professions work within challenging cognitive demands, such as:

1. A complex cognitive setting. This entails that cognition is distributed among a whole team of professionals, working together, sharing information and expertise between different people who jointly take care of a patient. In addition to the distributed

cognition at any one time, there is also a lack of cognitive temporal continuity with the change of caregivers and handovers.

2. A cognitively intense medical environment. Medical professionals sometimes work under time pressure, requiring them to quickly assess, diagnose and treat patients. Juggling and treating multiple patients at the same time and working in a noisy and distracting environment add a variety of additional cognitive demands.

3. Technological systems that are not always cognitively friendly. Medical professionals work with and rely on a variety of technological apparatus. However, these are not always suited and built to work effectively with their human users. Instead of supporting the human health professionals, they can interfere with and hinder their work. For example, monitors in the ICU are calibrated in a way that they go off so often that 'correct positives' are so rare (compared to the false alarms) that it renders them cognitively ineffective, and even detrimental.

When error-prone cognitive systems operate within such an environment, it is not a surprise that patient safety is an issue. But by understanding the cognitive weaknesses and how they are manifested in the medical profession, one can develop proper and effective teaching of patient safety.

Teaching patient safety

 Patient safety teaching must form mental representations that are not only long-lasting, but also cognitively salient.

Even with the good intentions of both the teachers and the learners (as well as administrators), it is hard to 'get the message home' when it comes to patient safety. There is huge pressure on the brain's resources, with many things continuously competing and fighting for its attention. Expecting that health professionals will have patient safety in the forefront of everything they do, at every moment, every time, during every action, just as a result of instructional learning is optimistic at best, if not naïve.

Even the most elaborate patient safety teaching that motivates and reinforces patient safety issues can easily be pushed aside by competing demands during actual patient care. Patient safety teaching must form mental representations that not only are long lasting, but also are cognitively salient. Training must encompass some pedagogical, cognitively effective ways to ensure (or at least encourage) that patient safety issues are well engrained in the learners' cognitive system. Such cognitive enhancement approaches have been used in training military fighter pilots (Dror et al 2008).

In this chapter I suggest an approach to teaching patient safety, a cognitively informed approach that is applicable across the medical curriculum and training. I will first explain the approach and then discuss practical ways and tools to achieve it.

To illustrate the approach, consider, for instance, that it is usually ineffective to teach by instructing people to 'save' their work while working on the computer, so as to avoid the loss of work in case the computer crashes. No matter how many times you teach them, explain to them, motivate them, people working on computers often do not save properly at regular intervals. How do people effectively learn to save properly? Not by directive instruction, but by experiencing failure! All it takes is one time for the computer to crash and for people to lose work. Then, they change, and learn: no matter how engaged they are, no matter how many competing tasks are fighting for their attention, they remember to save. This transformation occurs usually with a single crash, even if a small and insignificant amount of work is lost: quite impressive!

Even the most elaborate patient safety teaching that motivates and reinforces patient safety issues can easily be pushed aside by competing demands during actual patient care.

'Failures', and especially self-experienced ones, leave powerful and long-lasting impressions. Experiencing even a small and symbolic failure forms salient mental representations that shape future behaviour. Perhaps evolution and survival have taught us that it is critical to learn from mistakes, and therefore they are very effective ways of learning. Everyday life is full of personal examples of how well people remember mistakes they made, and how they shaped their future behaviour.

Errors can be an important tool for achieving learning (Marroua 1974), especially for elusive constructs and objectives, such as reliance on rigor rather than intuition (Ginat 2003), and – as suggested in this chapter – for teaching patient safety.

'Failures', especially self-experienced ones, leave powerful and long-lasting impressions.

The teaching approach: Learning from experiencing errors

The teaching of patient safety can capitalize on the cognitive power of errors. Harnessing this cognitive approach means that patient safety should be taught throughout the curriculum, teaching to avoid errors,

but not only by directive instructions (e.g. 'make sure to give the correct medication, to the correct patient', etc.), nor only by fostering and reinforcing a general 'culture of safety'. Patient safety should be continuously integrated into teaching by letting students make errors and 'burn' themselves, so as to create the more effective salient and long-lasting mental representations necessary for actually achieving patient safety.

The approach is to transform the teaching of patient safety by shifting the focus from understanding and trying to avoid errors to experiencing and recovering from errors.

Academically covering and teaching topics, such as what is patient safety, what is the human factor and why it is important for patient safety, understanding systems and the impact of complexity on patient care, and so forth (see WHO 2009, 'Patient Safety Curriculum Guide for Medical Schools', for a list of 11 suggested topics) is all well and good in theory, but will have (in my view) little real impact on increasing patient safety. A cognitively informed approach to teaching patient safety suggests that rather than teaching that poor communication can lead to adverse events, patient safety teaching should be transformed to having students actually experience poor communication errors, learning both to identify them and how to recover from them.

Patient safety teaching should not only allow learners to make patient safety-related errors, but also entrap them, setting them up to make these highly educational errors. Using 'sabotage' and other techniques (see below), teaching should ensure that students experience patient safety errors as a cognitively effective way to teach patient safety and 'get the message home'. The specific tools and ways to achieve this in practice are discussed below; in this subsection I focus on the logic and pedagogy underpinning this idea, as an overarching teaching approach, and then delve into the practicalities, details and practice of applying it.

The approach is to transform the teaching of patient safety by shifting the focus from understanding and trying to avoid errors to experiencing and recovering from errors. Teaching such an error recovery approach entails three main steps: inducing errors, identifying an error, and responding to the error by taking actions to counter and recover from the error.

INDUCING ERRORS

To teach error recovery, one must first ensure that errors occur within the controlled teaching environment. When unintentional and unplanned errors are made, as they do, both by instructors and by students, instructors should take advantage of them as an educational tool. Rather than a 'problem' to be buried quickly and discretely, errors offer a wonderful teaching opportunity which should be embraced.

Teaching patient safety should not rely only on spontaneous naturally occurring errors. In addition, errors should be carefully planned at critical learning junctions. The instructor should make errors during teaching (or have a confederate make them).

However, it is easier to identify errors in others than it is in oneself (Pronin et al 2002). This self-serving bias maintains and enhances one's self-identity and image. Furthermore, when regarding others, one is exposed only to their behaviour and thus has a clear focus and analysis only of their actions, whereas one's own behaviour is seen and judged within the internal context of motivation and mental states. Therefore, errors committed by instructors, or confederates, as part of teaching patient safety are important but not enough. One must make sure to induce errors to be committed by the learners themselves: there is nothing more effective than the learners experiencing it themselves, firsthand. The practical ways to induce such errors are discussed below in the practical section; here I focus on the pedagogical approach.

IDENTIFYING AN ERROR

Once an error has been committed (planned or not, by the instructor or by another), one must respond to it immediately. Not only will it have a greater educational value and be more cognitively effective, but one should never leave an error uncorrected, as this can be counterproductive, uneducational and dangerous. Therefore, the explicit identification of an error must take place soon after its occurrence.

If the error has been identified by a learner, then the teacher must take the following three steps:

1. Commend the person who identified the error, giving them proper recognition and praise. This is to encourage them and others to identify errors and to, de facto, foster a culture that promotes patient safety and being vigilant.

2. Emphasize the importance of error detection, making the following points:

   • Remind learners that all must be constantly alert and vigilant as to when errors occur

   • Emphasize that this is critical to patient safety and care

   • Give relevant statistics and prevalence of the specific type of error and its consequences

3. Move to teaching how to respond to the error and how best to recover from it.

If, however, the error has not been identified, and has gone by unnoticed, then the teacher must stop the activity and specifically ask if anyone has noticed any

problem or issue (thus 'throwing the ball to the learners', making them actively think).

• If a student says that he or she noticed the error when it occurred, then the instructor needs to question why the student did not point out the error earlier, when it actually happened. Clearly, the student did not want to interrupt the class, be rude by making the instructor look stupid or risk making themselves look stupid or foolish if an error did not actually happen. However, this is a critical junction in teaching patient safety, and the instructor must take on this paramount educational opportunity. Often patient safety is compromised when medical staff do not speak out. The pressures not to speak out in class when the instructor makes an error are minuscule compared to real clinical settings (Fischer et al 2006). However, such behaviour is an essential and integral part of patient safety, and the approach I am suggesting for teaching patient safety provides educational opportunities to teach this properly and effectively.

• If no one identifies the error, then:

   1. First, the instructor (or the confederate or student who committed the error) needs to re-enact it, giving the learners another opportunity to identify it.

   2. Second, the error now needs to be identified (either by the learners or by the instructor him- or herself).

   3. Third, the instructor needs to question the student about why the error was not identified in the first place, when it originally occurred.

Then the instructor should continue and follow steps 2 and 3 (above).

 Once an error has been committed (planned or not, by the instructor or by another), one must respond to it immediately.

RESPONDING TO THE ERROR BY TAKING ACTIONS TO COUNTER AND RECOVER FROM THE ERROR

Once the error is identified, then the learning must include the most effective actions, if any, that need to be taken. This will enable the learners to respond most appropriately to situations that do occur in the realities of clinical practice.

It is best for patient safety and care that teaching provides proper and detailed best actions to be taken when errors do happen. Rather than deny their existence by teaching only the correct treatment in the first place, or naively trying to avoid error with directive instructions, this approach deals with errors by teaching error recovery.

This approach not only prepares health professionals to deal with errors, and thus improve patient safety, but also solidifies salient mental representations. The time and effort spent learning how to identify and respond to the error and how best to recover from it during training involve a deeper level of cognitive processing. This is cognitively effective in avoiding the occurrence of errors actually happening in the future in clinical practice. It makes the learners more aware of, and pay more attention to, patient safety.

For teaching to be effective, it must be cognitively informed (Dror et al 2011). When it comes to teaching patient safety, this approach includes inducing errors, identifying an error and responding to the error by taking actions to counter and recover from the error. Now the question is how can one apply this approach in practice, which is the topic of the next section.

Practical ways to teach patient safety: Focus on error recovery rather than error avoidance

So, how do you achieve, in practice, this error recovery approach to teaching patient safety? Below, I specify some practical steps and best practices in applying this approach. This is not meant to be an exhaustive list but illustrations of how it should be done. I specify these practical elements, following the steps described in the approach section: inducing errors, identifying an error, and responding to the error by taking actions to counter and recover from the error.

INDUCING ERRORS

- **Selection of errors:** The teaching examples should reproduce the most commonly occurring errors in clinical practice and those errors with the most dire consequences. This is so patient safety will most benefit from training to avoid errors. If teaching relates to rare errors and those whose consequences are relatively negligible, then it can only minimally enhance patient safety. It is important to identify, based on data and clinicians, which errors are more problematic and therefore should be the focus.

- **Acting errors:** When instructors or confederates play out the errors (whether in class demos, videos, simulations, etc.), then these need to be as realistic as possible. However, for educational purposes, to allow different levels of difficulty and challenge (see below), teaching should include both obvious and explicit errors, and more subtle ones. Some errors should even be exaggerated and made very obvious (Dror et al 2008).

- **Inducing errors in the learners:** It is a difficult, but very important, challenge to make the learners experience errors themselves. This offers a unique and powerful tool for learning and can play a major role in teaching patient safety (Fischer et al 2006). The problem and challenge is obvious: How can one cause others to make errors? If and when they make spontaneous errors, from time to time, as everyone does, then one should use these as powerful examples. But one cannot rely and build patient safety teaching on such occurrences. First, they may or may not occur. Second, if and when they do occur, they may not be at the best time and may not be the most educational and beneficial examples. Therefore, it is important to try to set things up so the learners experience optimum firsthand educational errors. This can be achieved in a variety of ways. For example, a practical way to induce errors is to set up the wrong expectations. In practice this can be used to cause errors in diagnosis and treatment; for instance, when using simulations to increase patient safety in regards to sepsis, students coming to the simulation can be told that their training is in dealing with a drop in blood pressure (i.e. setting them up to miss the sepsis). Or one can induce the learners to make an error in administering a drug or using an instrument by swapping locations so as to cause a likely confusion. This, what I term 'sabotage', is intended to make errors more likely, to create dramatic and effective training opportunities for teaching patient safety.

IDENTIFYING AN ERROR

- **Gradual presentation:** The ultimate goal is that errors will be avoided and patient safety enhanced. But achieving these cognitive salient mental representations and focus is a gradual learning process. Therefore, it is suggested that initially one begins with more obvious, even exaggerated errors, committed by others. Then errors can become more and more subtle and hard to identify, requiring more focus, attention and awareness. Thereafter, move from identification of errors in others to identification of errors in one's own behaviour and actions.

- **Different usage of error identification:** Error identification can be used as a learning tool, as a means of practice and for informative as well as summative assessment.

- **Adding complexity and challenge:** Make error detection more realistic and challenging by adding noise and distractions that are typical in clinical settings. Challenge can be further added by measuring how quickly learners can detect an error, and by encouraging competition among learners to see who identifies the most errors, the most quickly, etc.

- *Platforms:* Presenting errors to be identified can take place in the most simple and low-technology environment, as well as with complex technological apparatus. On the simple end, a classroom, laboratory or any location can be used to act out or induce an error. All that is needed is that an inappropriate action is taken or that a needed action is not taken (e.g., it can be as simple as not washing your hands properly before approaching a patient). These types of errors do not require any specialized equipment that is not already needed for instructional teaching of the subject matter content. One can videotape errors and build up a library of how patient safety is compromised. However, since errors must be identified and corrected soon after their occurrence (see above), such videos should be interactive. Interactive videos require viewers to actively engage and respond. So, every time an error is presented, the viewer clicks on the error and receives feedback throughout the video (Dror et al 2011). Games, simulations and virtual realities are very effective and appropriate tools to use for this approach. They offer tools that enable learners to adopt and use the error recovery approach. And the error recovery approach offers a cognitively informed way to utilize these technological tools more effectively.

RESPONDING TO THE ERROR BY TAKING ACTIONS TO COUNTER AND RECOVER FROM THE ERROR

- *Gradual demands:* Initially, once an error is detected, then the correct recovery actions need to be presented to the learners. Then, rather than providing the correct responses, learners should be presented with multiple choice options to select the most appropriate actions. Finally, the learners themselves should be required to generate and execute the proper responses to recover from the errors.
- *Different usage of error recovery:* Error recovery can be used as a learning tool, as a means of practice and for informative as well as summative assessment.
- *Frequency:* If patient safety is to be taken seriously, then all teaching should include elements on this issue. This will not interfere with covering the topical subject materials because this approach to teaching patient safety is integrated within the subject matter content. If patient safety teaching consists of directive instructions to 'pay attention to detail', 'avoid making errors', etc., then repeating this throughout the curriculum is not effective, and will be boring to students (and instructors). Including errors, and expecting students to identify and respond to them, is engaging to the students and underpins this approach to teaching patient safety. Errors should not only be included at designated times, but also be unexpected, occurring at any time, anywhere. This will not only keep the students 'on their toes', but also play an important role in cognitively engraining patient safety, and therefore it is key to this teaching approach.

Summary

The importance of patient safety is self-evident and paramount. It is suggested that cognitively informed teaching will achieve a real impact and enhance patient safety. In such an approach, academically covering patient safety topics is not sufficient; for learners to form salient and long-lasting effective mental representations, teaching must emphasize errors. It is further suggested that rather than teaching about errors and how to avoid them, focus should shift to teaching error recovery. This training approach requires that throughout the curriculum errors are induced, errors are identified, and recovery actions are taken. Through actually experiencing and learning from errors, an effective approach to teaching patient safety can be achieved.

References

Dror IE: A novel approach to minimize error in the medical domain: Cognitive neuroscientific insights into training, *Medical Teacher* 33(1):34–38, 2011a.

Dror IE: The paradox of human expertise: Why experts can get it wrong. In Kapur N, editor: *The Paradoxical Brain*, Cambridge, 2011b, Cambridge University Press, pp 177–188.

Dror IE, Stevenage SV, Ashworth A: Helping the cognitive system learn: Exaggerating distinctiveness and uniqueness, *Applied Cognitive Psychology* 22(4):573–584, 2008.

Dror IE, Schmidt P, O'Connor L: A cognitive perspective on technology enhanced learning in medical training: Great opportunities, pitfalls and challenges, *Medical Teacher* 33(4):291–296, 2011.

Fischer MA, Mazor KM, Baril J, et al: Learning from mistakes: Factors that influence how students and residents learn from medical errors, *Journal of General Internal Medicine* 21(5):419–423, 2006.

Ginat D: *The greedy trap and learning from mistakes. Proceedings of the 34th ACM Computer Science Education Symposium – SIGCSE*, 2003, ACM Press, pp 11–15.

Landrigan CP, Parry GJ, Bones CB, et al: Temporal trends in rates of patient harm resulting from medical care, *New England Journal of Medicine* 363:2124–2134, 2010.

Marroua JR: The importance of making mistakes, *The Teacher Educator* 9(3):15–17, 1974.

Pape TM, Guerra DM, Muzquiz M, et al: Innovative approaches to reducing nurses' distractions during medication administration, *Journal of Continuing Education in Nursing* 36(3):108–116, 2005.

Payne JW, Bettman JR: The information-processing approach to decision making. In Koeler DJ, Harvey N, editors: *Blackwell Handbook of Judgement and Decision Making*, London, 2004, Blackwell Publishing, pp 110–132.

Pronin E, Lin DY, Ross L: The bias blind spot: Perceptions of bias in self versus others, *Personality and Social Psychological Bulletin* 28(3):369–381, 2002.

WHO (World Health Organization): *Patient Safety Curriculum Guide for Medical Schools*, Geneva, 2009, WHO Press.

Section 6

Assessment

Concepts in assessment

J. Norcini, M. Friedman Ben-David

Even a cursory review of the assessment literature reveals a bewildering array of dichotomies and concepts. These are often overlapping, and authors sometimes use them with less precision than is desirable, especially for the clinical teacher attempting to make sense of assessment for the first time. The purpose of this chapter is to identify some of these concepts and provide background to their meaning, development and use.

Test theories

Test theories or psychometric models seek to explain what happens when an individual takes a test (Crocker & Algina 1986). They provide guidance about how to select items, how long tests need to be, the inferences that can be drawn from scores and the confidence that can be placed in the final results. Each model makes different assumptions, and, based on those assumptions, different benefits accrue. There are many psychometric models, but three deserve attention here because they are used frequently in medical education.

CLASSICAL TEST THEORY (CTT)

CTT has been the dominant model in testing for decades, with roots in the late 19th and early 20th century (Lord & Novick 1968). It assumes that an individual's score on a test has two parts: true score (or what is intended to be measured) and error. To apply CTT to a practical testing situation, a series of very restrictive assumptions need to be made. The bad news is that these assumptions are often violated in practice, but the good news is that even when this happens, it seldom makes a practical difference (i.e. the model is robust with respect to violations of the assumptions).

A number of useful concepts and tools have been developed based on CTT (De Champlain 2010). Among the most powerful is reliability, which indicates the amount of error in observed scores. Also

very useful has been the development of item statistics, which helps with the process of test development. CTT has contributed significantly to the development of a series of excellent assessments, and it continues to be used and useful today.

GENERALIZABILITY THEORY (GT)

Although it has its roots in the middle of the 20th century, GT rose to prominence with the publication of a book by Cronbach et al in 1972. Like CTT (which is a special case of GT), it assumes that an individual's score on a test has two parts: true score and error. However, compared to CTT, GT makes relatively weak assumptions. Consequently, it applies to a very broad range of assessments and, like CTT, even when these assumptions are violated it usually makes little practical difference.

GT offers a number of advantages over CTT (Brennan 2001). For example, GT allows the error in a test to be divided among different sources. So in a rating situation, GT allows the error associated with the rater to be separated from the error associated with the rating form they are filling out. Likewise, GT supports a distinction between scores that are intended to rank individuals as opposed to scores that are intended to represent how much they know. Given these advantages, GT has special applicability to the types of assessment situations found in medical education.

ITEM RESPONSE THEORY (IRT)

With considerable interest starting in the 1970s, the use of IRT has grown substantially, especially among national testing agencies (Hambleton et al 1991). Unlike GT, IRT makes very strong assumptions about items, tests and individuals. These assumptions are difficult to meet, so there are a number of different IRT models, each with assumptions that are suitable for particular assessment situations.

When the assumptions are met, many practical benefits accrue (Downing 2003). For example, individual scores are independent of exactly which set of items are taken, and item statistics are independent of the individuals who take the test. So individuals can take completely different test questions, but their scores will still be comparable. As another example, IRT supports the creation of tests that are targeted to a particular score, often the pass–fail point. This permits a shorter test than would otherwise be the case.

 Compared to CTT, GT and IRT provide different but powerful advantages. However, for most practical day-to-day work any of the test theories are sufficient.

Score interpretation

A score is a letter or number that reflects how well an individual performs on an assessment. When a test is being developed, one of the first decisions to be made is how the scores will be interpreted: norm-referenced or criterion-referenced (Glaser 1963). This decision has implications for how the items or cases are chosen, what the scores mean when they are being used by students, teachers and institutions and how the reliability or reproducibility of scores is conceived (Popham & Husek 1969).

NORM-REFERENCED SCORE INTERPRETATION

When score are interpreted from a norm-referenced perspective they are intended to provide information about how individuals perform against a group of test takers. For example, saying that a student's performance was one standard deviation above the mean means that he or she did better than 84% of those who took the test. It says nothing about how many questions the student answered correctly.

Norm-referenced score interpretation is especially useful in situations where there are a limited number of positions and the need to select the best (or most appropriate) of the test takers. For example, in admissions decisions, there are often a limited number of seats and the goal is to pick the best of the applicants. Norm-referenced score interpretation aids in these types of decisions. However, it is not useful when the goal is to identify how much each individual knows or can do.

CRITERION-REFERENCED SCORE INTERPRETATION

When scores are interpreted from a criterion-referenced perspective (sometimes called domain-referenced) they are intended to provide information about how much an individual knows or can do given the domain of the assessment. For example, saying that a student got 70% of the items right on a test means that he or she knows 70% of what is needed. It says nothing about how the student performed in comparison to others.

Criterion-referenced score interpretation is particularly useful in competency testing. For example, an assessment designed to provide feedback intended to improve performance should yield scores interpreted from a criterion-referenced perspective. Likewise, an end-of-course assessment should produce scores that indicate how much material students have learned. However, criterion-referenced score interpretation is not useful when the goal is to rank students.

One common variation on criterion-referenced score interpretation is called a *mastery* test. In a mastery test, a binary score (usually pass or fail) connotes whether the individual's performance demonstrates sufficient command of the material for a particular purpose.

Score equivalence

When an assessment is given, there are many instances when it is desirable to compare scores among trainees, against a common pass–fail point and/or over time. Clearly, if all the trainees take exactly the same questions or encounter exactly the same patients, it is possible to compare scores and make equivalent pass–fail decisions. Some methods, like multiple-choice questions (MCQs) and standardized patients (SPs), were created in part to ensure that all trainees would face exactly the same challenges and their scores would mean exactly the same thing.

There are also a variety of important assessment situations when scores are not equivalent but where adjustments can be made. For example, in an MCQ or SP examination, the test items or cases are often changed over time and, despite maintaining similar content, these versions or forms of the same assessment differ in difficulty. With these methods of assessment, the issue can be addressed through test *equating* (Kolen & Brennan 1995, van der Linden & Hambleton 1997). Equating is a set of procedures, designs and statistics that are used to adjust scores so it is as if everyone took the same test. Although this provides a way to adjust scores, it is complicated, time intensive, and labour intensive. Consequently, it is used often in national assessments and less frequently for locally developed tests.

There are also a variety of important assessment situations where scores are not equivalent and where good adjustment is not practical or possible. For example, virtually all methods of assessment based on observed trainees' encounters with real patients yield scores (or ratings) that are not equivalent because patients vary in the level of challenge they present and observers differ in how hard they grade. Attempts to minimize these unwanted sources of influence on scores usually take the form of wide sampling of patients and faculty (to hopefully balance out the easy and difficult patients), training of observers, and certain IRT-based methods that statistically minimize some of the differences among observers (Linacre 1989). None of these are wholly satisfactory, however, and although these types of assessments are essential to the training and credentialing of doctors, the results must be interpreted with some caution when used for summative purposes. They are well-suited to formative assessment.

Standards

It is sometimes important to categorize performance on a test, usually as pass or fail (although there are times when more than these two categories are needed). The score that separates the passers from failures is called the standard or pass–fail point. It is an answer to the question, 'How much is enough?' There are two types of standards: relative and absolute (Norcini 2003).

RELATIVE STANDARDS

For relative standards, the pass–fail point is chosen to separate individuals based on how well they performed compared to each other. For example, a cutting score might be selected to pass the top 80% of students (i.e. the 80% of students with the best scores).

Relative standards are most appropriate in settings where a group of a particular size needs to be selected. For instance, in an admissions setting where the number of seats is limited and the purpose is to pick the best students, relative standards make the most sense. Relative standards are much less appropriate for assessments where the intention is to determine competence (i.e. whether a student knows enough for a particular purpose).

 The credibility of standards depends to a large degree on the standard setters and the method they use. The standard setters must understand the purpose of the test and the reason for establishing the cut score, know the content and be familiar with the examinees. The specific method chosen to set standards is not as important as whether it produces results that are fit for the purpose of the test, relies on informed expert judgment, demonstrates due diligence, is supported by a body of research and is easy to explain and implement.

ABSOLUTE STANDARDS

For absolute standards, the pass–fail point is chosen to separate individuals based on how much they know or how well they perform. For example, a cutting score might be selected to pass the students who correctly answer 80% of the questions.

Absolute standards are most appropriate in settings where there is a need to determine competence. For instance, in an end-of-year assessment where the purpose is to decide which students learned enough to progress to the next year, absolute standards make the most sense. Absolute standards are much less appropriate for assessments where the intention is to select a certain number or percentage of students for a particular purpose.

Types of assessment

Assessments can be classified in a variety of different ways and many of them are reasonable. One useful classification of assessments is as diagnostic, formative or summative (Hanauer et al 2009). Although some assessments are designed to simultaneously serve more than one purpose (e.g. be summative but also provide formative information), it is very difficult to do this well, and so one of the purposes usually dominates. In the end, it is better to develop a good *system* of assessment which incorporates different test methods, each of which serves a single purpose well.

DIAGNOSTIC ASSESSMENT

An assessment of trainees relevant to and before they are exposed to a particular educational intervention is generally referred to as diagnostic. Analogous to medicine, the purpose of these assessments is to determine the trainees' educational needs with the goal of optimizing learning. Often they produce a profile which identifies areas of strength and weakness.

Examples of this type of test are most common in continuing medical education, where participants select, or are assigned to, a particular educational experience based on their performance. In general, they are underutilized in formal training where the focus remains largely on educational process. With the movement to outcomes-based education, these types of assessments should increase in importance.

FORMATIVE ASSESSMENT

An assessment of trainees during an educational intervention is often referred to as formative. The purpose of these assessments is two-fold. First, they provide feedback to students and their teachers which is intended to guide learning. Second, there is recent work indicating that the act of assessment itself creates learning, so formative assessment is integral to education.

 Over the past 50 years, considerable energy has been devoted to the development of summative assessment. Although much work remains, good summative assessments of medical knowledge, clinical skills and other competencies are now readily available.

More recently, the focus has shifted to formative assessment and its focus on supporting and creating learning. We need to develop a much better understanding of how to build and use these types of assessments.

There are many examples of these types of assessments, like the workplace–based measures (e.g. Mini-CEX, direct observation of procedural skills). These often require some form of direct observation followed by assessment and then immediate feedback. Despite the fact that formative assessment is central to learning, insufficient attention has been paid to the development and refinement of these types of instruments.

SUMMATIVE ASSESSMENT

An assessment of trainees at the end of a period of time is generally referred to as summative. The purpose of these assessments is to determine whether the trainee has learned what has been taught. Consequently, summative assessments are usually cumulative and indicate whether the trainee is competent to move on in training or practice.

Examples of summative assessments are the examinations that occur at the end of units, courses, semesters and years. Also summative tests are for graduation, licensure, certification and so on. These tests are so pervasive, especially in medical school, that when most students are asked about it, they describe all assessments as summative.

Qualities of a good assessment

There are many ways to judge the quality of an assessment. Historically, there was emphasis on the measurement properties of the test alone (reliability and validity). More recently, van der Vleuten (1996) expanded the list of qualities, pushing beyond the traditional measurement characteristics to include issues related to the test's effect, acceptability and feasibility. These criteria were reaffirmed and added to in a consensus statement of the 2010 Ottawa Conference which resulted in the following criteria for good assessment (Norcini et al 2011):

• **Validity or coherence:** There is a body of evidence that is coherent ('hangs together') and that

supports the use of the results of an assessment for a particular purpose.

• **Reproducibility or consistency:** The results of the assessment would be the same if repeated under similar circumstances.

• **Equivalence:** The same assessment yields equivalent scores or decisions when administered across different institutions or cycles of testing.

• **Feasibility:** The assessment is practical, realistic and sensible, given the circumstances and context.

• **Educational effect:** The assessment motivates those who take it to prepare in a fashion that has educational benefit.

• **Catalytic effect:** The assessment provides results and feedback in a fashion that creates, enhances, and supports education; it drives future learning forward.

• **Acceptability:** Stakeholders find the assessment process and results to be credible.

 Over time, most of these criteria have been presented in detail by a variety of authors and their importance is clear. More recently, however, particular emphasis has been placed on the catalytic effect. This criterion refers to how well the assessment provides results and feedback in such a way that learning is created, enhanced and supported. It is central to the evolving view of assessment as means of generating learning as well as deciding the degree to which it has occurred.

Blueprints

The content included in an assessment is essential to the quality of the results and to establish both the validity and credibility of the scores and decisions emanating from it. A good assessment starts with a good blueprint (sometimes called a table of specifications), which specifies in appropriate detail what content needs to be covered (Downing & Haladyna 2006). This blueprint should be shared with anyone being assessed well in advance of the actual examination.

For example, the American Board of Internal Medicine publishes its blueprint for the certifying examination in internal medicine (www.abim.org). It specifies that at least 75% of the questions be patient based and, reflecting practice, 75% of the patient encounters be in an outpatient or emergency setting. More than 50% of the questions must require synthesis or judgement to reach the correct conclusion. The blueprint specifies in detail the percentage of the items devoted to each of the medical content categories (e.g.

cardiovascular disease is 14%, infectious disease is 9%, psychiatry is 4%), and there is a cross-cutting classification for areas like geriatric medicine (10%) and prevention (6%). Each item contributes to a primary content category and may contribute to a cross-cutting category as well (e.g. a prevention question in cardiovascular disease). Because this is a national assessment and there is so much at stake, the blueprint is very detailed. For local assessments and/or those based on fewer items or cases (e.g. an OSCE), this level of detail is unnecessary but a blueprint is still essential to ensure the validity of the results.

"For a credentialing examination, such as certification, the content and blueprint should be based on the nature of practice, not the nature of training. Consequently, the blueprints for such examinations are often based on a job analysis. This supports the validity of the scores by creating an explicit link between the test content and what is done in practice."

Colton et al 1991

The source of content for an assessment will depend on its purpose. For example, if it intended to determine what has been learned as part of a course, then the content should be drawn from the syllabus. However, if it is intended to indicate readiness for practice, then it should be based on the patient problems that constitute that practice. There are a variety of sophisticated designs and statistical methods for supporting the development of a blueprint that are suitable for assessments where the stakes are high (Downing & Haladyna 2006).

Self-assessment

Self-assessment has occupied a central role in medical education for some time. In general, it is assumed that the individual chooses what he or she believes is important to assess, selects how the assessment will be done, and then uses the results of the assessment to confirm strengths and address weaknesses. Within this context, virtually all methods of assessments can be used for self-assessment.

For society to grant doctors and other professionals the ability to self-regulate, it must assume that they are able to self-assess accurately. This ability has in turn been expected to drive day-to-day practice and lifelong learning. As important, accurate self-assessment is what allows doctors to limit their practices to areas of competence. Given this critical role, it is not surprising that medical education is expected to develop this ability in trainees and practitioners.

Despite its importance, there is good evidence that doctors and other professionals are not very good at self-assessment. A recent review of the literature by Davis and colleagues (2006) concluded that although the literature was flawed, doctors have a limited ability to self-assess accurately. Eva and Regehr (2005) added that self-assessment is 'a complicated, multifaceted, multipurpose phenomenon that involves a number of interacting cognitive processes'. Given its complexity, there is neither the research nor the educational strategies available at the moment to suggest that self-assessment in its purest form can be relied upon.

In a review of the literature, Davis and colleagues found that, "of the 20 comparisons between self- and external assessment, 13 demonstrated little, no or an inverse relationship, and 7 demonstrated positive associations. A number of studies found the worst accuracy in self-assessment among physicians who were the least skilled and those who were the most confident. These results are consistent with those found in other professions."

Davis et al 2006

Three important suggestions have been offered to make self-assessment more effective by ensuing that it is guided (Galbraith et al 2008). First, it is essential that the self-assessment be chosen to be be relevant to the learning or practice experience of the student or doctor; it should not be completely self-selected. Second, the self-assessment should be directly linked to educational experiences that can remediate difficulties. Third, the results of self-assessment should be periodically validated by external assessments.

Objective versus subjective assessments

In the literature, it is not unusual for authors to refer to some forms of assessment as 'objective' and others as 'subjective'. Generally speaking, objective assessments have one or more clearly correct or incorrect responses or behaviours that can be readily observed. Examples of objective assessments include MCQs and checklists. In contrast, subjective assessments often require judgements about a response or set of behaviours. Examples of subjective assessments include essay questions and rating forms.

"There is much research comparing checklists (seen as objective) and global ratings (seen as subjective). In fact, scores from checklists are slightly more reliable and global ratings are slightly more valid. But, the differences are relatively small so that using either methodology can produce good results."

Norcini & Boulet 2003

In many ways, this is not a useful dichotomy. MCQs are arguably the most objective of the assessment methods. Nonetheless, judgments are made through the test construction, scoring and standard-setting process. Creation of the blueprint requires a number of judgements about importance and frequency. When individual items are written, the author makes judgements about the patient's age, the site of care, which diagnostic tests and treatments are included among the potential responses and so on. For scoring, judgements need to be made about whether/how much to weight each response, how to aggregate those weights, what scale to report them on and where the pass–fail point will be.

All assessment requires judgement. The only difference among the various methods is the way in which those judgements are gathered and the number of experts involved. MCQs have an advantage because many experts can contribute to test creation so that items can be eliminated, various different perspectives can be represented and the product (i.e. the final test) can be validated by the group. In addition, many different clinical situations can be sampled efficiently. The exact same judgements are made in a bedside oral examination, but the method limits the number of experts and clinical situations that can be included. To the degree that the number of experts and patients can be increased, the 'objectivity' of the oral examination approaches that of MCQs.

Summary

The purpose of this chapter is to identify some of the concepts fundamental to assessment and to provide background to their meaning, development and use. The test theories underlying assessment have been briefly described, as have the types of assessment to which they apply and the criteria against which to judge their success. The importance of test content, as highlighted by the blueprint, plays a central role in the quality of an assessment, and more technical matters like score interpretation, equivalence and standards must be aligned with the purpose of assessments so they perform as intended. Finally, much is written about self-assessment and 'subjective' versus 'objective' measurement. The chapter has suggested some potential concerns and clarifications around these popular topics.

References

Brennan RL: *Generalizability Theory*, New York, 2001, Springer-Verlag.

Colton A, Kane MT, Kingsbury C, Estes CA: Strategies for examining the validity of job analysis data, *Journal of Educational Measurement* 28:283–294, 1991.

Crocker L, Algina J: *Introduction to classical and modern test theory*, Fort Worth, TX, 1986, Harcourt, Brace, & Jovanovich.

Cronbach LJ, Gleser CG, Rajaratnam N, Nanda H: *The dependability of behavioral measurements*, New York, 1972, Wiley.

Davis DA, Mazmanian PE, Fordis M, et al: Accuracy of physician self-assessment compared with observed measures of competence: a systematic review, *JAMA* 296(9):1094–1102, 2006.

De Champlain AF: A primer on classical test theory and item response theory for assessments in medical education, *Medical Education* 44(1):109–117, 2010.

Downing SM: Item response theory: applications of modern test theory in medical education, *Medical Education* 37(8):739–745, 2003.

Downing SM, Haladyna TM, editors: *Handbook of Test Development*, Mahwah, NJ, 2006, Erlbaum.

Eva KW, Regehr G: Self-assessment in the health professions: a reformulation and research agenda, *Academic Medicine* 80(10 Suppl):s46–s54, 2005.

Galbraith RM, Hawkins RE, Holmboe ES: Making self-assessment more effective, *Journal of Continuing Education in the Health Professions* 28:20–24, 2008.

Glaser R: Instructional technology and the measurement of learning outcomes: Some questions, *American Psychologist* 18:519–521, 1963.

Hanauer DI, Hatfull GF, Jacobs-Sera D: *Active Assessment: Assessing Scientific Inquiry*, New York, 2009, Springer.

Hambleton RK, Swaminathan H, Rogers HJ: *Fundamentals of Item Response Theory*, Newbury Park, CA, 1991, Sage Press.

Kolen MJ, Brennan, RL: *Test Equating: Methods and Practices*, New York, 1995, Springer-Verlag.

Linacre JM: *Many-Facet Rasch Measurement*, Chicago, 1989, MESA Press.

Lord FM, Novick MR: *Statistical Theories of Mental Test Scores*, Reading MA, 1968, Addison-Wesley.

Norcini JJ: Setting standards on educational tests, *Medical Education* 37:464–469, 2003.

Norcini J, Boulet J: Methodological issues in the use of standardized patients for assessment, *Teaching and Learning in Medicine* 15(4):293–297, 2003.

Norcini J, Anderson B, Bollela V, et al: Criteria for good assessment: Consensus statement and recommendations from the Ottawa 2010

Conference, *Medical Teacher* 33:206–214, 2011.

Popham WJ, Husek TR: Implications of criterion-references measurement, *Journal of Educational Measurement* 6:1–9, 1969.

van der Linden WJ, Hambleton RK, editors: *Handbook of Modern Item Response Theory*, New York, 1997, Springer-Verlag.

van der Vleuten C: The assessment of professional competence: Developments, research and practical implications, *Advances in Health Science Education* 1:41–67, 1996.

Standard setting

J. Norcini, D. W. McKinley

Introduction

In medical education, it is common to need to identify knowledge or performance that is 'just good enough' for a particular purpose. One example is a pass or fail multiple-choice examination, where a single score is chosen as the cutoff. Passing examinees achieve that cutoff score or higher, while failing examinees do not. Passing implies sufficient knowledge or skill given the purpose of the test, while failing implies insufficient knowledge or skill. Standard setting is the process of demarcating the level of knowledge and skill indicating proficiency and identifying a score on the examination that corresponds to it.

Unlike many medical tests, educational assessments only rarely have a gold standard against which to establish the validity of a cutoff score. The nature of a 'competent' physician or 'unsatisfactory' medical student varies over time, place and many other factors. Consequently, standards on educational tests are the expression of judgement in the context of a particular assessment, its purpose and the wider social-professional environment.

Because standards are based on judgement, methods for selecting them are not intended to discover an underlying truth. Instead, they are a means for gathering a variety of perspectives, blending them together and expressing them as a single score on a particular assessment. Consequently, the methods do not differ in the correctness of the standards they yield, but in their credibility and defensibility. This chapter describes the types of standards, specifies the important characteristics of the standard setters and the methods, reviews some of the common methods for setting standards and provides a framework for evaluating their credibility (Norcini & Shea 1997, Norcini 2003, Norcini & Guille 2002).

Types of standards

There are two types of standards:

- relative
- absolute.

Relative standards are expressed in terms of the performance of a group of examinees. For instance, a relative standard may be that the 120 examinees with the highest scores are admitted to medical school. This type of standard is appropriate for assessments intended to select a certain number or percentage of examinees, such as tests for admissions or placement.

Absolute standards are expressed in terms of the performance of examinees against the test material. For instance, a passing score may be that any examinee who correctly answers 75% or more of the questions knows enough anatomy to pass. This type of standard is appropriate for assessments intended to determine whether examinees have the necessary knowledge or skills for a particular purpose, such as course completion or graduation from medical school.

Important characteristics of the standard setters and standard setting methods

The characteristics of the standard setters are likely to have the biggest impact on the credibility of a standard. The standard setters must understand the purpose of the test and the reason for establishing the cut score, know the content and be familiar with the examinees. In a low-stakes setting like a course, a single faculty member is credible, but standards will vary over time, and he or she has a conflict of interest in being both the teacher and assessor. In a high-stakes setting like licensure, a significant number of standard setters need to be involved because this increases the reproducibility of standards and reduces the effects of 'hawks' and 'doves'. Ideally, the group would be free of conflicts of interest, include a mix of educators and practitioners and be balanced with regard to gender, race, geography and the like.

The specific method chosen to set standards is not as important as whether it produces results that are fit for the purpose of the test, relies on informed expert judgement, demonstrates due diligence, is supported by a body of research and is easy to explain and implement.

FIT FOR PURPOSE

The method must produce standards that are consistent with the purpose of the assessment. Methods that turn out relative standards are to be used when the purpose is to select a specific number of examinees. Methods that turn out absolute standards are to be used when the purpose is to judge competence.

BASED ON INFORMED JUDGEMENT

Methods for setting standards can be based entirely on empirical results (e.g. consequences, performance on criteria), entirely on expert judgement or on a blend of the two. There are only rarely instances in which it is possible to base a standard entirely on empirical results in medical education, with the exception of a few admissions testing situations (where outcome data, like successful completion of a course, are available and relative standards are being used).

Instead, most of the methods allow a standard to be based solely on the judgement of experts, without reference to performance data (e.g. the difficulty of the questions, the pass rate). Moreover, standard setters sometimes become uncomfortable when data are presented, thinking that it 'biases' their judgements.

In fact, methods for setting standards are not intended to discover an essential truth but to create a credible standard out of the judgements of experts. Such credibility derives from decisions that are based on all of the available information. Consequently, methods that permit and encourage expert judgement in the presence of performance data are preferable.

DEMONSTRATES DUE DILIGENCE

Methods that require the standard setters to expend thoughtful effort will demonstrate due diligence and this lends credibility to the final result. In contrast, methods that require quick, global judgements are less credible, and methods requiring several days of effort are unnecessary.

SUPPORTED BY RESEARCH

Methods supported by a research literature will produce more credible results. Ideally, studies should show that standards are reasonable compared to those produced by other methods, reproducible over groups of judges, insensitive to potentially biasing effects and sensitive to differences in test difficulty and content.

EASILY EXPLAINED AND IMPLEMENTED

Credibility is enhanced if the method is easy to explain and implement. This decreases the amount of training required for the judges, increases the likelihood of their compliance and consistency and assures examinees that they are being treated fairly.

Methods for setting standards

There is a host of methods for setting standards, and many have variations. Reviews and descriptions are available elsewhere (Berk 1986, Cusimano 1996), but according to Livingston and Zieky (1982) they fall into four categories:

- relative methods
- absolute methods based on judgements about assessment content (assessment-centred)
- absolute methods based on judgements about individual examinees (examinee-centred)
- compromise methods.

All of the methods require that several standard setters be selected and that they meet as a group. As the name implies, relative methods produce relative standards and thus judgements are made about what proportion of the examinees should pass. The two groups of methods for setting absolute standards differ in the type of judgements that are being collected. In one group, the standard setters consider whether individual examinees should pass, and these judgements are aggregated to derive the cutoff. In the other group, the standard setters consider individual test questions, and these judgements are combined to calculate the cutting score. The compromise methods require judgements about both what proportion of the examinees should pass and what score they need to achieve to do so. The final result is a compromise between these two types of judgements.

RELATIVE METHODS

In the fixed-percentage method, each standard setter announces what percentage (or number) of examinees is qualified to pass. Their judgements are recorded for all to see, and they then engage in a discussion, often led off by those with the highest and lowest estimates. All are free to change, and when the discussions are over the estimates are averaged. The standard is that score which passes the average percentage (or number) of examinees.

In the reference group method, the process is exactly the same except that the standard setters have a particular group of examinees in mind (e.g. graduates of a certain set of schools or examinees with specific educational experiences). The selection of this reference group is based on the fact that the standard setters are most familiar with them and able to make good judgements about them. The cutting score established for this reference group is applied without modification to all other examinees.

These methods are quick and easy to use, they only have to be repeated occasionally, the standard setters are comfortable making the required judgements and they apply equally well to all different test formats. However, the standards will vary over time with the ability of the examinees, and they are independent of how much examinees know and the content of the test.

ABSOLUTE METHODS BASED ON JUDGEMENTS ABOUT TEST QUESTIONS (TEST-CENTRED)

The two most popular methods in this category have been proposed by Angoff and Ebel. Both methods require that the standard setters specify the characteristics of a borderline group of examinees. The borderline group excludes examinees who would clearly pass or fail and is composed of those about whom the standard setters are uncertain.

In Angoff's method, the standard setters estimate the proportion of the borderline group that would respond correctly to an item. These are discussed with all being free to change their estimates, and the process is repeated for all items on the test. To calculate the standard, the estimates for each item are averaged and the averages are summed (see Table 36.1). Often, as a 'reality check', examinee performance is provided as well. In this example, the percentage of all examinees choosing the correct option (p value) is provided.

In Ebel's method, the standard setters build a classification table for the items in the test. For example, they might decide to classify items by difficulty (easy, medium and hard) and frequency with which encountered in practice (common and uncommon). The standard setters then assign each item to one of the categories. After all items are assigned, they estimate the proportion of items in a category that borderline examinees will answer correctly (see Table 36.2). As with Angoff's method, a discussion ensues, and estimates can be changed. To determine the standard, the estimates for each category are averaged, multiplied by the number of items in the category, and summed.

These methods are widely used in high-stakes testing situations and there is a considerable body of research supporting this method. The standard setters review every item on the test, resulting in more informed judgements. However, the standard setters sometimes have difficulty envisioning the performance of a borderline group and so feel that they are simply making up numbers. These methods can also be time consuming for long tests.

Table 36.1 Application of Angoff's method to an eight-item test

Question	Standard setter					Judges' mean	Percent choosing correct option
	1	2	3	4	5		
1	.90	.85	.80	.75	.85	.83	0.90
2	.60	.55	.40	.35	.50	.48	0.50
3	.70	.60	.65	.50	.55	.60	0.70
4	.85	.75	.80	.65	.70	.75	0.70
5	.95	.90	.85	.75	.80	.85	0.80
6	.50	.50	.45	.40	.50	.47	0.50
7	.65	.55	.45	.45	.60	.54	0.45
8	.85	.70	.80	.65	.75	.75	0.70
Standard (cut score)						**5.27**	

The meeting of five standard setters begins with a discussion of the characteristics of a borderline group of students. When the standard setters reach consensus, they turn to a consideration of the first item. The standard setters each estimate aloud what proportion of the hypothetical borderline group would respond correctly to the question. Their estimates are written on a board for all to see and a discussion ensues, led by the standard setters with the highest and lowest estimates. All standard setters are free to change their estimates. The standard setters proceed in this manner through all of the items on the test. The cut score is taken as the sum of the standard setters' mean estimates for each question.

1. If the test is very long and security is not a major issue, have the standard setters meet and judge 30–40 items. Then ask them to do the remainder at home.

2. A reliable standard will result even when subsets of standard setters make judgements about subsets of the items on a test, as long as there are enough doctors involved.

3. If the standard setters have not taken the assessment, they should take it before the meeting because it prevents overconfidence and unrealistically high standards.

4. Give the standard setters the correct answers during the meeting unless they are overconfident. It prevents embarrassment.

In addition to establishing standards for individuals, the Angoff method has been used to set school-level standards (Stern et al 2006). Standards could be set to evaluate the relative strengths and weaknesses of a medical school's programme in providing adequate training and experiences to students based on established competencies (e.g. Tomorrow's Doctors, UK; CANMeds, Canada; ACGME Core Competencies, United States). To set school-level standards, standard setters developed a profile of the borderline school, reviewed assessment materials involved in setting student-level standards, and then were asked to estimate the percentage of students who would receive passing scores on each of the measures at a borderline school. Variations in judgements were discussed, and then standard setters were provided with consequential data for applying their initial standard to eight unidentified schools, and were permitted to change their judgements. In this study, each of the assessments addressed one of six competency domains but the method could easily apply to standard setting for other outcomes (e.g. course objectives).

To simplify use of the Angoff with OSCEs, a variation is to have judges estimate the station score that would be attained by the borderline examinee. These scores would be averaged for each station and summed to determine the standard. Methods focusing on global judgements of examinee performance have been increasingly studied for OSCEs, and an overview to those methods is provided in the next section.

ABSOLUTE METHODS BASED ON JUDGEMENTS ABOUT INDIVIDUAL EXAMINEES (EXAMINEE-CENTRED)

In the contrasting groups method, a random sample of examinees is drawn before the meeting. The entire test paper of each member of this randomly selected group is taken to the meeting and given, one at a time, to the standard setters. They decide as a group whether each performance is passing or failing. To calculate the standard, the scores of the passers and failers are graphed separately but on the same piece

Table 36.2 Application of Ebel's method to a 100-item test

Category	Average proportion correct	No. of questions	Expected score
Common			
Easy	.95	20	19
Medium	.80	40	32
Hard	.70	10	7
Uncommon			
Easy	.70	15	10.5
Medium	.50	10	5
Hard	.30	5	1.5
Standard (cut score)			75

The standard setters begin with a discussion of how the test questions should be classified; they choose two dimensions, frequency and difficulty. As a group, they go through all of the questions on the test one by one and place them into one of the categories (e.g. easy and common). The standard setters then discuss the characteristics of a borderline group of students. When the group reaches consensus on these characteristics, they turn to a consideration of the first category of questions. The standard setters each estimate aloud what proportion of the hypothetical borderline group would respond correctly to the questions in the category. Their estimates are written on a board for all to see and a discussion ensues, led by the standard setters with the highest and lowest estimates. All standard setters are free to change their estimates. When done, the group proceeds through the rest of the categories. To derive the cut score, the average proportion correct is multiplied by the number of questions in each category to produce expected scores. These expected scores are summed to calculate the standard.

of paper. The cutting score can then be derived in a variety of ways. For example, the point where the curve of the passers overlaps least with the curve of failers could be taken as the standard. Figure 36.1 provides an illustration.

Standard setters are usually comfortable making the judgements required by this method, and it has the advantage of informing them with the actual test performance of examinees. Further, by shifting where the standard is set, it is possible to maximize or minimize false-positive and false-negative decisions. However, it is difficult for the standard setters to produce a balanced judgement when the test is relatively long. In addition, a large number of examinees need to be judged to produce precise results.

In a variation that makes the contrasting groups method more efficient for an OSCE, the standard setters consider the performances of a sample of examinees on each case. They sort them into 'acceptable' and 'unacceptable' groups, identify the score separating them, and then sum these scores across all of the stations to arrive at the standard for the test.

The contrasting groups method was applied to teacher evaluations (Shea et al 2009), and the standard setters in this study were familiar with teaching responsibilities and qualities needed for promotion and appointment. They reviewed data obtained from learners by department, faculty rank and setting (i.e. classroom, clinical). Their task was to sort dossiers of teacher performance into four groups: 'superior', 'excellent', 'satisfactory' and 'unsatisfactory'. Cut scores for each category were established by calculating the means of all judges and identifying the mean between the average scores of two adjacent groups. For example, if the average score for 'superior' dossiers was 85% and the average score for 'excellent' dossiers was 80%, the cut score for the 'superior' category would be 82.5%. For those concerned with promotion (or remediation) of faculty, standard setting may aid data interpretation.

A technique proposed by Dauphinee et al (1997) combines elements of both the Angoff and contrasting groups methods. When physicians are used to observe and score OSCE stations, they can be asked to rate each examinee in such a way that borderline performances are identified. The scores of the examinees with these borderline performances are averaged and then combined over all the stations in the assessment. One potential disadvantage is that for small-scale OSCEs, it may be impossible to secure enough judgements of borderline performance to define a valid standard. To avoid this potential shortcoming, a method using the entire score range has been studied. In the 'borderline regression method', checklist scores are regressed on the global ratings (Kramer et al 2003, Wood et al 2006). This approach has the advantage of using ratings for all examinees, and the midpoint of the rating scale was used to predict the cut score for each station and then averaged to derive the test standard.

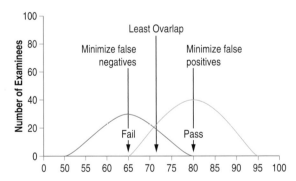

Fig. 36.1 Application of the contrasting groups method to a 100-item test. A sample of students is drawn at random, and the standard setters review the first student's answers to the entire test. After making a decision as a group about whether the performance merits a pass or a fail, the standard setters make similar decisions about the remaining students one by one. After judgements have been made about all the students, the scores of the failing group and passing group are graphed separately. The cut score is usually set at the point of least overlap between the two distributions, 72 in this example. If there is a need to minimize false negatives, the cut score is set at 65, and if there is a need to minimize false positives, it is set at 80.

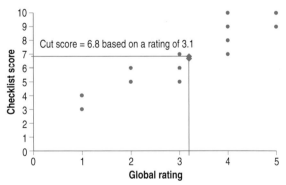

Fig. 36.2 Application of the borderline regression method to a single station. As part of scoring, judges (faculty members) provide a global rating of performance on the station (in this example, unacceptable, borderline, acceptable, good, superior). A regression analysis is run with ratings as the independent variable and checklist score as the dependent variable. The resulting equation is used to find the checklist score corresponding to a particular rating. In this case, the mean rating (3.1) was used, resulting in a station cut score of 6.81 out of 10.

A similar approach that has been studied involved having judges rate each performance as 'adequate' or 'inadequate'. A regression analysis was used to identify the station score at which 50% of the judges rated the peformance as 'adequate' and 50% rated the performance as 'inadequate' (McKinley et al 2005). An illustration of the borderline regression method for a single station is provided in Fig. 36.2. To the extent that the judgements are collected as part of the assessment, these methods are all simple to implement, provide consistent ratings, and have been shown to produce acceptable outcomes.

COMPROMISE METHODS

The Hofstee method is the most popular exemplar of this class of methods. The standard setters are asked to produce four judgements: the maximum and minimum acceptable pass rates and maximum and minimum acceptable cutoff scores. These judgements are discussed and changed, as with the other methods, and the final results for the four estimates are obtained by averaging across standard setters. The percentage of examinees who would pass for every possible value of the cut score on the test is graphed, and a rectangle is superimposed as defined by the four judgements of the standard setters. A diagonal is drawn through the box, and the standard is the point where it intersects the examinee performance curve. Figure 36.3 provides an illustration.

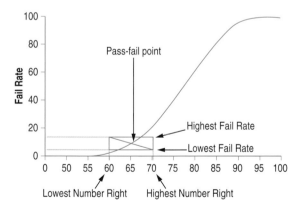

Fig. 36.3 Application of the Hofstee method to a 100-item test; the scores in this case are the numbers of items answered correctly. The standard setters are asked to answer four questions: What are the minimum and maximum acceptable fail rates, and what are the minimum and maximum acceptable cutoff scores? After a discussion where these estimates can be changed, means over all standard setters are calculated. These are graphed as a rectangle and a diagonal is drawn through it. The performance of the students is graphed, showing what the fail rate would be at each possible value for the cutoff.

This method is efficient, and the standard setters feel capable of making the judgements necessary for it. In some instances, however, the curve for examinee performance does not fall within the area circumscribed by the rectangle; in this case, the minimum or maximum acceptable pass rate is selected by default to provide a standard. Because it includes elements of a relative standard, this method is not ideal for regular use in a high-stakes setting. However, it is suitable occasionally, or for use in a low-stakes application.

 The contrasting groups method is especially useful when there is a need to directly manipulate the number of false-positive or false-negative decisions.

Putting it together

BEFORE THE MEETING

Prior to the meeting, the method for setting standards needs to be selected depending on the purpose of the test, the stakes and the resources available. Once this is done, the standard setters should be chosen to be broadly representative of the relevant perspectives. They should all review the assessment in detail so that they are familiar with the content and scoring. This is particularly important for the methods that do not require a review of the test as part of the standard setting process.

DURING THE MEETING

At the beginning of the meeting the methods should be explained to the standard setters. They should then engage in a discussion of the purpose and content of the test and the abilities of the examinees. These discussions are critical because they focus the standard setters on the task and guide them as they begin to make judgements. Once this discussion is completed, the standard setters should practise the method, where reasonable, with data that are not part of the test. Throughout the practice period and the remainder of the meeting, the standard setters should be given feedback about the consequences of their judgements (e.g. what percentage of examinees they would pass). It is important that all standard setters attend the entire meeting and that there are not interruptions. Absences, even for a short time, will generate missing data and could influence the standard more broadly by altering the discussion.

AFTER THE MEETING

Outliers

Common to all of the methods is the possibility that a standard setter with extreme views might significantly influence the results. Livingston and Zieky (1982) review methods for dealing with this problem, such as removing outlying judgements from the calculations or using the median instead of the mean. The removal of data should be a last resort, however, since it undermines the credibility of the process and the selection of standard setters.

Reliability

It is important to determine whether the results would be the same if the method was repeated with more or different standard setters. This is reliability or reproducibility; there are a variety of ways of calculating it, but generalizability theory offers a good alternative (Brennan & Lockwood 1980). If the results of this analysis are unacceptable given the purpose of the assessment, standard setters can be added in a second application of the method. The data from this second application should be combined with those of the first unless there were significant problems associated with it.

Outcomes

A standard that produces unreasonable outcomes (far too many or too few examinees pass) will not be viewed as credible regardless of the care with which it was derived. Therefore, it is important to collect data that support the fact that the stakeholders believe the standard is correct and that it has reasonable relationships with other markers of competence. For example, it would be supportive of the standard if the faculty generally believed that an appropriate number of students passed the summative assessment at the end of medical school. Moreover, it would be useful to gather evidence that the students who passed also performed well in the next phase of their training. In an assessment programme that continues over time, it is important to ensure that the stakeholders view the results as reasonable and that these results are related to the other indicators of proficiency.

Summary

A standard is a single score on a test that serves as the boundary between qualitatively different performances. These standards are an expression of judgement in the context of a particular assessment, its purpose and the wider social/professional environment. Consequently, methods for selecting them are a means for gathering a variety of perspectives, blending them together and expressing them as a single score. This chapter described the two types of standards, the characteristics that lead to their credibility, the more popular methods for setting standards and some efficient variations for use by medical educators.

References

Berk RA: A consumer's guide to setting performance standards on criterion-referenced tests, *Review of Educational Research* 56:137–172, 1986.

Brennan RL, Lockwood RE: A comparison of the Nedelsky and Angoff cutting score procedures using generalizability theory, *Applied Psychological Measurement* 4:219–240, 1980.

Cusimano MD: Standard setting in medical education, *Academic Medicine* 71:s112–s120, 1996.

Dauphinee WD, Blackmore DE, Smee S, et al: Using the judgements of physician examiners in setting standards for a national multi-center high stakes OSCE, *Advances in Health Sciences Education* 2:201–211, 1997.

Livingston SA, Zieky MJ: *Passing Scores: A Manual for Setting Standards of Performance on Educational and Occupational Tests*, Princeton, NJ, 1982, Educational Testing Service.

Kramer A, Muijtjens A, Jansen K, et al: Comparison of a rational and an empirical standard setting procedure for an OSCE. Objective structured clinical examinations, *Medical Education* 37:132–139, 2003.

McKinley DW, Boulet JR, Hambleton RK: A work-centered approach for setting passing scores on performance-based assessments, *Evaluation and the Health Professions* 28:349–369, 2005.

Norcini JJ: Setting standards on educational tests, *Medical Education* 37:464–469, 2003.

Norcini JJ, Guille RA: Combining tests and setting standards. In Norman G, van der Vleuten C, Newble D, editors: *International Handbook of Research in Medical Education*, Dordrecht, The Netherlands, 2002, Kluwer Academic, pp 811–834.

Norcini JJ, Shea JA: The credibility and comparability of standards, *Applied Measurement in Education* 10:39–59, 1997.

Shea JA, Bellini LM, McOwen KS, Norcini JJ: Setting standards for teaching evaluation data: An applicatin of the contrasting groups method, *Teaching and Learning in Medicine* 21:82–86, 2009.

Stern DT, Ben-David MF, Norcini JJ, et al: Setting school-level outcome standards, *Medical Education* 40:166–172, 2006.

Wood TJ, Humphrey-Murto SM, Norman GR: Standard setting in a small scale OSCE: a comparison of the modified borderline-group method and the borderline regression method, *Advances in Health Sciences Education Theory and Practice* 11:115–122, 2006.

Written assessments

L. W. T. Schuwirth, C. P. M. van der Vleuten

Introduction

Written assessments are probably the most widely used assessment methods in education. Their popularity is mainly due to their logistical advantages and their cost-effectiveness. In comparison with many other methods they are easy, they are cheap and they produce reliable scores. They are not a panacea, though; for comprehensive testing of competence a variety of written methods is needed.

 A variety of written and non-written methods of assessment are required to test medical competence comprehensively.

The purpose of this chapter is to provide some background information about the strengths and weaknesses of written assessment methods.

Question format

Often a distinction is made between open-ended and closed question formats.

 Response formats: Closed questions require candidates to select answers from a list of options. Open-ended questions require candidates to generate answers spontaneously.

Multiple-choice items are often deemed unfit for testing higher-order cognitive skills (e.g. medical problem solving) because the correct answer can be produced by mere recognition of the correct option (the so-called cueing effect). From the literature comparing response formats, however, it has become clear that the response format (open-ended or closed) is not so important, but that the stimulus (what you ask) is essential.

 "The positive cueing effect is considered as a disadvantage of the MCQ, and has been documented consistently. However, MCQs apparently also cue in the opposite direction: they can lead the examinee to choose the wrong answer."

Schuwirth et al 1996

Consider, for example, the following two questions regarding the response format:

You are a general practitioner, and you have made a house call on a 46-year-old patient. She appears to have a perforated appendix, and she shows signs of a local peritonitis. Which is the best next step in the management?

and

You are a general practitioner and you have made a house call on a 46-year-old patient. She appears to have a perforated appendix and she shows signs of a local peritonitis. Which of the following is the most appropriate next step in the management?

1. *Give pain medication and re-assess her situation in 24 hours.*
2. *Give pain medication and let her drive to the hospital in her own car.*
3. *Give no pain medication and let her drive to the hospital in her own car.*
4. *Give pain medication and call an ambulance.*
5. *Give no pain medication and call an ambulance.*

In these two questions there is very little difference in what is asked, whereas the way the response is recorded differs.

Now consider these two questions regarding stimulus format:

What is the most prevalent symptom of meningitis?

and

Make a SWOT analysis of the government's regulations to reduce the waiting lists in the healthcare system.

In these questions the response format is similar, but the content of the question is completely different. In the second question the expected thought processes are completely different from those evoked by the first.

 Stimulus formats: The content of a question will determine the thought processes required to answer it.

For the rest of this chapter we will therefore use the distinction between response formats and stimulus formats.

Quality control of items

No matter which assessment format is used, the quality of the examination is always related to the quality of the individual items. Therefore, it is of no use discussing strengths, weaknesses and uses of various item types if we cannot assume that optimal care has been taken to ensure their quality. One aspect of the quality of an item is its ability to discriminate clearly between those candidates who have sufficient knowledge and those who do not. So they are a 'diagnostic for medical competence'. This implies that when a student who has not mastered the subject matter answers a question correctly, this can be regarded as a false-positive result, and the opposite would signify a false-negative result. In quality control procedures, prior to test administration, the diagnosis and elimination of sources of false-positive and false-negative results are essential. In addition, the relevance of the items, the congruence between curricular goals and test content, and the use of item analysis and student criticisms are other important factors in quality control of assessment, but in this chapter we will focus on quality aspects of the individual items.

Response formats

SHORT-ANSWER OPEN-ENDED QUESTIONS

Description

This is an open-ended question type which requires the candidate to generate a short answer of often no more than one or two words. For example:

Which muscle origin is affected in the condition 'tennis elbow'?

When to use and when not to use

Open-ended questions generally take some time to answer. Therefore, fewer items can be asked per hour of testing time. There is a relationship between the reliability of test scores and the number of items, so open-ended questions can lead to less reliable scores per hour of testing time. Also, they need to be marked by a content expert, which makes them logistically less efficient and more costly. For these reasons the advice is to use short-answer open-ended questions preferably only if closed formats would not do.

A question such as:

Which kidney is positioned superior to the other one?

is not very sensible. Theoretically, there are only two possible answers, so the content prescribes a two-option multiple choice.

On the other hand, a question like:

In elderly people with vague complaints of fatigue, thirst and poor healing of wounds, which diagnosis should be thought of spontaneously?

would be odd in a multiple-choice format.

In general, the advice concerning the use of short-answer open-ended questions is not to use them unless the content of the question requires it.

Tips for item construction

Use clearly phrased questions. Reading errors may not be what you want to test, and may thus be a source of error. Therefore, use short sentences and avoid double negatives. If in doubt as to whether to use more words for clarity, or fewer words for brevity it is best to opt for more clarity.

Make sure a well-defined answer key is written. Correct and incorrect answers must be clarified and possible alternative answers must be identified (perhaps by a panel of examiners) beforehand. This is especially necessary if more than one person will be correcting the test papers.

Make sure that it is clear to the candidates what kind of answer is expected. A disadvantage of open-ended questions may be that it is unclear to the candidates what kind of answer is expected, for example, about the required level of detail. As an illustration, for a question on chest infection, the expected answer could be pneumonia, bacterial pneumonia or even pneumococcal pneumonia. There may also be a lack of clarity about what type of answer is expected, as for example in:

What is the main difference between the left and right lung?

Is the expected answer here that one is a mirror image of the other, the number of lobes, the angle of the main bronchus, the surface or the contribution to gas exchange?

Indicate a maximum length for the answer. Students often apply a 'blunderbuss' approach, which means that they will write down as much as they can in the hope that part of their response will be the correct answer. By limiting the length of the answer this can be prevented.

Use multiple correctors effectively. If more than one teacher is involved in correcting the test papers, it is better to have one corrector score the same item(s) for all students and another corrector score another set of items for all students than to have one corrector score the whole test for one group of students and another the whole test for another group of students. In the latter case a student can be advantaged by a mild corrector or be disadvantaged by a harsh one; in the former the same group of examiners will be used to produce the scores for all students, which leads to a better reliability with the same effort.

 For short-answer open-ended questions, it should be clear beforehand what would be correct answers and what would be incorrect answers.

ESSAY QUESTIONS

Description

Essay questions are open-ended types of questions that require a longer answer. Ideally, they are used to ask the candidate to set up a reasoning process, to evaluate a given situation or specifically to apply learnt concepts to a new situation. An example is:

John and Jim, both 15 years old, are going for a swim in the early spring. The water is still very cold. John suggests seeing who can stay under water longest. They both decide to give it a go. Before entering the water John takes one deep breath of air, whereas Jim breaths deeply about 10 times and dives into the cold water. When John cannot hold his breath any more he surfaces. Much to his shock he sees Jim on the bottom of the swimming pool. He manages to get Jim on the side, and a bystander starts resuscitation.

Explain at the pathophysiological level what has happened to Jim, why he became unconscious, and why this has not happened to John.

Of course, it is important that the situation of John and Jim is new to the students, and that it has not already been explained during the lectures or practicals. A question such as:

Explain the Bohr effect and how it influences the O_2 saturation of the blood.

is therefore less suitable as an essay type of question. Although the knowledge asked may be relevant, the question asks for reproduction of factual knowledge, which is more efficiently done with other formats.

When to use and when not to use

It is essential to use essay questions only for specific purposes. The main reason for this is the lower reliability and the need for hand-scoring. Essay questions are therefore best used when the answer requires spontaneous generation of information and when more than a short text is required. Examples are:

- Evaluating a certain action or situation, for example:

  Make a SWOT analysis of the government's new regulations to reduce waiting lists in the healthcare system.

- Application of learnt concepts on a new situation or problem, for example:

  During your course you have learnt the essentials of the biofeedback mechanism of ACTH. Apply this mechanism to the control of diuresis.

- Generating solutions, hypotheses, research questions

- Predicting or estimating

- Comparing, looking for similarities or discussing differences.

 It can be difficult to score answers submitted as an essay without being influenced by the student's literary style.

Tips for item construction

For essay questions, essentially the same item construction suggestions apply as for short-answer open-ended questions:

- The question must be phrased extremely clearly; the candidate must not be left in the dark as to what is expected.

- The answer key must be well-written, including alternative correct answers and plausible but incorrect answers. This must not be simply left to the corrector.

- The maximum length of the answer must be stipulated, to ensure a concise response and avoid the 'blunderbuss' approach.

A special type of essay question is the modified essay question. This consists of a case followed by a number of questions. Often these questions follow the case chronologically. This can lead to the problem of interdependency of the questions: if candidates answer the first question incorrectly, they are likely to answer all subsequent parts of the question incorrectly also. This is a psychometric problem which can only be avoided by an administrative procedure in which the candidates hand in the answers before they are allowed to proceed to the next question.

Currently, the key-feature approach of case-based assessment, which will be discussed below, is more popular.

TRUE–FALSE QUESTIONS

Description

True–false questions are statements for which the candidate has to indicate whether the given answer is true or false. For example:

> **Stem:** *For the treatment of a* Legionella pneumophila *pneumonia, a certain antimicrobial agent is most indicated. This is:*
> **Item:** *erythromycin True/False*

The first part, the stem, is information that is given to the candidate. It is always correct, so the candidates do not have to include it in their considerations. The item is the part for which the candidate has to indicate whether it is true or false.

When to use and when not to use

True–false questions can cover a broad domain in a short period of time, leading to broad sampling. They are often used for testing of factual knowledge, and this is probably what they are most suited for. Nevertheless, they have some inherent disadvantages. First, they are difficult to construct flawlessly. Careful item construction is needed to ensure that the answer is defensibly true or false. This often leads to artificial phrasing. For example:

> **Stem:** *Certain disorders occur together more often than is to be expected on the basis of pure coincidence. This is the case for:*
> **Item:** *diabetes and atherosclerosis True/False*

A second disadvantage is that when candidates answer a false-keyed item correctly, one can only conclude that they knew that the statement was untrue, and not necessarily that they would have known what would have been true. For example, the following question:

> **Stem:** *For the treatment of an acute gout attack in elderly patients, certain drugs are indicated. Such a drug is:*
> **Item:** *allopurinol True/False*

If a candidate answers 'false', one cannot conclude that they would have known which drugs are indicated.

Tips for item construction

Use stems when necessary. It is useful to put all information that is not part of the question in the stem. This way it is clear to the candidate what should and should not be considered. Also, with this method most item construction flaws are avoided.

Avoid semiquantitative terminology. Words such as 'often' and 'seldom' are difficult to define. Different people assign different meanings to those words, so whether the answer is 'true' or 'false' is then a matter of opinion and not of fact. In such cases one has to revert to statements indicating exact percentages, such as:

> **Stem:** *In a certain percentage of patients with acute pancreatitis the disease is self-limiting.*
> **Item:** *This percentage lies closer to 80% than to 50%.*

Avoid terms that are too open or too absolute. Words such as 'can', 'is possible', 'never' and 'always' lead test-wise students to the correct answer. The most probable answer to statements which are too open is 'true', and the most probable answer to statements which are too absolute is 'false'. The same applies to equality, synonymy, etc.

Make sure the question is phrased so that the answer is defensibly correct.

> **Stem:** *The cause of atherosclerosis is:*
> **Item:** *hypercholesterolaemia*

In this case one could argue that there are many causes or that there is a chain of aetiological factors that cause atherosclerosis. In such a case, for example, it would be better to ask for risk factors than causes.

Avoid double negatives. This is especially important in true–false questions, as the answer key 'false' can be seen as a negative also. Unfortunately, this cannot be avoided in all cases.

> **Stem:** *For patients with hypertension, certain drugs are contraindicated. Such a drug is:*
> **Item:** *corticosteroids False*

The double negative 'contraindicated' and 'false' (answer key) cannot simply be removed by using the combination 'indicated' and 'true', because then the question would not be correct.

MULTIPLE-CHOICE QUESTIONS

Description

This is certainly the most well-known item format. It is often also referred to as single-best-option multiple-choice or A-type. These questions consist of a stem, a question (called the lead in) and a number of options. The candidate has to indicate which of the options is correct.

> **Stem:** *During resuscitation of an adult, compressions of the thorax have to be performed to produce circulation. For this, one hand has to be placed on the sternum and the other has to be placed on this hand in order to give correct compressions.*

Lead-in: *Which of the following options indicates the most correct position of both hands?*
Options:

1. *the junction between manubrium and sternum*
2. *the superior half of the sternum*
3. *the middle of the sternum*
4. *the inferior half of the sternum*
5. *the xiphoid process of the sternum.*

When to use and when not to use

Multiple-choice items can be considered the most flexible question type. Although they may not always be simple to produce flawlessly, they are easy to administer. Answering and scoring are not time-consuming, and they are logistically efficient. They are best used if broad sampling of the domain is required and if large numbers of candidates are to be tested. They yield fairly reliable testing scores per hour of testing time. The two main situations in which multiple-choice questions should not be used are:

- when spontaneous generation of the answer is essential (this is explained in the paragraph on short-answer open-ended questions)
- when the number of realistic options is too large.

In all other cases, multiple-choice questions are a good alternative to open-ended questions.

Tips for item construction

The general tips mentioned in the preceding section all pertain to multiple-choice questions as well (clear sentences, defensibly correct answer key, etc.), but there are some tips that apply uniquely to multiple-choice questions. The first is to use equal alternatives.

Sydney is:

a. *the capital of Australia*
b. *a dirty city*
c. *situated at the Pacific Ocean*
d. *the first city of Australia.*

In this case the options all relate to different aspects. In order to produce the correct answer the candidate has to compare apples to oranges. A better and more focused alternative would be:

Which of the following is the capital of Australia?

a. *Sydney*
b. *Melbourne*
c. *Adelaide*
d. *Perth*
e. *Canberra.*

Use options of equal length. Often the longest option is the correct one, because often more words are needed to make an option correct than to make it incorrect. Students know this and will be guided by this hint.

Avoid fillers. Unfortunately, it is often prescribed to have four or five options where only three realistic ones can be found, leading to nonsense options (fillers). There is much to be said against this:

- Candidates will recognize the fillers and discard them immediately.
- You will underestimate the guessing chance.
- It will take a lot of item-writing time to find the extra option before you decide on the filler copy (this time would better be used for another question).
- Authors may use combination options ('all of the above' or 'none of the above') instead, which is ill-advised.

Use simple multiple-choice formats only.

The major symptoms associated with cardiovascular disease:

1. *are chest pain, dyspnoea, palpitations*
2. *appear to worsen during exertion*
3. *are fatigue, dizziness and syncope*
4. *appear during rest*
a. *(1), (2) and (3) are correct*
b. *(1) and (3) are correct*
c. *(2) and (4) are correct*
d. *only (4) is correct*
e. *all are correct.*

In this case the question is unnecessarily complicated. Not only can it lead to mistakes in choosing from all the combinations – which has nothing to do with medical competence – but the combinations could also give important clues as to which answer is correct simply by logic. The rule for these formats is simple: do not use them.

Try to construct the question in a way so that theoretically the answer could also be given without seeing the answer options. This ensures that there is a clear and well-defined lead in and that all the alternatives are aimed at the same aspect. So after a stem or case description, the lead in *Which of the following is true?* is too open, but the lead in *Which of the following is the most probable diagnosis?* is well-defined and could theoretically be answered as if it were an open-ended question.

MULTIPLE TRUE–FALSE QUESTIONS

Description

In this question format more than one option can be ticked by the candidate. There are two versions. In the first, candidates are told how many options they should select; in the second, this is left open. The former is used when there is no clear distinction between correct and incorrect, for example:

Select the two most probable diagnoses.

The latter version is used if there is a clear distinction, for example:

Select the drugs that are indicated in this case.

Scoring of such items can be done in various ways. The standard approach is to treat all options as true–false items and then regard a ticked option as 'true' and the others as 'false'. The score on the item is the total of correctly ticked and nonticked options divided by the total number of options. An alternative scoring system is to indicate a minimum of correct answers for a score of 1 and to score all other responses as 0.

When to use and when not to use

This format is best used when a selection of correct options from a limited number of options is indeed required, and when short-answer open-ended questions cannot be used.

Tips for item construction

There are no specific tips concerning this question type other than those applying to multiple-choice and short-answer open-ended questions.

Stimulus formats

EXTENDED-MATCHING QUESTIONS

Description

Extended-matching items consist of a theme description, a series of options (up to 26), a lead in and a series of short cases or vignettes.

Theme: *diagnosis*
Options:

a. *hyperthyroidism*

b. *hypothyroidism*

c. *prolactinoma*

d. *hyperparathyroidism*

e. *phaeochromocytoma*

f. *Addison's disease*

g. *…etc.*

Lead in: *For each of the following cases, select the most likely diagnosis.*
Vignettes: *A 45-year-old man consults you because of periods of extensive sweating. One or two times per day he has short periods during which he starts sweating heavily. His wife tells him that his face is all red. He feels very warm during this period.*

He has had this now for over 3 weeks. At first he thought the complaints would subside spontaneously, but now he is not sure any more. Pulmonary and cardiac examination reveal no abnormalities. His blood pressure is 130/80, pulse 76 regular.

When to use and when not to use

Because the questions ask for decisions and the stimuli are cases, extended-matching items focus more on decision making or problem solving. The large number of alternatives reduces the effect of cueing. Because the items are relatively short and can be answered quickly, extended-matching questions cover a large knowledge base per hour of testing time. They are best used in all situations where large groups of candidates have to be tested in a logistical and feasible way.

Tips for item construction

First, determine the theme. This is important because it helps to focus all the alternatives on the same element. To minimize the influence of cueing it is important that all the options could theoretically apply to all vignettes.

The options should be short. The shorter and clearer the options, the less likely it is that any hints as to the correct answer may be given. It is best to avoid using verbs in the options.

The lead in should be clear and well-defined. A lead in such as 'for each of the following vignettes select the most appropriate option' is too open and often indicates that the options are not homogeneous or the vignettes are not appropriately related to the options.

 In constructing extended-matching questions:

- Determine the theme first.

- Keep the individual options short.

- Ensure that the lead in is clear and well-defined.

KEY-FEATURE APPROACH QUESTIONS

Description

Another format is the key-feature approach. It consists of a short, clearly described case or problem and a limited number of questions asking essential decisions. Such tests can consist of many different short cases, enabling a broad sampling of the domain and thus fairly reliable test results per hour of testing time. They have also been demonstrated to be valid for the assessment of medical decision making or problem solving. Sometimes, certain response formats are prescribed, but they can also be used with various response formats depending on the content of the question.

For key-feature approach questions:

- All the important information must be presented in the case.
- The question must be directly linked to the case.
- The question must ask for essential decisions.

Tips for item construction

Apart from all the tips concerning the other question types, some tips are specifically pertinent to key-feature tests.

Make sure all the important information is presented in the case. This means not only relevant medical information, but also contextual information (where you see the patient, what is your function, etc.). After you have written the questions, it is a good idea to re-address the case to check whether all the necessary information is provided.

Make sure the question is directly linked to the case. It should be impossible to answer the question correctly if the case is not read. Ideally, all the information in the case must be used to produce the answer, and the correct answer is based on a careful balancing of all the information.

The question must ask for essential decisions. An incorrect decision must automatically lead to an incorrect management of the case. In certain instances the diagnosis may not be the key feature, for example, if different diagnosis would still lead to the same management of the case. Another way to check this is to see whether the answer key would change if certain elements of the case (such as location of the symptoms or age of the patient) were to be changed.

"It has proven to be ill-advised to make up cases without consulting others."

Schuwirth et al 1999

SCRIPT CONCORDANCE TEST QUESTIONS

Description

Based on cognitive expertise theory, Charlin and co-workers (2000) developed the script concordance test (SCT). Such tests use ill-defined problems and a method called aggregate scoring that takes expert variability into account. A clinical scenario in which not all data are provided for the solution of the problem is presented, and a menu of options is presented from which the candidate may score the likelihood of each option in relation to the solution of the problem on a +2 to −2 scale. An example is:

A 25-year-old male patient is admitted to the emergency room after a fall from a motorcycle

with a direct impact to the pubis. Vital signs are normal. The X-ray reveals a fracture of the pelvis with a disjunction of the pubic symphysis.

If you were thinking of:

Urethral rupture

And then you find:

Urethral bleeding

This hypothesis becomes:

−2 −1 0 +1 +2

SCT tests have good reliability per hour of testing time and good validity for its purpose. SCT has been specifically designed to test clinical reasoning.

Tips for item construction

Many of the tips mentioned above are relevant to constructing SCT items. Clear phrasing of the vignettes is essential, as well as careful selection of the considered diagnoses and associated symptoms. The developers of this format recommend the use of expert teams to construct such items and the scoring key.

"A final piece of advice would be the suggestion . . . to look for the possibility of cooperation with other departments or faculties since the production of high quality test material can be tedious and expensive."

Schuwirth et al 1999

Summary

It must be stressed again that there is no one single best question format; for a good and comprehensive assessment of medical competence, a variety of instruments is needed. This chapter has provided a brief overview of various written question formats with some of their strengths and weaknesses and some hints for their use. The reference and further reading lists suggest more detailed literature.

References

Charlin B, Rogh, Brailovsky, et al: The script concordance test: a tool to assess the reflective clinician, *Teaching and Learning in Medicine* 12:185–191, 2000.

Schuwirth LWT, van der Vleuten CPM, Donkers HHLM: A closer look at cueing effects in multiple-choice questions, *Medical Education* 30:44–49, 1996.

Schuwirth LWT, Blackmore DB, Mom EMA, et al: How to write short cases for assessing problem-solving skills, *Medical Teacher* 21:144–150, 1999.

Further reading

Bordage G: An alternative approach to PMPs: the 'key-features' concept. In Hart IR, Harden R, editors: *Further Developments in Assessing Clinical Competence. Proceedings of the Second Ottawa Conference*, Montreal, 1987, Can-Heal Publications, pp 59–75.

Cantillon P, Hutchinson L, Wood D, editors: *ABC of Learning and Teaching in Medicine*, London, 2003, BMJ Publishing Group.

Case SM, Swanson DB: Extended-matching items: a practical alternative to free-response questions, *Teaching and Learning in Medicine* 5:107–115, 1993.

Case SM, Swanson DB: *Constructing Written Test Questions for the Basic and Clinical Sciences*, Philadelphia, 1998, National Board of Medical Examiners.

Farmer EA, Page G: A practical guide to assessing clinical decision-making skills using the key features approach, *Medical Education* 39:1188–1194, 2005.

Schuwirth LWT: *An Approach to the Assessment of Medical Problem Solving: Computerised Case-Based Testing*, Maastricht, 1998, University of Maastricht.

Swanson DB, Norcini JJ, Grosso LJ: Assessment of clinical competence: written and computer-based simulations, *Assessment and Evaluation in Higher Education* 12:220–246, 1987.

Performance and workplace assessment

L. Etheridge, K. Boursicot

Introduction

The apprenticeship model of medical training has existed for thousands of years: the apprentice learns from watching the master, and the master, in turn, observes the apprentice's performance and helps them improve. Therefore, performance assessment is not a new concept. However, in the modern healthcare environment, with its discourse of accountability, performance assessment has an increasing role in ensuring that professionals maintain the knowledge and skills required for practice. A number of international academic and professional bodies have incorporated performance assessment into their overall assessment frameworks for licensing, training and continued professional development. In the United States, the Medical Licensing Examination (USMLE) makes use of a structured test of clinical skills in the second stage of the licensing assessment. In the UK and Australasia, the main Royal Colleges have assessment frameworks for trainees that include a portfolio of workplace-based assessment (WPBA) tools.

The terms performance and competence are often used interchangeably. However, competence should describe what an individual is *able to do*, while performance should describe what an individual *actually does in clinical practice*. Clinical competence is the term being used most frequently by many of the professional regulatory bodies and in the educational literature. There are several dimensions to competence, and a wide range of well-validated assessments have been developed examining these. Traditional methods focus on the assessment of competence in artificial settings built to resemble the clinical environment. However, more novel methods of performance assessment concentrate on building up a structured picture of how the individual practitioner acts in his or her everyday working life, in interactions with patients and other practitioners, using technical, professional and interpersonal skills. Miller's model, shown in Fig. 38.1, provides a framework for understanding the different facets of clinical competence and the assessment methods that test these.

 "Competence describes what an individual is able to do... while performance should describe what an individual actually does in clinical practice."

Boursicot et al 2011

In this chapter we will look at the different methods used to assess clinical performance, which we will define as the assessment of clinical skills and behaviours in both academic and workplace settings. These methods fall in the top two layers of Miller's pyramid. We will discuss how and why they are used and some of the practical aspects to be considered for educators wishing to make use of them. We will also explore the strengths and weaknesses of the various tools and consider some of the outstanding issues concerning their use.

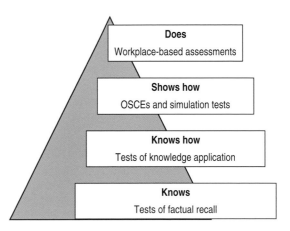

Fig. 38.1 Miller's model of competence (adapted from Miller: *Academic Medicine* 65(suppl):S63–S67, 1990.).

Choosing the right assessment

When planning assessments, it is important to be aware of the purpose of the assessment and where it fits into the wider educational programme: a tool is only as useful as the system within which it resides. Considerations would include how to make pass/fail decisions, how to give feedback to candidates, effects on the learning of candidates and whether the assessment is 'high-stakes'. For example, assessments for the purpose of certification may require different criteria than some medical school assessments, where the primary purpose is to encourage and direct the learning of students (Downing 2003).

In considering the best tools for the purpose of a particular assessment system, educators need to evaluate their validity, reliability, educational impact and acceptability (Schurwith & van der Vleuten 2009).

Validity has been classically regarded as the answer to the question 'Does this assessment tool measure what it is intended to measure?' Evidence to support the validity of an assessment has to be gathered from various sources to support the use of the assessment in any particular context. Evidence includes:

- Demonstrating that the content of the assessment relates meaningfully to the learning outcomes

- Demonstrating that the quality of the items has been rigorously appraised

- Demonstrating that the results (scores) accurately reflect the candidates' performance

- Demonstrating that the statistical (psychometric) properties of the assessment are acceptable. This includes the reproducibility of the assessment, as well as item analyses (such as the difficulty of each item and the discrimination index).

Reliability is a measure of the reproducibility of the scores of an assessment, so that the outcome is the same if the assessment is repeated over time. There are various mathematical models for calculating a reliability coefficient, the commonest being Cronbach's alpha.

Generalizability is a form of reliability measure which takes into account the conditions of a typical objective structured clinical examination (OSCE), where not all the candidates see the same patients, and are not all examined by the same examiners.

Educational impact is important to consider, as inevitably assessments will influence students' learning strategies. Aligning the content of any assessment to the desired learning objectives would be a useful way to encourage students to attend to the most important outcomes. Other factors such as timing, outcomes (e.g. pass/fail) and format of the assessment will also influence student behaviours.

Acceptability and cost-effectiveness are important features to consider when setting up an assessment system. The administrative setup required to manage a robust and defensible system must be planned and supported, with due regard for costs. The issue of having sound educationally based systems and high quality has to be balanced against such costs. Acceptability extends to not only whether the candidates and examiners believe in the system of assessment, but also other stakeholders such as regulatory bodies, employers and members of the public.

Assessments of clinical competence

Assessments of what a student or doctor is *able to do* can take place in artificial settings and have the advantage of being able to examine a number of individuals at the same time. The best known of these types of assessment is the OSCE.

OBJECTIVE STRUCTURED CLINICAL EXAMINATION (OSCE)

What is it? An OSCE consists of a series of structured stations around which a candidate moves in sequence. At each station specific tasks have to be performed, usually involving clinical skills such as history taking, clinical examination or practical skills. Different degrees of simulation may be used to test a wide range of psychomotor and communication skills, using simulated patients, part-task trainers, charts and results, resuscitation manikins or computer-based simulations. There is a time limit for each station, and the marking scheme is structured and determined in advance.

 When designing an OSCE, the fundamental principle is that every candidate completes the same task in the same amount of time and is marked using the same schedule.

How is it used? The OSCE is typically used in high-stakes summative assessments at both the undergraduate and postgraduate level. The main advantages are that large numbers of candidates can be assessed in the same way across a range of clinical skills. High levels of reliability and validity can be achieved in the OSCE due to four main features (Newble 2004):

- Structured marking schedules, which allow for more consistent scoring by assessors

- Multiple independent observations collected by different assessors at different stations, so individual assessor bias is lessened

- Wider sampling across different cases and skills, resulting in a more reliable picture of overall competence
- Completion of a large number of stations, allowing the assessment to become more generalizable

Overall, candidate scores are less dependent on who is examining and which patient is selected than in traditional long case or *viva voce* examinations. The key to reliability is the number of stations; the more stations marked by different examiners there are, the more reliable the OSCE will be. However, this has to be balanced with practicality, as clearly the longer an OSCE, the more onerous it will be for all involved.

Organization: OSCEs can be complex to organize. Planning should begin well in advance of the examination date, and it is essential to ensure that there are enough patients, simulated patients, examiners, staff, refreshments and equipment to run the complete circuit for all candidates on the day of the exam. Careful calculations of the numbers of candidates, the length of each complete circuit and how many circuits have to be run need to be made. The mix of stations is chosen in advance and depends on the curriculum and the purpose of the assessment. A blueprint should be drawn up which outlines how the assessment is going to meet its goals. An example of a simple blueprint, detailing the different areas of a curriculum and how the stations chosen will cover these, can be seen in Fig. 38.2. Development of a blueprint ensures adequate content validity, the level to which the sampling of skills in the OSCE matches the learning objectives of the whole curriculum. It is also necessary to think about the timing of the stations. The length of the station should fit the task requested as closely as possible. Ideally, stations should be practised in advance to clarify this and anticipate potential problems with the setup or the mark sheet. Thought also has to be given to the training of assessors and standardized or simulated patients.

 "To allow insufficient time for the preparation of an OSCE is to court disaster and if the examination is to be successful advanced planning is essential."

Harden & Gleeson 1979

Outstanding issues: The OSCE has been developed and adapted since it was originally described. The last 10 years has seen an increase in the development of high-fidelity simulation technology for use in medical education. This permits reproduction of complex conditions at any time and allows individuals and teams to practise their skills and management and gain formative feedback. However, the use of complex simulators in high-stakes summative assessment is still being evaluated. The original description of OSCE marking schemes advocated checklist style mark sheets, where assessors ticked off the various elements of the task as they were performed. The advantage of this method is the reduction of assessor bias and improvement of inter-rater reliability. However, recent debate has questioned the suitability of this for expert practitioners, who are more likely to have moved away from strictly prescribed and regimented practice (Hodges et al 1999). Global rating scales are increasingly being developed, which take a more holistic approach to scoring and allow for variation in practice and style. The consensus currently is that checklists are more suited to the early novice stage of practice and global ratings are better at capturing increasing levels of clinical expertise (Boursicot et al 2011). Thought is also being given to who is best placed to do the scoring. In most parts of the world clinician assessors

	History	Examination	Health promotion	Practical skills
Cardiovascular	History of palpitations			ECG interpretation
Respiratory	History of breathlessness		Smoking cessation advice	
Gastro		Abdominal examination	Explain high-fibre diet	
Neuro		Gait examination		Lumbar puncture on manikin

Fig. 38.2 Example of an OSCE blueprint.

will complete the mark sheets. However, in some countries, such as the United States, scoring by standardised patients is common practice. As with all elements of assessment, consideration needs to be given to the purpose of the test and what is being assessed. If the main goal of the station is to test communication skills with patients, then a patient assessor may be the most appropriate person to judge this. However, if a complex practical task is being assessed, then a clinician with knowledge of the procedure will be better placed. Some institutions will combine clinician and patient assessments in their scoring method.

OTHER ASSESSMENTS OF CLINICAL COMPETENCE

A disadvantage of the OSCE is that candidates only spend short amounts of time at each station and undertake part tasks rather than complete clinical encounters. The Objective Structured Long Case Examination Record (OSLER) attempts to address this by holistic appraisal of the candidate's ability to interact, assess and manage a real patient without the bias and variability associated with the traditional long case (Gleeson 1997). In the OSLER candidates are assessed throughout history, examination and communication with a standardized patient. Two examiners review the case in advance and use a structured marking schedule. The OSLER is more reliable than the traditional long case, but a large number of different cases are needed to achieve the sort of reliability required for a high-stakes summative assessment.

Assessing performance in the workplace

Assessment of what a doctor *does in practice* requires assessment within the workplace. This raises a number of issues, as clearly traditional tests of competence cannot be transplanted easily into busy clinical environments. It is vital that these assessments are feasibly carried out without too much disruption to clinical work or patient care. Using a wide range of WPBA tools helps identify strengths and weaknesses in different areas of practice, such as technical skills, professional behaviour and team working. The main tools described in the literature and in use in medical education are outlined here, although individual institutions have developed a variety of other tools to fit their own specific needs.

 "There has been concern that trainees are seldom observed, assessed, and given feedback during their workplace-based education. This has led to an increasing interest in a variety of formative assessment methods that require

observation and offer the opportunity for feedback."

Norcini & Burch 2007

MINI CLINICAL EVALUATION EXERCISE (MINI-CEX)

What is it? The Mini-CEX was developed by the American Board of Internal Medicine to assess the clinical skills of residents, particularly focused history taking and physical examination. An assessor directly observes the practitioner's performance in 'real' clinical encounters with patients in the workplace. He or she then discusses diagnosis and management with the practitioner and gives them feedback on the encounter. The practitioner is judged in a number of clinical domains and on his or her overall clinical care. The average Mini-CEX encounter takes around 15–25 minutes. Immediate feedback is then given, which helps identify strengths and weaknesses and improve skills (Norcini 2003).

How is it used? As part of a programme of WPBA, the Mini-CEX should be performed on multiple occasions with different patients and different assessors. There have been several studies in different clinical specialties looking at the optimum number of Mini-CEX encounters to reliably assess performance. While there is good evidence of its reliability, most studies have looked at use of the Mini-CEX in experimental rather than real-life settings. This makes it possible for one performance to be assessed by multiple assessors, something that is not practical in real clinical settings. Generally, between 10 and 14 encounters are needed to show good reliability, if assessed by different assessors and on multiple patients (Boursicot et al 2011). However, the number of encounters possible in real clinical practice settings needs to be balanced against the need for reliability.

Strengths and weaknesses: High satisfaction rates have been reported by both assessors and assessees. The perceived educational impact of the Mini-CEX is high due to its ability to provide opportunities for structured feedback, giving practitioners the potential to correct their weaknesses and develop as professionals (Weller et al 2009). Increasing the interaction between junior and senior doctors may also enable monitoring of progress and identification of educational needs.

 "Feedback can change physicians' clinical performance when provided systematically over multiple years by an authoritative, credible source."

Veloski et al 2006

The Mini-CEX appears able to discriminate effectively between junior and senior trainees, with more senior doctors attaining higher clinical and global competence scores (Norcini et al 1995). In addition, it is relatively feasible within the workplace, being centred on real patients and clinical encounters. However, scheduling a Mini-CEX does require commitment by both the trainee and the senior doctor. Time constraints and lack of motivation in busy clinical settings may make completing assessments difficult and stressful. The reported inter-rater reliability of the Mini-CEX is variable, even among same assessor groups. There is also variation in scoring across different grades of assessor, with studies showing that trainees tend to score Mini-CEX encounters more leniently than consultants (Kogan et al 2003). Inter-rater variations can be reduced, with more assessors rating fewer encounters, rather than few assessors rating multiple encounters. Formal assessor training may also help, but the evidence for this is variable, with some studies showing that training makes very little difference to scoring consistency and others reporting more stringent marking and greater confidence following assessor training (Boursicot et al 2011). Finally, the purpose of the Mini-CEX within a programme of WPBA needs to be clarified. If the goal of the programme is to demonstrate satisfactory progress only, then fewer encounters will be needed. However, if the goal is to discriminate sufficiently between trainees to allow ranking, then a greater number of encounters is required, limiting feasibility.

CASE-BASED DISCUSSION (CBD) OR CHART-STIMULATED RECALL (CSR)

What is it? The CBD in the UK and Australasia, or CSR in North America, is a structured interview in which practitioners discuss aspects of a case in which they have been involved in order to explore their underlying reasoning, decision making and ethical understanding. It can be used in a variety of settings, such as clinics, wards or assessment units, and different clinical problems can be discussed. The practitioner selects suitable cases and gives his or her written records of these to the assessor in advance. It is expected that the practitioner will select cases of varying complexity. He or she then presents the case to the assessor, who asks questions to probe his or her clinical reasoning and professional judgement. The practitioner is scored in a number of domains, mapped to the competencies expected within the programme of training. A CBD will usually take around 15–20 minutes for presentation and discussion with 5–10 minutes afterwards for feedback (Davies et al 2009).

How is it used? As with other WPBA tools, repeated encounters are required to obtain a valid picture of a practitioner's level of development. Again, though, this has to be balanced with the practicalities of a busy clinical setting. The Royal College of General Practitioners in the UK asks trainees to complete a minimum of six CBDs in each of the first 2 years of training and 12 in the final year, but other Royal Colleges require different numbers. There are data available for the CSR which show good reliability. A comparison with different assessment methods has shown that assessment carried out using the CSR is able to differentiate between doctors in good standing and those identified as poorly performing (Boursicot et al 2011).

Strengths and weaknesses: As with all WPBAs, the evidence regarding the true costs of the CBD is scarce. Direct costs include training of all assessors and central administration of WPBA records, but there are also costs associated with assessor and practitioner time in theatres, clinics and wards. There is also little published research on the educational impact of the CBD. However, as with other WPBAs, the opportunity for specific and timely feedback is thought to be valuable in helping learners progress.

DIRECT OBSERVATION OF PROCEDURAL SKILLS (DOPS)

What is it? DOPS is a method of assessment developed by the Royal College of Physicians in the UK specifically for assessing practical skills. The practitioner is directly observed by an assessor while undertaking a procedure on a real patient. Specific components of the procedure are judged and then feedback is given after the event. The mean observation time for DOPS varies according to the procedure assessed and, on average, feedback time takes an additional third of the procedure observation time (Wilkinson et al 1998).

How is it used? Many of the UK Royal Colleges now incorporate DOPS into their programmes of WPBA. Some use a generic score sheet, looking at overall aspects of procedural skill, while others have developed specific score sheets related to the procedure under assessment. There is a wide variety of skills that can be assessed with DOPS, from simple procedures such as venepuncture to more complex procedures such as endoscopy. Again, organizations vary in their expectations of trainees and which type of procedures should be assessed and how often.

Strengths and weaknesses: As with the Mini-CEX and CBD/CSR, DOPS needs to be repeated on several occasions for it to be a reliable measure of performance. Scores have been shown to increase between the first and second half of a training year, indicating validity (Davies et al 2009). In surveys, the majority of practitioners feel that DOPS is a fair method of assessing procedural skills and that it is practical and feasible (Wilkinson et al 1998). There is little current research on the educational impact of DOPS, but again the opportunity for feedback gives it important potential as an educational tool.

MULTISOURCE FEEDBACK (MSF)

What is it? The goal of MSF, or 360° assessment, is to collect the structured judgements of those who work with, or have experience of, the practitioner and feed these back in a systematic way, building up a picture of individual practice. Judges can include both senior and junior colleagues, nurses, administrative staff, medical students and patients, depending on the tool used. All judges remain anonymous, and their scores and comments are fed back to the trainee. Comparable assessment tools have been used in industry for nearly 50 years.

How is it used? Two similar instruments have been used in the UK to evaluate doctors in training. The Sheffield Peer Review Assessment Tool (SPRAT) was validated in paediatric trainees (Archer et al 2005). The mini Peer Assessment Tool (mini-PAT) was developed for more junior doctors based on the SPRAT and has been used by the UK Foundation School. The aim of the mini-PAT is to assess behaviours and attitudes such as communication, leadership, team working and reliability (Archer et al 2008). It is these sorts of attributes that are often best judged by multisource feedback tools. The mini-PAT is primarily meant as a formative form of assessment, allowing the doctor to reflect on the feedback received in order to improve his or her clinical performance.

Strengths and weaknesses: One of the main advantages of MSF is its anonymity, encouraging honest opinions. The main criticisms are that feedback is delayed and lacking specificity because of the anonymous nature. Inter-rater variance has been reported, with consultants tending to give lower scores. However, the longer the consultants have known the doctor, the more likely they are to score them higher. Senior doctors achieve a small but statistically significant higher overall mean score compared to more junior doctors, demonstrating construct validity (Lockeyer 2003). There are potential disadvantages to MSF tools as well, including risk of discrimination and potentially damaging feedback, which may need to be managed. However, MSF can be used as part of a programme of WPBA to inform personal development, especially regarding professional and interpersonal skills.

 To be of the most value, assessments within the workplace should capitalize on the rich diversity of clinical practice and build up an authentic picture of the practitioner over time.

Outstanding issues in WPBA

 "Workplace-based assessment brings a unique set of challenges to medical education and requires fresh thinking about how we consider and construct assessment programmes."

Swanwick & Chana 2009

WPBA tools are now well-described in many different areas of medicine, and a number of institutions make use of these in their programmes of assessment. However, a number of issues remain unresolved, and there continues to be some resistance amongst practising clinicians to their use. Although the goal of WPBA is to assess what a clinician does in practice, formalizing practitioner observation in a structured way does have the effect of reducing practice to the 'shows how' level of Miller's pyramid and may not reflect real life. This, to some extent, seems unavoidable, but as WPBA becomes more integrated into clinical life this effect may be diminished. However, there is still work to be done on how to incorporate the practice of WPBA into busy clinical environments with minimal disruption and maximum benefit and ensure its acceptability to all stakeholders. While most of the research on reliability and validity of WPBA has been done in experimental settings, it remains difficult to determine how it is best used in real-life settings, in different grades and different clinical specialties. Institutions need to be clear about the purpose of their programmes of WPBA: are they purely for formative purposes, or will the results be used to guide progression? Is their goal to ensure the 'bare minimum' level of performance, or are they being used to rank trainees? Without clarity from institutions, both trainees and trainers will feel confusion. Research so far is focused on their use as formative rather than summative tools, although it is not always clear that this is how they are being used in practice. There is some evidence that trainees are finding the culture shift in assessment hard to adapt to. There is an expectation that all WPBAs should be clearly 'passed' from the start, rather than using them to demonstrate competency progression over time. This can lead to trainees fitting all their assessments into the end of a placement rather than using the assessment and its accompanying feedback as a tool to facilitate improvement over the course of a placement.

While all the tools described above are widely used in postgraduate assessment around the world, their use is becoming more widespread in the undergraduate arena. The issues here remain largely the same, with a need for clarity of purpose and use of a battery of tools over time to build up a holistic picture of the student's strengths, weaknesses and progression.

Summary

The valid and reliable assessment of performance requires the use of a number of different assessment methods, each with its own strengths and weaknesses, which enable a complete picture of the practitioner to be developed. This is becoming increasingly important in a world where professionals are required to demonstrate competence. In undergraduate and postgraduate academic settings, the OSCE is a well-validated method that is widely used in high-stakes, summative assessment for licensing and progression. In the workplace, a number of instruments have been developed which offer insight into different aspects of clinical performance and can be used for formative feedback to guide professional development. Institutions need to consider their assessment strategies and goals and make the best use of the different methods available, in order that educators can be trained and guided in their use.

References

Archer J, Norcini J, Davies H: Use of SPRAT for peer review of paediatricians in training, *British Medical Journal* 330(7502):1251–1253, 2005.

Archer J, Norcini J, Southgate L, et al: Mini PAT: A valid component of a national assessment programme in the UK? *Advances in Health Sciences Education* 13(2):181–192, 2008.

Boursicot K, Etheridge L, Setna Z, et al: Performance in assessment: Consensus statement and recommendations from the Ottawa conference, *Medical Teacher* 33:370–383, 2011.

Davies H, Archer J, Southgate L, Norcini J: Initial evaluation of the first year of the Foundation Assessment Programme, *Medical Education* 43:74–81, 2009.

Downing S: Validity: on the meaningful interpretation of assessment data, *Medical Education* 37(9): 830–837, 2003.

Gleeson F: Assessment of clinical competence using the objective structured long examination record (OSLER), *Medical Teacher* 19:7–14, 1997.

Harden R, Gleeson F: Assessment of clinical competence using an objective structured clinical examination (OSCE), *Medical Education* 13(1): 39–54, 1979.

Hodges B, Regehr G, McNaughton N, et al: OSCE checklists do not capture increasing levels of expertise, *Academic Medicine* 74(10):1129–1134, 1999.

Kogan J, Bellini L, Shea J: Feasibility, reliability, and validity of the mini-clinical evaluation exercise (mCEX) in a medicine core clerkship, *Academic Medicine* 78(10):33–35, 2003.

Lockeyer J: Multisource feedback in the assessment of physician competencies, *Continuing Education in the Health Professions* 23(1):4–12, 2003.

Newble D: Techniques for measuring clinical competence: Objective structured clinical examinations, *Medical Education* 38(2):199–203, 2004.

Norcini J: Work based assessment, *British Medical Journal* 326(5):753–755, 2003.

Norcini J, Blank L, Arnold G, Kimball H: The mini-CEX (clinical evaluation exercise): A preliminary investigation, *Annals of Internal Medicine* 123(10):795–799, 1995.

Norcini J, Burch V: Workplace-based assessment as an educational tool: AMEE Guide No. 31, *Medical Teacher* 29:855–871, 2007.

Schurwith L, van der Vleuten C: How to design a useful test. In: *Understanding Medical Education: Evidence, Theory and Practice*, Dundee, 2009, Association for the Study of Medical Education.

Swanwick T, Chana N: Workplace based assessment, *British Journal of Hospital Medicine* 70(5):290–293, 2009.

Veloski J, Boex J, Grasberger M, et al: Systematic review of the literature on assessment, feedback and physicians clinical performance: BEME Guide No. 7, *Medical Teacher* 28(2):117–128, 2006.

Weller J, Jolly B, Misur M, et al: Mini-clinical evaluation exercise in anaesthesia training, *British Journal of Anaesthesia* 102(5):633–641, 2009.

Wilkinson J, Crossley J, Wragg A, et al: Implementing workplace-based assessment across the medical specialties in the United Kingdom, *Medical Education* 42(4):364–373, 1998.

Chapter

39

Section 6:
Assessment

Portfolio assessment

E. W. Driessen, S. Heeneman, C. P. M. van der Vleuten

Introduction

In less than two decades, portfolios have gained a prominent position in medical education. The portfolio owes its popularity to its suitability for attaining goals that are difficult to achieve with other educational methods: monitoring and assessing competency development and nontechnical skills, such as reflection. In this way the portfolio is in keeping with recent developments in education, such as outcome-based education and competency-based learning. This chapter discusses the lessons we have learned from 20 years of experience with portfolios in medical education. We will focus on four topics:

- the objectives and contents of portfolios
- success factors for portfolios
- portfolio assessment
- a concrete example of an assessment procedure.

We will especially focus on the assessment of portfolios. In an earlier publication we focused on the portfolio as a coaching method (Driessen et al 2010). The assessment principles and strategies we will describe in this chapter not only apply to portfolios but have broader applications. They can also be used for other complex assessments, such as assessment of projects or papers, such as a master's thesis.

 The objective of the portfolio, and consequently its format and content, can vary markedly.

The objectives and contents of portfolios

Learners, residents, doctors and teachers are regularly asked to compose a portfolio. The objective of the portfolio, and consequently its format and content, can vary markedly. We distinguish the following main objectives for portfolios:

- *Guiding* the development of competencies. The learner is asked to include in the portfolio a critical reflection on his or her learning and performance. The minimal requirement for this type of portfolio is the inclusion of reflective texts and self-analyses.

- *Monitoring* progress. The minimum requirement for this type of portfolio is that it must contain overviews of what the learner has done or learned. This may be the numbers of different types of patients seen during a clerkship or the competencies achieved during a defined period.

- *Assessment* of competency development. The portfolio provides evidence of how certain competencies are developing and which level of competency has been achieved. Learners often also include an analysis of essential aspects of their competency development and indicate in which areas more work is required. This type of portfolio contains evidential materials to substantiate the level that is achieved.

 Most portfolios are aimed at a combination of goals.

Most portfolios are aimed at a combination of goals and therefore comprise a variety of evidence, overviews and reflections (Fig. 39.1). Portfolios thus differ in objectives, and the objectives determine which component of the portfolio content is emphasized. Portfolios can also differ in scope and structure (Van Tartwijk et al 2003). Portfolios can be wide or narrow in scope. A limited scope is appropriate for portfolios aimed at illustrating the learner's development in a single skill or competency domain or in one curricular component. An example is a portfolio for communication skills of undergraduate students. A portfolio with a broad scope is aimed at demonstrating the learner's development across all skills and competency domains over a prolonged period of education.

At the end of this chapter we will describe an example of this type of portfolio.

Portfolios also differ in the degree of structuring or guidance that is provided to the learner in composing the portfolio. This dimension is characterized by the contrast between an open and a closed portfolio. A closed portfolio has to comply with detailed guidelines and regulations and offers relatively little freedom to learners with respect to the format and content of the portfolio. As a consequence, portfolios of different learners are highly comparable and the portfolios are easy to navigate.

 Portfolios with a closed structure are highly comparable while portfolios with an open structure allow learners the opportunity to display their individual learning trajectories and competencies.

A more open portfolio gives general directions, but allows the learners freedom with respect to the actual contents and format of the portfolio. The framework is described in such a way that learners are given a choice about how they present their individual learning process and learning results. A uniform basic structure is nevertheless important, because teachers and peers who have to view several portfolios should be able to easily follow the general structure of the materials. An advantage of an open portfolio is that it offers learners the opportunity to reveal their individual learning trajectories and competency development.

We have explained that portfolios can contain overviews, evidential materials and reflection. We have

located these elements on the corners of a triangle (Fig. 39.1). We will now focus on the format and place of each of these elements in the portfolio.

OVERVIEWS

When learners are following more distinct routes in a curriculum it becomes increasingly difficult for learners, teachers and supervisors to keep track of their progress. In order to facilitate this, many portfolios contain overviews to be used by learners to show what they have done, where they have done it, what they have learned as a result and how they are planning to proceed. Overviews may contain the following information:

- Procedures or patient cases. Which procedures? What was the level of supervision? Which types of patients? What was learned? Were the activities assessed? Plans?

- Prior work experience. Where? When? Which tasks? Strengths and weaknesses? Which competencies or skills were developed? Evaluation by the learner?

- Prior education and training. Which courses or programmes? Where? When? What was learned? Completed successfully? Evaluation by the learner?

- Experiences within and outside the course/programme. Where? When? Which tasks? What was done? Strengths and weaknesses? Which competencies or skills were developed? Evaluation by the learner? Plans?

- Components of the course/programme. Which attended at this point? Which not (yet) attended? When? What was learned? Completed successfully? Evaluation by the learner? Plans?

- Competencies or skills. Where addressed? Level of proficiency? Plans? Preferences?

MATERIALS

Portfolios can contain a variety of of materials. We distinguish three different types:

- Products, such as reports, papers, patient management plans, letter of discharge, critical appraisals of a topic

- Impressions, such as photographs, videos, observation reports

- Evaluations, such as test scores, feedback forms (e.g. Mini-CEX), letters from patients or colleagues expressing appreciation, certificates.

The nature and diversity of the materials determine the richness of the picture learners present of their learning and progress. It can be tempting for learners to include a vast amount of materials, leaving it up to the assessor to determine their value. This not

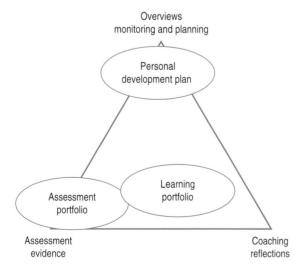

Fig. 39.1 Purposes and content of portfolios.

only increases the assessors' workload, but also can mean that assessors are unable to see the wood for the trees. It is therefore important for learners to be selective. A good selection criterion is that materials should provide insight into the student's learning and progress. We will discuss the size and feasibility of portfolios later in this chapter.

 Learners can use captions to indicate the context in which the material was collected or produced, its relevance and why it was included.

REFLECTIONS

Many portfolios contain reflections. These are often organized around the competencies to be demonstrated by the learner in the portfolio. They can relate to one or more strengths and areas requiring more work for one competency, or they can be extensive reflective essays describing the learner's personal profile. The latter type of reflection can pertain to the learner's motivation for attending the programme, the objectives the learner wishes to attain and/or the learner's views of him- or herself as a doctor/professional. These reflections can be used by learners as a long-term agenda. Learners support their reflections by referring to materials and overviews in the portfolio. This is important not only to convince others of the validity of the reflections, but also to focus the reflections, because learners are likely to aim for consistency of reflections and evidential materials. This makes the reflections less noncommittal. It is, for instance, not acceptable for learners to simply state that they have learned how to give a clinical presentation. They will have to substantiate this statement by evidential materials and overviews demonstrating why and how they have done this.

Success factors for portfolios

 Mentoring is of the essence for portfolio use.

Despite the simplicity of the portfolio concept – a learner documents the process and results of his or her learning activities – the portfolio has proved to be not invariably and automatically effective. The literature on portfolios shows mixed results. The key question here is what makes a portfolio successful in one situation and less successful in another situation? A number of reviews have shed light on some key factors (Buckley et al 2009, Driessen et al 2007, Tochel et al 2009).

MENTORING

Mentoring is of the essence for portfolio use. The mentor gives feedback on the portfolio, ensures depth of learning and helps the learner to identify learning needs and formulate learning objectives. Learners tend to stop working on their portfolio when they receive no feedback or when they are not questioned about their analyses. The mentor may be a teacher or a peer. Mentoring can take place in one-on-one meetings or in mentor groups. It is important that mentors are prepared for their task. Mentoring requires a coaching approach, which is different from the approach customarily taken by teachers when they are teaching and/or supervising patient contacts.

FEASIBILITY

Feasibility should also be considered. Learners and teachers can easily come to see work on the portfolio as burdensome paperwork. Portfolios can be sizeable, and the work for portfolios often comes on top of other tasks. Excessive workload can be prevented by a number of simple precautions. Firstly, learners should be stimulated to be selective in including materials in their portfolio. Portfolio content is only informative if it is relevant to learning and competency development. This requires that it is clearly explained to learners what is expected from them. The competencies to be achieved, the criteria, the content and purpose of the portfolio must be clearly communicated to both learners and teachers. Modern electronic portfolios sometimes aggregate information from the portfolio to the different competencies, giving users a quick overview of competency development. One mouse click suffices to view the original materials. An example is an electronic portfolio for work-based assessment (www.epass-maastricht.nl).

PERCEIVED USEFULNESS

The learner must experience direct benefit from working on the portfolio. When self-direction is required in a programme, the usefulness of the portfolio will be self-evident to learners. Residents, for instance, are largely responsible for their own learning in the clinical workplace. Using the portfolio as a starting point for discussing their work and progress can support that learning. Residents can ask for feedback and arrange for more time to be scheduled for matters that are relevant to their learning. This will motivate them to work on their portfolio. If little self-direction is required, for instance, when the programme consists of lectures and working groups, learners can only too easily come to the conclusion that the portfolio is of little real use to them.

Perceived usefulness also depends on how well the portfolio is embedded in the overall programme. If the portfolio is an integral part of the curriculum and is purposefully used for learning, it will have more value in the eyes of the learners than when it is just another educational activity. A final factor that can contribute to the educational value of the portfolio is the degree to which it accommodates differences between learners. When learners can present their individual profiles in the portfolio, they are more likely to value its usefulness.

 Learners must experience direct benefit from working on their portfolio

Portfolio assessment

If there is one area in which the portfolio has shown remarkable development in recent years, it is in the way it is assessed. The traditional, psychometric approach to assessment, characterized by standardization and analytical assessment criteria to achieve objective judgements, has proved incompatible with the non-standardized nature of portfolios. Content and format of portfolios vary with the learners, and this runs counter to standardization.

In addition to numerical information (scores), portfolios also contain a variety of qualitative information. Besides technical skills, portfolios are used to assess the softer skills. Weighing the information in a portfolio to assess a competency, such as professionalism, demands of assessors that they use their own judgement to interpret the information. This kind of judgement task is difficult to translate to an analytical assessment procedure using a standardized checklist with numerous strictly defined criteria.

To match assessment with the characteristics of the portfolio, we advocate an approach based on the methodology of qualitative research (Driessen et al 2005). Qualitative research also requires interpretation of different kinds of qualitative information in order to arrive at meaningful statements about ill-defined problems.

The concept of trustworthiness is at the centre of qualitative research: various procedural measures can ensure that the research is sufficiently rigorous to justify confidence that the conclusions are supported by the data. The principles and methods for evaluating the quality of qualitative research can be translated to principles and procedures for assessing portfolios (Driessen et al 2005). The following assessment strategies can be used with portfolios.

INCORPORATE FEEDBACK CYCLES

Incorporate in the procedure intermittent feedback cycles to ensure that the final judgement does not come as a surprise to the learners. Since the contents of a portfolio are usually collected over a longer period of time, it is inadvisable to wait until the end of the period to make pronouncements about the quality of the portfolio. Intermediate formative assessments, such as feedback from a mentor, allow learners to adapt and improve their portfolio. Not only from an assessment perspective but also from a mentoring perspective, is it advisable to give feedback at various stages of the portfolio. As we remarked earlier, users will be tempted to stop working on their portfolio if they do not receive feedback.

 Incorporate intermittent feedback cycles to ensure that the final judgement does not come as a surprise to the learners.

OBTAIN MULTIPLE SOURCES OF FEEDBACK

Information for the assessment should be obtained from different people who are involved in the portfolio process one way or another. In addition to the assessors who judge the portfolio at the end of the period, others can be involved in the assessment as well. This enables triangulation of different judgements for the final assessment. We already mentioned that a portfolio is usually the result of work done over a longer period of time. In fact, the portfolio is not just a finished product – a file or web page containing materials – but it is first and foremost a process during which learners document their development over a (prolonged) period of time.

Different people who are involved in the portfolio process can also contribute to the assessment. It is the mentor who first advises about the quality of the portfolio. He or she often knows the learner best, is able to determine the authenticity of the materials and is familiar with the learner's work habits. Peers are another group that can be involved in the assessment. The advantage of peer assessment is that peers know from experience what it means to produce a portfolio, and by engaging in peer assessment they can familiarize themselves with the assessment standards for the portfolio.

Learners can also be asked to judge the quality of their own portfolios. They could, for instance, be asked for their reaction to the mentor's recommendation and/or to self-assess their different competencies. Self-assessment by learners supported by recommendations from the mentor can lead to better validated self-assessments. From the self-assessment literature we know that self-assessments tend to be biased. Eva and Regehr therefore recommended that learners should be encouraged to actively seek information about their performance to arrive at well-validated self-assessments (Eva & Regehr 2008).

SEPARATE THE ROLE OF THE MENTOR AND ASSESSOR

Separate the multiple roles of assessors by removing the summative assessment decisions from the coaching task. In relation to the previous item, we argued the wisdom of involving the mentors in portfolio assessment, because they possess relevant information. However, learners should also have a safe learning climate in which they feel free to discuss the weaknesses of their portfolio with their mentor. It is therefore advisable that mentors should not be required to make the final summative decisions. Such decisions should be the responsibility of a separate assessment committee. In an earlier publication, we described four scenarios for the role of the mentor in assessment (Van Tartwijk & Driessen 2009). This role can range from full responsibility for assessment to a role that is strictly limited to coaching.

- *The teacher* This is the most common assessment scenario in education. Just like most teachers in primary, secondary and higher education, mentors discuss their learners' performance and progress and assess their level of competence at the end of a course.

- *PhD supervisor* In some scenarios the role of the mentors in the assessment procedure of portfolios is comparable to the role of the supervisors of PhD students. In many countries, formal assessment of theses/portfolios is the responsibility of a committee. Supervisors invite their peers to sit on the committee, of which they themselves are not a member. A negative assessment of the thesis/portfolio would harm their reputation among their peers. For this reason they are highly unlikely to invite their peers to sit on the committee unless they are convinced the portfolio meets the criteria. As a consequence, mentors and learners have a shared interest: to produce a thesis or portfolio that merits a positive judgment.

- *Driving instructor* In this model the roles of the mentor and the assessor are strictly separated. The mentor/driving instructor coaches the learner in achieving the required competencies, which are shown in the portfolio. If the mentor thinks the learner is sufficiently competent, he or she invites an assessor from a professional body (e.g. the examiner from the Driver and Vehicle Licensing Agency) to assess the competencies of the learner. It is also possible for learners to take the initiative to approach the licensing agency themselves.

- *Coach* In this model, the learners take the initiative. They can, for instance, ask a senior colleague to coach them until they have achieved the required level of competence. This scenario is appropriate, for instance, when a professional wants to obtain an additional qualification. The assessor would be someone from an external body.

 Separate the multiple roles of assessors by removing the summative assessment decisions from the coaching task.

TRAIN THE ASSESSORS

Organize a meeting of the assessors (before the assessment round and at an intermediate stage of the portfolio period) in which they can calibrate their assessments and discuss the assessment procedure and its results. Assessing the vast amounts of very diverse information in portfolios hinges on professional judgement. Assessors use assessment criteria idiosyncratically. Judgement depends, for instance, on prior experience with assessment and individual notions and beliefs about education and the competencies to be judged. Differences between assessors can be reduced by organizing discussions between assessors. As a result of discussing a benchmark portfolio, assessors' interpretations of assessment criteria will tend to converge, and a joint understanding of the procedure to be followed can emerge. It is advisable to organize such discussions not only immediately before an assessment round but also at an intermediate stage of the portfolio period when assessors can compare their own portfolio judgements with those of their colleagues and discuss differences of interpretation. After the final assessment the assessors can be given information about all the assessments to gain a better understanding of the entire process.

 Differences between assessors can be reduced by organizing discussions between them.

USE A SEQUENTIAL PROCEDURE

Organize a sequential assessment procedure in which conflicting information necessitates the gathering of more information. At Maastricht Medical School a procedure has been developed to optimize efficient use of the time available for assessment (Driessen et al 2005). The mentor makes a recommendation for the assessment of the portfolios of his or her students. The learner and an assessor decide whether they agree with this recommendation. If they agree, the assessment procedure is completed. If they do not agree, the portfolio is submitted to a larger group of assessors. In this way, when there is doubt about the assessment of a portfolio, the portfolio is judged more carefully than portfolios whose assessment is straightforward. This gives stronger guarantees of trustworthy assessment, because, in cases of doubt, more judges are consulted. The discussions between the assessors will also promote clarity with respect to the application of the criteria (see also under the heading training of assessors).

REQUEST NARRATIVE INFORMATION

Incorporate in the portfolio requests to provide qualitative, narrative feedback and give this information substantial weight in the assessment procedure.

Narrative comments offer learners and judges much richer information than quantitative, numerical feedback. A score of 7 on a 10-point scale, for instance, gives little insight into what a learner has done well and what he or she has not done well. Only when strengths and weaknesses of performance are supported by narrative feedback does assessment become truly informative. An additional problem with workplace assessment is rater leniency. There are various reasons why low scores are rarely given in practice. As a result, scores do not discriminate well, and narrative feedback will often provide better information about the learner's competency development. Narrative feedback can be facilitated by providing a blank space at the top of the assessment form to insert descriptions of strengths and weaknesses.

PROVIDE QUALITY ASSURANCE

Quality assurance must be built into the procedure:

- Offer learners the possibility to appeal against assessment decisions.
- Carefully document the different steps of the assessment procedure (a formal assessment plan approved by an examination board, overviews of results).
- Organize quality assessment procedures with an external auditor.

USE RUBRICS

Education institutions often put a great deal of energy into formulating competency profiles. The important thing is to strike a balance between long lists of concrete criteria detailing all the things a learner must be able to do (can-do statements) on the one hand, and global descriptions offering a general outline but little practical guidance on the other hand. In other words, the trick is to find the right balance between analytical and global criteria. This can be done by giving learners and assessors an idea of the expected level for each global competency. Rubrics are very useful in this respect (an example is given in Table 39.1). They typically contain descriptions of each competency at different levels, such as the level to be expected from a novice, from a competent professional and from an expert.

An example of a portfolio assessment procedure

From our own experience with portfolios we have learned that many people do not feel comfortable with the high level of abstraction of some of the assessment principles, and as a consequence have difficulty applying them in their own practice. Below we illustrate how the principles can be applied by

Table 39.1 Rubrics used for the assessment of final-year medical students

	Below expectation	As expected	Above expectation
Clinical performance (for instance as judged by Mini-CEX)	Slow in taking a history and performing a physical examination. Considers irrelevant aspects. Slow in making a diagnosis. Misses important conclusions. Frequently unable to formulate management plan and needs considerable guidance.	Adequate speed in taking a history and performing a physical examination. Relevant aspects are considered. Adequate speed in making a diagnosis. Diagnosis contains important conclusions. Formulates an adequate management plan for simple clinical presentations. Needs some guidance. Achieves these goals in the second half of the internship.	Conducts an adequate and efficient history and physical examination. Arrives at an accurate diagnosis within adequate time. Formulates an adequate management plan for simple clinical presentations. Needs little guidance. Has achieved these goals at the start of the internship.
Professionalism (for instance, as judged by 360-degree feedback)	Does not keep appointments. Occasionally fails to ask for supervision when this is necessary. Reacts defensively to feedback. Is unable to cope with stress. Does not pay attention to his or her personal appearance. Frequently shows inappropriate behaviour or behaves disrespectfully.	Keeps appointments. Asks for supervision when this is necessary. Needs help in reflecting and considering alternatives and responds adequately to feedback. Occasionally needs help in coping with stress. Appropriate personal appearance; behaves respectfully.	Keeps appointments. Asks for supervision when this is necessary. Is able to reflect critically; responds adequately to feedback and is prepared to acknowledge errors. Is able to cope with stress adequately. Looks well cared for and behaves respectfully.

Source: Maastricht University

teachers in the practice of portfolio assessment. We do so by giving a concrete description of an assessment procedure based on the assessment principles outlined above.

We will use the portfolio of the Maastricht research master Physician–Clinical Investigator as an example of an assessment procedure based on the principles of qualitative research. The procedure is inspired by the Cleveland Clinic Lerner College of Medicine portfolio and the Maastricht Medical School portfolio (Dannefer & Henson 2007, Driessen et al 2005). The portfolio in question is broad in scope. During the whole study period it is the central point for coaching, monitoring and assessing students. All assessments go into the portfolio, and all summative decisions are taken with the help of the portfolio. This means that per study year all credit points for assessments are linked to the portfolio assessment. The portfolio is labour intensive, but all the information about assessment, monitoring of progress and mentoring is collected in this one portfolio. The portfolio is completely integrated into the learning environment. It is not an activity that is simply added on to the normal work for students and teachers.

The student collects all (narrative) feedback, evaluations, judgements and assessments in the electronic portfolio. In Box 39.1 we present the feedback, evaluations and assessments collected by the student during a given period. The student regularly uses the information in the portfolio to write a reflection on his or her competency development. The student discusses the portfolio with his or her mentor. The mentor is an experienced teacher trained to coach students. The mentor attends regular peer debriefing meetings for mentors. Halfway through each study year, a second mentor is present at the student–mentor meeting. This serves several purposes:

- peer debriefing for the mentor
- independent feedback for the student from another mentor
- an intermediate recommendation for the final assessment at the end of the year (based on the content of the portfolio at the time of the meeting).

Near the end of the final semester, the mentor makes a recommendation for the final assessment of the portfolio. The student indicates whether and why he or she agrees or disagrees with the recommendation. The team of mentors, excluding the student's mentor, assesses the student's portfolio, taking into account the mentor's recommendation and the student's reaction. The recommendation of the mentor team is submitted to the independent Portfolio Examination Committee. Two members of this committee independently assess the portfolio. If they disagree, the portfolio is discussed in the full committee, consisting of four or five members with a clinical or research background. The committee decides on the final assessment of the portfolio (fail, satisfactory, good). The procedure is documented in an assessment plan that is formally approved by the Committee of Exams of the University. Figure 39.2 presents an overview of this assessment procedure.

Summary

Portfolios serve different purposes in medical education. These purposes can be summarized as guiding, monitoring and assessing the development of students' competencies. Portfolios often combine several objectives. Apart from differences in objectives, portfolios also differ in scope: a brief versus a long education period, a limited competency domain versus a comprehensive competency profile and an open versus a closed structure. A portfolio is not automatically effective. A number of conditions must be met to ensure that a portfolio makes a meaningful contribution to the learning of students. Mentoring, feasibility and immediate benefits to learners are key factors for portfolio success. Assessing portfolios requires a different approach than is customarily used by most teachers. An approach based on principles from qualitative research is more appropriate than a psychometric one. A number of strategies to ensure rigour of assessment are described: incorporate feedback cycles in the procedure, involve mentor and learners in the assessment, separate the role of the mentor and the assessor, train assessors, use a sequential procedure, use narrative information, provide quality assurance and make use of rubrics. These strategies are also suited to other complex assessment situations, such as the assessment of projects and theses.

Box 39.1 Example of feedback, evaluations, judgements and assessments of thorax module in Year 1

- Report on child and development, feedback from peer and teacher
- Report on risk of fine dust assignment, with presentation, feedback from peer and teacher
- Feedback on professionalism from teacher and peers in tutorial group halfway and at the end of the module
- Assessment of medical skills heart and lung (qualification and feedback)
- SWOT analysis by the student
- Feedback on SWOT by mentor
- Analysis of progress test results.

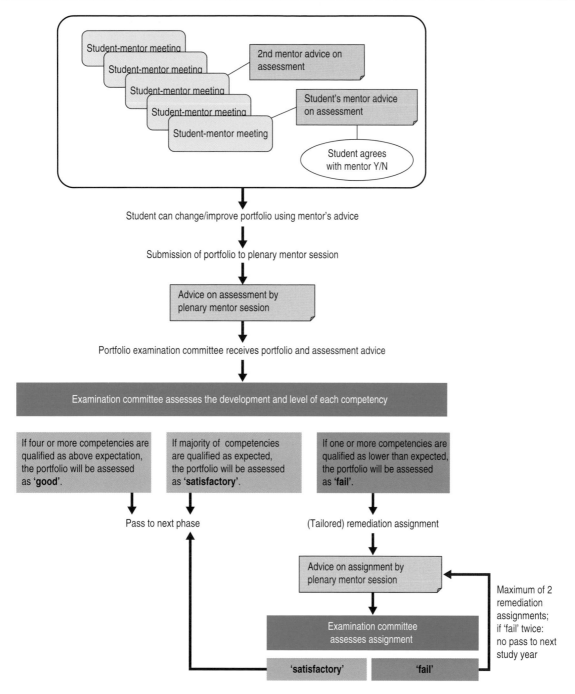

Fig. 39.2 Portfolio assessment procedure.

References

Buckley S, Coleman J, Davison I, et al: The educational effects of portfolios on undergraduate student learning: a Best Evidence Medical Education (BEME) systematic review. BEME Guide No. 11, *Medical Teacher* 31:282–298, 2009.

Dannefer EF, Henson LC: The portfolio approach to competency-based assessment at the Cleveland Clinic Lerner College of Medicine, *Academic Medicine* 82:493–502, 2007.

Driessen E, van der Vleuten C, Schuwirth L, et al: The use of qualitative research criteria for portfolio assessment as an alternative to reliability evaluation: a case study, *Medical Education* 39:214–220, 2005.

Driessen E, van Tartwijk J, van der Vleuten C, Wass V: Portfolios in medical education: why do they meet with mixed success? A systematic review, *Medical Education* 41:1224–1233, 2007.

Driessen E, Overeem K, Van Tartwijk J: Learning from practice: mentoring, feedback, and porfolios. In Dornan T, Mann K, Scherpbier A, Spencer J, editors: *Medical Education: Theory and Practice*, Edinburgh, 2010, Churchill Livingstone Elsevier.

Eva KW, Regehr G: "I'll never play professional football" and other fallacies of self-assessment, *Journal of Continuing Education for Health Professionals* 28:14–19, 2008.

Tochel C, Haig A, Hesketh A, et al: The effectiveness of portfolios for post-graduate assessment and education: BEME Guide No 12, *Medical Teacher* 31:299–318, 2009.

Van Tartwijk J, Driessen EW: Portfolios for assessment and learning: AMEE Guide no. 45, *Medical Teacher* 31:790–801, 2009.

Van Tartwijk T, Driessen E, et al: Werken met een elektronisch portfolio (To Work with an Electronic Portfolio), Groningen, 2003, Wolters-Noordhoff.

Giving feedback

S. K. Krackov

Introduction and background

Feedback is an essential component of the teaching and learning process. Constructive feedback from the teacher gives the learner insight into his or her actions and their consequences. Feedback allows the learner and teacher to successfully achieve both personal and course or programme objectives. The ideas and strategies in this chapter are intended to help make feedback a more productive experience for both the teacher and the learner.

WHAT IS FEEDBACK?

"Information describing students' or house officers' performance in a given activity that is intended to guide their future performance in that same or a related activity."

Ende 1983

FORMATIVE FEEDBACK VERSUS SUMMATIVE ASSESSMENT

Formative feedback and summative assessment are different. The teacher should tell the learner in advance which one he or she is providing.

- **Feedback.** The purpose of feedback is *formative*: to provide insights that help the learner make mid-course adjustments in performance and demonstrate improvement. The language of feedback is descriptive and neutral. Formative feedback should be task-orientated and given frequently and as soon as feasible after the performance so the learner has time to make changes. (Perera et al 2008).

- **Summative assessment.** Summative assessment occurs at the conclusion of a course of study and communicates a decision about performance. This assessment should follow formative feedback and subsequent remedial actions and should express a judgement about whether the learner has achieved the expected outcomes. Summative assessment is often given as a grade or the learner's ranking in

comparison to other learners or to a standard, for example, 4.2/5 on clinical skills.

THE INTENT OF A FEEDBACK SESSION

Feedback sessions can vary:

- **Brief ongoing feedback.** Brief feedback sessions (5–10 minutes) occur frequently, in the context of regular work activities, while the learner is demonstrating findings on physical examination or during the presentation of the patient's history. On these occasions, the teacher might say, 'I'd like to give you some pointers about another way to examine the spleen'.

- **Formal mid-course feedback.** A formal feedback session is scheduled in advance, and both learner and teacher plan ahead. The session may last from 10–30 minutes and addresses the teacher's observations over a period of time. This allows for improvement prior to the summative evaluation.

- **End-of-course feedback.** Summative assessment should be accompanied by feedback, reflection, and mentoring to help the learner improve (Krackov & Pohl 2011).

WHY IS FEEDBACK IMPORTANT?

Ericsson (2004) maintains that the 'acquisition of expert performance requires engaging in *deliberate practice* and that "continued deliberate practice is necessary for maintenance of many types of professional performance'. Feedback is an essential component of the deliberate practice concept. In Ericsson's framework, the following conditions lead to improvement through deliberate practice:

- Well-defined tasks or objectives

- Detailed and immediate feedback on performance

- Opportunities to improve by performing the same or similar tasks repeatedly.

Feedback plays a critical role for the learner, the teacher and the educational programme.

For the learner

Feedback helps the learner achieve course or programme goals. It reinforces good performance and provides a basis for correcting mistakes. Feedback serves as a reference point for summative assessment. It offers insights into actual performance and demonstrates commitment to the learner as a person (Box 40.1)

Learners value teachers who facilitate their learning by giving constructive feedback that is adapted to their professional needs. King (1999) asked learners for their views on feedback.

Negative feedback experiences are characterized by:

- public humiliation
- comments about personality
- one-way discussion
- lack of personal interest in the learner
- feedback that is too general
- feedback that is too brief and/or too long after the event to be useful.

Positive feedback experiences involve:

- active listening
- mutual respect
- specific praise or criticism
- genuine desire to help
- spending adequate time.

Box 40.1 Why is feedback important to the learner?

- Clarifies goals and expectations
- Reinforces good performance
- Provides a basis for correcting mistakes (formative assessment)
- Serves as a reference point for ultimate (summative) evaluation at the conclusion of the educational programme
- Offers insight into *actual* performance and consequences versus what the learner *thought or intended*
- Reduces reliance on self-validation
- Reduces anxiety and insecurity about performance
- Demonstrates interest about the learner as a *person*
- Promotes two-way communication
- Provides guidance

For the teacher

Giving feedback is a critical component of a teacher's role. Feedback links teaching and assessment of the learner's performance and demonstrates the teacher's commitment to help the learner achieve course or programme goals. Most teachers recognize the importance of feedback but find it difficult to do, particularly when the feedback is negative. When they are asked to suggest specific educational training activities that they would find useful, most teachers say they would like to have help with feedback.

For the educational programme

Making feedback a regular part of the educational experience encourages the development of expertise (Ericsson 2004, Krackov & Pohl 2011). A culture that accepts and promotes feedback supports a feeling of positive improvement in the school or training programme.

Feedback is also a requirement. Medical schools and post-graduate training programmes are accountable to external agencies. These agencies foster the belief that the institutions should build the learner's competence instead of penalizing learners who have not achieved the objectives that have been set out.

In the United States and Canada, the agency with responsibility for the accreditation of medical schools, the Liaison Committee on Medical Education (LCME), establishes *standards* for the structure and function of the school:

> *"Each student in a medical education program should be assessed and provided with formal feedback early enough during each required course or clerkship… to allow sufficient time for remediation."*
>
> LCME Standard ED31 2011

In the UK, the General Medical Council (GMC) plays an important role in defining educational standards:

> *"Students must receive regular information about their development and progress. This should include feedback on both formative and summative assessments."*
>
> General Medical Council 2009

Why is giving feedback difficult to do?

Both learners and teachers recognize the importance of feedback; yet most learners say their feedback is inadequate and many people have difficulty giving feedback, particularly when it centres on problem areas.

BARRIERS

Despite the acknowledged importance of feedback, a wide range of impediments may prevent or limit the giving or receiving of feedback:

- *Time and place.* The teacher and learner are 'too busy' for a feedback session; this can lead to an excessive delay before feedback is given or prevent it from happening at all. There may be no appropriate space for a feedback session in the area where the teacher and learner interact.

- *Knowledge base.* Both teacher and learner may be unclear about the purpose or use of feedback. The teacher may lack first-hand data about the learner's performance or may not be certain what feedback is appropriate in a given situation.

- *Ability.* The teacher may not know how to give feedback or have had little practice giving feedback.

- *Affective factors.* A variety of elements play a role:
  - Poor rapport between the learner and teacher may affect or prevent feedback sessions.
  - The teacher may be concerned about the impact of negative feedback on the learner or on their relationship, or the ability of the learner to receive and respond appropriately to feedback.
  - Ende (1983) believes the concern that negative feedback can elicit an unwanted emotional reaction from the learner may lead the teacher to use unclear, indirect statements or avoid giving feedback at all.

- *Different perceptions about feedback.* Learners and teachers differ in their perceptions about feedback. Teachers believe they provide feedback more frequently than learners say they received it.

- *The culture.* The traditional culture of medicine requires that the learner acquire extensive knowledge and skills in a highly structured hierarchical environment. It promotes a one-way flow of information from teacher to learner and can form an experience in which the learner feels like a 'victim' rather than a partner in a collegial activity. In this culture, the learner may consider negative feedback as an overall assessment of worth.

CONSEQUENCES

The consequences of ineffective or nonexistent feedback can be significant. A learner may learn about substandard performance only after receiving the summative evaluation at the end of a period of learning. In the absence of constructive feedback, other forms of assessment, such as written examinations, may assume inflated importance.

 "Without feedback, mistakes go uncorrected, good performance is not reinforced, and clinical competence is achieved empirically or not at all. The sense of being adrift in a strange environment is amplified and learners may 'generate their own feedback by attaching inappropriate importance to internal and external cues'."

Ende 1983

Principles of effective feedback:

Attention to important principles of effective feedback will help set the stage for an effective session (Ende 1983, Hesketh & Laidlaw 2002, Pendleton et al 1984).

- *A culture that values constructive improvement.* The educational climate should foster constructive improvement in an atmosphere of trust and concern. Both learner and teacher should expect feedback to be a regular and frequent occurrence. From the outset it should be clear that they will work together toward a common goal of improving performance. Providing feedback about the course and instructors should be an expected responsibility of learners. The learner might also be asked to provide feedback to the teacher in the context of the feedback session. All of this will foster a climate of mutual trust.

- *Attention to time and location.* Formal feedback sessions should be scheduled so they are mutually convenient for the teacher and the learner and both should have adequate time to prepare. Either the teacher or the learner can initiate a feedback session. The session should take place in a private setting where the learner will feel more relaxed and comfortable discussing sensitive issues.

- *Use of standards.* The learner's performance should be measured against well-defined outcome goals and objectives.

- *First-hand observation.* Whenever possible, the teacher should observe the behaviours first-hand and not relate feedback observed by somebody else. Passing along feedback based on data collected from another person may send mixed messages and produce defensiveness.

- *Use of positive communication strategies.* Giving effective feedback requires attention to a range of dynamics: some observable and others unseen.
  - *Communicating effectively.* Feedback involves active listening, asking open-ended reflective, facilitative questions and responding. These key skills help the learner gain insight into strengths and weaknesses.

- *Making it a two-way process.* The teacher should treat the learner as an ally who is expected to participate in the feedback session. The learner should take an active part in the feedback process by initiating and responding to questions.

- *Using precise, descriptive and objective language.* The information given should be specific, be nonevaluative and contain real examples. Global statements do not help build ability. 'Your history was complete and you showed a concern for Mr Wench's struggle with his weight' is preferable to 'You did a great job!'

- *Focusing on the behaviour, not the person.* It is easier to change behaviours than personalities. 'You were standing, a position of power, which may have made the patient uncomfortable', instead of 'You tend to act superior with patients.'

- *Monitoring the learner's background, temperament, personality and response.* It is important to be aware of the learner's mores, perspectives and responses. 'I noticed that you did not take part in the group's discussion of coronary artery disease. Were you uncomfortable? I'd like to help you increase your participation.'

- *Being selective.* Limit the feedback to what the learner can absorb in one session. 'Today, I think we should concentrate on your examination of the chest.'

- *Awareness of the 'process' of the encounter.* Body language, the tone of your voice and subtle evidence of judgement in words or affect can make the experience less effective.

- *Use of 'I' statements.* Using 'I' instead of 'you' can defuse subjective feedback, for example, 'I noticed that you appeared to be falling behind by the end of the day', instead of 'You work too slowly.'

- *Encouraging reflection.* Reflection can create insights into behaviour, move the discussion to a more complex level and form the basis for improvement (Sargeant et al 2008). 'Let's reflect on what happened with Mr Stratus. How could you play a role in helping him deal with this complex ethical issue?'

- *Keeping cool.* It is important to keep personal feelings and tell-tale nonverbal expressions out of the session. If the learner did something that made you angry, delay the feedback session until you have had a chance to cool down. Your feedback will be more effective if it is not emotion-laden.

- *Giving positive feedback, too.* A learner may not be aware of exactly which components of his or her effort were correct and why. Specific positive feedback will improve the chances that the learner will repeat desirable actions and will retain the learner's motivation and desire to learn and to receive more feedback. 'You identified the most important elements of the problem in your presentation. Good work!'

- *Focusing on decisions and actions.* Feedback should provide insights and guide future performance. Concentrate on actions with specific examples. 'What are the options for evaluating Mr Yonge's injury? Have you considered doing an MRI?' (See Box 40.2.)

Template for effective feedback sessions

The following guide will help produce a successful feedback encounter.

PREPARE IN ADVANCE

- *Collect data.* The teacher's direct observation of the learner provides the most valuable data for a feedback session. Giving attention to this step will improve the quality of the session.

- *Know what to look for.* Be familiar with the content and process you will be assessing. Observe and record specific examples to share with the learner. For example, when observing an interaction with a patient, notice the learner's respect for the patient's privacy and comfort. When listening to a presentation, consider the learner's organization, thoroughness and ability to identify and interpret changes.

- *Write it down.* Brief written notes will support and reinforce your observations. Include specific examples to share with the learner, for example, the greeting to the patient, draping of the patient during examination.

- *Invite the learner to the feedback session* and agree on time, location and agenda. 'Let's take a little time for a feedback session. How is eight o'clock tomorrow morning in my office?'

- *Explain the purpose of the session* and suggest that it would be useful to reflect on the learner's performance in preparation. 'When we meet, our purpose will be to discuss your clinical skills.'

MAKE THE FEEDBACK SESSION INTERACTIVE

These essential components of an interactive session balance support with a stimulus for improvement:

- *Review the purpose of the session.* Call it feedback. Explain the distinction between feedback

Box 40.2 Important principles of feedback

Feedback should be:

- Timely, frequent and expected by both teacher and learner
- Based on first-hand data: personal observation by the teacher
- Labelled clearly as feedback so the learner has no doubt about receiving feedback
- Descriptive: not evaluative
- Constructive
- Specific, including examples not generalizations
- Nonjudgemental
- Balanced, giving positives and negatives
- Objective, focused on behaviour, performance, and not on personality traits
- Directed to behaviour that can be changed
- Selective: addressing one or two key issues
- Focused on helping the learner come to a better understanding of the problem and ways in which he or she can address it more effectively
- Monitored to the learner's temperament, personality and response
- Two-way process between learner and teacher
- Designed to address decisions and actions

and summative assessment and label the purpose of the session. 'We have discussed how feedback differs from your final assessment. Today I am going to give you some feedback about your clinical skills.'

- **Get agreement on goals.** At the outset make certain that you and the learner have the same goals for the session. 'Today, I would like to discuss your physical examination skills when you saw Ms Jasper. Is that plan acceptable to you?'

- **Invite the learner to self-assess.** Use open-ended questions. This approach begins the session as a conversation, promotes reflective practice and gives insights into the learner's awareness of his or her strengths and weaknesses. The learner may bring up the same points you had planned to discuss. 'What aspects of your meeting with Ms Symme do you think went well? Which ones can be improved? Have you seen patients like this before?'

- **Listen actively to the learner's response.** Show that you are interested and involved by making eye contact and using positive body language.

- **Respond.** Reinforce or correct the learner's self-assessment. Frame the discussion in the context of the session's goals.

- *Begin by acknowledging and reinforcing positive behaviours.* This will help ensure that these behaviours continue. 'Your examination of the patient's abdomen correctly identified the enlarged spleen.'

- *Correct when necessary.* Provide specific examples where improvement is needed. 'When you did/said that, I was concerned because…' is more helpful than a general statement like, 'Your work is not up to par.'

- *Offer specific constructive suggestions for improvement.* If the learner made an error, tell him or her how to do it right. 'Let me show you how to examine the head and neck.'

- **Confirm the learner's understanding.** 'Would you like to ask any questions?' 'Based on our discussion, what would you do?'

- **Conclude with actions.** Create an action plan that both parties feel is acceptable: 'Let's develop a plan.'

- *Invite the learner to generate ideas.* 'How do you think you could improve the skills we identified?'

- *Endorse or modify the learner's statements and outline new strategies.* 'I agree with your assessment of Mrs Hutch's problem, but I would modify the treatment you suggested by…'.

- *Summarize the meeting.* Include the learner's strengths and a plan to improve weaknesses. 'To recap our meeting, your communication skills are very good. In order to strengthen your physical examination skills, we agreed that you would…'.

- *Set a timeline for the plan and a follow up feedback session.* 'Let's meet again next week to review your progress.'

RESPOND TO A DEFENSIVE REACTION

Some learners may become defensive about negative feedback and deny, rationalize or blame somebody else for the problem. The following strategies may help (King 1999):

- *Identify and explore the issues.* 'You seem to be concerned/angry. Can you tell me why?'

- *Keep a positive focus.* Identify the learner's strengths and use them to help resolve the defensive reaction. 'You have good motor skills, which will help you master this procedure.'

- **Ask the learner to own part of the problem.** 'Would you agree that it was difficult for you to communicate with that patient in a positive way?'

- *Negotiate and ask the learner to take responsibility* for the problem and for improvement: 'In order to work on this, first you should commit to…'.
- *Offer time out.* 'Would you like to have some time to think about these things? Let's meet again next week.'

REFLECT

Reflecting on your feedback session can create helpful insights that will strengthen your feedback skills (see Table 40.1).

- What went well? What techniques seemed effective?
- What can you do differently next time?
- What are your strategies for future feedback sessions?

Some other approaches

Some alternatives to the traditional feedback session between learner and teacher are described below.

CHECKLISTS

Checklists are being used regularly as the basis for a teacher-led feedback session. Clay et al (2007) reported the successful use of checklists to provide formative feedback and foster reflection. They developed checklists for five core competencies encountered by house officers in the intensive care unit at Duke University, United States. The checklists defined explicit steps and behaviours for each competency. House officers were alerted that the checklists were on the critical care website. Following a patient encounter, the fellow (physician supervisor) completed a checklist before a debriefing session with the house officer in which the checklist was used to guide discussion about the house officer's performance. The house officer was encouraged to reflect on his or her performance, and the debriefing was documented on an electronic version of the checklist. The authors concluded that the checklists enabled the house officer to compare performance against a 'gold standard' and enabled a 'high-fidelity' learning experience based on actual patient encounters.

COMPUTER-BASED FEEDBACK

Computer-based feedback is also becoming part of the feedback tool kit. Porte et al (2007) compared the effectiveness of two types of feedback on the ability of medical students at the University of Toronto, Canada, to perform a basic technical skill: computer-based feedback (with and without a criterion standard) and feedback from an expert that included constructive ways to improve performance. The computer-based method was initiated in an effort to provide an alternate method of giving feedback that would relieve clinical faculty time. All groups showed improvement from pre- to post-test. However, only the group that received verbal feedback from an expert teacher showed lasting improvement. The authors suggested that the additional information

Table 40.1 Feedback examples

Ineffective feedback	High-quality feedback
Vague, not descriptive, may include sweeping generalizations	**Specific, descriptive**
'Your performance was disappointing'	'You addressed Ms Taylor's concerns. But, it is also important to consider her history of diabetes, which plays a role in today's visit'
'Good job'	'You take time with patients and answer their questions'
Unnecessarily harsh/focuses on negative	**Fair, even-handed, constructive**
'You can't prioritize!'	'The issues you raise about Mrs Wynch's smoking are important, but today I think it is more important to address her hypertension'
'Undistinguished'	'Preparing an outline of your reading may help you solidify concepts'
Focused on personality traits	**Focused on behaviour/performance**
'You are too competitive'	'Your viewpoints are valuable, but it is important to hear from the rest of the team, too'
'Good mind'	'During rounds, you continually identify the important elements of the case'
Based on rumour, hearsay	**Based on personal observation**
'Dr X told me that you have problems with this material'	'I see you are having problems with your formulations'

from an expert increased the learner's cognitive understanding and resulted in better performance.

PEER FEEDBACK

Feedback from peers is being used more frequently. Gukas et al (2008) studied student views of feedback from persons in their anatomy student-selected study module. Most students were comfortable giving and receiving feedback, and their attitudes towards peer feedback were generally positive. Hughes et al (2008) used eMed Teamwork, a computer-based system to collect feedback from peers in project groups. Formative feedback from peers was available to the recipient and became part of the portfolio of both the feedback giver and the recipient.

Training faculty to give feedback

ROLE OF FACULTY TRAINING

Faculty training activities are designed to improve the teacher's knowledge and skills in specific target areas. The feedback skills described in this chapter call for a variety of training opportunities for faculty and can involve a wide range of individual and group activities:

- Ongoing reflection by the teacher after feedback sessions
- Review of learner evaluations about feedback practices with a skilled educator to help interpret the results and suggest new strategies
- Workshops that provide opportunities to practise and build skills
- Longer in-depth programmes that feature immersion
- Peer coaching programmes in which more experienced colleagues provide assistance
- Small-group discussions.

Henderson et al (2005) make the case that faculty training should address two areas: improving feedback skills and changing the culture that underlies the application of those skills. They advocate a culture that supports giving and receiving both positive and negative feedback, regardless of the position of the person in the hierarchy. Using adult learning principles, the authors developed a longitudinal, iterative 'strand' for students at the University of Cambridge, UK, in which feedback is taught conceptually and practically throughout the course of an entire year.

GUIDE FOR A FACULTY-TRAINING WORKSHOP ON GIVING FEEDBACK

A workshop is an effective mechanism for training faculty about feedback. Workshops can be scheduled at the faculty's convenience. They offer an opportunity to present basic theory and information and they involve active learning.

The example workshop that appears below includes several elements:

- Brainstorming, so participants can describe their personal experiences of why feedback is important and why it is so difficult
- An interactive lecture by the workshop faculty to describe how to do it well
- Videos, to provide real-life examples
- Role-play, so participants can practise feedback skills. These sessions:
  - inject realism into the learning process
  - demonstrate desirable and undesirable behaviours
  - enhance an exchange of ideas about the process
- Follow-up simulation session, so workshop participants can demonstrate retention and increase and integrate their feedback skills. Here, the workshop participant/teacher gives feedback to a 'standardized student'. Following the encounter, the 'student' completes a checklist about the teacher's feedback skills. Workshop faculty review the checklist, watch a video of the interaction and conduct a debriefing session. This process enables the workshop participants to assess their strengths and weakness and strengthen their feedback skills (Pohl H, personal communication, 2008).

The faculty-training workshop and follow-up activity outlined here incorporate fundamental elements of learning and use a variety of methods. This comprehensive approach will have a beneficial impact on improving teachers' feedback skills.

Summary

The feedback literature in medical education focuses on feedback in clinical training. However, the principles and suggestions in this chapter apply to any situation in a learning or work environment. Feedback is a formative tool that reinforces behaviour and enables changes that improve abilities. When feedback is given skilfully, the teacher and learner work as allies toward a common goal. Good communication skills are essential to giving effective feedback. Faculty training can support and enable exemplary feedback techniques. As we look toward the future, we can use feedback as an important instrument in moving the traditional culture of medical education to one that fosters improvement in an environment of trust and responsibility.

Workshop feedback

The following example depicts a feedback workshop.

WORKSHOP OBJECTIVES AND INTENDED OUTCOMES

At the end of this activity, participants will be able to:

1. Describe important components of an effective feedback session.
2. Choose an appropriate setting and language for giving feedback.
3. Observe and practise giving and receiving feedback.
4. Develop an action plan for improving feedback in their own setting.
5. Demonstrate retention; increase and integrate the new feedback skills.

INSTRUCTIONS FOR ROLE PLAY

- Divide into small groups of three or more people per group.
- Remain in the same group for the duration of the exercise.
- At the outset, the group should read the role play and resolve any questions.

Role play (5 minutes)

- Each group member will play an assigned role as described in the scenario:
  - Learner (student, house officer)
  - Teacher (faculty, house officer)
  - Observer: the observer gives feedback to the learner and teacher about the performance in the role play.
- Each person should prepare for the role he or she will play.
- One group member should volunteer to keep time.

It is important to stay in role during the entire exercise.

Debrief (5 minutes)

Begin with self-assessment by the learner and teacher:

- What went well?
- What problems did you encounter?
- What other strategies could have been used?

Additional questions for the teacher:

- What was the most difficult thing to discuss?
- What was the easiest?

Additional questions for the learner:

- How did you feel when you received this feedback?
- What was your reaction?

Workshop agenda and format	
10 minutes:	**Introduction** (workshop faculty) *Workshop overview* *Rationale*
20 minutes:	**Why is feedback important and why is it so difficult?** Brainstorming (all)
15 minutes:	**What is effective feedback?** Brainstorming (all) *Workshop faculty and participants identify characteristics of effective feedback.*
20 minutes:	**Video vignettes:** (all) *Participants identify effective and ineffective feedback demonstrated in the videos.*
15 minutes:	**How to do it well:** (workshop faculty) *Workshop faculty describe an effective location, steps and techniques for giving feedback.*
15 minutes:	Break
45 minutes:	**Role play** (small groups) *Participants convene in groups of three or four to practise feedback techniques.*
20 minutes:	**Report back** (plenary) *Participants share ideas gained from role play.*
20 minutes:	**Action plan** (plenary) *Participants identify three things they will do differently in the future.* *Workshop evaluation*

NOTE: A follow-up activity using 'standardized students' will be scheduled at a later date to demonstrate retention and increase and integrate the new feedback skills.

The observer should offer feedback on what he or she observed.

- What went well?
- What problems did you notice?
- What other strategies could have been used?
- Were they in a private location?
- Was the feedback specific, descriptive, nonjudgemental?

After the role-play and debrief, participants can rotate (change) roles and replay the simulation.

MID-COURSE VERBAL FEEDBACK: TEACHER VERSION

You have to schedule a mid-course feedback session with your student in the physical diagnosis course.

You have noticed that the student appears to enjoy learning about the physical exam and problem solving the differential diagnosis. You also noticed a lack of interest in being with patients and hearing them talk about their problems. In fact, a few patients have complained that the student is abrupt and cuts them off.

The student has told you of plans for a research career after graduation. Nonetheless, this student will have to communicate with patients throughout medical school and may even decide against a research career. You think it is important to address this issue.

The form you received says that the feedback session should involve the following elements:

Approach to the patient

History taking

Physical exam

Write-ups

What will you say?

MID-COURSE VERBAL FEEDBACK: STUDENT VERSION

You know that your mid-course feedback session in physical diagnosis is coming up and you wonder what your teacher will have to say.

You enjoy performing a physical exam and problem solving the issues in the differential diagnosis. However, you plan to have a research career after you graduate from medical school. You are not particularly interested in being with patients and listening to them talk about their problems. Some of the patients seem to go on forever! In fact, a few times you had to cut in to stop the wandering and focus the patient back on the important topics.

A few patients complained that you were abrupt and not interested, but you expect the teacher will recognize your academic abilities and overlook comments like this. After all, you have mentioned your career in research several times.

You were told that the feedback session would involve the following elements:

Approach to the patient

History taking

Physical exam

Write-ups

What will you say?

MID-COURSE FEEDBACK SESSION: OBSERVER VERSION

You are observing the teacher give a student mid-course feedback about his performance in the physical diagnosis course.

The student enjoys learning about the physical exam and problem solving the issues in the differential diagnosis but plans to have a research career after graduation and is not terribly interested in being with patients and discussing their problems.

The feedback session involves the following elements:

Approach to the patient

History taking

Physical exam

Write-ups.

References

Clay AS, Que L, Petrusa ER, et al: Debriefing in the intensive care unit: a feedback tool to facilitate bedside teaching, *Critical Care Medicine* 35(3):738–754, 2007.

Ende J: Feedback in clinical medical education, *JAMA* 250:777–781, 1983.

Ericsson KA: Deliberate practice and the acquisition and maintenance of expert performance in medicine and related domains, 2003. Research in Medical Education invited address, *Academic Medicine* 79(10):S70–S81, 2004.

General Medical Council: *Tomorrow's Doctors. Recommendations on undergraduate medical education, Domain 5-Design and delivery of the curriculum, including assessment,* London, 2009, General Medical Council.

General Medical Council: Tomorrow's Doctors, Recommendations on undergraduate medical education, Domain 5, Design and delivery of the curriculum, including assessment; Assessment in undergraduate medical education: Advice supplementary to Tomorrow's Doctors, London, 2011, General Medical Council.

Gukas ID, Miles S, Heylings DJ, Leinster SJ: Medical students' perceptions of peer feedback on an anatomy student-selected study module, *Medical Teacher* 30(8):812–814, 2008.

Henderson P, Ferguson-Smith AC, Johnson MH: Developing essential professional skills: a framework for teaching and learning about feedback. *BioMed Central Medical Education* 5:1–6, 2005.

Hesketh E A, Laidlaw J M: Developing the teaching instinct: 1, *Feedback, Medical Teacher* 24(3): 245–248, 2002.

Hughes C, Toohey S, Velan G: eMed Teamwork: a self-moderating system to gather peer feedback for developing and assessing teamwork skills, *Medical Teacher* 30(1):5–9, 2008.

King J: Giving feedback, *BMJ* 318(7200):1–3, 1999.

Krackov SK, Pohl H: Building expertise using the deliberate-practice curriculum-planning model, *Medical Teacher* 33(7):570–575, 2011.

Liaison Committee on Medical Education (LCME). Available at: http://www.lcme.org/functions, 2012.

Pendleton D, Schofield T, Tate P: A method for giving feedback. In: *The Consultation: An Approach to Learning and Teaching*. Oxford, 1984, Oxford University Press, pp 68–71.

Perera J, Lee N, Win K, et al: Formative feedback to students: the mismatch between faculty perceptions and student expectations, *Medical Teacher* 30: 395–399, 2008.

Porte MC, Xeroulis G, Reznick RK, Dubrowski A: Verbal feedback from an expert is more effective than self-accessed feedback about motion efficiency in learning new surgical skills, *American Journal of Surgery* 193:105–110, 2007.

Sargeant JM, Mann KV, Van der Vleuten CP, Metsemaker JK: Reflection: a link between receiving and using assessment feedback, *Advances in Health Science Education* 13(3):275–288, 2008.

Evaluating professionalism

S. Ginsburg

Evaluating professionalism in medical education has become much more explicit over the past decade. All important regulatory and accreditation bodies (such as the Royal College of Physicians and Surgeons of Canada, the Accreditation Council of Graduate Medical Education in the United States, Frank & Danoff 2007 and the Accreditation Council for Graduate Medical Education 2010) mandate that professionalism be taught and evaluated during training. However, since professionalism is a difficult construct to define – and therefore evaluate – no clear consensus exists as to the best methods to use. Further, issues of reliability and validity are difficult to resolve, as there is no gold standard. This chapter describes the difficulties in defining professionalism, some common pitfalls in evaluating it, and outlines some useful approaches from the research literature.

One important recent resource is the report from the International Ottawa Conference working group on the assessment of professionalism (Hodges et al 2011). This international working group was tasked with developing a consensus statement on the evaluation of professionalism and elected to conduct a 'discourse analysis' to help categorize and understand the dominant perspectives on assessment from the published literature. The group suggested that the evaluation of professionalism can be viewed from three different yet complementary perspectives: the individual, the relational and the organizational.

"The evaluation of professionalism can be viewed from three different yet complementary perspectives: the individual, the relational, and the organizational."

Hodges 2011

- The individual perspective focuses on an individual's characteristics, attributes or behaviours. This is useful for evaluation purposes (most of which focus on single individuals) and for personal accountability. Most of the focus has shifted towards behaviours, as they appear to be more objective than attitudes or traits; however, behaviours are not always good indicators of motivations or intent and should be interpreted carefully. This perspective does not adequately consider or account for the context that is so powerful in shaping behaviours.

- The relational perspective considers professionalism as arising from (and affecting) relationships between individuals. This is helpful in broadening our understanding of context and in understanding how unprofessional behaviour may arise. However, it may not adequately be able to address individuals' problematic behaviours, or the macro-social forces that act upon relationships.

- The institutional or organizational perspective allows one to consider how policies and power hierarchies can influence or even constrain individuals' actions. This is helpful in understanding how and why people don't always act according to their stated beliefs. However, it can obscure individual responsibility and accountability.

All three perspectives have important things to offer, but all can give rise to blind spots. It is important to think about these issues when planning evaluations; however, in most cases it is recognized that individual-level evaluations are desired. The Ottawa group also stated, importantly, that the 'overall assessment programme is more important than the individual tools'. What this means is that rather than relying on a single tool or measure of professionalism, it is important to gather relevant information from multiple assessments and stakeholder perspectives and triangulate these data to result in an integrated assessment of individuals.

The "overall assessment programme [for professionalism] is more important than the individual tools."

Hodges 2011

Defining professionalism

Although defining professionalism is not the focus of this chapter by any means, most would agree that it is impossible to evaluate something without first declaring what it is. In this case the definition is particularly important, as disagreement persists about what professionalism actually is, and what it encompasses. The Ottawa report states that the concept of professionalism varies across historical time periods and cultural contexts and that there is a need to develop or adopt concrete and operationalizable definitions from which to teach and evaluate professionalism. Further, these definitions should be negotiated with the public, as the practice of medicine relies on a social contract between the profession and society.

In practical terms this means that before a programme intends to evaluate professionalism, it should choose a definition that resonates with its members and should make this explicit so that teaching and evaluation can follow. See, for example, Wilkinson and colleagues' efforts (2009) to blueprint professionalism assessment by considering aspects of its definition.

Why evaluate professionalism?

The evaluation of professionalism has, until relatively recently, been largely implicit rather than explicit like other domains of knowledge and skills. However, over the past couple of decades there has been a move to consider professionalism as a distinct entity that is evaluated, for several important reasons. For one thing, it signals to all stakeholders (the programme, students, patients and the public) that it is being taught and evaluated with the same importance (and consequences) as other knowledge and skills. It is assumed that this attention may help counteract effects of the hidden curriculum, along with the reported decrease in empathy that often occurs during training. And if professionalism issues are identified early in training, the logical outcome would be remediation (or removal).

Interestingly, it is only recently that evidence has been published to support this last point, but it is now clear that some professionalism issues identified early in training may predict disciplinary actions in practice (Papadakis et al 2005, Papadakis et al 2008). That said, these authors and others have pointed out that these red flags account for only a small proportion of attributable risk (i.e. most students do not go on to have documented difficulties in practice) so should be interpreted with caution. Other researchers have found that certain behaviours in the first 2 years of medical school can predict professionalism issues in clerkship: behaviours such as turning in course evaluations or being up to date on immunizations that some have referred to collectively as conscientiousness (McLachlan et al 2009, Stern et al 2005).

What to evaluate

There has also been debate about what exactly belongs in a definition of professionalism. As described above, there is no clear consensus on how to define professionalism, and therefore there is disagreement even among experts over what to include in an evaluation. As an example, the issue of communication, while certainly important for professionalism, is usually covered elsewhere or in separate evaluations entirely. The literature and research on evaluating communication skills do not often intersect with those on professionalism. The same is true of ethics and some other domains. Thus it is important when planning evaluation to consider what might be consistent with the programme's conceptualization of professionalism but that might already be evaluated by other means.

Pitfalls to consider in evaluation

When evaluating professionalism one must consider a few important caveats, some of which apply to many areas of evaluation and some of which are particular to professionalism. In an article written over 10 years ago, for example, we argued that the assessment of professionalism should focus on behaviours rather than attitudes and should incorporate and acknowledge the importance of context, value conflicts and resolution (Ginsburg et al 2000). These issues are still important, and although some have been modified (based on new research) the basic principles are worth briefly revisiting.

 Understanding the context in which behaviours are enacted is critical to interpreting professionalism.

The context in which behaviour occurs is extremely important to consider. We can all recognize that there is a time and a place in which some behaviours may seem appropriate and others in which the exact same behaviour would be viewed as inappropriate. Some important contextual influences include the microculture created by the clinical environment (e.g. the emergency department or operating room environments compared to psychiatry wards) and expectations and norms existing for different cultural or ethnic groups.

 Unprofessional behaviour often arises from a conflict between equally worthy values or principles.

Similarly, when unprofessional behaviour arises it is often as the result of conflict between competing principles (each of which may be completely worthy), e.g. honesty versus confidentiality, individual patient advocacy versus stewardship of resources, efficiency versus comprehensiveness, and a limitless combination of any values. In evaluation, it is important to consider which values have come into conflict, under which particular context, and then to consider how and why the individual chose to act in the way he or she did.

Although we began with a call to focus on behaviours, as they seem more objective, it is important to note that research in other domains has provided abundant evidence that an individual's behaviour, and how we interpret it, is largely shaped by environmental factors (Regehr 2006, Rees & Knight 2007). With this understanding it has been argued that we should modify our approach to evaluating professionalism, and in particular in remediating it. It no longer makes sense to evaluate an individual as if he or she acted in a vacuum; rather, we should acknowledge the factors that shape these behaviours and work to create environments that foster, rather than hinder, professional behaviour (Hodges et al 2011, Lesser et al 2010, Lucey & Souba 2010).

That said, programmes still have to evaluate individuals. What follows is a brief overview of commonly used evaluation methods that are well-described in the literature. A full explication of each would be beyond the scope of this practical chapter; however, for the interested reader, several review articles, chapters and books have been published that review these in much greater detail (Lynch et al 2004, Stern 2006, van Mook et al 2009). There is also an excellent review by Clauser and colleagues (2010) of how to consider – and build – evidence for validity when it comes to evaluating professionalism.

It is well worth considering a final word of advice from the Ottawa consensus group: that it may be 'more important to increase the depth and quality of the reliability and validity of a programme' of existing measures in various contexts 'than to continue developing new measures for single contexts' (Hodges et al 2011). In other words, use what's 'out there' already and modify if needed, rather than building a new assessment from scratch.

Common methods of evaluation

IN-TRAINING EVALUATION REPORTS (ITERS)

ITERs and their variants (ward evaluations, faculty evaluations, etc.) are the mainstay of evaluation in most educational settings. Their advantages include familiarity, feasibility and comprehensiveness. However, they are also plagued by issues of unreliability and have not

often been shown to be valid. Some issues are related to the fact that these evaluations are meant to be based on observation, yet it is widely recognized that the evaluators often do not directly observe performance; rather, they observe snippets of performance and then extrapolate, or use information from other sources (such as residents, students, nurses, etc.) (Clauser et al 2010, Mazor et al 2008).

Another problem is that they are often filled out at the end of a rotation and thus suffer from recall bias. Often the elements of professionalism are explicit on evaluation forms, but it can be difficult to decide whether a particular behaviour (e.g. poor communication with allied health) is an issue of professionalism, communication, collaboration or some combination (as modelled on the CanMEDs roles). Thus documentation can be inconsistent.

Another significant issue is the fact that clinician attendings and supervisors have repeatedly been shown to be reluctant to provide constructive or negative feedback – on any issue, in fact – but particularly on professionalism. This is despite every good intention to do so. Faculty report feeling unprepared, uncomfortable, unsure (of what they are witnessing) and, in many cases, unwilling (due to the difficulty involved, lack of support, fear of appeals or reprisals, etc.) (Burack et al 1999, Cleland et al 2008, Dudek et al 2005). These issues should not be ignored, but should be addressed with proper education, faculty development and training.

Despite these issues, there is some evidence in the literature of the utility of ITER type evaluations in picking up issues in professionalism (Colliver et al 2007, Frohna & Stern 2005, Stern et al 2005). It is also worth noting that the comments on these forms can be an even more fruitful source of information although they are not often analysed or reported systematically (Frohna & Stern 2005, Ginsburg et al 2011).

 Evaluations are more reliable and valid when based on direct observation of trainees and when rating scales are tailored to relevant performance.

A final point to consider is whether the evaluation of professionalism can be included on the existing instruments for evaluation of competence or whether a separate form is required. For example, in our institution a separate form for evaluating professionalism was instituted across all pre-clerkship and clerkship rotations, for several reasons. For one, it was felt that the existing forms did not adequately emphasize professionalism as compared to other knowledge and skills. Further, the decision was made to make professionalism a requirement for every course; that is, a student had to pass professionalism in addition to all other elements of performance in order to pass. We also wanted a way to track issues in professionalism throughout training, between courses, etc., so a separate form used by all courses made this easier. However, despite fulfilling most of these goals, the main drawbacks have been 'evaluation fatigue', as there are sometimes multiple forms to be filled out, and a concern (because the form focuses on behavioural expectations and lapses) that it does not adequately consider exemplary professionalism.

Points for optimizing this type of evaluation:

- Decide whether the assessment of professionalism will be included in the existing evaluation form or if a separate form is required, and consider pros and cons to each approach.
- Promote direct observations by faculty.
- Provide training in the use of rating instruments.
- Include behaviours that are relevant to the clinical setting, and avoid those that are not.
- Ensure that the language is clear and unambiguous.
- Use a rating scale that is based on performance and not simply on expectations.
- Provide ample space for comments and consider evaluating these systematically.

MULTI-SOURCE FEEDBACK AND EVALUATION

Following on the above, many programmes are using multi-source methods of evaluation, sometimes called '360s', in which feedback is systematically sought from peers, students, residents, attendings as well as others, such as nurses, allied health professionals and patients. (Peer assessment will be considered separately below.) The National Board of Medical Examiners has developed an approach focused on 360° feedback, and that has demonstrated feasibility and some evidence of validity (National Board of Medical Examiners 2011). The main strength of this approach is that it provides for more frequent observations from more (and different) perspectives. This would logically lead to a more 'accurate' picture of any single individual. The biggest drawback is that it can be difficult to integrate or reconcile differences when they occur, which they often do. Decisions should be made up front about how the different elements will be weighted and considered. There are also feasibility and cost issues when collecting data from multiple sources. Finally, one group reported that a 360° evaluation process in a surgical residency represented 'increased work, with little return' (Weigelt et al 2004). These points should be kept in mind before developing a new system.

Points for optimizing this type of evaluation:

- Gather data from groups who have the most contact with learners, across multiple settings.
- Conduct a formal orientation to the system and its elements, especially if groups have never used these before.
- Be clear about how information gathered will be used, integrated and weighted.
- Consider the pros and cons of anonymity.
- Develop an administrative structure to distribute and collect these evaluations in a systematic way.

PEER ASSESSMENT

Peers offer a unique perspective from which to assess professionalism. They interact with each other in intense, varied and often informal ways, such as on the wards, in teaching sessions and in study groups. They are often the only ones present during each others' behaviours. This, of course, provides advantages when trying to get an overall picture of a student or resident's performance and abilities. However, there are obvious drawbacks, such as a fear of damaging friendships and reputations, fear of reprisal and concerns that the information gathered will be used for purposes not intended. Arnold and colleagues (2005) determined that most students would be willing to participate in peer assessment if their preferences are taken into account. A further multi-institutional study found that students prefer a system that is anonymous, provides immediate feedback, focuses on positive and negative behaviours (i.e. isn't just about lapses) and provides for rewards as well as action for unprofessional behaviour (Arnold et al 2007).

There are two basic methods of peer assessment: ratings and nominations. In rating systems students are assigned (either randomly or by some other systematic approach) to evaluate their peers. This can be simple, such as asking all members of a small group to evaluate each other, or can be more complicated, e.g. asking students to choose peers whom they feel they are in a position to evaluate. Standard types of assessments can be used for this purpose (e.g. student-orientated versions of the forms that faculty use). Every student would receive ratings from several peers. By contrast, in a nomination method, students may be asked, for example, to nominate, select or vote for a certain number of classmates who they feel are exemplary in their professionalism or whom they would want as a colleague or physician for a loved one. Alternatively, they may be asked to select peers whom they would never want to work with again or would never send a relative to. These methods are good at picking up the outliers at both ends, with demonstrated reliability. One recent study found that positive nominations were predictive of better clinical competence and higher empathy scores when compared with non-nominated students (Pohl et al 2011). However, a large proportion of students will not be nominated (i.e. are not at either end of the scale) and thus it would not be as useful as a contribution to overall assessment.

Interestingly, it may not matter whether students choose the peers to evaluate them or whether they are assigned (Lurie et al 2006). Thus this decision can be based on practicality or student preferences.

The following points have been suggested by Norcini, Arnold and others in articles exploring peer assessment in general and with respect to professionalism (Arnold et al 2005, Norcini 2003) (Box 41.1).

 Peer assessment can be very useful and powerful if conducted in a sensitive and supportive manner.

STANDARDIZED PATIENTS AND OSCES

Standardized patients (SPs) have been used in a multitude of settings to evaluate all sorts of clinical skills and areas of performance (see Chapter 26). SPs can be reliably trained to observe and evaluate behaviour on multiple dimensions, including aspects of professionalism such as empathy, communication, dealing with uncertainty and conflict management. There are interesting reports in the literature of OSCE stations being developed specifically to evaluate professionalism (e.g. a scenario involving a boundary crossing) (Gaufberg & Fitzpatrick 2008), although

most commonly elements of professionalism are embedded in 'regular' stations. These then take the form of scales focused on communication, tolerance of differing viewpoints, cultural sensitivity, etc. Some OSCEs have even been developed solely to focus on elements of professionalism (e.g. the ethics OSCE) (Singer et al 1996) but these suffer from issues of context-specificity and the requirement of a large number of stations to ensure reliability.

Two recent articles found that although it is feasible to train and use SPs to evaluate professionalism during OSCEs, they tend to rate differently than faculty, by showing greater variability in scores (although similar rank-orderings of residents) and by attending to different types of behaviours (Mazor et al 2007, Zanetti et al 2010). A further interesting study reported that unprofessional behaviour was observable during both, a regular clinical skills OSCE, and the remediation process for students (Hauer et al 2009). Two of the more frequent issues identified (diminished capacity for self-improvement and irresponsibility) corresponded to the higher-risk types of behaviours that had previously been linked to unprofessional behaviour in practice. Thus there may be some utility in paying attention to these sorts of issues during the exam process.

At this point, given the above areas of uncertainty, these types of assessments may best be used for formative assessment or teaching rather than for high-stakes exams.

Points for optimizing this type of method:

- Consider whether professionalism will be the focus of a station or embedded in several (or all) stations.

- Use behavioural scales and anchors that are clearly worded.

- Train all raters.

WRITTEN EXAMS

We don't often think of written exams as being useful for assessing professionalism, but some have suggested that this can be a very effective way to test the knowledge base required for appropriate professional behaviour (Cruess & Cruess 2009). Even multiple-choice exams may be useful to assess, for example, learners' knowledge and understanding of legal and regulatory frameworks, basic ethical and professional principles and even their approach to professional dilemmas. One study presented in 2009 found that multiple-choice questions about professionalism actually performed better than other types of questions on a high-stakes licensing exam (Lee et al 2009).

Another approach to written exams involves assessing learners' responses to professional or ethical dilemmas. This is a feasible approach, with some

---

Box 41.1 Tips for optimizing peer assessment

- Define the purpose (e.g. to identify positive and/or negative behaviours) and communicate it clearly

- Consider whether to use ratings (of all students) or a nomination method

- Consider how to select who should assess whom: random assignment, student selection, etc.

- Consider pros/cons of anonymity versus confidentiality versus an open system

- Develop solid, defensible and transparent assessment criteria

- Train participants in conducting the ratings and in giving/receiving feedback

- Monitor the results as they unfold to detect anomalies or misuse

- Provide remediation and counselling for those who receive low ratings

caveats. For one, it can be difficult for raters to reach consensus on what would constitute the correct response (Ginsburg et al 2009), even for purportedly 'simple' dilemmas (Goldie et al 2004). And, of course, one has to consider that responses during an exam may not correlate with behaviours in practice.

That said, written exams are relatively inexpensive and can be standardized so should have a place in evaluating at least knowledge around professionalism issues.

Newer methods

P-MEX

The P-MEX, or Professionalism Mini-Evaluation Exercise, is an evaluation instrument modelled on the Mini-CEX which was developed to evaluate professionalism. It was developed in a multi-step process beginning with broad input from relevant groups as to what professionalism entails in the clinical setting (Cruess et al 2006). It is designed to be used for single, observed encounters and provides for immediate feedback. It is in the process of being validated in several settings and cultures (Tsugawa et al 2009). Its advantages include the requirement for direct observation, the provision of immediate feedback and the inclusion of multiple observations in different settings. However, it can be challenging to employ in real-life settings where supervisors already feel overburdened with other evaluations, and it can be difficult to collect and collate data from multiple sources. It does, however, provide for a relatively simple and useful tool for feedback purposes.

CONSCIENTIOUSNESS INDEX

Some researchers have explored the idea of using less-obvious student behaviour as a proxy measure for professionalism. Building on research data that suggested that professionalism issues in clerkship might be predictable based on students' compliance with things like handing in course evaluations or documenting that their immunizations are up to date (Stern et al 2005), some groups have developed measures of what they call conscientiousness. In two studies at one institution, conscientiousness index (CI) scores correlated with faculty ratings of professionalism and with peer nominations for professionalism (Finn et al 2009, McLachlan et al 2009). The benefits are that the points awarded along the way can be recorded by faculty or administrative staff (e.g. attendance) and are objective, in that they require no value judgement. However, these results would need to be replicated in other contexts and settings before widespread use, especially as there are issues of acceptability to students who already feel they are under enough scrutiny.

Final considerations

As one plans assessment of professionalism, a final point worth considering is that professionalism develops along with other knowledge and skills; that is, there is a trajectory, and pre-clinical students should be taught and evaluated differently than their clinical counterparts. Further, some students have reported feeling 'harassed' by all the attention paid to their professional and unprofessional behaviour compared, for example, to the behaviour displayed by their faculty (Humphrey et al 2007). And especially with the advent of social media there are many more opportunities for learners (or faculty, for that matter) to be observed, and therefore monitored, so any new evaluations or policies developed should be sensitive to these issues and take the opportunity to educate students, not just discipline them (Ellaway 2010).

 Evaluation will be most useful if it incorporates "multiple kinds of measures, by multiple observers synthesized over time with data gathered in multiple, complex and challenging contexts."

Hodges 2011

Summary

As can be seen from the preceding, many methods exist that can be used or modified to assess learners' professionalism. Workplace-based assessments including ward evaluations or in-training evaluation reports are likely the most common in education settings, but the use of peer-assessment, 360° evaluations and other creative methods like the conscientiousness index are increasing in popularity. It is important to keep in mind that one method will not be sufficient: as the Ottawa consensus group recommended, 'triangulation of multiple kinds of measures, by multiple observers, synthesized over time with data gathered in multiple, complex and challenging contexts' is likely to be most useful (Hodges et al 2011). And it is worth restating that the overall programme of assessment is more useful than any one individual tool. 'The best programmes use a variety of tools in a safe climate; provide rich feedback, anonymity (where appropriate)' and follow-up behaviour over time.

References

Arnold L, Shue CK, Kritt B, et al: Medical students' views on peer assessment of professionalism, *Journal of General Internal Medicine* 20(9):819–824, 2005.

Arnold L, Shue CK, Kalishman S, et al: Can there be a single system for peer assessment of professionalism among medical students? A multi-institutional study, *Academic Medicine* 82(6):578–586, 2007.

Burack JH, Irby DM, Carline JD, et al: Teaching compassion and respect. Attending physicians' responses to problematic behaviors, *Journal of General Internal Medicine* 14(1):49–55, 1999.

Clauser BE, Margolis MJ, Holtman MC, et al: *Validity considerations in the assessment of professionalism,* 2010, Advances in Health Sciences Education.

Cleland J, Knight LV, Rees CE, et al: Is it me or is it them? Factors that influence the passing of underperforming students, *Medical Education* 42(8):800–809, 2008.

Colliver JA, Markwell SJ, Verhulst SJ, Robbs RS: Editorial: The prognostic value of documented unprofessional behavior in medical school records for predicting and preventing subsequent medical board disciplinary action: The Papadakis Studies revisited, *Teaching and Learning in Medicine* 19(3):213–215, 2007.

Cruess R, Cruess S: The cognitive base of professionalism. In Cruess R, Cruess S, Steinert Y, editors: *Teaching Medical Professionalism,* New York, NY, 2009, Cambridge University Press, pp 7–30.

Cruess R, McIlroy J, Cruess S, et al: The Professionalism Mini-evaluation Exercise: a preliminary investigation, *Academic Medicine* 81(10 Suppl):S74–78, 2006.

Dudek NL, Marks MB, Regehr G: Failure to fail: the perspectives of clinical supervisors, *Academic Medicine* 80(10 Suppl):S84–87, 2005.

Ellaway R: Digital professionalism, *Medical Teacher* 32(8):705–707, 2010.

Finn G, Sawdon M, Clipsham L, McLachlan J: Peer estimation of lack of professionalism correlates with low Conscientiousness Index scores, *Medical Education* 43(10):960–967, 2009.

Frank JR, Danoff D: The CanMEDS initiative: implementing an outcomes-based framework of physician competencies, *Medical Teacher* 29(7):642–647, 2007.

Frohna A, Stern DT: The nature of qualitative comments in evaluating professionalism, *Medical Education* 39(8):763–768, 2005.

Gaufberg E, Fitzpatrick A: The favour: a professional boundaries OSCE station, *Medical Education* 42(5):529–530, 2008.

Ginsburg S, Regehr G, Hatala R, et al: Context, conflict, and resolution: a new conceptual framework for evaluating professionalism, *Academic Medicine* 75(10 Suppl):S6–S11, 2000.

Ginsburg S, Regehr G, Mylopoulos M: From behaviours to attributions: further concerns regarding the evaluation of professionalism, *Medical Education* 43(5):414–425, 2009.

Ginsburg S, Gold W, Cavalcanti R, et al: Competencies 'plus': The nature of written comments on internal medicine residents' evaluation forms, *Academic Medicine* 86(10 Suppl):s34, 2011.

Goldie J, Schwartz L, McConnachie A, et al: Can students' reasons for choosing set answers to ethical vignettes be reliably rated? Development and testing of a method, *Medical Teacher* 26(8):713–718, 2004.

Hauer KE, Lovett M, O'Sullivan P, Teherani A: Categorization of unprofessional behaviours identified during administration of and remediation after a comprehensive clinical performance examination using a validated professionalism framework, *Medical Teacher* 31(11):1007–1012, 2009.

Hodges BD, Ginsburg S, Cruess R, et al: Assessment of professionalism: Recommendations from the Ottawa 2010 Conference, *Medical Teacher* 33(5):354–363, 2011.

Humphrey HJ, Smith K, Reddy ST, et al: Promoting an environment of professionalism: The University of Chicago 'roadmap', *Academic Medicine* 2007.

Lee RS, Boulais A-P, Bennett T: Professionalism assessment with multiple-choice questions: Believe it or not? In: *AMEE 2009 Final Abstract Book,* AMEE, 2009.

Lesser CS, Lucey C, Egener B, et al: Behavioral and systems view of professionalism, *JAMA* 304(24):2732–2737, 2010.

Lucey C, Souba W: Perspective: the problem with the problem of professionalism, *Academic Medicine* 85(6):1018–1024, 2010.

Lurie SJ, Nofziger AC, Meldrum S, et al: Effects of rater selection on peer assessment among medical students, *Medical Education* 40(11):1088–1097, 2006.

Lynch DC, Surdyk PM, Eiser AR: Assessing professionalism: a review of the literature, *Medical Teacher* 26(4):366–373, 2004.

Mazor KM, Zanetti ML, Alper EJ, et al: Assessing professionalism in the context of an objective structured clinical examination: an in-depth study of the rating process, *Medical Education* 41:331–340, 2007.

Mazor KM, Canavan C, Farrell M, et al: Collecting validity evidence for an assessment of professionalism: findings from think-aloud interviews, *Academic Medicine* 83(10 Suppl):S9–12, 2008.

McLachlan JC, Finn G, Macnaughton J: The conscientiousness index: a novel tool to explore students' professionalism, *Academic Medicine* 84(5):559–565, 2009.

Norcini J: Peer assessment of competence, *Medical Education* 37(6):539–543, 2003.

Papadakis MA, Teherani A, Banach MA, et al: Disciplinary action by medical boards and prior behavior in medical school, *New England Journal of Medicine* 353(25):2673–2682, 2005.

Papadakis MA, Arnold GK, Blank LL, et al: Performance during Internal Medicine Residency Training and Subsequent Disciplinary Action by State Licensing Boards, *Annals of Internal Medicine* 148(11):869–876, 2008.

Pohl CA, Hojat M, Arnold L: Peer nominations as related to academic attainment, empathy, personality, and specialty interest, *Academic Medicine* 86(6):747–751, 2011.

Rees CE, Knight LV: Viewpoint: the trouble with assessing students' professionalism: theoretical insights from sociocognitive psychology, *Academic Medicine* 82(1):46–50, 2007.

Regehr G: The persistent myth of stability. On the chronic underestimation of the role of context in behavior, *Journal of General Internal Medicine* 21(5):544–545, 2006.

Singer PA, Robb A, Cohen R, et al: Performance-based assessment of clinical ethics using an objective structured clinical examination, *Academic Medicine* 71(5):495–498, 1996.

Stern DT, editor: *Measuring Medical Professionalism*, New York, NY, 2006, Oxford University Press.

Stern DT, Frohna A, Gruppen LD: The prediction of professional behaviour, *Medical Education* 39(1):75–82, 2005.

Tsugawa Y, Tokuda Y, Ohbu S, et al: Professionalism Mini-Evaluation Exercise for medical residents in Japan: a pilot study, *Medical Education* 43(10):968–978, 2009.

Van Mook WN, Gorter SL, O'Sullivan H, et al: Approaches to professional behaviour assessment: tools in the professionalism toolbox, *European Journal of Internal Medicine* 20(8):e153–157, 2009.

Weigelt JA, Brasel KJ, Bragg D, Simpson D: The 360-degree evaluation: increased work with little return? *Current Surgergy* 61(6):616–626, 2004.

Wilkinson TJ, Wade WB, Knock LDA: Blueprint to assess professionalism: results of a systematic review, *Academic Medicine* 84(5):551–558, 2009.

Zanetti M, Keller L, Mazor KM, et al: Using standardized patients to assess professionalism: a generalizability study, *Teaching and Learning in Medicine* 22(4):274–279, 2010.

Websites

Assessment of Professional Behaviors. Available at: http://www.nbme.org/schools/oa/APB/index.html

Common Program Requirements 2011. Available at: http://www.acgme.org/acgmeweb/Portals/0/dh_dutyhoursCommonPR07012007.pdf

Section 7

Staff and students

Medical education leadership

J. McKimm, S. J. Lieff

Introduction

Medical educators are involved in a wide range of activities including teaching, facilitating learning, curriculum design and development, assessment, evaluation and managing teams, departments and programmes. All these activities require some form of leadership, whether this is leading a team on a project, ensuring that you provide the right learning environment on a ward or in clinic or leading the development of a new programme or curriculum. We often think of 'leadership' as associated with senior management, with deans or principals or about people other than ourselves. However, Drucker (1996) suggests that effective leaders are people who have followers, who do the right things and achieve results, who set examples and are visible and who take responsibility. Leadership can therefore be found at all levels.

Medical educators take both leadership and followership roles, which can be:

- 'big L' Leadership: leading big projects or leadership at senior levels

- 'little l' leadership: leading teams, classroom leadership

- 'active' followership: independent critical thinkers, actively engaged in creating positive energy for the organisation

- 'passive' followership: look to the leader to do their thinking, passive involvement, negative energy.

Kelley 1988

Evidence from all sectors of industry, public, private or third sector, shows that good leadership is vital in ensuring organizational success. And, conversely, that poor leadership and management have been shown to play a major part in failing organizations (Kotter 1990). From an educational standpoint, health professionals are increasingly required to engage in clinical leadership, and medical students and doctors are no exception. Internationally, doctors are being called upon to take more active engagement in the leadership and management of clinical services, which has led to an increased emphasis on ensuring that medical students 'learn leadership' in their undergraduate programmes. This requires medical educators to be much more aware not only of the practice of leadership as it relates to their educational work, but also of planning and delivering education that includes leadership concepts and examples. In this chapter we focus specifically on medical educational leadership, but many articles and books on general leadership (drawn mainly from industry) and educational leadership (particularly in the schools sector) and a growing literature on clinical leadership are all highly relevant to medical education, which straddles both education/training and health services.

A massive leadership literature has growing emphasis on whether (and if so, what) specific qualities, attributes, knowledge or skills are most effective in different organizational and professional contexts. Identifying specific issues, challenges and opportunities in medical education helps to strengthen capacity of organizations, improve individual leaders' performance and enhance the experience for those who work within organizations and our clients or customers (i.e. students and the end users of medical education: patients).

Medical education leadership involves:

- Roles played out in a highly visible, regulated and complex environment: a 'crowded stage'

- Working across boundaries and organizations (higher [tertiary] education environments, community settings and complex health services) continually in a state of flux and reconfiguration

- Producing highly skilled, socially accountable professionals.

Leadership and management

"No-one is terribly enthusiastic about managers who don't lead: they are boring, dispiriting. Well, why should we be any more enthusiastic about leaders who don't manage: they are distant, disconnected. Hence I shall argue for leading embedded in managing, by recognizing its true art and respecting its true craft."

Mintzberg 2009

In this chapter, we have subsumed 'management' under the topic of leadership. Although many writers in the past have clearly differentiated between leadership and management, this approach tends to reinforce the difference between the two sets of activities, with management somehow being seen as secondary to leadership, thus promoting the idea that it is preferable to be a leader than a manager. Leadership theories in the 1950s and 1960s identified 'transactional leadership' as similar to a managerial approach in that the leader/manager engaged in transactions with subordinates. So a leader might motivate people by offering rewards for a job well done or imposing sanctions for non-compliance or failing to deliver. Contemporary theory emphasizes that effective leaders require managerial skills and vice versa. Whilst many of the (copious) lists of leadership qualities emphasize the importance of vision, strategic thinking, setting direction and communication, if the vision cannot be translated into activities that work on the ground and make a difference to improving the performance of an organization or learners' experience, then the vision is illusory. The most effective leaders know their strengths and weaknesses and build a team who can deliver the shared vision.

"The challenge of modern organisations requires the objective perspective of the manager as well as the brilliant flashes of vision and commitment wise leadership provides."

Bolman & Deal 1997

Our current understanding of medical education leadership

Much has been written about leadership characteristics, behaviours, mind-sets and competencies in academic medical and education settings. In academic medicine, practising and aspiring leaders identify knowledge of academic role-related and health professional practice, interpersonal/social skills, vision and organizational orientation as desired abilities of academic physicians (Taylor et al 2008). Rich et al's (2008) literature review of desirable qualities of medical school deans identifies a variety of management and leadership skills and attitudes as well as specific knowledge regarding academic medical governance, processes of medical education, legal issues and challenges and expectations of faculty. Leithwood et al (2009) found that successful school leaders engaged in four sets of core practices: setting directions, developing people, redesigning the organization and managing the teaching programme.

The literature surrounding medical education leadership is, however, still in its infancy. Bland et al (1999) were among the first to empirically study specific education leadership behaviours for successful university-community collaborations related to curricular change. In successful collaborative curriculum change projects, leaders most frequently used participative governance and cultural value-influencing behaviours: communicating vision, goals and values, creating structures to achieve goals, attending to members' needs and development, and creating and articulating symbols and stories representing dominant values. Lieff and Albert (2011) extended these findings by studying the leadership practices (what they do and how they do it) of a diversity of medical education leaders in a faculty of medicine in their daily work.

 Medical education leaders' practices fall into four domains:

- intrapersonal (e.g. role modelling, communication)
- interpersonal (e.g. value relationships, soliciting support)
- organisational (e.g. sharing vision, facilitating change)
- systemic (e.g. political navigation, organisational understanding).

Lieff & Albert 2011

This framework of practices aligns with the primarily relational and complex nature of leadership work in an ever-changing medical education system that must simultaneously attend to education and healthcare service needs. It also creates an opportunity for identifying enabling competencies for effectiveness in these multiple practices.

Bordage et al (2000) set out to identify the desirable competencies, skills and attributes of prospective educational programme directors in a variety of health professions as judged by potential employers. They identify being a competent practitioner as well as educational, decision-making, communication, interpersonal, teamwork and fiscal management skills. The top personal attributes were being visionary, flexible, open-minded, trustworthy and value-driven.

McKimm's (2004) study of health and social care education leaders in the UK describes similar skills and attributes, but adds self-awareness, self-management, strategic and analytic thinking skills, tolerance of ambiguity, being willing to take risks, professional judgement and contextual awareness.

 The Academy of Medical Educators (2012) in the UK sets out a framework of professional standards for medical educators. Within the theme of educational management and leadership, three elements of management, leadership and governance are defined in terms of graded levels of competence:

- an ability to manage personal time and resources effectively to the benefit of the educational faculty and the needs of the learners

- a consolidated understanding of his or her role in the work of an educational faculty

- an ability to describe the roles of relevant bodies in the provision of medical education.

 "Managing is a tapestry of the threads of reflection, analysis, worldliness, collaboration and proactiveness, all of it infused with personal energy and bonded by social integration."

Mintzberg 2009

Mintzberg's 'threads' require deliberate attention in order to be effective. Effective leaders know how to think and make decisions in complex environments, which are dynamic and constantly evolving in response to internal processes as well as external demands that cannot be predicted. For complex issues, leaders are encouraged to act and learn at the same time by conducting small experiments with tight feedback loops that illuminate the path forward (Snowden & Boone 2007). Education leaders must realize that fragmentation is a natural tendency of a complex system; therefore, their role is to enable coherence making. They must keep their eye on the central focus of student learning and ideas that will further the thinking and vision of the school as a whole (Fullan 2002).

 When leading education change: "never a checklist, always complexity."

Fullan 2002

Lieff and Albert's study (2010) of medical education leaders' mind-sets shows that, while these leaders employed Bolman and Deal's 'four frames' for understanding organizational work, they favour the human resource frame followed closely by the political and symbolic frames. From the political frame perspective, they recognize, understand and engage with stakeholders' interests in order to be informed, advocate and cultivate support. They identify and leverage diverse sources of power and appreciate the complexity of resource and political issues as underpinning tensions in educational work. From a symbolic perspective, they work at ensuring a vision or direction that people can engage with in order to commit. They attend to the importance of credibility and modelling values and messages in behaviours, activities, structures and policies of programmes. They also appreciate that histories, traditions and belief systems can impede or enable change. Additionally, they deliberately appraised others' interpersonal and work style in order to understand how to socially situate people in the organization so they can work to their strengths.

 Education leaders need to invest in valuing, supporting and caring for faculty and students and think carefully about the alignment of faculty interests with organizational needs in order to engage people (a human resource frame).

Lieff & Albert 2010

Leadership theory and practice

In this section, we describe theories and models that are most relevant to medical education leadership and give examples of how these might apply in practice for contemporary medical education leaders. Table 42.1 summarizes a wider range of leadership theories and key features (with different approaches, underpinning perspectives or discourses) found in the literature.

As its name suggests, the situational leadership model proposes that how a leader behaves should depend on the situation. Hersey and Blanchard (1993) suggest that leaders should flexibly shift amongst four behaviours: directing, coaching, supporting and delegating in response to the followers or group context and goals. If followers are less confident, capable or willing, a directing or coaching approach is appropriate. With increased capability and confidence, leaders need to shift to more supporting or delegating styles. Laiken (1998) proposes that these behaviours map onto Tuckman's stages of group development: forming, storming, norming, performing and adjourning. In the early stages of a team's work, leaders need to be more directive to facilitate forming. As the group moves into storming and norming, leaders shift to a coaching style and so on. This model can be useful for medical education leaders in appreciating the need for flexibility in their leadership of individuals, committees, task forces or teams. Often medical education leaders prefer the coaching and supporting roles, where they

Table 42.1 Leadership theories and approaches

Leadership theory	Key features	Indicative theorists
Adaptive leadership	This leader facilitates people to wrestle with the adaptive challenges for which there is no obvious solution.	Heifetz & Linsky 2004
Affective leadership	Involves expressed emotion, the 'dance of leadership'. Leaders rapidly assess the affective state of the other, analyse their affective state and select the appropriate affect to display in order to achieve the desired (or best achievable) outcome.	Denhardt & Denhardt 2006, Newman et al 2009
Authentic leadership	Extends from authenticity of the leader to encompass authentic relations with followers and associates. These relationships are characterized by transparency, trust, worthy objectives and follower development.	Luthans & Avolio 2003
Charismatic leadership Narcissistic leader	Hero leader, strong role model, personal qualities important, 'leader as messiah'. Organization invests a lot in one senior person, often seen as rescuer, doesn't recognize human fallibility. Leader fails to distribute/share power and can lead organization to destruction.	Maccoby 2007a,b
Complex adaptive leadership	Views leadership work as embedded in systems of interdependence that are constantly changing in response to internal and external forces. Diversity of perspectives and experimentation are the norm.	Zimmerman et al 1998
Collaborative leadership	Ensure all those affected are included and consulted. Work together (networks, partnerships) to identify and achieve shared goals. The more power we share, the more power we have.	Bradshaw 1999
Contingency theories	Leadership varies according to (contingent on) the situation or context in which the leader finds him- or herself.	Goleman 2000
Dialogic leadership	Promotes inquiry and advocacy practices in order to explore possibilities and stimulate creative thinking.	Isaacs 1999
Distributed, dispersed leadership	Informal, social process within organizations, open boundaries, leadership at all levels, leadership is everyone's responsibility.	Kouzes & Posner 2002
Eco leadership	Connectivity, interdependence and sustainability. Socially responsive and accountable.	Western 2012
Emotional intelligence (EI)	Comprises self-awareness; self-management; social awareness; social skills: can be learned.	Goleman 2000
Engaging leadership	Nearby leadership, based on relationship between leaders and followers. Effective style for public services.	Alimo-Metcalfe & Alban-Metcalfe 2008
Followership	Followers are as important as (if not more than) leaders. All have different styles and behaviours (active, passive, independent thinkers, critical, negative, star followers, pragmatists, yes people) that impact on leadership. A mix of followers is helpful; take care not to stereotype.	Kelley 1988, 1992, Collinson 2006
Leader-member-exchange (LMX) theory	Every leader has a unique, individual relationship with each follower. These relationships differ in terms of the quality of the interactions based on whether the follower is part of the 'in-group' or 'out-group'.	Graen & Uhl-Bien 1995, Seibert et al 2003
Ontological leadership	'Being' a leader is central, in terms of process, actions and impact on others and self.	Erhard et al 2011

Table 42.1 Leadership theories and approaches–cont'd

Leadership theory	Key features	Indicative theorists
Relational leadership	Emerged from human relations movement. Leaders motivate through facilitating individual growth and achievement.	Binney et al 2004
Servant leadership	Leader serves to serve first, then aspires to lead; concept of stewardship is important.	Greenleaf 1977
Situational leadership	Leadership behaviour needs to adapt to readiness or developmental stage of individuals or the group, e.g. directing, coaching, supporting, delegating. Attention equally on task, team, individual.	Adair 2004, Hersey & Blanchard 1993, Laiken 1998
Trait theory 'Great man' theory	Based on personality traits and personal qualities, e.g. 'big five' personality factors: extraversion, agreeableness, conscientiousness, neuroticism, openness to new experience	Judge et al 2002, Maccoby 2007a,b
Transactional leadership	Similar to management, relationships seen in terms of what the leaders can offer subordinates and vice versa. Rewards (and sanctions) contingent on performance.	Burns 1978, Bass 1996
Transformational leadership	Leads through transforming others to reach higher order goals or vision. Used widely in public services, e.g. the UK National Health Service *Leadership Qualities Framework*.	Bass & Avolio 1994
Value-led Moral leadership	Values and morals underpin approaches and behaviours.	Collins 2001

still have a hand in the work, but leaders need to delegate once the group or individual seems willing and capable enough to perform independently. Succession planning is a critical issue in leadership, so leaders need to find ways to provide leadership experiences and exposure to others.

The contingent leader assesses the context to determine what leadership style would be most appropriate. Goleman (2000) proposes six leadership styles based on emotional intelligence:

- Coercive
- Authoritative
- Pacesetting
- Affiliative
- Democratic
- Coaching.

Leaders create resonance by being attuned to others and moving them in a positive direction. Emotionally intelligent leaders fluidly and consciously choose the most relevant leadership style, are flexible and can adapt their style to context and situation. Leaders who use the authoritative, affiliative, democratic and coaching styles outperform those who use fewer and other styles. The authoritative style has the most strongly positive impact on organizational climate. The authoritative leader presents a compelling future vision and clear articulation of the actions required to achieve the desired future, maximizes commitment to the organization's goals and structures, invites people to join him or her and generates trust. The affiliative, democratic and coaching styles emphasize emotional harmony, consensus and support and development, respectively.

Leaders need to reflect on context prior to selecting their leadership style. Often medical education leaders have little formal power or authority, so engaging people around aspirations, valuing them and ensuring that voices are heard can be an effective way of meaningfully involving and motivating others.

 Importantly for medical education leaders (who are often high-performing clinicians or academics) pacesetting leadership can have a negative impact on organizational performance and can lead to the leader becoming alienated and resented by colleagues as they struggle to keep up to (sometimes) unrealistic standards or pace of work.

Dialogic leadership evolved from the field of dialogue (Bohm et al 1991). In the knowledge and networked world of medical education, the ability to communicate and think together well is critical to team and organizational effectiveness. Dialogue requires an inquiry that surfaces ideas, perceptions and understanding. The dialogic leader uncovers, through conversations, people's untapped wisdom, collective insights and creative potential (Isaacs 1999), particularly when leaders are dealing with issues to which no one has clear answers. The leader's role is to ensure that people are transparent about their ideas, build on and do not judge others' ideas and resist the inclination to make decisions. The leader must evoke people's genuine voices, listening deeply, holding space for and respecting others' legitimate views and broaden awareness and perspective. This leader embodies these attributes and activates them in others. In medical education, this leader would try to ensure that committee and task force members appreciate the necessity for their group members to share responsibility for four action capabilities:

- initiating ideas and offering direction
- supporting and helping others clarify their thoughts
- respectfully challenging what is being said
- providing perspective on what is happening.

Transformational leadership focusses on stimulating the 'followers' in the organization to transcend their own self-interest for a perceived greater organizational good or goal (Bass 1996). This approach emphasizes motivating members of a group by raising their awareness of the importance of idealized goals and values and moving them to address higher-order needs. This is achieved through role modelling, influencing skills and providing leadership tailored to enabling people to see the alignment of their own personal and professional goals with those of the organization to effect positive change.

"The four 'I's' of transformational leadership:
- Idealized influence
- Inspirational motivation
- Intellectual stimulation
- Individualized consideration."

Bass 1996

Kouzes and Posner describe five practices: model the way, inspire a shared vision, challenge the process, enable others to act and encourage the heart (Kouzes & Posner 2002). Both these approaches align closely with findings on the mind-sets and practices of medical education leaders, suggesting that this is a popular implicit model (Lieff & Albert 2010, Lieff & Albert 2011). These leaders are keenly aware of the need to role model the values and moral standards, leading others to trust and respect them. They believe in creating a shared vision that arises from the collective and inspire through motivation to become part of these great expectations. Critical to this discourse is

the leader's role in creating a supportive climate by nurturing, coaching and developing people to collaborate to achieve these goals. Programme and course directors can appeal to their faculty members' growth needs of esteem, self-respect and self-actualization. It can be exciting for people to have the opportunity to stretch themselves (with appropriate development) to create and contribute to something that is greater than the local and immediate needs. Such enterprises include curriculum development, health improvement initiatives or other educational innovations or adaptations that feel meaningful.

Increasingly, the world of medical schools and their curricula is being recognized as a complex adaptive system (Mennin 2010) which includes collections of individual agents who have the freedom to act in ways that are not always totally predictable and whose actions are interconnected such that one agent's actions change the context for others (Westley et al 2006). Complex systems are dynamic and constantly evolving in response to internal or external influences. Complex issues have unknown answers with little agreement or certainty on how to approach them (Stacey 1992), and medical education leaders need to let go of notions of control and work with others to identify patterns and shared meaning.

 Effective medical education leaders:

- Recognize that they, their organization, department, programme or team needs to interact with and adapt to the environment with minimal constraints
- Embrace acting and learning at the same time
- Encourage education 'experiments' in curricula, assessment, etc. with tight feedback loops to ensure learning and evolution
- Develop informal networks around shared interests
- Bring together heterogeneous mind-sets and viewpoints whilst enabling emergence of innovative ideas and approaches
- Hold alternate viewpoints and facilitate the communication and development of relationships within diverse perspectives.

For the adaptive leader, leadership is an improvisational and experimental art (Heifetz et al 2009) in which leaders discern whether challenges can be solved with known expertise or whether new learning and pattern of behaviours are required. Technical problems reside in the head; adaptive challenges lie in the stomach and the heart (Heifetz & Linsky 2004). Changing curricula demands, clinical capabilities and healthcare innovations are adaptive challenges that require new learning. The leaders' work is to mobilize people to wrestle with these issues in order to be able to adapt. This leader is a facilitator who, while keeping the picture of the whole education system in mind (school, programme), must identify the issue and relevant stakeholders. Leaders must create a holding environment which regulates and puts enough stress on the group so that they are sufficiently motivated, but not so much that they cannot focus, or so little that they become complacent (Heifetz & Laurie 2003).

The adaptive leader maintains focus on issues by asking difficult ('wicked') questions that enable conflicts and sensitive issues to surface. The leader–follower relationship is similar to that of the physician–patient relationship when dealing with a complex management issue such as the diagnosis and management of a poor prognosis carcinoma (Heifetz 1994). The role of the physician is not to tell the patient how to manage the last 10 months of their life. Rather, the physician assists the patient and their family in receiving the information they need to know as they are ready to receive it and asks the difficult questions that enable them to make decisions about their present and their future.

The authentic leader is someone who is deeply aware of how they think and behave. They:

- Demonstrate a passion for their purpose
- Lead based on their personal convictions and values
- Lead who they are (like teachers, who 'teach who they are')
- Are aware of others' values, perspectives and strengths
- Establish long-term meaningful relationships connected through a common purpose
- Are resilient
- Know they are fallible, demonstrate humility and are not complacent

George et al 2007, Palmer 2006

Authentic leaders are equally aware of the context in which they operate (Shamira & Eilam 2005). In the unpredictable and ever-changing world of medical education, extrinsic motivators such as material reward and recognition are insufficient to motivate and engage people. Authentic leaders are needed who attend to people's search for meaning and connection, genuinely relate to others, support optimism and display resilience (Avolio et al 2004). This contributes to the building of trust, engagement and commitment in others (Avolio & Gardner 2005, George et al 2007). Members of this leader's team are motivated by the leader's example, support of authenticity and

self-determination in others as well as emotional contagion and positive social exchanges.

The relational leader takes a 'leader as therapist' role, an approach derived from the human relations movement as a contrasting model and discourse to the charismatic, transformational and heroic leader: 'leader as messiah', or to the more managerial or transactional 'leader as controller' (Western 2012). In these models, 'being a leader' (the ontological nature of leadership) and 'living leadership' is central (Erhard et al 2011).

 "A focus on individual personal growth and self-actualisation was readily translated to the workplace, through techniques to motivate individuals and teams, through job re-design and job satisfaction to make work more satisfying and produce group cohesion."

Western 2012

The leaders' personal qualities include values (value-led leadership) of moral purpose, of authenticity in everyday interactions and spirituality. The relational leader is 'post-heroic', works with people in an authentic way, displays emotional congruence, humility, emotional intelligence and quiet authority. In this model, there are elements and echoes of affective leadership, servant leadership, collaborative leadership and dispersed or distributed leadership. Much of the recent focus of leadership development activities on coaching and personal development reflects this approach.

In reality, leaders often fulfil many roles and operate within multiple discourses and realities. This is the challenge for the postmodern leader, trying to achieve a balance whilst operating in complex and constantly changing environments, managing as well as leading, being as well as doing, and doing all this with compassion, authenticity and efficiency. Western's (2012) discussion of the prevalent discourses that define leadership offers us a new paradigm of eco-leadership. Again, this model has elements and echoes from other approaches (particularly that of the change literature and of complex adaptive systems) but takes an ecological perspective. The eco-leader works within open systems, within networks and connectedness.

 "Eco-leadership is about connectivity, interdependence and sustainability, underpinned by an ethical, socially responsible stance ... it is fuelled by the human spirit, for some this is underpinned by spirituality, for others not."

Western 2012

Summary

"Educators carry the double burden of managing and leading teams and institutions in a rapidly changing educational environment whilst working in close collaboration with a range of healthcare professionals to deliver safe and high-quality patient care."

McKimm & Swanwick 2011

Medical education leadership is characterized by its ultimate goal: to benefit today's and tomorrow's patients, yet leaders work in a complex system which includes university environments, healthcare organizations and other regulatory and professional bodies. Navigating through this complexity requires understanding of policy agendas, strategy, systems and organizations as well as knowledge of operational management processes and procedures, without which change and quality improvements will not happen. Educators and managers at all levels provide leadership to their learners, colleagues and others. Effective leaders are change agents who are comfortable with working in uncertain and rapidly changing environments, holding onto and communicating core vision and values, adapting strategy to external and internal change. Being able to negotiate across and within organizational, professional, department and team boundaries and to work within the 'spaces between' (which is where change is effected) is a vital characteristic.

But leadership is also about knowing yourself and 'people work': emotional labour (Held & McKimm 2011). So authentic and consistent personal leadership and 'modelling the way' is vital. This is where leadership most closely intersects with where medical education and the practice of medicine are moving: into an arena where the social accountability role of medical schools is being questioned and co-created, where the concept of being and becoming a doctor and a professional is debated, researched and challenged, and where the importance and impact of emotional labour is acknowledged. Here is where the most recent discussions of leadership in terms of values, relations, authenticity, complexity and eco-leadership can inform the day-to-day practice of all medical educators, whether or not they are in formal leadership roles.

References

Academy of Medical Educators: Professional Standards, 2012. Available at http://www.medicaleducators.org/index.cfm/profession/profstandards/

Adair J: *The John Adair Handbook of Leadership and Management*, London, 2004, Thorogood.

Alimo-Metcalfe B, Alban-Metcalfe J: *Engaging Leadership: Creating Organizations That Maximise the Potential of Their People*. London, 2008, CIPD.

Avolio BJ, Luthans F, Walumba FO: Authentic leadership: Theory building for veritable sustained performance. Working paper: Gallup Leadership Institute, University of Nebraska-Lincoln, 2004.

Avolio BJ, Gardner WL: Authentic leadership development: Getting to the root of positive forms of leadership, *The Leadership Quarterly* 16: 315–338, 2005.

Bass BM: *Transformational Leadership*, ed 2, Mahwah, NJ, 1996, Lawrence Erlbaum.

Bass BM, Avolio B: *Improving Organisational Effectiveness through Transformational Leadership*, Thousand Oaks, NJ, 1994, Sage.

Binney G, Wilke, G, Williams C: *Living Leadership: A Practical Guide for Ordinary Heroes*, London, 2004, Pearson Books.

Bland CJ, Starnaman S, Hembroff L, et al: Leadership behaviours for successful university-community collaborations to change curricula, *Academic Medicine* 74:127–1237, 1999.

Bohm D, Factor D, Garrett P: Dialogue – A proposal, 1991. http://www.david-bohm.net/dialogue/dialogue_proposal.html

Bolman I, Deal T: *Reframing Organisation: Artistry, Choice and Leadership*, San Francisco, 1997, Jossey Bass.

Bordage G, Foley R, Goldyn S: Skills and attributes of directors of educational programmes, *Medical Education* 34(3):206–210, 2000.

Bradshaw L: Principals as boundary spanners: Working collaboratively to solve problems, *NASSP Bulletin* 83(611):38–47, 1999.

Burns JM: *Leadership*, New York, 1978, Harper & Row.

Collins J: *Good to Great*, London, 2001, Random House.

Collinson D: Rethinking followership: A poststructural analysis of follower identities, *The Leadership Quarterly* 17:179–189, 2006.

Denhardt B, Denhardt V: *The Dance of Leadership: The Art of Leading in Business, Government, and Society*, Armonk, NY, 2006, M.E. Sharpe.

Drucker P: Foreword: Not enough generals were killed. In Hesselbein F, Goldsmith M, Beckhard R, editors: *The Leader of the Future*, San Francisco, 1996, Jossey Bass.

Erhard WH, Jensen MC, Granger KL: Creating leaders: an ontological model. Harvard Business School Negotiation, Organisations and Markets Research

Papers No. 11-037, 2011. Available at: http://ssrn.com/abstract=1681682

Fullan M: The change leader. *Educational Leadership* (May):16–20, 2002.

George B, Sims P, McLean AN, Mayer D: Discovering your authentic leadership, *Harvard Business Review* (Feb):129–138, 2007.

Goleman D: Leadership that gets results, *Harvard Business Review* (March):78–90, 2000.

Graen GB, Uhl-Bien M: The relationship-based approach to leadership: Development of LMX theory of leadership over 25 years: Applying a multi-level, multi-domain perspective, *Leadership Quarterly* 6(2):219–247, 1995.

Greenleaf RK: *Servant Leadership: A Journey into the Nature of Legitimate Power and Greatness*, Mahwah, NJ, 1977, Paulist Press.

Heifetz RA: *Leadership without Easy Answers*, Cambridge, MA, 1994, Harvard University Press.

Heifetz RA, Laurie DL: The leader as teacher: creating the learning organization, *Ivey Business Journal* (Jan/Feb):1–9, 2003.

Heifetz RA, Linsky M: When leadership spells danger. *Educational Leadership* (April):33–37/August:62–69, 2004.

Heifetz RA, Grashow A, Linsky M: Leadership in a (permanent) crisis. *Harvard Business Review* (July):2009.

Held S, McKimm J: Emotional intelligence, emotional labour and affective leadership. In Preedy M, Bennett N, Wise C, editors: *Educational Leadership: Context, Strategy and Collaboration*, Milton Keynes, 2011, The Open University.

Hersey P, Blanchard K: *Management of Organizational Behaviour: Utilizing Human Resources*, ed 6, Englewood Cliffs, NJ, 1993, Prentice Hall.

Isaacs I: Dialogic leadership, *The Systems Thinker* 10(1):1–5, 1999.

Judge TA, Bono JE, Ilies R, Gerhardt MW: Personality and leadership: a qualitative and quantitative review, *Journal of Applied Psychology* 87(4):765–780, 2002.

Kelley R: *The Power of Followership*, New York, 1992, Doubleday.

Kelley RE: In praise of followers, *Harvard Business Review* 66:142–148, 1988.

Kouzes JM, Posner BZ: *The leadership challenge*, ed 3, San Francisco, 2002, Jossey-Bass.

Kotter JP: *A Force for Change: How Leadership Differs from Management*, New York, 1990, Free Press.

Laiken M: *The Anatomy of High Performing Teams: A Leader's Handbook*, ed 3, Toronto, 1998, University of Toronto Press.

Leithwood K, Day C, Sammons P, et al: *Successful school leadership: what it is and how it influences pupil learning. Research report 800. National College for School Leadership*, 2009, University of Nottingham.

Lieff SJ, Albert M: The mindsets of medical education leaders: how do they conceive of their work? *Academic Medicine* 85:57–62, 2010.

Lieff S J, Albert M: What do I do? Practices and learning strategies of medical education leaders. Abstract from the Proceedings of the International Conference on Faculty Development, Toronto, 2011.

Luthans F, Avolio BJ: Authentic leadership: A positive developmental approach. In Cameron KS, Dutton JE, Quinn RE, editors: *Positive Organizational Scholarship*. San Francisco, 2003, Barrett-Koehler, pp 241–261.

Maccoby M: *Narcissistic Leaders: Who Succeeds and Who Fails*, Boston, 2007a, Harvard Business School Press.

Maccoby M: *The Leaders We Need and What Makes Us Follow*, Boston, 2007b, Harvard Business School Press.

McKimm J: *Special Report 5. Case Studies in Leadership in Medical and Health Care Education*, York, 2004, The Higher Education Academy.

McKimm J, Swanwick T: Educational leadership. In Swanwick T, McKimm J, editors: *The ABC of Clinical Leadership*, London, 2011, Wiley Blackwell.

Mennin S: Self-organisation, integration and curriculum in the complex world of medical education, *Medical Education* 44:20–30, 2010.

Mintzberg H: *Managing San Francisco*, 2009, Berett-Koehler.

Newman MA, Guy ME, Mastracci SH: Beyond cognition: affective leadership and emotional labour, *Public Administration Review* 69:6–20, 2009.

Palmer P: An undivided life. podcast, 2006. http://www.couragerenewal.org/podcast

Rich EC, Magrane D, Kirch DG: Qualities of the medical school dean: insights from the literature, *Academic Medicine* 83:483–487, 2008.

Seibert SE, Sparrowe RT, Liden RC: A group exchange structure approach to leadership in groups. In Pearce CL, Conger JA, editors: *Shared Leadership: Reframing the Hows and Whys of Leadership*, Thousand Oaks, CA, 2003, Sage Publications.

Shamira B, Eilam T: What's your story? A life-stories approach to authentic leadership development, *The Leadership Quarterly* 16:395–417, 2005.

Snowden DJ, Boone ME: A leader's framework for decision-making, *Harvard Business Review* (Nov):68–76, 2007.

Stacey R: *Managing the Unknowable*, San Francisco, 1992, Jossey-Bass.

Taylor CA, Taylor JC, Stoller JK: Exploring leadership competencies in established and aspiring physician leaders: an interview-based study, *Journal of General Internal Medicine* 23(6):748–754, 2008.

Western S: An overview of leadership discourses. In Preedy M, Bennett N, Wise C, editors: *Educational Leadership: Context, Strategy and Collaboration*, Milton Keynes, 2012, The Open University.

Westley F, Zimmerman B, Patton M: *Getting to Maybe: How the World Has Changed*, Toronto, 2006, Random House.

Zimmerman B, Lindberg C, Plsek P: Edgeware: Insights from Complexity Science for Healthcare Leaders, Irving, TX, 1998, VHA Publishing.

Additional reading

Doyle ME, Smith MK: Classical leadership. In *The Encyclopedia of Informal Education*, 2001. http://www.infed.org/leadership/traditional_leadership.htm

Introduction

Selection seems deceptively easy: if there are more applicants than places, then simply choose the best applicants. In practice, things are rather more complicated. Selection may be:

- of dubious validity
- statistically unreliable
- a vulnerable process legally and ethically
- open to challenge on grounds such as discrimination
- criticized by society at large
- under-resourced given the implicit expectations of society, the profession and medical schools.

Although student selection is traditionally concerned with entry to medical school, recent years have seen a growing interest in postgraduate selection, where similar problems apply and similar principles and methods can be used.

"For a man to be truly suited to the practice of medicine, he must be possessed of a natural disposition for it, the necessary instruction, favourable circumstances, education, industry and time. The first requisite is a natural disposition, for a reluctant student renders every effort vain."

Hippocrates

Why select?

"Selection is of key importance to medical education. What sort of students are recruited at the beginning is a major determination of what kind of doctors come out at the end."

Downie & Charlton 1992

Selection programmes must clearly state their reasons for selecting. If the *only* reason were reduction of numbers, then a lottery would suffice. In reality, selection has multiple components occurring at different stages.

SELECTION OF STUDENTS BY THE MEDICAL SCHOOL

The straightforward reason is to choose the best students. Although seemingly simple, that little word 'best' hides many subtleties and complexities.

SELECTION BY APPLICANTS OF MEDICINE AS A CAREER

The pool of medical school applicants only contains those who have selected medicine as a career. The very many individuals who did not apply cannot be selected, even if they might have made excellent doctors.

"Although there are reasons for being anxious about medical school selection, not all of the blame can be laid at the door of the selectors. Self-selection and preselection out of the applicant pool is extensive."

Johnson 1971

IMPLICIT SELECTION OF THE MEDICAL SCHOOLS BY APPLICANTS

While schools are selecting students, they are also selecting us, studying a range of schools and deciding which to apply to. An excellent selection system is of little use if the best applicants apply elsewhere. Effective selection begins by encouraging the right students to apply.

EXPLICIT SELECTION OF MEDICAL SCHOOLS BY APPLICANTS

When applicants receive offers from two or more medical schools, it is they who select medical schools, not vice versa.

SELECTION FOR A PARTICULAR COURSE

Increasingly, medical schools are developing courses with different emphases. Courses with large components of problem-based learning in small groups might prefer students who work together cooperatively rather than competitively.

SELECTION BY STAFF FOR STAFF

Staff who are actively involved in selection feel ownership of selection, developing a relationship with future students, who themselves feel that by staff selection they have become accepted into membership of the institution.

The limits of selection

"*Unfortunately the qualities which count for most in medicine are not precisely measurable. The measurable − examination performance at school − neither necessarily relates to these quantities nor guarantees intellectual potential. … In this sea of uncertainty it is not surprising that selection processes are imperfect and open to criticism or that the remedy is not immediately apparent.*"

Richards 1983

A common misconception is that medical schools receive numerous applications. In practice, particularly in the UK, the ratio is typically about two and a half applicants for every place, although admissions officers may feel the ratio is much higher as each candidate makes multiple applications. The power of selection ultimately depends on the 'selection ratio', the number of applicants for each place. As the ratio grows, selection can be more effective. A ratio of less than one means a school is recruiting, not selecting.

The limits of selection are easily shown mathematically. If selecting on a single criterion (such as intellectual ability) which has a normal distribution of ability, and with a selection ratio of two applicants per place, the optimal selection is shown in Fig. 43.1. The candidates are placed in rank order, and those above the median are selected.

The limits of selection become apparent when two or more criteria are introduced, for example, intellectual ability and communication skills, which are essentially uncorrelated. The distribution is now bivariate normal (see Fig. 43.2) and the aim is to select the best 50% of candidates on the joint criteria. The dashed lines indicate the median for each of the separate distributions.

Selecting candidates to be above a particular threshold on *both* criteria means they are in the top right-hand corner of the figure. The key point to realize is that the threshold on either criterion will be substantially below the median. In fact, with two independent criteria, selected candidates are only in the top 71% of the ability range, rather than the top 50%, and hence are less able on average than if either criterion on its own had been used. The same conclusion applies also if one allows compensation between the separate abilities (McManus & Vincent 1993). If medical student selection is based predominantly on academic achievement, then for nonacademic factors to be taken substantially into account, academic standards must be lowered.

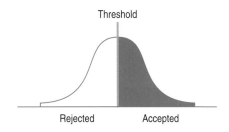

Fig. 43.1 A simple model of selection when there is a single characteristic on which selection is taking place; those above the threshold are accepted, and those below are rejected.

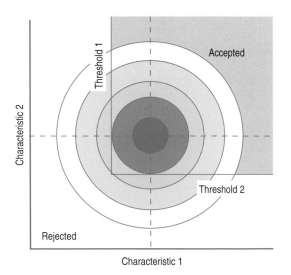

Fig. 43.2 Example showing two criteria.

Medical schools considering nonacademic attributes for selection rapidly develop long lists of desiderata, often containing 5, 10, 20 or even 50 components. The model of Fig. 43.2 can easily be extended to three, four, five or many criteria, when the limits of selection appear with a vengeance. Assuming the criteria are statistically independent, then Table 43.1 shows that as the number of criteria rise, so the proportion of candidates eliminated *on any single criterion* (shown in the second column) becomes ever smaller. To put it bluntly, 'if one selects on everything, one selects on nothing.'

Therefore:

- Selection should aim at a relatively small number of what can be called 'canonical traits' – the three or four stable characteristics that are likely to predict future professional behaviour and can be assessed reliably at medical school application.

- If schools currently select almost entirely on academic ability, then they will have to reduce academic standards in order to select effectively on nonacademic criteria.

- Selection should be recognized as being limited in its power. The really powerful tools for affecting change are education and training (McManus & Vincent 1993).

Table 43.1 The effects of selection on the basis of multiple criteria (assuming two applicants for every place)

Number of independent selection criteria	Proportion of applicants rejected on any single criterion
1	Bottom 50%
2	Bottom 29.3%
3	Bottom 20.6%
4	Bottom 15.9%
5	Bottom 12.9%
6	Bottom 10.9%
10	Bottom 6.7%
20	Bottom 3.4%
50	Bottom 1.4%
N^*	Bottom $100 \cdot (1 - r^{(-1/N)})$%

$^*N$: number of criteria; r: selection ratio (e.g. if $r = 3$, there are 3 applicants for each place and 1/3 applicants are accepted).
Reproduced from McManus IC, Vincent CA: Selecting and educating safer doctors. In Vincent CA, Ennis M, Audley RJ, editors: *Medical Accidents*, Oxford, 1993, Oxford University Press, pp 80–105.

What are the canonical traits in selection?

 "'A' levels tell us nothing about some of the most desirable attributes of the doctor. The four desiderata are technical competence, human sympathy, wisdom and experience."

McKeown 1986

Attempts have been made to identify canonical traits for selection (McManus & Vincent 1993).

INTELLECTUAL ABILITY

Doctors probably cannot be too intelligent. Meta-analyses of selection in many different occupations show that general mental ability is the best predictor both of job performance and of the ability to be trained (Schmidt & Hunter 1998). Although claims are often made for some minimum threshold ability level which is 'good enough', systematic research suggests that 'more is better' (Arneson et al 2011).

LEARNING STYLE AND MOTIVATION

Students study as university students for many different reasons, and those motivations mean they adopt particular study habits and learning styles. In Biggs's typology (Table 43.2), both deep and strategic learning (but not surface learning) are compatible with the self-directed, self-motivated approach to learning that is required in the lifelong learning needed in medical practitioners.

COMMUNICATIVE ABILITY

Most complaints about doctors involve communication problems, and so it makes sense to include it in selection. Communicative ability has been developing throughout life, so those with poor communication skills even at age 17 will probably respond well to training. Assessment is not straightforward, but interviews, multiple mini interviews, questionnaires and situational judgement tests can all assess communication.

PERSONALITY

Many studies have examined the 'big five' personality traits of extroversion, neuroticism, openness to experience, agreeableness and conscientiousness. Schmidt and Hunter's (1998) meta-analysis showed that the best predictor of job performance and trainability, after intellectual ability, was integrity or conscientiousness, not least because highly conscientious people tend to work harder and be more efficient and so gain more and better experience. Conscientiousness may, though,

Table 43.2 Summary of the differences in motivation and study process of the surface, deep and strategic approaches to study

Style	Motivation	Process
Surface	Completion of the course	Rote learning of facts and ideas
		Focusing on task components in isolation
	Fear of failure	Little real interest in content
Deep	Interest in the subject	Relation of ideas to evidence
	Vocational relevance	Integration of material across courses
	Personal understanding	Identification of general principles
Strategic/Achieving	Achieving high grades	Use of techniques that achieve
	Being successful	highest grades

Based on the work of Biggs 1987, 2003.

not be a good predictor when creativity or innovation is important. At medical school, conscientiousness better predicts achievement in basic medical sciences, rather than clinical studies or postgraduate activities such as research output (McManus et al 2003).

SURROGATES FOR SELECTION

Although intelligence, learning style, communication and personality should probably form the basis of selection, it is often sufficient to select on measures that correlate highly with them. School-leaving examinations are such a surrogate, as high grades are the result of adequate intelligence, appropriate learning styles and a systematic approach to study (and hence school-leaving exams are better predictors of career outcomes than pure tests of intelligence; McManus et al 2003). A person of lower intellect may pass exams by prodigious rote learning, conscientiously carried out, but that becomes increasing difficult at higher levels of achievement. Playing in an orchestra or for a sports team also implies conscientiousness at practising, good communicative ability when collaborating and an interest in the deeper aspects of a skill (intrinsic motivation). Good selection processes do not use such surrogates uncritically, but must ask what underlying psychological traits are being assessed by such biographical data (biodata).

Methods and process of selection

 "A multitude of ad hoc policies implemented by miscellaneous admissions officers of various medical schools cannot be properly evaluated or criticized, and is open to considerable abuse. Selection itself is problematic enough, without trying to make it a panacea for the world's ills. If selectors are trying to do too much too well, they will end by failing to do anything properly."

Downie & Charlton 1992

The process of selection and the methods used to carry it out are entirely separate (Powis 1998). Medical schools should have a selection policy which clearly states how selection takes place, how information is collected and how decisions are based on the information, including the weighting of the various components. Although it might seem absurd at first sight, decision making itself should be an entirely administrative process, as that ensures good practice and avoids suggestions of discrimination, unfairness, or apparent inconsistencies in selection. Academic and educational inputs to the system should be in deciding the protocol and, where necessary, making subtle judgements about the information (such as evaluating aspects of the application form or interviewing). A corollary of the principle is that the separate items of information should be assessed separately. If interviewers are asked to judge a candidate's knowledge of medicine as a career, then that is what they should do; information about interviewees' examination results, hobbies, etc. may result in a 'halo effect'.

ASSESSING METHODS OF SELECTION

 "We have found dissatisfaction in many quarters with the basis on which applicants are selected for admission to the undergraduate medical course. Many headmasters and headmistresses believe, for example, that in at least some universities the selection of medical students is not based on clearly equitable criteria."

Royal Commission on Medical Education 1968

The many methods of selection each have their strengths and weaknesses. Each should be assessed in terms of:

• *Validity.* All selection assessments are implicit predictions of a candidate's future behaviour. If there is no correlation with future behaviours, then methods are not useful, however much assessors may like them.

- **Reliability.** If different selectors disagree about a characteristic, or reassessment gives different answers, then the information is probably unhelpful.
- **Feasibility.** If an assessment involves too great a cost, either financially or in staff effort, then the gain may not be worth the expenditure.
- **Acceptability.** Candidates, and their teachers, friends and relations, and the public in general, must feel selection methods are appropriate.

DIFFERENT METHODS OF SELECTION

Open admissions and lotteries

Systems for avoiding the hard decisions of selection are the former Austrian 'open admissions' system and in Holland the weighted lottery used since 1972. Myths abound about both. Selection has recently been introduced in both countries, and detailed comparisons show that selected students perform better academically and are better motivated than those admitted by an open system or lottery (Reibnegger et al 2010, Urlings-Strop et al 2011). Such findings are probably the death knell for solving problems of selection by not selecting.

Administrative methods

These are typically carried out by office staff who assess relatively objective information from application forms, primarily for rejecting unsuitable candidates. While usually reliable, cheap and acceptable, its validity depends on the information being used.

Assessment of application forms

Unstructured personal statements and referees' reports on application forms (so-called 'white-space boxes') are often assessed by short-listers who try to determine a candidate's motivation and experience of medicine as a career.

Like interviewing, it is subjective and often of moderate or even poor reliability and of dubious validity. It is, however, cost-effective and acceptable to applicants. Reliability is improved by training and the use of structured assessment protocols, clear criterion referencing and carefully constructed descriptors of the various characteristics to be identified. The rise of the internet, however, does mean that statements can be heavily plagiarized (see quotation below).

> "Ever since I accidentally burnt holes in my pyjamas after experimenting with a chemistry set on my eighth birthday, I have always had a passion for science."
>
> Plagiarised quotation used by 234 UK medical school applicants in 2007, detected using specialist software (http://news.bbc.co.uk/1/hi/education/6426945.stm)

Biographical data (biodata)

Biodata can be assessed from an open-ended application form (e.g. the 'personal statement') or from a semi-structured questionnaire. Its utility derives from the psychological principle that the best predictor of future behaviour is past behaviour. Generally, it is reliable, valid (Cook 1990), cost-effective and acceptable, although verification may be needed to present dissimulation.

Referees' reports

If honest, these can be useful, but referees often feel greater loyalty to the candidate (whom they know) than to the medical school (whom they don't know). Experienced head teachers say that medical schools should 'read between the lines', so that what matters is not what is said, but what is left unsaid or understated. Reliability is inevitably low, validity dubious and acceptability ambiguous. They are expensive in terms of referees' time but not the medical school's. No doubt with effort, and if standardized, they could be far more effective.

Interviewing

> "The personal character, the very nature, the will, of each student had far greater force in determining his career than any helps or hindrances whatever. … The time and the place, the work to be done, and its responsibilities, will change; but the man will be the same, except in so far as he may change himself."
>
> *Sir James Paget 1869*

Although most UK medical schools now hold interviews, that has not always been the case, suggesting genuine uncertainty about their usefulness. Although credited as being unreliable, they can sometimes be reliable (Kreiter et al 2004), with Marchese and Muchinsky (1993) reporting that reliability and validity depend mostly on interviewer training and a clear structure. Behavioural interviewing, which emphasizes the candidate's actual, previous behaviour in concrete situations, is typically more effective than questions about hypothetical unknown situations in the remote future. Although expensive in terms of staff time, interviews are highly acceptable to the general public, who are not happy with doctors being selected purely on academic grounds, but are often criticized after the event by candidates and teachers, and may not actually be effective (Goho & Blackman 2006).

Multiple Mini-Interviews (MMIs)

Developed originally at McMaster, MMIs are effectively OSCEs (objective structured clinical examinations) used for selection, typically with 12 or so short stations. Reliability is good, certainly better than for conventional interviews, and good claims are also made for predictive validity (Eva et al 2009). It seems likely that they will be used much more in the future.

Psychometric testing

Pscyhometric tests are of several types. Measures of motivation and personality, and of psychomotor characteristics such as manual dexterity, are often used in industry where they can have good predictive validity, but are little used at present in medicine. In medicine, psychometric tests can be time-consuming and expensive to administer and can be unpopular with candidates who worry that there are 'trick' questions and that the content does not seem relevant to a career in medicine. Tests of attainment, such as the biological sciences scale of the American MCAT, have good predictive validity (Donnon et al 2007), but inevitably correlate with school-based measures of educational attainment. Tests such as BMAT, UMAT, GAMSAT and UKCAT have become popular in the UK, Australia and elsewhere, despite being introduced without evidence of predictive validity (McManus et al 2005). Recent studies of UMAT (Mercer & Puddey 2011) and GAMSAT (Wilkinson et al 2008) suggest that predictive validity is low, particularly when educational attainment is taken into account. When psychometric tests are predictive, it mainly seems to be due to assessing attainment rather than ability or aptitude (McManus et al 2011).

Situational judgement tests

Situational judgement tests are multiple-choice assessments in which a range of options are ranked in order, often involving not merely factual knowledge but also an holistic awareness of the social processes and organizational needs of modern health care (Weekley & Ployhart 2006). Their use is rapidly increasing in selection for postgraduate training, and it is also being suggested that they may be effective for selection into medicine. An interesting theoretical question concerns why they may work. One possibility is that they demonstrate candidates' ability imaginatively to place themselves in novel situations and anticipate the consequences (so that perhaps they are assessing situational empathy).

Assessment centres

"Prolonged observation of candidates in different situations by trained selectors makes the final ... decision relatively easy. This contrasts with the brief interviews done by ... medical schools where dubious decisions are often based on inadequate evidence. The experience of assessment centres is that early opinions may be suspect ... The time has come to establish on an experimental basis a Medical Selection Board along the lines of the assessment centres of the Army, Civil Service and British Airways."

Roberts & Porter 1989

Assessment centres are the core selection method of the army, civil service and major companies. Candidates are brought together in groups of 4–12, for 1–3 days, and carry out a series of novel exercises, often involving group work (Roberts & Porter 1989). They are particularly appropriate if the emphasis is upon assessing ability under competitive time stress or when collaborating in group activities. Their reliability is good since assessors are highly trained, but they are expensive and time-consuming.

The costs of selection

"It is impossible to separate selection from training. In this country the only case I know of a thoroughly validated selection procedure from first to last was one in which selection and training were treated as a single problem."

Sir Frederick Bartlett 1946

The direct costs of selection for a medical school are difficult to assess, but are probably about £2000+ per entrant, mostly accounted for by staff time. The unstated and unmeasured criterion of success is that graduates practise high-quality medicine in the National Health Service until retirement, perhaps 40 years later. In contrast, major British companies typically spend about 50 times as much, with a typical criterion of success being that a graduate stays with the company for 5 years.

Little is spent on medical student selection at present for two reasons. Student selection is currently an 'open-loop' system, without feedback. Bad doctors may cost society very dearly, but none of that cost comes back to the medical school. Good, effective selection therefore benefits an institution little, and the temptation is to minimize costs. If the loop were closed, so that graduates incurred costs and provided rewards to their medical school throughout their careers, then selection and subsequent training would be at the core of a medical school's activities, instead of at its margins.

"The stakes for selection are every bit as high as for assessment for competence within a programme, if not higher."

Prideaux et al 2011

Routine monitoring of selection

Selection is vulnerable to criticism and even to legal challenge, making it essential that clear policies are in place, and that routine data are collected for monitoring the process, particularly of what the UK Equality Act of 2010 refers to as 'protected characteristics' (age/disability/gender reassignment/marriage and civil partnership/pregnancy and maternity/race/religion or belief/sex/sexual orientation). Simple head counts are not sufficient, since groups may differ in relevant background factors, making multivariate techniques necessary for identifying possible disadvantage and understanding its locus (McManus et al 1995).

Widening access

Monitoring of the demographics and social background of medical students and doctors has resulted in concern about widening access to the medical profession, with attempts to increase participation of students from low socioeconomic backgrounds or particular ethnic or geographical groups. There can be a tension if it is felt that candidate selection is based on quotas rather than quality or ability as such. Prideaux et al (2011) have suggested the importance of 'political validity' in selection.

"Widening access is a values question, not a technical question of choosing one selection method over another. Widening access is driven by socio-political concerns. These are real concerns. ... Social accountability requires responsiveness to the communities the medical school serves and ensuring that the communities are represented in the student population. From this derives the concept of political validity."

Prideaux et al 2011

Studying selection and learning from research

Medicine can be notoriously insular. Research and experience outside of medicine are often ignored, and there are medical schools which will not even consider experience gained at other medical schools, never mind in industry, commerce and the public sectors in general. Personnel selection has been much studied

and there is a vast literature. A good place to start is the regular series of articles in the Annual Review of Psychology, which are frequently updated (see Sackett & Lievens 2008).

EVIDENCE-BASED MEDICINE AND THE SCIENTIFIC STUDY OF SELECTION

Evidence-based medicine is the current dogma in medicine, and student selection should be no different. However the limitations of the purely evidence-based approach should be recognized. If only 'gold-standard' randomized controlled trials were accepted as evidence, then most of medical education would have no evidence base; then, the inevitable result is that opinion, prejudice and anecdote become the bases for action. Observational studies and epidemiology's powerful methods are also useful, as elsewhere in the social sciences, particularly when embedded in robust theories developed in psychology, education and other basic sciences. A particularly infuriating error occurs in evaluating methods of selection, when arguments of the following form are used simultaneously:

- 'These students have only been followed up for 5 years, but our selection process was assessing who would become good practising doctors in the future. These results do not look far enough into the future.'
- 'This study was carried out over 5 years ago, and since then we have changed our selection process and our undergraduate curriculum, and the doctors will be working in a medical system that has also changed. These results are only of historical interest.'

Put thus, the sophistry is obvious: prospective, longitudinal studies for N years must, of necessity, have been started more than N years ago. Of course, the same arguments are not used in medical practice: chemotherapeutic regimens looking at 5-year survival must be subject to the same problems, but the trials are still done.

A further problem with studying selection is the vulnerability of the egos of those doing the selection. No one wants to feel that their actions have been wasted or their best-considered schemes are worthless. Nor do institutions want to publish results suggesting they are not doing a perfect job. A typical reflex response is to demand an unreasonably high criterion of evidence that is a paragon of perfection. The best is, however, the enemy of the good. The scientific study of selection is no different from any other science. One is not searching for proof of absolute truth, but identifying working explanatory hypotheses, compatible with evidence, which have acceptable methodology, take known problems into account and are therefore robust against straightforward refutation and make useful predictions. That is then a basis for practical action and further research. Just like medicine, in other words.

 "We hope that research will in the course of time lead to the establishment of reasonably objective criteria of professional performance, valid in the many different fields and kinds of medical practice, and thereby make possible an objective evaluation of student selection. This is a long-term aspiration however."

Royal Commission on Medical Education 1968

Summary

Selection is an important but under-resourced aspect of medical school activity. Medical schools select applicants but also applicants select medical schools.

Many selection methods can be used by schools, from a purely administrative review, reading of application forms, assessment of biodata, psychometric testing, interviews, multiple mini-interviews, situational judgements tests, and assessment centres.

Whatever process is used, it will have its costs and its benefits and needs to be routinely monitored, evaluated and compared with examples of best evidence-based practice.

References

Arneson JJ, Sackett PR, Beatty AS: Ability-performance relationships in education and employment settings: Critical tests of the more-is-better and good-enough hypotheses, *Psychological Science* 22:1336–1342, 2011.

Biggs JB: *Study Process Questionnaire: Manual*, Melbourne, 1987, Australian Council for Educational Research.

Biggs JB: *Teaching for Quality Learning at University*, Milton Keynes, 2003, SRHE Open University Press.

Cook M: *Personnel Selection and Productivity*, Chichester, 1990, John Wiley.

Donnon T, Paolucci EO, Violato C: The predictive validity of the MCAT for medical school performance medical board licensing examinations: A meta-analysis of the published research, *Academic Medicine* 82:100–106, 2007.

Downie RS, Charlton B: *The Making of a Doctor: Medical Education in Theory and Practice*, Oxford, 1992, Oxford University Press.

Eva KW, Reiter HI, Trinh K, et al: Predictive validity of the multiple mini-interview for selecting medical trainees, *Medical Education* 43:767–775, 2009.

Goho J, Blackman A: The effectiveness of academic admission interviews: an exploratory meta-analysis, *Medical Teacher* 28:335–340, 2006.

Johnson ML: Non-academic factors in medical school selection: a report on rejected applicants, *BMJ* 5:264–268, 1971.

Kreiter C, Solow C, Brennan R: Investigating the reliability of the medical schools admissions interview, *Advances in Health Science Education* 9:147–159, 2004.

Marchese MC, Muchinsky PM: The validity of the employment interview: a meta-analysis, *International Journal of Selection and Assessment* 1:18–26, 1993.

McKeown T: Personal view, *British Medical Journal* 298:200, 1986.

McManus IC, Vincent CA: Selecting and educating safer doctors. In Vincent CA, Ennis M, Audley RJ, editors: *Medical Accidents*, Oxford, 1993, Oxford University Press, pp 80–105.

McManus IC, Richards P, Winder BC, et al: Medical school applicants from ethnic minorities: identifying if and when they are disadvantaged, *British Medical Journal* 310:496–500, 1995.

McManus IC, Smithers E, Partridge P, et al: A levels and intelligence as predictors of medical careers in UK doctors: 20 year prospective study, *British Medical Journal* 327:139–142, 2003.

McManus IC, Powis DA, Wakeford R, et al: Intellectual aptitude tests and A levels for selecting UK school leaver entrants for medical school, *British Medical Journal* 331:555–559, 2005.

McManus IC, Ferguson E, Wakeford R, et al: Predictive validity of the BioMedical Admissions Test (BMAT): An evaluation and case study, *Medical Teacher* 33:53–57, 2011.

Mercer A, Puddey IB: Admission selection criteria as predictors of outcomes in an undergraduate medical course: A prospective study, *Medical Teacher* 33:997–1004, 2011.

Powis D: How to do it: select medical students, *British Medical Journal* 317:1149–1150, 1998.

Prideaux D, Roberts C, Eva K, et al: Assessment for selection for the health care professions and specialty training: Consensus statement and recommendations from the Ottawa 2010 conference, *Medical Teacher* 33:215–223, 2011.

Reibnegger G, Caluba H-C, Ithaler D, et al: Progress of medical students after open admission or admission based on knowledge tests, *Medical Education* 44:205–214, 2010.

Richards P: *Learning Medicine: An Informal Guide to a Career in Medicine*, London, 1983, British Medical Association.

Roberts GD, Porter AMW: Medical student selection – time for change: discussion paper, *Journal of the Royal Society of Medicine* 82:288–291, 1989.

Royal Commission on Medical Education: *Royal Commission on Medical Education (Todd Report), Cmnd 3569*, London, 1968, HMSO.

Sackett PR, Lievens F: Personnel selection, *Annual Review of Psychology* 59:419–450, 2008.

Schmidt FL, Hunter JE: The validity and utility of selection methods in personnel psychology: practical and theoretical implications of 85 years of research findings, *Psychological Bulletin* 124:262–274, 1998.

Urlings-Strop LC, Themmen APN, Stijnen T, Splinter TAW: Selected medical students achieve better than lottery-admitted students during clerkships, *Medical Education* 45:1032–1040, 2011.

Weekley JA, Ployhart RE: *Situational Judgment Tests: Theory, Measurement, and Application*, Hove, 2006, Psychology Press.

Wilkinson D, Zhang J, Byrne GJ, et al: Medical school selection criteria and the prediction of academic performance: Evidence leading to change in policy and practice at the University of Queensland, *Medical Journal of Australia* 188:349–354, 2008.

Student support

R. J. Duvivier, J. A. Dent

Introduction: Student well-being

Medical students are exposed to a variety of pressures, many of which may cause stress. Although this is true for all university students, medical students have higher anxiety scores than their non-medical peers (Buchman et al 1991, Sherry et al 1998). It seems that the first year of medical school is particularly stressful, with depression levels increasing significantly throughout that year (Stewart et al 1999). In later years, medical students frequently spend periods of time away from the university campus while studying in clinical placements elsewhere. This social isolation, compounded by unsocial hours of study, contributes to an ongoing cause of chronic stress (Schmitter et al 2008). Moffat and colleagues (2004) reported recent introduction of curriculum change as a further source of stress. Several studies have shown that the intense pressures and demands of medical school can have detrimental effects on the academic performance, physical health and psychological well-being of the student (Dyrbye et al 2006).

 Medical students are exposed to a variety of pressures, many of which may cause stress.

Stress may also harm trainees' professional effectiveness: it decreases attention, reduces concentration, impinges on decision-making skills, and reduces trainees' abilities to establish strong physician–patient relationships (Dyrbye et al 2005). With regards to the physician–patient relationship, empathy declines during medical school and may even decline further during residency (Hojat et al 2004, Newton et al 2008, Toews et al 1997). It is worrisome that this decline of empathy, also called 'ethical erosion', seems to worsen when students' activities are shifting towards patient care, as this is when empathy is most essential (Feudtner et al 1994).

Associations between medical students' stress, academic performance and personal and mental health underscore the importance of successful adaptation to the medical school environment, while maladaptive skills developed during medical school may lead to later professional maladjustment (Stern et al 1993). The inability to cope with the demands of medical school may lead to a cascade of consequences at both a personal and a professional level. Stress may affect trainees at all levels (students, interns, residents) with harmful outcomes such as alcohol and drug abuse, interpersonal relationship difficulties, depression, anxiety or even suicide (Dyrbye et al 2005).

During their undergraduate years students are subjected to different kinds of stressors, such as the pressure of academic life with an obligation to succeed, an uncertain future and difficulties of integrating into the system (Robotham & Julian 2006). In addition, several factors peculiar to the medical profession have been found to contribute to a decline in students' well-being as the years progress including exposure to patient suffering and deaths, sleep deprivation, financial concerns and workload (Davis et al 2001, Griffith & Wilson 2003, Hojat et al 2004, Woloschuk et al 2004).

Factors influencing student well-being

Problems and pressures experienced by students in general fall into six domains:

1. **Personal:** social, health, lack of time for recreation, relationships and family (Folse et al 1985)
2. **Professional:** coping with healthcare structures and life and death issues as seen in the working/learning environment, student abuse (verbal, emotional, etc.) (Silver & Glicken 1990)
3. **Academic:** course work, examinations (Kidson & Hornblow 1982), recent introduction of curriculum change

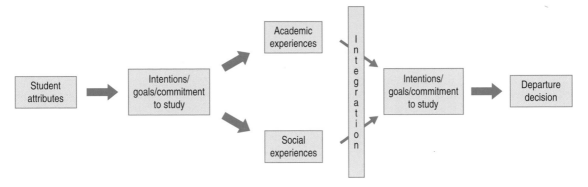

Fig. 44.1 Simplified form of departure model. (Adapted from Tinto V: Stages of student departure: Reflections on the longitudinal character of student leaving, *Journal of Higher Education* 59:438–455, 1988.)

4. **Administrative:** anxiety relating to timetable and teaching venue changes or meeting curriculum deadlines

5. **Financial:** the ongoing problem of increasing student debt

6. **Careers:** choosing a specialty, application process, demands of residency (Gill et al 2001).

Because students face such a wide range of potentially stressful factors, it is important to think of a stress-management system as an appropriate facility for all students to be aware of, a resource for maintaining academic performance, not just for helping students having problems. As stress is an aspect of a doctor's professional life, it is important that all students develop coping skills as undergraduates (Stewart et al 1999).

 "Appropriate interventions may be required to reduce student stress in revised curricula."

Moffat et al 2004

Role of medical teachers

As Dyrbye put it: 'Medical school should be a time of personal growth, fulfilment and well-being – despite its challenges' (Dyrbye et al 2006). Based on epidemiological and observational studies quoted earlier, it is clear that this statement does not hold true for all medical students in all aspects or stages of their training. Negative experiences trigger different coping strategies amongst medical students. Those coping strategies – whether adaptive or maladaptive – can lead students either to express resilience and perseverance in their academic programme or to drop out. Students may arrive at the conclusion that the academic, social, emotional and/or financial costs of

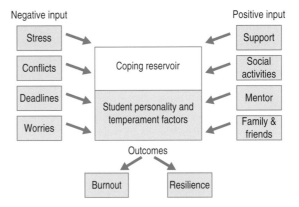

Fig. 44.2 Conceptual model: Coping reserve tank. (Adapted from Dunn LB, Iglewicz A, Moutier C: A conceptual model of medical student well-being: promoting resilience and preventing burnout, *Academic Psychiatry* 32:44–53, 2008.)

staying on are greater than the benefits (Tinto 1975), at which point they withdraw from academic or social integration (Yorke 1999).

Tinto (1975, 1988) produced an integrative theory and model of student dropout. His model had six progressive phases: student pre-entry attributes, early goals/commitments to study, institutional experiences, integration into the institution, goals/commitments to the institution and ending in a departure decision (Fig. 44.1).

This model described a longitudinal process of interactions between the individual and the academic and social systems of the university environment. It is against this background that we discuss possible ways of student support in this process and how to integrate them in medical schools. Dunn and colleagues (2008) developed a model of medical student coping which he termed the 'coping reservoir' (Fig. 44.2).

This model is used to highlight the dynamic nature of students' experiences and the effect on enhanced resilience and mental health versus distress and burnout. The reservoir itself consists of the individual students' personal traits, temperament and coping style. It is replenished or drained by various experiences. Formal and informal input within the medical schools can help fill the reservoir, while negative factors will drain it. With adequate support students can monitor their coping reservoir, cultivate the skills to refill it and so sustain their well-being.

The internal structure of the reservoir represents the students' own personal traits, temperament and coping style and their ability to use adaptive/maladaptive coping strategies.

The input of either positive factors (filling or replenishing the reservoir) or negative factors (draining the reservoir) combined with the internal structure of the reservoir itself can lead, on the one hand, to resilience and enhanced mental health or, on the other hand, to burnout and cynicism. A good tutor can help a student monitor their coping reservoir and provide positive resources to fill it.

 Tutors are not required to:

- have a specialist knowledge of the content of each part of the course
- have firsthand experience of the training requirements of all specialties
- be a health, financial or marital counsellor
- have a degree in psychotherapy
- understand the administrative details of the medical school.

(Dent & Rennie 2009)

Role of the student: Coping strategies

Students who have experienced academic or mental health problems before will deal with current concerns differently from those who have no history of academic problems, depression or anxiety. Those with no prior history will present with new onset anxiety. Students with a prior history have a relative additional risk in terms of lowered sense of confidence in own abilities, increased self-doubt on future goals (becoming a doctor) and recurrence of depressive/anxiety symptoms. Awareness of students' prior mental health history is useful in recognition of normal reaction versus impending relapse in mood or anxiety disorder. However, issues of confidentiality and voluntary disclosure need to be considered by student counsellors (Chew-Graham et al 2003). Their support should be tailored to the individual student's need.

Parkes (1986) described three common methods of coping in student nurses in initial ward placements: general coping, direct coping and suppression. General coping refers to a tendency to use cognitive and behavioural coping strategies. Direct coping means using rational problem-orientated strategies to change or manage the situation and avoidance of emotionally based items such as fantasy, wishful thinking and hostility. By using suppression as the main coping strategy, students suppress thoughts of the situation and display behaviour that inhibits action, i.e. carrying on as if nothing has happened.

Role of the institution

A recent synthesis of the literature (Prebble et al 2005) suggested 13 propositions aimed at policy makers in tertiary institutions to improve student outcomes (Box 44.1). Although the research on which these propositions are based stems from a wide variety

---

Box 44.1

1. Institutional behaviours, environment and processes are welcoming and efficient
2. The institution provides opportunities for students to establish social networks
3. Academic counselling and pre-enrolment advice are readily available to ensure that students enrol into appropriate programmes and papers
4. Teachers are approachable and accessible inside and outside of class times for academic discussions
5. Students experience good quality teaching and manageable workloads
6. Orientation/induction programmes are provided to facilitate both social and academic integration
7. Students working in academic learning communities have good outcomes
8. A comprehensive range of institutional services and facilities are available
9. Supplemental instruction is provided
10. Peer tutoring and mentoring services are provided
11. The institution ensures there is an absence of discrimination on campus, so students feel valued, fairly treated and safe
12. Institutional processes cater for diversity of learning preferences
13. The institutional culture, social and academic, welcomes diverse cultural capital and adapts to diverse students' needs

of academic settings, we believe it has implications for the specific context of medical schools. A student support system in a medical school should therefore be based on these propositions, and aiming to facilitate students' development.

How can students be supported?

PREVENTATIVE MEASURES

A self-coping questionnaire (Folkman & Lazarus 1988) can help students identify personal resources and coping mechanisms (Fig. 44.3).

FAMILY SUPPORT

Students often quote family, friends and peers as the first and most readily available source of positive help. Students with good family support were found to be able to cope better with academic stress (Klink et al 2008).

PEER SUPPORT AND PAL (COLLABORATIVE LEARNING)

The university's orientation week (often referred to as freshers' week) at the start of each academic year introduces new students to a number of unofficial student-support activities as well as providing answers to common questions. These student interest groups contribute to student support with a wide range of social, sports, religious, musical or social activities and promote interdisciplinary integration. Extracurricular work may also enhance integration into the wider community.

'Senior–junior', 'big sibs', 'parenting', 'buddy-system': all these systems for pairing new students with a more senior student are very common and popular. Either individually or in a group, junior students are provided with a senior student 'parent'. They act as advisers for incoming students, based on personal experience as they have encountered similar problems and concerns as a junior themselves. They may also be a good source of specific information about electives, housing and securing jobs.

The Medical Student Council and similar associations provide an academic focus and a means of essential communication between staff and students including useful tips on administrative and logistical issues such as books required, event locations and grant awarding bodies.

MEDICAL SCHOOL SUPPORT

Study skills tutor

A study skills tutor may be able to guide students with time management skills, study methods and skills in revision and examination techniques. A list of specialty advisors willing to provide subject-specific support may be available.

Tutor schemes

Staff volunteers within the faculty are allocated groups of students to see either individually or on a group basis. The groups may include students from several years or be all from the same year. It is possible to link these tutor meetings with some academic activity by using them to review or supervise recent learning activity within the course. Some tutors feel this gives their meetings more substance, facilitates interaction and encourages student participation in the scheme. However, recruiting sufficient tutors who are able to positively engage informally with students is often difficult (Cotterel et al 1994).

Mentors

A mentoring scheme enables continuity by following students through the whole course. Mentor and student develop a relationship through educational and social activities. While keeping track of an individual student's academic performance the mentor can offer informal help and advice with academic, career, professional, personal or administrative problems. He or she may be able to oversee the construction of the student's portfolio or provide a stimulus for personal development. Of course, the student may have chosen an unofficial mentor with no formally defined relationship to them to act as a role model or to provide career advice (see Chapter 17, Mentoring).

"The best advisers are individuals who are warm, empathetic and spontaneous, who have constructive, sound judgement, and who get satisfaction out of watching medical students grow into mature adults as well as competent physicians."

Eckenfels et al 1984

Mentors can also facilitate the onward referral to other resources for more professional help if appropriate (see Fig. 44.4). This model indicates how there

| Healthy Coping | Sharing Objective Externalizing | Not sleeping Working over night | Unhealthy Coping |

Fig. 44.3 Coping strategies spectrum.

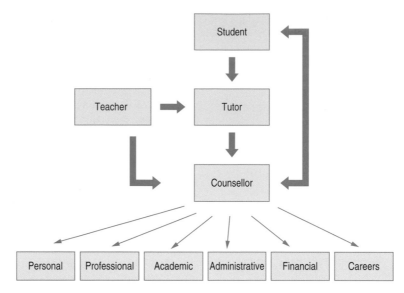

Fig. 44.4 Routes to student guidance.

can be a two-way communication pathway between students and counsellors. The latter can be notified by teachers or tutors who are concerned about one individual student's progress or mental health, and the counsellor can choose to call them in for a friendly chat and perhaps some more formal advice or referral.

Internet

One central email address for students to communicate with the support services facilitates access and should to be given to all students and adequately administered by staff to provide prompt responses (e.g. support@nameofuniversity.org).

Email is good for answering administrative problems; websites provide announcements and an overview of available services while discussion/bulletin boards or electronic learning environments such as BlackBoard provide an additional learning and administrative resource. Social networking sites such as Facebook and other mobile apps give students innovative ways of communicating with each other and a source of collaborative 'anywhere/anytime' learning support (see Chapter 28, Mobile learning).

UNIVERSITY SUPPORT

'Freshers' week', mentioned above, is a university-wide orientation event providing students with an overview of many resources for student welfare. The university counselling service and the chaplaincy services are usually prominently represented.

The student advisory office, staffed by professional advisors within the university, will be able to use a variety of strategies, tailored to student needs. They can filter student problems to the appropriate specialist, e.g. career guidance, GP or accommodation officer.

EXTERNAL SUPPORT

Finally, outside of the university, the Citizens' Advice Bureau, the Samaritans and the individual student's GP may all have a role to play in student support and may be accessed directly or on behalf of the student.

Implementation

HOW TO ORGANIZE A MENTOR SYSTEM

 "The relationship that is formed between students and tutors is the most important factor contributing to the success of the scheme."
Malik 2000

To be successful, tutors must be seen as credible by the students and will need to gain their trust and respect. They should be enthusiastic and committed, accessible to students and sensitive to the particular stresses of medical school and the student's stage of life. They should be trustworthy and reliable, capable of handling confidential issues appropriately and following institutional policy. They should also have an understanding of the faculty system and curriculum and their role in it.

Six commons areas of knowledge required include (see Fig. 44.4):

- **Academic:** learning style, study technique, structure or content curriculum components, objectives, additional assignments, possibilities for electives
- **Career:** available options after graduation, understanding of junior doctor system, tips on how to get into specialty of choice, help with making decisions, alternative careers, specific career counsellor
- **Professionalism:** guidance and advice; help with portfolio, address issues of misconduct
- **Personal:** active listening, show empathy, refer to mental health professional if needed
- **Administrative:** understand organization of faculty, responsible persons, administrators, course secretaries, have knowledge of examination rules, help with appeals, advocate on student behalf for examination board.
- **Financial:** an understanding of and straightforward advice on budgeting.

Staff development resources will often be required to provide this knowledge/skills set:

- **Academic:** list of key people, content teachers, coordinators on all levels (block, phase, year)
- **Career:** available training programmes, entry requirements, application process, contact details of specialty career advisors, postgraduate deans also outside own region, international opportunities
- **Professional:** rules and regulations pertaining to professional behaviour, guidelines on dealing with misconduct (e.g. plagiarism)
- **Personal:** availability of university support services regarding accommodations, financial, health problems, contact details for professional counselling services, mental health unit
- **Administrative:** admission office, secretaries, coordinators
- **Financial:** information on student loans, banking and investment, National Union of Students advice on financial management.

Summary

Student support is required in relation to six areas of potential stress: personal worries, academic problems, financial issues, career advice, professional issues and administrative questions. Support can be provided in a variety of ways by tutor schemes, students' advisory offices, university and external support services, peer support groups or via the internet. Individual medical schools can make a selection of an appropriate mixture of several of the methods described so that all students can use these services to the extent that they require.

References

Buchman BP, Sallis JF, Criqui MH, et al: Physical activity, physical fitness, and psychological characteristics of medical students, *Journal of Psychosomatic Research* 35:197–208, 1991.

Chew-Graham CA, Rogers A, Yassin N: 'I wouldn't want it on my CV or their records': Medical students' experiences of help-seeking for mental health problems, *Medical Education* 37:873–880, 2003.

Cotterel DJ, McCrorie P, Perrin F: The personal tutor system: an evaluation, *Medical Education* 28:544–549, 1994.

Davis BE, Nelson DB, Sahler OJ, et al: Do clerkship experiences affect medical students' attitudes toward chronically ill patients? *Academic Medicine* 76:815–820, 2001.

Dent JA, Rennie S: Student support. In Dent JA, Harden RM, editors: *A Practical Guide for Medical Teachers*, ed 3, 2009. Elsevier Limited.

Dunn LB, Iglewicz A, Moutier C: A conceptual model of medical student well-being: promoting resilience and preventing burnout, *Academic Psychiatry* 32:44–53, 2008.

Dyrbye LN, Thomas MR, Shanafelt TD: Medical medical student distress: causes, consequences, and proposed solutions, *Mayo Clinic Proceedings* 80:1613–1622, 2005.

Dyrbye LN, Thomas MR, Shanafelt TD: Systematic review of depression, anxiety, and other indicators of psychological distress among U.S. and Canadian medical students, *Academic Medicine* 81:354–373, 2006.

Eckenfels EJ, Blacklow RS, Gotterer GS: Medical student counseling: the Rush medical college adviser program, *Journal of Medical Education* 59:573–581, 1984.

Feudtner C, Christakis DA, Christakis NA: Do clinical clerks suffer ethical erosion? Students' perceptions of their ethical environment and personal development, *Academic Medicine* 69:670–679, 1994.

Folkman S, Lazarus RS: *Ways of Coping Questionnaire*, Palo Alto, CA, 1988, Consulting Psychologists Press.

Folse ML, Darosa DA, Folse R: The relationship between stress and attitudes towards leisure among first year medical students, *Journal of Medical Education* 60:610–617, 1985.

Gill D, Palmer C, Mulder R, Wilkinson T: Medical student career intentions at the Christchurch School of Medicine: the New Zealand Wellbeing, Intentions, Debt and Experiences (WIDE) survey of medical students pilot study: results part II, *New Zealand Medical Journal* 114:465–467, 2001.

Griffith CH, Wilson JF: The loss of idealism throughout internship, *Evaluation and the Health Professions* 26:415–426, 2003.

Hojat M, Mangione S, Nasca T, et al: An empirical study of decline in empathy in medical school, *Medical Education* 38:934–941, 2004.

Kidson M, Hornblow A: Examination anxiety in medical students: experiences with the visual analogue scale for anxiety, *Medical Education* 16:247–250, 1982.

Klink JL, Byars-Winston A, Bakken LL: Coping efficacy and perceived family support: potential factors for reducing stress in premedical students, *Medical Education* 42:572–579, 2008.

Malik S: Students, tutors and relationships: the ingredients of a successful student support scheme, *Medical Education* 34:635–641, 2000.

Moffat KJ, McConnachie A, Ross S, Morrison JM: First-year medical students' stress and coping in a problem-based learning medical curriculum, *Medical Education* 38:482–491, 2004.

Newton BW, Barber L, Clardy J, et al: Is there hardening of the heart during medical school? *Academic Medicine* 83:244–249, 2008.

Parkes KR: Coping in stressful episodes: the role of individual differences, environmental factors, and situational characteristics, *Journal of Personality and Social Psychology* 51(6):1277–1292, 1986.

Prebble T, Hargraves H, Leach L, et al: Impact of Student Support Services and Academic Development Programmes on Student Outcomes in Undergraduate Tertiary Study: A Synthesis of the Research Report to the Ministry of Education, Government of New Zealand, 2005.

Robotham D, Julian C: Stress and the higher education student: a critical review of the literature, *Journal of Further and Higher Education* 30:107–117, 2006.

Schmitter M, Liedl M, Beck J, Rammelsberg P: Chronic stress in medical and dental education, *Medical Teacher* 30:97–99, 2008.

Sherry S, Notman MT, Nadelson CC, et al: Anxiety, depression, and menstrual symptoms among freshman medical students, *Journal of Clinical Psychiatry* 49:490–493, 1998.

Silver HK, Glicken AD: Medical student abuse: incidence, severity, and significance, *JAMA* 263(4):527–532, 1990.

Stern M, Norman S, Komm C: Medical students' differential use of coping strategies as a function of stressor type, year of training, and gender, *Behavioral Medicine* 18:173–180, 1993.

Stewart SM, Lam TH, Betson CL, et al: A prospective analysis of stress and academic performance in the first two years of medical school, *Medical Education* 33:243–250, 1999.

Tinto V: Dropout from higher education: A theoretical synthesis of recent research, *Review of Educational Research* 45:89–125, 1975.

Tinto V: Stages of student departure: Reflections on the longitudinal character of student leaving, *Journal of Higher Education* 59:438–455, 1988.

Toews, JA, Lockyer JM, Dobson DJ, et al: Analysis of stress levels among medical students, residents, and graduate students at four Canadian schools of medicine, *Academic Medicine* 72:997–1002, 1997.

Woloschuk W, Harasym PH, Temple W: Attitude change during medical school: a cohort study, *Medical Education* 38:522–534, 2004.

Yorke M: Leaving Early. Undergraduate Non-completion in Higher Education, London, 1999, Falmer Press.

Staff development

Y. Steinert

Introduction

Staff development, or faculty development as it is often called, has become an increasingly important component of medical education. Staff development activities have been designed to improve teacher effectiveness at all levels of the educational continuum (e.g. undergraduate, postgraduate and continuing medical education) and diverse programmes have been offered to healthcare professionals in many settings.

For the purpose of this discussion, staff development will refer to that broad range of activities that institutions use to renew or assist faculty in their roles (Centra 1978). That is, staff development is a planned activity designed to *prepare* institutions and faculty members for their various roles (Bland et al 1990) and to *improve* an individual's knowledge and skills in the areas of teaching, research and administration (Sheets & Schwenk 1990). The goal of staff development is to teach faculty members the skills relevant to their institutional and faculty position, and to sustain their vitality, both now and in the future.

> "It goes without saying that no man can teach successfully who is not at the same time a student."
>
> *Sir William Osler*

Although a comprehensive staff development programme includes attention to all faculty roles, including research, writing, and administration, the focus of this chapter will be on staff development for teaching improvement. The first section will review common practices and challenges; the second section will provide some practical guidelines for individuals interested in the design, delivery and evaluation of staff development programmes.

Common practices and challenges

Knowledge of key content areas, common educational formats, frequently encountered challenges, and programme effectiveness will help to guide the design and delivery of innovative staff development programmes. These topics are discussed below.

KEY CONTENT AREAS

The majority of staff development programmes focus on teaching improvement. That is, they aim to improve teachers' skills in clinical teaching, small-group facilitation, large-group presentations, feedback and evaluation (Steinert et al 2006). They also target specific core competencies (e.g. the teaching and evaluation of professionalism), emerging educational priorities (e.g. social accountability; cultural awareness and humility; patient safety), curriculum design and development and the use of technology in teaching and learning. In fact, many of the chapters in this book can become the focus of a staff development programme.

At the same time, less attention has been paid to the personal development of healthcare professionals, educational leadership and scholarship and organizational development and change. Although instructional effectiveness at the individual level is critically important, a more comprehensive approach to staff development should be considered. That is, we need to develop individuals who will be able to provide leadership to educational programmes, act as educational mentors and design and deliver innovative educational programmes. Staff development also has a significant role to play in promoting teaching as a scholarly activity and in creating an educational climate that encourages and rewards educational leadership, innovation and excellence. Irrespective of the specific focus, we should remember that staff development can serve as a useful instrument in the promotion of organizational change and that medical schools can play a fundamental role in the design and delivery of this essential activity. As McLean and colleagues (2008) have said, 'Faculty development is not a luxury. It is an imperative for every medical school.'

To date, the majority of staff development programmes have focused on the medical teacher. Staff development initiatives should also target curriculum planners responsible for the design and delivery of educational programmes, administrators responsible for education and practice, and all healthcare professionals involved in teaching and learning. Moreover, although staff development is primarily a voluntary activity, some medical schools now require participation in this type of professional development as they increasingly recognize the 'professionalization' of teaching.

> *"The one task that is distinctively related to being a faculty member is teaching; all other tasks can be pursued in other settings; and yet, paradoxically, the central responsibility of faculty members is typically the one for which they are least prepared."*
>
> *Jason & Westberg 1982*

Staff development also needs to target the organization that supports teaching and learning. For example, staff development can work to promote a culture change by helping to develop institutional policies that support and reward excellence in teaching, encourage a re-examination of criteria for academic promotion and create networking opportunities for junior faculty members. Clearly, we need to target the organizational climate and culture in which teachers work in order to be successful.

EDUCATIONAL FORMATS

The most common staff development formats include workshops and seminars, short courses, sabbaticals and fellowships (Steinert et al 2006). Workshops are one of the most popular formats because of their inherent flexibility and promotion of active learning. In fact, faculty members value a variety of teaching methods within this format, including interactive lectures, small-group discussions, individual exercises, role plays and simulations, and experiential learning. However, given the ever-changing needs and priorities of medical schools and healthcare professionals, we should consider a variety of formats for staff development, including integrated longitudinal programmes, decentralized activities, peer coaching, mentoring, self-directed learning and computer-aided instruction, all of which are outlined below. We should also remember that staff development can occur along two dimensions: from individual (independent)

experiences to group (collective) learning, and from informal approaches to more formal ones (Steinert 2010). That is, many healthcare professionals learn through experience, by 'doing' and reflecting on that experience; others learn from peer or student feedback, while work-based learning and belonging to a community of practice is key for others. Although the medical school (as an institution) is primarily responsible for the organization of more formal (structured) activities, we must be aware of the powerful learning that can occur in informal settings.

> *"The greatest difficulty in life is to make knowledge effective, to convert it into practical wisdom."*
>
> *Sir William Osler*

Integrated longitudinal programmes

Integrated longitudinal programmes have been developed as an alternative to fellowship programmes. These programmes, in which faculty members commit 10–20% of their time over 1–2 years, allow healthcare professionals to maintain most of their clinical, research and administrative responsibilities while furthering their own professional development. Programme components typically consist of a variety of methods: including university courses, monthly seminars, independent research projects and involvement in a variety of staff development activities. Integrated longitudinal programmes, such as a Teaching Scholars Program (Steinert et al 2003), have particular appeal because teachers can continue to practise and teach while improving their educational knowledge and skills. As well, these programmes allow for the development of educational leadership and scholarly activity in medical education.

Decentralized activities

Staff development programmes are often departmentally based or centrally organized (i.e. faculty-wide). Given the increasing use of community preceptors and ambulatory sites for teaching, staff development programmes should be 'exported' outside of the university setting. Decentralized, site-specific activities have the added advantage of reaching individuals who may not otherwise attend staff development activities and can help to develop a departmental culture of self-improvement.

Peer coaching

Peer coaching as a method of faculty development has been described extensively in the educational literature. Key elements of peer coaching include the identification of individual learning goals (e.g. improving specific teaching skills), focused observation of teaching by colleagues, and the provision of feedback, analysis and support (Flynn et al 1994). This underutilized approach, sometimes called co-teaching or peer observation, has particular appeal because it occurs in the teacher's own practice setting, enables individualized learning and fosters collaboration. It also allows healthcare professionals to learn about each other as they teach together.

Mentorship

Mentoring is a common strategy to promote the socialization, development and maturation of academic medical faculty (Bland et al 1990). It is also a valuable, but underutilized, staff development strategy. Daloz (1986) has described a mentorship model that balances three key elements: support, challenge and a vision of the individual's future career. This model can serve as a helpful framework in staff development. The value of role models and mentors has been highlighted since Osler's time, and we should not forget the benefits of this method of professional development despite new technologies and methodologies.

 "Mentoring is vital to create new leaders and new kinds of leadership."

Anderson 1999

Self-directed learning

Self-directed learning initiatives are not frequently described in the staff development literature. However, there is clearly a place for self-directed learning that promotes 'reflection in action' and 'reflection on action', skills that are critical to effective teaching and learning (Schön 1983). As Ullian and Stritter (1997) have said, teachers should be encouraged to determine their own needs through self-reflection, student evaluation and peer feedback, and they should learn to design their own development activities. Self-directed learning activities have been used extensively in continuing medical education (CME); staff development programmes should build on these experiences.

Computer-aided instruction

Computer-aided instruction is closely tied to self-directed learning initiatives. As time for professional development is limited, and the technology to create interactive instructional programmes is now in place, the use of computer-based staff development should be explored. Web-based learning can allow for individualized programmes targeted to specific needs and the sharing of resources, as long as we do not lose sight of the value and importance of working in context, with our colleagues.

 "We must find new ways to help faculty adapt to their new roles and responsibilities while coping with the day-to-day demands that these changes bring."

Ullian & Stritter 1997

FREQUENTLY ENCOUNTERED CHALLENGES

Staff development programmes cannot be designed or delivered in isolation from other factors that include institutional support, organizational goals and priorities, resources for programme planning and individual needs and expectations. These critical factors can also become challenges. Common challenges faced by faculty developers include defining goals and priorities; balancing individual and organizational needs; motivating faculty to participate in staff development initiatives; obtaining institutional support and 'buy in'; promoting a 'culture change' that reflects renewed interest in teaching and learning; and overcoming limited human and financial resources. As motivating faculty to participate in staff development is one of the key challenges, it will be discussed in greater detail.

Teachers differ from students and residents in a number of ways. They have more life experiences, they have more self-entrenched behaviours, and change may be seen as a greater threat. In addition, motivation for learning cannot be assumed and time for learning is not routinely allocated. Staff development programmes must address these challenges. Teachers do not participate in staff development activities for a variety of reasons. Some do not view teaching – or teaching improvement – as important; others do not perceive a need for improvement or feel that their institution does not support or value these activities. Many are not aware of the benefits (or availability) of staff development programmes and activities. We must be cognizant of all these factors in programme planning.

To motivate faculty, we need to develop a culture that promotes and encourages professional development, consider multiple approaches to achieving the same goal, tailor programmes to meet individual and organizational needs and ensure relevant and 'high-quality' activities. We must also build a network of interested individuals, encourage the dissemination of information, utilize student feedback to illustrate need, recognize participation in staff development and, if possible, provide 'release time'. Whenever possible, it is also helpful to link staff development activities with ongoing programmes (e.g. hospital rounds, CME events), to provide a range of activities and methods and to offer free and flexible programming. Organizational support for these initiatives is also critical, as are staff development strategies that target organizational norms and values (e.g. recognizing the importance of teaching and learning).

> *"The goal of faculty development is to empower faculty members to excel in their role as educators and, in so doing, to create organizations that encourage and reward continual learning."*
>
> *Wilkerson & Irby 1998*

PROGRAMME EFFECTIVENESS

Despite numerous descriptions of staff development programmes, there has been a paucity of research demonstrating the effectiveness of most faculty development activities (Steinert et al 2006). Few programmes have conducted comprehensive evaluations to ascertain what effect the programme is having on faculty, and data to support the efficacy of these initiatives have been lacking. Of the studies that have been conducted in this area, most have assessed participant satisfaction; some have explored change in cognitive learning or performance; and several have examined the long-term impact of these interventions. Although most of the research has relied on self-report rather than objective outcome measures or observations of change, methods to evaluate staff development programmes have included end-of-session evaluations, follow-up survey questionnaires, pre- and post-assessments of cognitive or attitudinal change, direct observations of teaching behaviour, student evaluations and faculty self-ratings of post-training performance. Common problems have included a lack of control or comparison groups, heavy reliance on self-report measures of change and small sample sizes.

Despite these limitations, we do know that staff development activities have been rated highly by participants and that teachers rate the experience as useful, recommending participation to their colleagues. A number of studies have also demonstrated an impact on teachers' knowledge, skills and attitudes, and several have shown changes in student behaviour as a result of staff participation in faculty development programmes (Steinert et al 2006). Other benefits have included increased personal interest and enthusiasm, improved self-confidence, a greater sense of belonging to a community and educational leadership and innovation (Steinert et al 2003).

> *"My view of myself as a teacher has changed, from an information provider to a 'director' of learning."*
>
> *McGill Teaching Scholar*

The challenge in this area is to conduct more rigorous evaluations of staff development initiatives from the outset, to consider diverse models of programme evaluation, to make use of qualitative research methods and to broaden the focus of the evaluation itself. In no other area is the need to collaborate or transcend disciplinary boundaries greater.

> *"I leave rejuvenated and ready to go out and teach a thousand students again!"*
>
> *McGill Teaching Scholar*

Designing a staff development programme

The following guidelines are intended to help individuals design and deliver effective staff development programmes. They are also based on the premise that the medical school has a critical role to play in providing institutional leadership, appropriate resource allocation and recognition of teaching excellence (McLean et al 2008).

UNDERSTAND THE INSTITUTIONAL/ ORGANIZATIONAL CULTURE

Staff development programmes take place within the context of a specific institution or organization. It is imperative to understand the culture of that institution and to be responsive to its needs. Staff developers should capitalize on the organization's strengths and work with the leadership to ensure success. In many ways, the cultural context can be used to promote or enhance staff development efforts. For example, staff development during times of educational or curricular reform can take on added importance (Rubeck & Witzke 1998). It is also important to assess institutional support for staff development activities and lobby effectively. Staff development cannot occur in a vacuum.

 Capitalize on the institution's strengths, and promote organizational change and development.

DETERMINE APPROPRIATE GOALS AND PRIORITIES

As with the design of any other programme, it is imperative to clearly define goals and priorities. What is the programme trying to achieve? and why is it important to do so? Carefully determining goals and objectives will influence the choice of activity, programme content and methodology. Moreover, although determining priorities is not always easy, it is essential to balance individual and organizational needs.

CONDUCT NEEDS ASSESSMENTS TO ENSURE RELEVANT PROGRAMMING

As stated earlier, staff development programmes should base themselves on the needs of the individual as well as the institution. Student needs, patient needs and societal needs may also help to direct relevant activities. Assessing needs is necessary to refine goals, determine content, identify preferred learning formats and assure relevance. It is also a way of promoting early 'buy in'. Common methods include written questionnaires or surveys, interviews or focus groups with key informants (e.g. participants, students, educational leaders), observations of teachers 'in action', literature reviews and environmental scans of available programmes and resources. Whenever possible, it is worth acquiring information from multiple sources and distinguishing between 'needs' and 'wants'. Clearly, an individual teacher's perceived needs may differ from those expressed by their students or peers. Needs assessments can also help to further translate goals into objectives, which will serve as the basis for programme planning and evaluation of outcome.

 Assess needs to refine goals, determine content, identify preferred learning formats and promote 'buy in'.

DEVELOP DIFFERENT PROGRAMMES TO ACCOMMODATE DIVERSE NEEDS

Different educational formats have been described in an earlier section. Clearly, medical schools must design programmes that accommodate diverse goals and objectives, content areas, and the needs of the individual and the organization. For example, if the goal is to improve faculty members' lecturing skills, a half-day workshop on interactive lecturing might be the programme of choice. On the other hand, if the goal is to promote educational leadership and scholarly activity among peers, a Teaching Scholars Programme or educational fellowship might be the preferred format. In this context, it is also helpful to remember that staff development can include development, orientation, recognition and support, and different programmes are required to accommodate diverse objectives. Programme content and methods must also change over time to adapt to evolving needs.

INCORPORATE PRINCIPLES OF ADULT LEARNING AND INSTRUCTIONAL DESIGN

Adults come to learning situations with a variety of motivations and expectations about teaching methods and goals. Key principles of adult learning (e.g. Knowles 1988) include the following:

- Adults are independent.
- Adults come to learning situations with a variety of motivations and definite expectations about particular learning goals and teaching methods.
- Adults demonstrate different learning styles.
- Much of adult learning is 'relearning' rather than new learning.
- Adult learning often involves changes in attitudes as well as skills.
- Most adults prefer to learn through experience.
- Incentives for adult learning usually come from within the individual.
- Feedback is usually more important than tests and evaluations.

Incorporation of these principles into the design of a staff development programme can enhance receptivity, relevance and engagement. In fact, these principles should guide the development of all programmes, irrespective of their focus or format, as physicians and other healthcare professionals demonstrate a high degree of self-direction. They also possess numerous experiences that should serve as the basis for learning.

 Incorporate principles of adult learning to enhance receptivity, relevance and engagement.

Principles of instructional design should also be followed. For example, it is important to develop clear learning goals and objectives, identify key content areas, design appropriate teaching and learning strategies and create appropriate methods of evaluation (of both the students and the curriculum) (Fig. 45.1). It is equally important to integrate theory with practice (e.g. Kaufman et al 2000) and to ensure that the learning is perceived as relevant to the work setting

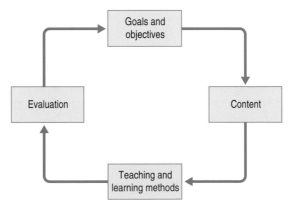

Fig. 45.1 The educational cycle.

and to the profession. Learning should be interactive, participatory and experientially based, using the participants' previous learning and experience as a starting point, and a positive environment for learning should be maintained. Detailed planning and organization involving all stakeholders are also critical.

OFFER A DIVERSITY OF EDUCATIONAL METHODS

In line with principles of adult learning, staff development programmes should try to offer a variety of educational methods that promote experiential learning, reflection, feedback and immediacy of application. Common learning methods include interactive lectures, case presentations, small-group exercises and discussions, role plays and simulations, videotape reviews and live demonstrations. (Many of these methods are described in earlier sections of this book.) Practice with feedback is also essential, as is the opportunity to reflect on personal values and attitudes. Computer-aided instruction, debates and reaction panels, journal clubs and self-directed readings are additional methods to consider. In line with our previous example, a workshop on interactive lecturing might include interactive plenaries, small-group discussions and exercises and opportunities for practice and feedback. A fellowship programme might include group seminars, independent projects and structured readings. Whatever the method, the needs and learning preferences of the participants must be respected, and the method should match the objective.

 Promote experiential learning, reflection, feedback and immediacy of application.

PROMOTE 'BUY IN' AND MARKET EFFECTIVELY

The decision to participate in a staff development programme or activity is not as simple as it might at first appear. It involves the individual's reaction to a particular offering, motivation to develop or enhance a specific skill, being available at the time of the session and overcoming the psychological barrier of admitting need (Rubeck & Witzke 1998). As faculty developers, it is our challenge to overcome reluctance and to market our 'product' in such a way that resistance becomes a resource to learning. In our context, we have seen the value of targeted mailings, professionally designed brochures and 'branding' of our product to promote interest. Continuing education credits, as well as free and flexible programming, can also help to facilitate motivation and attendance. 'Buy in' involves agreement on importance, widespread support, and dedication of time and resources at both the individual and the systems level and must be considered in all programming initiatives.

WORK TO OVERCOME COMMONLY ENCOUNTERED CHALLENGES

Common implementation problems, such as a lack of institutional support, limited resources, and limited faculty time have been discussed in an earlier section. Faculty developers must work to overcome these problems through creative programming, skilled marketing, targeted fundraising, and the delivery of high-quality programmes. Flexible scheduling and collaborative programming, which address clearly identified needs, will also help to ensure success at a systems level.

PREPARE STAFF DEVELOPERS

The recruitment and preparation of staff developers are rarely reported. However, it is important to recruit carefully, train effectively, partner creatively and build on previous experiences. Faculty members can be involved in a number of ways: as co-facilitators, programme planners or consultants. In our own setting, we try to involve new faculty members in each staff development activity and conduct a preparatory meeting (or 'dry run') to review content and process, solicit feedback and promote 'ownership'. We also conclude each activity with a 'debriefing' session to discuss lessons learned and plan for the future. Whenever possible, staff developers should be individuals who are well-respected by their peers and have some educational expertise and experience in facilitating groups. It has been said that 'to teach is to learn twice'; this principle is clearly one of the motivating factors that influence staff developers.

 "I was given new tools to teach. Not only were they described to me in words, but they were also used in front of me and I was part and parcel of the demonstration."

McGill Teaching Scholar

EVALUATE – AND DEMONSTRATE – EFFECTIVENESS

The need to evaluate staff development programmes and activities is clear. In fact, we must remember that the evaluation of staff development is more than an academic exercise, and our findings must be used in the design, delivery and marketing of our programmes. It has been stated earlier that staff development must help to promote education as a scholarly activity; we must role model this approach in all that we do.

In preparing to evaluate a staff development programme or activity, we should consider the goal of the evaluation (e.g. programme planning versus decision making; policy formation versus academic inquiry), available data sources (e.g. participants, peers, students or residents), common methods of evaluation (e.g. questionnaires, focus groups, objective tests, observations), resources to support assessment (e.g. institutional support, research grants) and models of programme evaluation (e.g. goal attainment, decision facilitation). Kirkpatrick's levels of evaluation are also helpful in conceptualizing and framing the assessment of outcome (Kirkpatrick 1994). They include the following:

- **Reaction:** participants' views on the learning experience
- **Learning:** changes in participants' attitudes, knowledge or skills
- **Behaviour:** changes in participants' behaviour
- **Results:** changes in the organizational system, the patient or the learner.

At a minimum, a practical and feasible evaluation should include an assessment of utility and relevance, content, teaching and learning methods and intent to change. Moreover, as evaluation is an integral part of programme planning, it should be conceptualized at the beginning of any programme. It should also include qualitative and quantitative assessments of learning and behaviour change, using a variety of methods and data sources.

 Evaluate effectively and ensure that research will inform practice.

Summary

Academic vitality is dependent upon faculty members' interest and expertise. Staff development has a critical role to play in promoting academic excellence and innovation. In looking to the future, we should focus on content areas that go beyond the improvement of specific teaching skills (e.g. educational leadership and scholarship, academic and career development); adopt diverse educational formats such as integrated longitudinal programmes, decentralized activities and self-directed learning; consider the benefits of work-based learning and communities of practice in promoting staff development as well as the value of staff development in fostering a sense of community; use staff development programmes and activities to promote organizational change and development; and evaluate the effectiveness of all that we do so that practice informs research and research can inform practice. We should also remain innovative and flexible so that we can accommodate the ever-changing needs of our teachers, our institutions and the healthcare systems in which we work.

 "A medical school's most important asset is its faculty."

Whitcomb 2003

References

Anderson PC: Mentoring, *Academic Medicine* 74(1): 4–5, 1999.

Bland CJ, Schmitz C, Stritter F et al: *Successful Faculty in Academic Medicine: Essential Skills and How to Acquire Them*, New York, 1990, Springer Publishing Company.

Centra JA: Types of faculty development programs, *Journal of Higher Education* 49(2):151–162, 1978.

Daloz LA: *Effective Teaching and Mentoring*, San Francisco, 1986, Jossey-Bass.

Flynn SP, Bedinghaus J, Snyder C, Hekelman F: Peer coaching in clinical teaching: a case report, *Family Medicine* 26(9):569–570, 1994.

Jason H, Westberg J: *Teachers and Teaching in US Medical Schools*, Norwalk, CT, 1982, Appleton-Century-Crofts.

Kaufman DM, Mann K, Jennett PA: *Teaching and Learning in Medical Education: How Theory Can Inform Practice*, Edinburgh, 2000, Association for the Study of Medical Education.

Kirkpatrick DL: *Evaluating Training Programs*, San Francisco, 1994, Berrett-Koehler Publishers.

Knowles MS: *The Modern Practice of Adult Education: From Pedagogy to Andragogy*, New York, 1988, Cambridge Books.

McLean M, Cilliers F, Van Wyk JM: Faculty development: yesterday, today and tomorrow, *Medical Teacher* 30(6):555–584, 2008.

Rubeck RF, Witzke DB: Faculty development: a field of dreams, *Academic Medicine* 73(9 Suppl):S32–S37, 1998.

Schön DA: *The Reflective Practitioner: How Professionals Think in Action*, New York, 1983, Basic Books.

Sheets KJ, Schwenk TL: Faculty development for family medicine educators: an agenda for future activities, *Teaching and Learning in Medicine* 2(3):141–148, 1990.

Steinert Y: Faculty development: from workshops to communities of practice, *Medical Teacher* 32(5):425–428, 2010.

Steinert Y, Nasmith L, McLeod PJ, Conochie L: A teaching scholars program to develop leaders in medical education, *Academic Medicine* 78(2): 142–149, 2003.

Steinert Y, Mann K, Centeno A, et al: A systematic review of faculty development initiatives designed to improve teaching effectiveness in medical education: BEME Guide No. 8, *Medical Teacher* 28(6): 497–526, 2006.

Ullian JA, Stritter FT: Types of faculty development programs, *Family Medicine* 29(4):237–241, 1997.

Whitcomb ME: The medical school's faculty is its most important asset, *Academic Medicine* 78(2):117–118, 2003.

Wilkerson L, Irby DM: Strategies for improving teaching practices: a comprehensive approach to faculty development, *Academic Medicine* 73(4):387–396, 1998.

Academic standards and scholarship

S. Mennin

 "We believe that it is time to move beyond the tired old 'teaching versus research' debate and give the familiar and honorable term 'scholarship' a broader, more capacious meaning, one that brings legitimacy to the full scope of academic work. Surely, scholarship means engaging in original research. But the work of the scholar also means stepping back from one's investigation, looking for connections, building bridges between theory and practice, and communicating one's knowledge effectively to students."

Boyer 1990

Introduction

Academic standards are what the academy and society mutually agree upon as benchmarks of quality that shape and frame the roles, responsibilities and actions of the professoriate. Education and the scholarship of education are not neutral. They are political, social and historical (Freire 1993) and involve choices about setting the agenda for what and how future health professionals will learn and whom they will serve, and how teachers will live and work in the academic world. Scholarship is a cornerstone of university life that can guide the future of medical education and the development of teachers in the health professions. In most parts of the world, opportunity for academic advancement is limited.

Standards, like culture, are slow to adapt to changing circumstances. There continues to be a need for adaptive change in medical education, to modernize curricula to be more socially responsible, incorporate other pedagogies, introduce early and sustained clinical experiences, promote viable community-based education and use new technologies in the learning/assessment process. At the same time, strained economies and the migration of health professionals are pushing already overburdened health systems to adapt. The pressures on faculty and staff to do more with less are greater than ever before. Monetary

pressures have pushed academic medical centre leaders to adopt values and fiscal policies more attuned to the entrepreneurial world of business than to the primary goals of health, learning and scholarship. There is a danger that the core values of learning and scholarship are being subjugated to a profit-oriented world. The internet, diseases without borders, conflicts and other international events emphasize the essential role of collaboration in the face of complex regional and transnational issues. The call for international or global standards in medical education that respect regional cultural integrities grows stronger.

Brazil, India, Australia, the United States, many parts of Africa and Asia have published national requirements and standards for the implementation of core (standard) competencies for medical education. Paradoxically, one observes in medical curricula less attention and time devoted to discussion, reflection and problem solving related to failure of healthcare systems and the millions of people who are without access to basic attention and healthcare.

Double standard: Research, patient care and teaching

 "The scholarly enterprise of teaching includes the creative development of innovative pedagogic practices and course materials, and aims to encourage independent learning and critical thinking. Scholarly teaching requires enthusiastic, intellectually engaged faculty who are well informed about the latest advances in their disciplines."

Marks 2000

There is a double standard: one for research and patient care and another one for education. Research and patient care have clear, well-established rules, expectations and standards and formal preparation for professional roles and responsibilities. The ability to generate outside funding from research and/or clinical care confers influence and status in academic and political processes. The culture of research and patient care is highly developed and almost universally accepted. Not so for scholarly work in education. Unlike research and patient care activities, teachers in the health professions rarely receive formal preparation for the teaching–learning process, education and assessment of learners. Poor teaching performance is tolerated, whereas poor quality in research and substandard patient care are not. Peer review is well established for research and patient care activities, yet still remains relatively undeveloped in teaching and other educational activities. Teachers at medical schools are well aware that the rewards and recognition for research and patient care are substantive and those for teaching and education much less so.

The absence of a common language in education and related shared values presents a major barrier to the coherent integration of scholarship and teaching. Few teachers can accurately describe how people learn, what is known about the development of expertise or the application of basic concepts and approaches to assessing learners. Even fewer can formulate and pursue research questions related to health professions education. It is a disturbing observation that those who are entrusted with the care and preparation of their successors are ill-informed about contemporary approaches to learning, teaching and education. We profess, but are we professional?

Professionalizing teaching

It is time to professionalize teaching and education; to have agreed-upon standards for teaching that are part of, rather than separate from, scholarly work and to hold teaching to the same high standards as research and patient care. How can this be done? Broadening the definition of scholarship to include the scholarship of discovery, application, integration and teaching (Boyer 1990) makes it feasible to articulate and reward all forms of excellence and to support an enriched culture for education and teaching in health professions schools.

Broadening the definition of scholarship

 "What we urgently need today is a more inclusive view of what it means to be a scholar – a recognition that knowledge is acquired through research, through synthesis, through practice and through teaching."

Boyer 1990

The traditional academic definition of scholarship applied by health professions schools to the work of the professoriate is exclusive; reserved only for those who conduct research and publish in peer reviewed journals. Large areas of legitimate academic activity and productivity vital to fulfilling the educational mission in the health professions are excluded by this definition. The work of the professoriate essential to the success of educational change and innovation is at risk of failing to be recognized because it lies outside the purview of the traditionally accepted forms of scholarship. A broader and more inclusive definition of scholarship goes beyond the discovery of new ways of knowing and new knowledge to include integration, application and teaching. It enables educators to pose important questions (Table 46.1) (Boyer 1990, Glassick et al 1997). This broader approach to scholarship is *inclusive*, establishing criteria for and recognizing the value of teaching as part of the merit and promotion process at a time when changes in education are needed (McGaghie 2009).

Table 46.1 Four arenas of scholarship

Category of scholarship	Description	Questions posed
Discovery	Knowledge for its own sake	What is known? What is yet to be found?
Integration	Making connections across disciplines, illuminating data in a real way, interpreting, drawing together and bringing new insight to bear on original work	How do these findings fit together … with what is already known?
Application	Engagement with society to apply what is known	How can what is known be responsibly applied to consequential problems? How can it be helpful to individuals, society and institutions?
Teaching	To make accessible and to participate in the transformation of what can be known with others	How can what is known be shared? How can what is known be transformed?

From Boyer EL: *Scholarship Reconsidered: Priorities of the Professoriate.* The Carnegie Foundation for the Advancement of Teaching. San Francisco,1990, Jossey-Bass.

Criteria for scholarship in education

Criteria for scholarship (Boyer 1990, Glassick et al 1997, Hutchings & Schulman 1999) require that:

- Educational activities be informed by both the latest ideas in the subject field and the most current ideas in the field of teaching
- Be open and accessible to the public
- Be subject to peer review critique and evaluation using acceptable criteria
- Be accessible in a form upon which others can build.

 "Inspired teaching keeps the flame of scholarship alive. Almost all successful academics give credit to creative teachers – those mentors who defined their work so compellingly that it became, for them, a lifetime challenge. Without the teaching function, the continuity of knowledge will be broken and the store of human knowledge dangerously diminished."

Boyer 1990

Most teachers in the world work in an environment where day-to-day activities leave little time for scholarship. Strategies for linking everyday educational activities and scholarship through a relative value, stepwise process have been developed by Morahan and Fleetwood (2008). This is especially important in places where resources are limited and opportunities for academic advancement few.

 "A teacher has a scholarly approach when he/ she uses best available practices and documents a systematic approach to the planning, implementation and evaluation of educational activities based on the literature."

Simpson et al 2007

When an anatomist or a paediatrician reads the latest literature on a topic, adds relevant contemporary findings, and places his or her teaching in a clinical context relevant to learners he or she is building on existing knowledge and is said to be taking a scholarly approach. A deeper level, educational scholarship, occurs when a teacher produces a work that is shared publicly with the education community in a form such that others can build on it. Being in the public domain, educational work is subject to peer review using accepted criteria for assessing scholarship. When a teacher makes his or her work available to other teachers, presents it at a peer reviewed professional meeting, has it accepted by an approved peer reviewed clearing house, or disseminates it on a website, he

or she has demonstrated educational scholarship. The teacher has engaged with and contributed to the broader educational community. Other forms of scholarship may consist of the production and sharing of syllabi, web-based instructional materials, fellowship programmes, continuing medical education programmes, performance data about learners, accomplishments of advisees and educational leadership programmes (Morahan & Fleetwood 2008, Simpson et al 2007). How can the teacher's department and school recognize and count this work toward merit and promotion?

Assessing scholarly teaching and educational scholarship

 "Academics feel relatively confident about their ability to assess specialized research, but they are less certain about what qualities to look for in other kinds of scholarship, and how to document and reward that work."

Glassick et al 1997

Academic standards for recognition and promotion based on scholarship and scholarly activities require credible documentation that includes (1) the quantity and (2) the quality of the educational activities and (3) a description of the nature of the person's engagement with the wider educational community (Simpson et al 2007). Quantity refers to the types and frequencies of educational roles and activities. Quality refers to measures of the effectiveness and excellence of the educational activity. Engagement with the education community occurs when the educational activity is informed by what is known in the field (scholarly approach) and educational scholarship when the educator contributes to the knowledge in the field. Table 46.2 illustrates the application of the criterion from Glassick et al (1997) to scholarship in lecturing, precepting, small-group facilitation and educational administration (Fincher et al 2000).

Institutional support for scholarly teaching and education

 "The effort to broaden the meaning of scholarship simply cannot succeed until the academy has clear standards for evaluating this wider range of scholarly work. After all, administrators and professors accord full academic value only to work they can confidently judge."

Glassick et al 1997

Table 46.2 Illustrative applications of the scholarship criteria of Glassick et al (1997) to lecturing, precepting, group work and educational administration

Six criteria for scholarship (Glassick et al 1997)	Criteria for quality teaching (Fincher et al 2000)	Documentation of evidence (Simpson et al 2007)			
		Quantity	Quality	Draws from field to inform own work (*scholarly approach*)	Contributes to field to inform others' work (*educational scholarship*)
Clear, achievable goals that are important to the field	Establish clear, achievable, measurable, relevant objectives	Teaching role, how long (duration and frequency)	Awards with criteria, evaluation by students, peers, consultants	How teaching approach is informed by the literature	List of interactive learning exercises is accepted in peer-reviewed repository
Adequate preparation, including an understanding of the existing work in the field	Identify and organize key materials appropriate to audience level and objectives	Where (required courses, venue)	Evidence of learning (self-reports, performance on standardized tests)	Impact of colleague discussions on subsequent practice	List of invitations to present teaching approach at regional, national and/or international conferences
Appropriate methods relative to goals	Select teaching methods and assessment measures to achieve and measure objectives	Formats, number and level of learners			
Significant results that contribute to the field	Assess learner performance				
Effective communication of work to intended audiences	Assess quality of presentation–instruction				
Reflective critique to improve quality of future work	Critical analysis of teaching that results in change to improve it				

From Fincher RME, Simpson DE, Mennin SP, et al: Scholarship as teaching: an imperative for the 21st century, *Academic Medicine* 75:887–894, 2000, with permission.

Mechanisms exist to support peer-reviewed basic and clinical science research, while those for teaching are variable and intermittent. The support of departments, medical schools, universities and professional organization sis required to elevate teaching to the level of scholarship by providing resources equivalent to those that support traditional basic and applied research. Table 46.3 presents an outline useful to assess an organization's infrastructure related to the scholarship of teaching and education.

The change process and the scholarship of teaching

 "Adaptive leadership consists of mobilizing people to do work that consists of the learning required to address conflicts in the values people hold, or to diminish the gap between the values people stand for and the reality they face. Adaptive work requires a change in values, beliefs or behavior."

Heifetz 1994

Leadership can be top-down (traditional hierarchical leadership) or bottom-up (emergent). It is important to be able to recognize this and know when and where they fit best (Hazy et al 2007). Experience teaches us that the role of leadership is critical before, during and after change and innovation in medical education. Insight into the dynamical nature of change as a process and the sociopolitical and economic interactions related to academic life, teaching/learning, healthcare and health are essential if the scholarship of teaching is to become part of the structural and cultural reality in medical schools (Bloom 1988, Mennin & Krakov 1998).

Change requires a disturbance of the status quo. The scholarship of teaching, for most medical schools, has relatively little impact. However, it can be linked to larger issues like promotion and merit. The status quo can be disturbed when new information and information-seeking activities about scholarship are present at multiple levels within the institutional organization (Departments, clinics, hospitals, deans, etc.). Important strategies are to provide information iteratively, have frequent formal and informal discussions, inform leadership and opinion leaders and clarify issues (if possible via research in medical education) by posing questions about scholarship such as:

- What is it?
- How does it work?
- Why do we need it?
- What's wrong with the way things are now?
- What are some advantages and disadvantages?

The adoption of a curriculum change and of different standards in medical education and the implementation of scholarship in teaching are unlikely to happen unless the leadership and teachers feel that they will resolve some crisis or uncertainty that affects them directly and that they will improve the quality of their daily work life. Some important strategic approaches at this stage involve embedding the scholarship of teaching into larger institutional and societal needs such as the introduction of community-based medical education in service of regional health needs or national and international movements to improve health professions education.

Academic organizations, like other living organisms, establish boundaries, rules and values based on individual and institutional history, context and initial conditions. In a bounded organization, change is more likely to occur when an environmental change makes living within the current boundaries unworkable, when the institution fails to achieve its stated and desired goals or when it is thought that the goals can be better satisfied in another way (Levine 1980). An internal review at the University of Kentucky School of Medicine revealed that its faculty recruitment, development, retention and promotion processes were not working optimally, particularly in the clinical departments (Nora et al 2000). A task force, including a broad representation of senior basic and clinical scientists, as well as nontenured faculty and others, collected data, developed procedures, examined policies and perceptions, kept in close contact with the larger faculty community, the university administration and governing bodies and reported findings publicly to the general faculty. These activities represent normal academic processes. Although the mission of the school embraced all four areas of scholarship outlined by Boyer (1990), the majority of the faculty perceived that only the scholarship of discovery mattered in the promotion process. Subsequently the university clarified promotion guidelines and implemented new mechanisms to support faculty in all forms of scholarly work. They also reaffirmed their support for the basic values in all forms of scholarship, including teaching (Nora et al 2000).

 "Most individuals do not evaluate an innovation on the basis of scientific studies of its consequences; instead, most people depend mainly upon a subjective evaluation conveyed to them from other individuals like themselves who have already adopted the innovation."

Rogers 2003

The implementation of the scholarship of teaching will require careful attention to how education is perceived by both individuals and groups of teachers

Table 46.3 Key infrastructure features of medical schools and professional organizations supportive of the scholarship of teaching/education

Department/medical school	Professional organization
[Frame 1: Structural]	
Educational leadership positions listed on organizational chart • Equivalent to research and/or clinical practice positions	Formal affiliation opportunities for medical educators • Committees, sections, special interest groups, leadership positions related to education
School-wide medical education office, committee or individual	Peer review committees/panels
Medical school library/website to access literature and websites specific in medical education	Society publishes peer-reviewed education papers
Education facilities and support personnel	Education clearinghouse/bookstore
[Frame 2: Human resources]	
Orientation programmes about medical education • For new faculty, course directors, clerkship directors, committee members	Fellowships in medical education • Teaching-career advancement, fellowships
Education handbooks/web-based materials • 'How-tos' for course and programme directors; relevant skills, resources, policies for education programmes	Educational resource materials • Society-support guidelines and materials for education-based work • How to document activities for promotion
Faculty development programmes/workshops • Curriculum development, teaching skills, preparation of promotion materials as educational scholarship, mentoring from senior faculty • Hiring process for educational positions	Faculty development workshops/programmes • Annual skills workshops, refresher courses related to educational skills
[Frame 3: Policies]	
Selection/election/appointment process for key positions and committees	Selection/election/appointment process for key positions
Educators in leadership positions • Chairs of key committees, working groups, promotion and tenure groups, budget process	Educators in leadership positions • Key decision-making positions, resource allocation, policy and by-law decisions
Educator coalitions to influence decisions • Influence resource allocation	Educator coalitions to influence decisions • Resource allocation, presence on organization website
[Frame 4: Symbolic]	
Public documents • Department/medical school committee agendas have a standing education line item	Public documents • Education is featured in multiple venues
Rituals/traditions/ceremonies • Awards, recognition for education scholarship	Ritual/traditions/ceremonies
Department/medical school-wide public forums • Visiting or distinguished lectureship on education attended by leaders • Education periodic focus of grand rounds or conferences	Public forums • Annual lectureship • Listservs for educators

From Fincher RME, Simpson DE, Mennin SP, et al: Scholarship as teaching: an imperative for the 21st century, *Academic Medicine* 75:887–894, 2000, with permission.

(McGaghie 2009). Some characteristics of innovations valued by potential adopters of innovations (Rogers 2003) include:

- **Relative value.** To what degree is the scholarship of teaching perceived as an opportunity for career advancement? Is it socially prestigious? Is it more satisfying? One advantage of introducing a broader definition of scholarship and recognizing it as part of the promotion process is to the retention of faculty vital to the success of a school's education mission in a rapidly changing world.

- **Compatibility.** Is the scholarship of teaching consistent with existing individual and institutional values, past experiences, the needs of potential adopters as well as societal values? Expanding the definition of scholarship to include application, integration and teaching in addition to discovery creates a more inclusive environment without lowering the standards of the scholarship of discovery. It fits well with teachers who produce educational materials and innovations and who are recognized for that work when it meets the criteria of scholarship. Promotion criteria based on a narrow interpretation of scholarship (publications, grants and awards) are inconsistent with the rising demands of clinical work and can result in the loss of outstanding clinicians and educators. The educator's portfolio can be an institutional strategy for clinical teachers to meet the criteria for promotion by providing acceptable evidence of the scholarship of teaching (Simpson et al 1994).

- **Degree of difficulty.** How difficult is it to grasp and implement the idea of the scholarship of teaching (McGaghie 2009)? For some faculty, education is not the most important part of their day-to-day activities. Few people give their best effort to activities for which they are insufficiently prepared or do not fully understand and for which they receive insufficient recognition. The University of Louisville, like many institutions, found itself caught in economic difficulty: having to earn more clinical income to support teachers and to subsidize other activities. The administration found itself using a research-focused promotion and reward system to evaluate clinician educators (Schweitzer 2000), something that is very common in the developing world. Further, structural changes requiring post-tenure review stimulated a reconsideration of the best way to maximize faculty resources and talent. The university adopted the Boyer approach, broadening the definition of scholarship to include the scholarship of teaching. However, the faculty had difficulty in understanding how scholarship applied to a variety of faculty activities, as did the promotion and tenure committee in seeing how the model could be adapted to their school. The model was too difficult and burdensome and was not adopted by the faculty (Schweitzer 2000).

- **Trialability.** To what extent can teachers or institutions experiment with the scholarship of teaching on a limited basis? Educational approaches that can be pilot tested have a much better chance of succeeding than those for which a small-scale trial is not possible. Teaching, when perceived as not being appropriately rewarded, can result in teachers choosing not to pursue their interests in the educational process. The adoption of criteria for scholarship applied universally without regard to the forum in which the activity or the subject occurred can promote a shared understanding of scholarship applied to education.

- **Observability.** To what extent will the results of the scholarship of teaching be observable? If faculty can see it working in a department or with someone they respect (opinion leader), they will be more likely to adopt it. Visibility stimulates peer discussion and helps spread the innovation to others.

Summary

The definition of scholarship has been expanded beyond discovery and creation of new findings and their public presentation and publication in peer-reviewed media to include the scholarship of integration, application and teaching. The criteria for educational scholarship, like other forms of scholarship, require that activities be informed by both the latest ideas in the subject field and the most current ideas in the field of teaching; be open and accessible to the public; be subject to peer review critique and evaluation using acceptable criteria; and be accessible in a form upon which others can build. Teachers engaged in routine teaching activities can take a scholarly approach when they draw from the established literature and known practices in their subject area. Teaching becomes educational scholarship when teachers make original contributions to the existing peer-reviewed resources in their field. Academic standards for recognition and promotion based on scholarship and scholarly activities require credible documentation that includes the quantity and the quality of the educational activities and a description of the nature of the person's engagement with the wider educational community. The challenge is to promote the development and acceptance of documentation of scholarship as an important part of an educator's portfolio in support of merit and promotion.

Successful movements in medical education, such as the current expansion of the definition of scholarship and the refinement of documentation of evidence for recognition and promotion, depend on an understanding of the practical and theoretical aspects of adaptive leadership. The introduction of educational scholarship requires dedicated staff and teachers capable of expanding the boundaries of education, together with a system capable of recognizing and supporting those who do so. Academic health science centres, medical education, and healthcare systems are part of a complex ecology that emerges from the local dialogues and activities we have with one another. It is up to each of us to engage with those around us so that an understanding and application of educational scholarship can emerge as part of a 'new traditional' institutional fabric supportive of academic careers in health professions education and the priority health needs of society.

References

Bloom SW: Structure and ideology in medical education: an analysis of resistance to change, *Journal of Health and Social Behavior* 29:294–306, 1988.

Boyer EL: *Scholarship Reconsidered: Priorities of the Professoriate. The Carnegie Foundation for the Advancement of Teaching*, San Francisco, 1990, Jossey-Bass.

Fincher RME, Simpson DE, Mennin SP, et al: Scholarship as teaching: an imperative for the 21st century, *Academic Medicine* 75:887–894, 2000.

Freire P: *Pedagogy of the Oppressed*, New York, 1993, The Continuum International Publishing Company.

Glassick CE, Huber MT, Maeroff GI: *Scholarship Assessed: Evaluation of the Professoriate*, San Francisco, 1997, Jossey–Bass.

Hazy JK, Goldstein JA, Lichtenstein BB, editors: Complex systems Leadership Theory: New Perspectives from Complexity Science on Social and Organizational Effectiveness. Exploring Organizational and Complexity Series, Vol. 1, Mansfield, MA, 2007, ISCE Publishing.

Heifitz RA: *Leadership Without Easy Answers*, Cambridge, MA, 1994, Belknap Press of Harvard University Press.

Hutchings P, Shulman LS: The scholarship of teaching: new elaborations, new developments, 1999. Change September/October:11–15.

Levine A: *Why Innovation Fails*, Albany, 1980, State University of New York Press.

McGaghie WC: Scholarship, publication, and career advancement in health professions education: AMEE Guide No. 43, *Medical Teacher* 31:574–590, 2009.

Marks ES: Defining scholarship at the Uniformed Services University of the Health Sciences School of Medicine: a study in cultures, *Academic Medicine* 75:935–939, 2000.

Mennin SP, Krackov SK: Reflections on relatives, resistance, and reform in medical education, *Academic Medicine* 73(suppl):S60–S64, 1998.

Morahan PS, Fleetwood J: The double helix of activity and scholarship: building a medical education career with limited resources, *Medical Education* 42: 34–44, 2008.

Nora LM, Pomeroy C, Curry TE Jr, et al: Revising appointment, promotion, and tenure procedures to incorporate an expanded definition of scholarship: The University of Kentucky College of Medicine experience, *Academic Medicine* 75:913–924, 2000.

Rogers EM: *The Diffusion of Innovations*, ed 5, New York, 2003, Free Press.

Schweitzer L: Adoption and failure of the 'Boyer model' in the University of Louisville, *Academic Medicine* 75:925–929, 2000.

Simpson D, Morzinski J, Beecher A, Lindemann J: Meeting the challenge to document teaching accomplishments: the educator's portfolio, *Teaching and Learning in Medicine* 6:203–206, 1994.

Simpson D, Fincher RM, Hafler JP, et al: Advancing educators and education: defining the components and evidence of educational scholarship. Proceedings from the American Association of Medical Colleges Group on Educational Affairs Consensus Conference on Educational Scholarship, 9–10 February 2006, Charlotte, NC. Washington, DC, 2007, AAMC, 2007 Available at: https://members.aamc.org/eweb/DynamicPage.aspx?webcode=PubHome.

Publishing

J. Bligh, J. Browne

Publishing in medical education: Joining the conversation

As a clinical teacher, you belong to a huge and diverse international community of medical educators engaged in managing, researching and delivering education and training to medical students and doctors. Members of this community are in constant conversation, sharing, discussing, debating, exploring and finding solutions to the everyday challenges they face. Where these conversations are recorded and made available to others interested in the same issues, they become 'the medical education literature'.

It goes without saying that, if you are reading this book, you already take a scholarly approach to your work as a clinical teacher. You are engaged in following the worldwide conversation as a reader, and therefore you almost certainly have something to say as a writer. There's no time like the present: so why not start writing?

This chapter will discuss the various publishing options open to you as an author, describe the advantages of publishing in a high-quality journal, offer some advice on developing a strategic approach to writing and publication and outline some practical things that you can do to maximize your work's chance of acceptance, and, above all, we hope that it will encourage you to get involved in the worldwide medical education conversation.

Where to start?

There was once a time, not so long ago, when people would have understood the phrase 'medical education literature' to mean simply 'the academic books and journals within library collections'. To some extent this is still true, but nowadays, the explosion in digital and desktop publishing gives you more opportunities and choice than ever before.

There are many different publication formats and media, so pick the one that you feel is best suited to your message. The most important thing is to engage in that conversation with the community; once you get started, you will find that opportunities and ideas start to flow (Box 47.1).

These are exciting times and clinical teachers everywhere are taking advantage of the opportunities the digital age offers to share their work with a variety of audiences. If your aim is simply to get your work out to other clinical teachers, it's relatively easy to do it

---

Box 47.1 Possible ways in which clinical teachers can join debates in medical education

- Abstracts, conference presentations, posters
- Book chapters
- Book reviews
- Books (authored or co-authored)
- Books (edited or co-edited)
- Conference reports
- Educational case reports or 'teaching moments'
- Lecture notes and presentations
- Literature reviews and meta-analyses
- Online repositories of teaching materials such as the AAMC's MedEdPortal (www.mededportal.org)
- Opinion pieces, editorials or commentaries
- Pilot research reports; provisional or interim findings
- Reports of curricular developments and policy
- Research studies (both experimental and qualitative)
- Responses, rejoinders or critiques of previously published work, usually in the form of a letter to the editor
- Social media: tweets, blogs, etc.
- Textbooks and monographs

yourself, provided you have access to the necessary tools and a reasonable internet connection. You can publish virtually anything you like from the comfort of your own desk. You don't even need to trouble yourself to set up your own website: it is a relatively simple matter to upload and share text, images, sound and video files using a vast array of providers and sites. Any format is open to you; the level of sophistication and audience involvement is up to you, from a simple Word document to a highly interactive multi-media resource. You can invite comments, open discussions and provide online links to further resources and references. You can manipulate images and text until they are barely recognizable when compared with their original source. You can set up information exchanges such as blogs and wikis, use social networking sites and post pictures and clips that may attract worldwide attention.

REPORTS OF THE DEATH OF THE PUBLISHER ARE PREMATURE

The fact that digital formats make self-publication so easy has led to fears that academic publishers as we know them will one day become obsolete (Thompson 2005). In fact, at present the reverse seems to be true: publishers are going from strength to strength, new academic journals are being launched all the time, and editors report that the numbers of papers being submitted to their journals are continuing to increase. So it's worth pausing to consider why it is that journal publication – online or in paper – continues to be seen as the gold standard and why, if you are a scholarly teacher, you should aim to submit your work for publication in a high quality peer-reviewed journal. Box 47.2 explains some of the benefits of having your work published by a professional publisher.

Whatever format and medium you eventually decide to publish in, the advice which follows in this chapter holds good, but it is particularly aimed at helping you to publish your education research in one of the high-quality academic journals.

PLAN YOUR SUBMISSION STRATEGY IN ADVANCE

Academic publishing is a huge and fast-changing field, and journals need to be competitive. Whilst editors are by the nature of their role dedicated to serving the academic community in which they work, they have to set publishing priorities, and one of their chief concerns must be to maintain and, if possible, increase their readership.

When making decisions about journal content, therefore, an editor will almost inevitably place the needs and wishes of the reader ahead of those of the author. You may be convinced that the world needs your particular article, but the editor's job is to question whether his or her readers want to read it. The challenge is to make your work stand out amongst the hundreds or even thousands of other manuscripts that the journal receives each year. To persuade the editor

---

Box 47.2 Some ways in which professional peer-reviewed publication adds value

- **Academic recognition**. Publication in high-impact journals is still recognized by universities, awarding bodies and employers as the ultimate scholarly achievement and will enhance your career resume.

- **Reassurance for authors and readers regarding the quality of the review and publication process.** Editors and editorial staff are increasingly professional or semi-professional and increasingly undertake training. Many journal editors are members of professional editors' groups and adhere to ethical codes. Journal owners usually provide a range of support services to editors including administrative support, sophisticated electronic peer review systems including plagiarism detection software and advice on insurance, legal liabilities and business strategy.

- **Profile-raising.** Publishers' marketing departments publicize journals, issues and even individual papers. It will be easier for your work to appear in collections, such as themed issues or series, where it will benefit from being marketed alongside similar publications. Publishers can target your work at specific groups; some journals are distributed to professional groups and learned societies as part of their membership subscriptions.

- **Authors' services such as copy editing, typesetting and proofreading**. Publishers will prepare your manuscript for publication. They will typeset and design your publication, sometimes using a distinctive 'house style' which will be familiar to readers. Some journals and publishers also offer technical editing and translation services.

- **Archiving and indexing**. The big journal publishers will ensure that your work is archived permanently and retrievably with a unique digital object identifier (DOI) number and that it is linked to various indexes, databases, libraries and repositories. This is important to research assessment exercises, and it will increase the likelihood of your work being cited. Publishers also fiercely protect copyright and administer user licensing on their own (and therefore on your) behalf.

that your paper is exactly what his or her readers are looking for, you need to plan your submission carefully.

CHOOSE YOUR JOURNAL CAREFULLY

Journals vary considerably both in scope and in the quality of work they publish, so it's worth doing a bit of homework before deciding where to submit your manuscript. Naturally, you will be looking for a high-quality journal. One indicator of prestige is the impact factor; most of the older, well-established journals are ranked by this. Research assessment exercises, employers and grant funders are increasingly influenced by impact factors. Papers in a journal with a high impact factor are cited more frequently than those in a low-impact journal, so there are clear benefits to publishing in higher-impact journals.

 You can find out more about impact factors and other bibliometric measures of journal quality from Thomson ISI's website www.isinet.com

Put simply, the impact factor is a measure of how often the 'average article' in a journal has been cited in a particular year. The impact factor is calculated by dividing the number of current citations to articles published in the two previous years by the total number of articles published in the two previous years. Other measures of a journal's quality are more subtle, but a bit of research can help you to predict which journals are most likely to offer their authors good service (Box 47.3).]

TAKE AN OBJECTIVE LOOK AT YOUR WORK

Big, high-impact international journals may give a less personal service and your risk of rejection is much higher, but the prestige of being published in one is considerable, and if it gets accepted, your article is more likely to be extensively cited. For authors, it's a decision that has to be weighed very carefully. You will need to think objectively about the academic rigour, originality and significance of your work and ask yourself how far you are prepared to risk rejection in order to get it published in a really high quality journal: always remembering that (a) rejection is the very worst that can happen; (b) whatever the final outcome, you will learn something from the process; and (c) you may actually be successful!

Whatever you ultimately decide about the potential impact of your work, there is a good deal you can do to give it the best possible chance of publication, and we will discuss this in more detail below.

READ YOUR TARGET JOURNAL

Ensuring that your work is a good fit for your desired journal is absolutely crucial. We cannot stress this

---

Box 47.3 Some questions to ask to help you decide on a target journal

- What is its readership? Who reads it and how widely?
- Is it indexed, and by which indexes?
- What is its impact factor, and how does it compare with other journals in the field? Is it rising or falling?
- Is it peer reviewed? Open or blinded review?
- How quickly does it make decisions? How much feedback can authors expect?
- Who is the editor? Who is on the editorial board?
- Is it the journal of an academic association? If so, which one? How old is the journal?
- Is the publisher well established? What other journals does it publish? What is its marketing like?
- Does the journal declare its ethical standards? Does it have a policy of openness, and is it clear about its processes? Is it a member of the Committee on Publication Ethics or one of the other editors' organizations?
- Are there print and electronic versions? What added value is there in the electronic version (e.g. dynamic referencing, early online publication, supplementary material, interactive reader responses)?
- Is it 'open access' or subscription-only? If it is an open-access journal (that is, free to all readers without a subscription), are authors expected to pay a publication fee at any point?

---

strongly enough. Ideally, you should be thinking about who you want to read your work and where you want to publish it before you start any research project, and certainly before you begin writing up.

Reading several recent issues is the only way to get a good idea of what a journal is publishing. You can see what debates are going on in its pages, and editorials, calls for papers and mission statements in particular can sometimes give you a clue as to what the editor is looking for. Look at the various papers in the journal. What do they have in common? Would your paper look out of place among them? Will it add anything to what has already been published on the subject?

Do not underestimate the importance of this background research. Editors can always tell when someone has not bothered to read their journal before submitting a paper. This is not very flattering, of course, but, much more significantly, it indicates that the author is out of touch with the current debates and that the reference list will be lacking important recent citations.

READ THE JOURNAL'S ADVICE TO AUTHORS

Guidelines for authors are usually available on the journal's website. Read them carefully. Then read them again. If something is not clear, do not guess; ask the editorial office. Author guidelines are there for a reason, and a little time spent getting the formatting of your paper correct in the initial stages may save you a great deal of time later.

As we mentioned before, research papers are not the only way to get your message across, and you may stand more chance of getting a shorter piece accepted, particularly in paper journals where publication space is limited. So ask yourself if your work would be better presented in one of the other formats offered by your target journal. These may include commentaries, case reports, letters to the editor, short communications, discussion papers, review articles and personal accounts. Or the journal may be willing to publish a short report of your work in the paper edition with other sections such as references, figures or tables published online only. The journal, in its advice to contributors, will tell you about the options available to you and outline its standard word lengths and formats.

Start to write

ADOPT A CLEAR AND ECONOMICAL WRITING STYLE

Editors are usually looking for a paper that has real substance and, regardless of research methodology, tells a good clear story about:

- what you did and why you did it (background and introduction)
- how you did it (methods)
- what you found out (results)
- what it means (discussion)
- and what you think should be done next (conclusions)

Although we are not proposing that you should 'dumb down' your key messages, there is no point in making your article unnecessarily difficult for the reader by adopting an inflated and wordy writing style. A paper needs to be worth the space it takes up in a journal; the clearer and more succinct it is, the more likely it is to capture and hold readers' attention (Eva 2010).

Writing well is a key tool for any medical teacher, and it is worth investing time in improving your style. There are plenty of courses and learning resources available, but the important thing to bear in mind is that you can really only improve your writing skills by actually writing and getting feedback. If you postpone writing until you think your skills are good enough, you may never get around to it.

 "Writing is a self-taught craft; the more you work at it, the more skilled you become. And when you're not writing, READ."

Lois Duncan

REVIEW, REVIEW, REVIEW

Sometimes, especially when you have been working on a paper for a long time, you may start to lose confidence in what you are writing and how you are writing it. That is the time to seek advice and feedback from someone you can trust. Experienced authors always seek feedback on their work before submitting it.

Try to get feedback from several colleagues. It is very important that they are honest with you. If they think your manuscript is boring, over-technical or difficult to follow, the likelihood is that the editor will also have problems with it. It is much better to get constructive advice before you submit so you have a chance to nip any potentially fatal flaws in the bud.

Consider asking someone who is not an expert in the field to look at your manuscript for readability. Remember that not all of your readers – and sometimes not even the editor or peer reviewers – will be fully conversant with your specialist field of research or your methodology, and a substantial number will be 'interested amateurs'. Your work needs to be accessible to as wide a range of people as possible, so try it out on a non-expert who may be better able to spotlight areas where concepts, methods and technical terms need clarification.

Don't forget to review your work for detail. Give the best possible impression by avoiding spelling and grammatical errors, unreadable figures and misplaced and missing references and tables. Check your target journal's technical requirements for reporting; this is particularly important where you are presenting quantitative data.

IF ENGLISH IS NOT YOUR FIRST LANGUAGE

It is becoming increasingly important to write and to publish in English, whatever your country of origin. This puts writers whose first language is not English at an unfair disadvantage in a highly competitive market. While editors may be sympathetic to the difficulties faced by non-English speaking authors, most do not have the resources to spend time deciphering and rewriting an article written in very poor English.

It is therefore essential, if English is not your first language, to get your manuscript read by someone fluent in English. If that person is not an expert in the field in which you are working, you will also need the advice of someone with excellent English who has a good grasp of the technical complexities of your research. If you use writing assistants or technical editors to help you prepare your manuscript, it is unlikely that they will qualify for full authorship, but you should acknowledge their contribution when submitting your final manuscript.

ETHICAL CONSIDERATIONS: A WARNING

Unethical practice in medical education research and publication is dangerous because it damages the academic record by misleading readers and distorting the evidence. It also wastes valuable time and resources and may lead to a general loss of confidence in the academic rigour of the published archive. While institutional review boards and ethics committees are there to remind research staff about the need to make ethical considerations a priority when designing projects, ethical issues surrounding publication are more easily overlooked by authors in the rush to get published.

Authors who commit any of the 'big three' infractions – fraudulent use of data, fabrication of results and data, and plagiarism – may rightly anticipate serious consequences if they are caught. However, there is growing concern among editors about the threat posed by other types of unethical practice which are perhaps more insidious and widespread. Journals have increasingly sophisticated ways of detecting misconduct. They are becoming much less inclined to accept pleas of ignorance from authors who have failed to match up to the required standards, and they are increasingly likely to take action, including contacting authors' institutions, when they suspect misconduct (Brice et al 2009).

It is therefore your responsibility as an author to make yourself familiar with, and to apply, the highest possible standards in publication ethics. Behaviours expected of an author include, but are not restricted to:

- Ensuring that all authors are credited, and that those who are credited really are authors (which is usually understood to mean that they have (1) made a substantial contribution to the study design, data collection and analysis; (2) made an important intellectual contribution to the writing; (3) agreed with the final version)
- Acknowledging contributors and revealing any potential competing interests
- Giving 'value for money' in publication terms: this means not recycling old work, nor trying to eke out

> **Box 47.4 Sources of guidance on research and publication ethics**
>
> - American Psychological Society (APA): www.apa.org/research
> - Committee on Publication Ethics (COPE): http://publicationethics.org/
> - EQUATOR Network: www.equator-network.org
> - International Committee of Medical Journal Editors (ICJME): www.icmje.org
> - Office of Research Integrity (ORI): http://ori.hhs.gov/

your data into as many thin and repetitive papers as possible

- Being honest and proportionate in your interpretation of data
- Being frank with editors about previous or related publications, and making sure that you submit to only one journal at a time.

A list of ethics resources is shown in Box 47.4.

Although current systems for obtaining ethics committee (or institutional review board) approval for studies in medical education have frequently been criticized for being bureaucratic, slow and sometimes inappropriate for this type of research, journal editors will almost certainly reject your paper outright if you attempt to bypass the required processes (Ten Cate 2009). You must also make a statement somewhere in your work about how ethical considerations were addressed; if approval was waived or unnecessary, you should still let the editor know why.

GIVE YOUR MANUSCRIPT A GOOD TITLE AND ABSTRACT

The title and abstract of your manuscript are the first things that the editor and reviewers will read, and are crucial to 'selling' your paper, so they ought to be the last parts you write. Some busy editors read no further than the abstract before making their decision on whether an article is worth further review, so do not under any circumstances rush this important writing task. If your abstract is inaccurate, boring, wordy, vague or unoriginal, it may give an unfairly bad impression of the content and readers will skip past your work without reading further. Finally, keep the title as short as you can while making sure it tells readers as much as possible about what they can expect to find in the article; look at other titles in the journal to get ideas. For more detailed advice on writing titles and abstracts, see Cook et al (2007).

PREPARE A COVERING NOTE TO THE EDITOR

The covering note is your chance to tell the editor why your paper is important, but authors who are in a hurry to submit their manuscript sometimes try to get by without writing one. This is a wasted opportunity. If you have (a) read the literature in the field, (b) thought about why your research matters and (c) targeted your journal carefully, it should be easy to prepare a good case for publication. Tell the editor what your work adds to what has previously been published on the subject and – most importantly – *why you think readers of his or her journal will want to read it*. If there's anything special about your paper that you want to bring to the editor's attention, the covering note is the place to do it (Brice & Bligh 2005).

Submit your manuscript

Allow plenty of time for submitting your manuscript, because it always takes longer than you expect. If you are writing with co-authors, choose a time to submit when you know you will be able to contact them if questions arise. There is nothing more frustrating than starting to submit a manuscript, only to find that you are missing vital information from a co-author who happens to be away.

Most biomedical journals use electronic submission and review. When submitting electronically, try to ensure you have access to a reliable internet connection, keep copies of everything and save your work regularly. Once you have submitted, you will get a receipt from the journal with a reference number in case you want to follow the progress of your submitted work.

Understand how peer review actually works

 "The purpose of peer review is to keep egg off authors' faces."

Drummond Rennie (Goldbeck-Wood 1998)

Although it may feel as if your manuscript vanishes into a black hole when you submit it, a great deal in fact happens to it once it has entered the editorial process. Each journal has its own style and requirements, but the basic procedures for handling, processing, selecting and publishing papers are broadly similar. Once you understand how your manuscript will be assessed for publication, then you will find the process of submitting it and waiting for a result much easier to bear.

Editors usually base their decisions on advice from other people working in the same field. This is what is meant by 'peer review' (Jefferson & Godlee 2003). It is an intensive process and takes time. In most journals, your work will be assessed by one or more staff editors, including section and specialist editors. It may also receive statistical review from a staff statistician. You may be sent a firm decision at this point, but if initial scrutiny is favourable most journals will then send your work to academic colleagues in other institutions for more detailed feedback.

The review process is done with varying degrees of anonymity; you may be told the reviewers' names, they may know yours, or peer review may be carried out 'double-blinded' so that neither side is aware of the other's identity. The process of peer review takes anywhere from a few days to a couple of months depending on the speed with which the reviewers respond. You should have been told how long a decision will take, so don't worry that nothing is happening if you don't hear anything during that period. However, once the deadline for a decision is past, do not be afraid to ask what is happening. Delays are almost always due to slow reviewers, and a polite enquiry may help the process along.

Once all the reviewers' reports are available, they will be assessed, sometimes by an editorial committee, and a decision letter containing varying amounts of feedback prepared. You will receive one of three decisions: a rejection, an offer to reconsider the paper provided you revise it to a greater or lesser degree or an acceptance.

Don't get upset: Rejection is not the end

When you receive a final decision, there is a strong probability that you will be disappointed. Remember that in most journals, many more papers are rejected than accepted, and in some specialist and high-prestige journals such as *Medical Education*, nine out of ten authors will eventually receive a rejection letter.

Despite knowing the odds, it can still dent your confidence severely to receive a rejection or request for a major rewrite, especially if you feel that the comments are unfair or unnecessarily harsh. But peer review is there to help you improve your work, so the sooner you calm down, consider the comments you have received as objectively as you can, revise your paper in the light of that feedback and resubmit it, the sooner you will get your paper published.

It sometimes happens that a reviewer suggests a revision that you feel is unnecessary or just plain wrong. Sometimes reviewers will ask for amendments that are mutually exclusive (for example, one may suggest you cut a section out, while another suggests you expand it). Sometimes they will ask you to do things you feel would fundamentally change the nature of your research, or to supply information or data that you don't have. You do not have to follow their advice slavishly, but nor should you dismiss their comments as ill-informed or prejudiced. In the end, it's your paper and your choice what you do with it next; but the reviewers were carefully chosen for their expertise and they made their comments for a reason, so it is wise to reflect calmly on what they have said and respond constructively rather than simply dismissing their views.

Even when you feel that the reviewers have completely missed the point of your paper, ask yourself the following questions:

- What didn't they understand about my work?
- Could I have explained it more clearly?
- Was this really the right journal for my manuscript?

Try to respond to these points in any revision, either within the manuscript itself or in the covering note to the editor. If submitting to a new journal, it helps if you include copies of previous reviews and an explanatory note so that the editor can see exactly what you have done to improve your work.

You may have to revise your manuscript several times and resubmit it to more than one journal before it is accepted. It can be a frustrating process, but each time you revise your paper, you are simply making it better and therefore improving its chances of acceptance.

So keep trying, working your way down your list of suitable journals, and sooner or later, you will have the very satisfying experience of seeing your work in print.

Summary

The medical education community is in constant conversation with itself through a wide variety of media. Clinical teachers who take a scholarly approach to their work can participate in current debates, not just as readers but also as authors. New technologies provide more options for publication than ever before.

Publication in a peer-reviewed academic journal is still seen as the 'gold standard' at present. In order to write a paper which will be acceptable to the most highly regarded journals, successful authors develop a strategic approach to writing and publishing. This involves selecting and targeting the most appropriate journal, checking its quality and performance against that of other journals in the field. It is important to understand how peer review works and what the editor and reviewers want. Experienced authors study the medical education literature, paying particular attention to their target journal. They are careful to read both the content and the guidelines for authors to make sure that their work will fit comfortably within the scope and format of the journal.

Successful authors are good writers; they understand that their aim is to communicate a clear message to their readers, so they work hard to develop a simple and direct style. Less experienced writers sometimes adopt an overly formal style, which is superficially impressive but can obscure the message and will make the paper less acceptable to the editor. Experienced authors seek feedback from colleagues, both expert and non-specialist, on their work's quality and also on its readability and clarity. When preparing to submit their manuscripts, successful authors take their time and don't rush the process because they know that errors and missing information can be more time-consuming in the long run.

Once a final decision is made, it can be very discouraging to receive a rejection, but successful authors don't give up; they revise and reformat their manuscripts in the light of editor and reviewer feedback and carry on submitting. Sooner or later their paper will be accepted, but only if they persist.

References

Brice J, Bligh J: 'Dear Editor': advice on writing a covering letter, *Medical Education* 39(9):876, 2005.

Brice J, Bligh J, Bordage G, et al: Publishing ethics in medical education journals, *Academic Medicine* 84(13):S1–S3, 2009.

Cook DA, Beckman TJ, Bordage G: A systematic review of titles and abstracts of experimental studies in medical education: many informative elements missing, *Medical Education* 41(11):1074–1081, 2007.

Eva KW: Enough rope to hang yourself: word limits in medical education, *Medical Education* 44(5): 432, 2010.

Goldbeck-Wood S: What makes a good reviewer of manuscripts? *BMJ* 316(7125):86, 1998.

Jefferson T, Godlee F: *Peer Review in Health Sciences*, ed 2, London, 2003, BMJ Books.

Ten Cate O: Why the ethics of medical education research differs from that of medical research, *Medical Education* 43(7):608–610, 2009.

Thompson JB: Books in the Digital Age, Cambridge, 2005, Polity.

Educational environment

S. McAleer, S. Roff

Introduction

The environment or climate in the meteorological context is a key topic for discussion on a daily basis. It is impossible not to watch a news bulletin or read a newspaper without reference to global warming, the ozone layer or the disappearance of the rain forests. 'Look after the planet, or the planet will soon cease to exist' is the recurring message. The environment in the context of an educational setting has also become an issue for debate. If we do not foster a nurturing climate in which to learn, then how can we expect to maximize the educational input? If our medical schools are subject to an educational tsunami, then the outcome will not be in terms of 'lives lost' but of 'careers ruined'.

 "Wet spring had merged imperceptibly into bleak autumn. For months the sky had remained a depthless grey. Sometimes it rained, but mostly it was dull … It was like living inside Tupperware."

Bill Bryson, The Lost Continent (1989)

Surely we would hope that life as an undergraduate medical student would not be viewed as a colourless, boring experience. It should be a major aim of every medical school to have a vibrant, effective 'learning site'.

Defining educational environment

Genn (2001) has stated, 'Students experience or perceive the educational environment of the overall medical school as the climate. It is the climate that influences behaviour.' The educational environment as perceived by the students becomes the climate. In many instances the terms environment and climate are viewed as synonymous. In this chapter let us view climate as the environment seen through the eyes of the undergraduate or postgraduate student.

 "School climate refers to the impressions, beliefs and expectations held by members of the school community about their school as a learning environment, their associated behaviour, and the symbols and institutions that represent the patterned expression of behaviour"

Homana et al 2005

From the above quote we can see that the climate is how we feel about the environment. Each of us will have our own unique view of what is happening around us. For example, student A may feel that Dr Kildare is a warm and empathetic individual, whereas student B may not be too impressed with said doctor. The resulting climate will be different in the eyes of the two students.

The key components of educational climate

When students arrive at university, one of the first interactions they have is with their teachers. How are students being taught, and what subjects are they being taught? These two aspects will have an immediate influence on whether they have a positive view of their initial experience in medical school. If their teachers are seen as authoritarian figures and if the teaching methods are making learning difficult, then it will be likely that the climate is far from healthy. Table 48.1 provides a list of some of the variables that can have an impact on how the environment is perceived.

We have listed only 20 elements but there is really no limit as to what could be included. What is important in the educational environment will be ever changing. Variables will take on different importance within different educational institutions. The primary school, the high school and the university will have certain things in common, but there may also be features which will be at the forefront in one establishment but not so important in another.

Table 48.1 Elements of an educational environment

Teachers' skills	Assessment methods
Classroom	Accommodation
Size of class	Food
Learning materials	Personal safety
Teaching methods	Transport availability
Timetable	Library
Social life	Leisure facilities
A sense of belonging	Clinical experience
Student support	Access to computers
Clear learning outcomes	Study skills

 Aspects of the learning environment will change over time. Remember that what is important for a first-year student may be of no concern to a final-year student and vice versa.

Climate can be looked at from a macro viewpoint. For example, what do first-year students think about their first term in medical school? Their perceptions will probably be based on their evaluation of many of the items included in Table 48.1. Alternatively, a more micro approach to climate might be applied. A good example of this is described by Homana et al (2005) when they list the characteristics associated with a positive climate for citizenship education in schools: meaningful learning of civic knowledge, cooperation and collaboration in civic-related learning, mutual trust among staff and students, student input, deliberation and dialogue, engagement within the school and community and official recognition of the civic purpose of education that is conveyed to all involved in the process. These characteristics would form a different list from the one in Table 48.1.

The link between environment and curriculum is a strong one, as the quote from Genn below illustrates. The curriculum is more than just a syllabus with a series of learning outcomes attached.

 "It has come as something of a surprise to some teachers and administrators in medical education to hear that curriculum comprises, in part, students chatting over lunch in the Medical Club, staff greeting students out of class, student union meetings, pictures on the walls, sculptures, landscaping, gardens, medical students' reaction to the death of a patient, conversations of staff, students and patients at the Health Centre, and so on and so forth, almost ad infinitum, one could say."

Genn 2001

Learning environment applies to a vast range of settings, both formal and informal. Primary, secondary and tertiary education each has its own specific environment. At the postgraduate level it might be the hospital ward, the operating theatre or a general practice surgery. Each of these potential training sites should be linked to a curriculum (see Chapter 7, The hidden curriculum). The Postgraduate Medical Education and Training Board (PMETB) (2005) in the UK defined the curriculum as:

A statement of the intended aims and objectives, content, experiences, outcomes and process of an educational programme including:

- *a decision of the training structure (entry requirements, length and organization of the programme including its flexibilities, and assessment system),*
- *a description of expected methods of learning, teaching, feedback and supervision*

The curriculum should cover both generic professional and specialty areas.

From the above definition one could begin to tease out the various key areas that would be important for a good educational climate. A more specific view of the training involved would be required to determine discrete elements. Such an exercise would probably produce a core set of characteristics, e.g. the quality of the trainer, the range of conditions, the trainer–trainee rapport. Such a list could be applied to a number of training scenarios.

 Each educational environment will have its own special characteristics. In order to establish what these are, you must look at the purpose of the training as well as the setting in which it takes place. Look at what your learning outcomes are and also the social and physical geography of the surrounds. This will help you determine the relevant aspects of the environment.

Why is it important to gauge the educational climate?

 "A cloudy day or a little sunshine have as great an influence on many constitutions as the most real blessings or misfortunes."

Joseph Addison

The quote from Joseph Addison, the English essayist and poet, is a good reminder that the weather can have a major impact on the well-being of the individual. There is no reason to suspect that the environs of the workplace or learning habitat cannot have an equally important effect.

Cross et al (2006) underline the importance of the perceived environment, i.e. climate, in establishing a successful career choice. They state, 'the pace of change demanded by central policy on medical education and healthcare delivery and the uncertainty this entails make it important that postgraduate deaneries keep the learning environment constantly under review.' The emphasis placed on regular monitoring is a key to ensuring that the level of postgraduate and undergraduate training never dips into dangerous waters. The training environment is obviously crucial in attracting young doctors into a particular specialty, and having a 'healthy climate' is the first step in this process.

Jefferys and Elston (1989) made a similar point in relation to undergraduate teaching and emphasize the importance of the medical school environment since it can have a significant influence on the students' progress in becoming doctors and even determine their attitudes towards medical specialization. Genn and Harden (1986) also provided a comprehensive account of the underlying reasons for measuring the environment. It acts as the basis for the diagnosis of practices or situations within an institution. In addition, since the environment is changeable, the measurement will also act as a platform for making the necessary modifications towards better educational practices in line with the institution's own goals.

 If you have to make changes within your medical school, then it is usually best to do so when the general atmosphere is perceived as healthy. Be proactive – to use a sporting analogy – the best time to make changes to a team is when it is successful. It is difficult to bring new faces into a 'beaten' team and expect a sudden change.

The educational environment is of importance to each individual who is part of the training programme, whether at the undergraduate or postgraduate level, or as part of continuing professional development. If there is a respect for the teaching and a confidence in the teachers, then motivation of the learners will not be a problem and the end product will mean 'better professionals'.

In an educational system that is extremely competitive, it is essential to provide evidence that the training is of high quality. Measuring the educational climate will allow institutions to show that their school is 'ticking all the right boxes'. It will indicate exactly where they are quality wise, in very specific terms, and will point out clear targets to pursue in order to achieve overall excellence. School climate shows a significant positive correlation with student performance, with staff retention, with staff–student

Box 48.1 Reasons for measuring educational climate

- Improved student performance
- Higher staff morale
- Increased motivation among students
- A positive institutional profile
- Quality teaching
- Evidence of positive changes

satisfaction indices and with the ability of institutions to introduce positive changes. Box 48.1 encapsulates some of the main reasons for looking at the educational climate.

 "A healthy school climate will contribute to effective teaching and learning. These instruments for assessing climate can help schools make informed and meaningful changes for the better."

Freiberg 1998

What is involved in measuring the learning environment?

If you aim to evaluate a learning environment, where should you start? How should you determine the key features? The process can be viewed in three stages: (1) planning, (2) collecting the data and (3) interpreting the findings.

PLANNING

The first thing that needs to be made clear is the reason for the study. Why do you want to find out about the educational climate? For example, is it part of a curriculum evaluation process? You will also need to clearly define the environment you want to assess. For instance, are you looking at the teaching aspects, or is it perhaps only the educational materials and backup facilities? What resources have you available to help with the process, e.g. the manpower, the time that you have available?

DATA COLLECTION

This involves selecting the subjects. Are you going to target the entire student population, or will you use a sample? It is important to have knowledge of the various sampling techniques available. Will cluster sampling be more appropriate than, say, simple random sampling? Perhaps it is the clinical staff in a hospital that will be the main data source. If so, will you be able to access everyone, or will you have difficulty getting a list of names and addresses? You will also have to decide on how to collect the information needed. The type of response and the number of respondents will determine to a large extent the method used. For instance, you may well use a questionnaire or inventory if your target audience is the complete undergraduate population. This may mean designing your own survey, or you may decide to use one of the inventories already in use. We will look at the various tools available later in the chapter. Alternatively, you may opt for entrance and exit interviews, which can be effective ways of measuring school climate from the students' perspective. For example, Freiberg (1998) gives four questions which were asked of graduating students to elicit information about the environment:

1. What do you like about your school?

2. What was your most memorable experience?

3. What area would you like to have improved in your school?

4. What is one message you would like to give to your teachers?

If you are using your own data-gathering tool, you must ensure that it is a valid and reliable device and has been piloted.

 Determine what climate you wish to assess. It may be on a large scale such as an entire medical school, or it may be something less imposing such as a small department or a small-group session. This will determine the type of measuring tools needed and give you an idea of the cost in terms of resources and finance

INTERPRETING THE FINDINGS

There is little point in measuring the educational climate if nothing happens as a result of the assessment. You will be restricted in what you can do by the sensitivity of the data-gathering tool. If it is a finely tuned inventory which can pick up on specific details, then the information will be very select. If, on the other hand, the report is based on a few general questions to an unrepresentative group of students, then there is not a lot you can do with the results. Whatever type of data you collect, the findings must be reported back to the appropriate people, e.g. curriculum development committees or hospital boards. Dissemination of the results is all important.

 Listen to what your students are saying about their learning experience. Talk to your colleagues and find out what they think. This will give you pointers as to what are the pressing needs.

How is the educational climate measured?

 "There will be a rain dance Friday night, weather permitting."

George Carlin

Unlike the rain, we can be sure that you will always get a reading for educational climate, be it good, bad or indifferent. In assessing perceptions of the environment, either qualitative or quantitative methods can be employed. Quantitative methods usually involve the administration of a validated instrument or inventory to the target group. How well the educational environment is perceived will be reflected by the scores measured by the inventory. The qualitative approach involves collecting data mainly through interviews, focus group discussions, observational techniques and reflective diaries. It allows for a more in-depth exploration of the learning experience. However, in terms of cost, time, physical and human resources, the quantitative method is the more efficient.

 Before creating your own learning environment questionnaire, check the literature to see what is available. There are a variety of tools to choose from.

Soemantri et al (2010) reviewed the instruments that have been developed in recent years to measure the educational climate. The inventories are listed in Table 48.2.

The most suitable instruments for each setting have been identified. The Dundee Ready Educational Environment Measure (DREEM), the PHEEM, Clinical Learning Environment and Supervision (CLES) and Dental Student Learning Environment Survey (DSLES) are likely to be the most suitable instruments for undergraduate medicine, postgraduate medicine, nursing and dental education, respectively. The content validity of these instruments was established through the clear and detailed description of the instruments' development process. Some instruments had established their construct validity. These instruments were also proven to be reliable throughout their applications.

Remember, when we speak of measuring the climate we are talking about the perceptions of the learners: 'the perceived climate'. Of course, perception and reality may result in two entirely different profiles. The perceived environment is crucial in that it impacts on how the learners feel about their experiences. It can have physical, psychological and motivational repercussions.

"In Scotland there is no such thing as bad weather – only the wrong clothes."

Billy Connolly

Educational climate is a given. Our job is to ensure that we have the right 'clothes' available to suit the changes in the 'weather'. The answer to the question of how to measure the climate will relate to the reasons why the climate is being measured. It may be that it is a comparative study. Are there differences between medical school A and medical school B? One of the inventories listed in Table 48.2 could be distributed to students from both schools and scores compared. Alternatively, some may be interested in looking to see if there are any differences between perceived environment and ideal environment. For such a study it would be necessary not only to have a perceived score on a number of items but also to ask the students what they see as an ideal rating for each of these items. In a good educational environment the difference between perceived and ideal should be

Table 48.2 Tools to measure the educational climate

No.	Instrument/Inventory	Setting
1	MSLES (Medical School Learning Environment Survey): modified (Feletti & Clarke 1981)	Medicine
2	LEQ (Learning Environment Questionnaire) (Rothman & Ayoade 1970)	Medicine
3	Questionnaire from Parry et al (2002)	Medicine
4	Veteran Affairs Learners' Perceptions Survey	Medicine (postgraduate [PG])
5	LEA (Learning Environment Assessment)	Medicine (PG)
6	MSEQ (Medical School Environment Questionnaire) (Wakeford 1981)	Medicine
7	Questionnaire from Robins et al (1997)	Medicine
8	MSEI (Medical School Environment Inventory) (Hutchins 1961)	Medicine
9	Questionnaire from Rotem, Godwin and Du (1995)	Medicine (PG)
10	CVI (Course Valuing Inventory)	Medicine
11	DREEM (Dundee Ready Education Environment Measure) (Roff et al 1997)	Medicine (undergraduate and PG), nursing, dental, chiropractic
12	OREEM (Operating Room Educational Environment Measure)	Medicine (PG)
13	Instrument from Pololi and Price (2000)	Medicine
14	STEEM (Surgical Theatre Educational Environment Measure)	Medicine (PG)
15	ATEEM (Anaesthetic Theatre Educational Environment Measure)	Medicine (PG)
16	Practice-based Educational Environment Measure	Medicine (PG)
17	PHEEM (Postgraduate Hospital Educational Environment Measure)	Medicine (PG)
18	Questionnaire from Patel and Dauphinee (1985)	Medicine
19	Learning Climate Measure (from Wangsaturaka 2005)	Medicine
20	Questionnaire from Orton (modified)	Nursing
21	Questionnaire from Hart and Rotem (1995)	Nursing
22	CLE (Clinical Learning Environment) Scale	Nursing
23	CLEI (Clinical Learning Environment Inventory)	Nursing
24	CUCEI (College and University Classroom Environment Inventory)	Nursing
25	CLES (Clinical Learning Environment and Supervision)	Nursing
26	CPCLES (Clinical Post-Conference Learning Environment Survey)	Nursing
27	Questionnaire from Gerzina, McLean and Fairley (2005)	Dentistry
28	ClinEd IQ (Clinical Education Instructional Quality)	Dentistry
29	LES (Learning Environment Survey)	Dentistry
30	DSLES (Dental Student Learning Environment Survey)	Dentistry

Adapted from Soemantri D, Herrera C, Riquelme A: Measuring the educational environment in health professions studies: A systematic review, *Medical Teacher* 32:947–952, 2010.

small. Another area which may be of some interest to an institution is the comparison between staff and student scores. Are there elements of the environment that both groups rate highly or poorly? Are there specific issues which show up differences? Individual item and subscale scores would be of particular interest in such situations.

The quote below encapsulates the main ingredients of a good approach to measuring the educational environment.

 If you wish to ensure a good assessment process then
- target trends across academic years
- use a variety of data gathering techniques
- use the information in a practical way
- look at the progress made
- revaluate the educational environment using contributions from key stakeholders.

Educational climate plays a meaningful part in maximizing learning. It is therefore essential that all educational establishments have a valid and reliable approach to measuring the various components that make up the environment.

The DREEM has been used with strong statistical reliability for the following purposes:

Institutional profiles: to generate a 'profile' of a particular healthcare profession institution's strengths and weaknesses as perceived by a particular cohort of students at the time of administration of the inventory. It can be analysed according to a range of variables such as gender, course level, mode of entry to course or ethnicity.

Comparative studies: the DREEM can be used to make comparative analyses of students' perceptions of educational environments both within an institution and between institutions, or between different cohorts (e.g. students on different courses) within an institution.

Perceptions of educational environment and learning styles in relation to grade point averages or other assessments: the DREEM has been administered in conjunction with learning styles inventories to assess the correlation with academic results in terms of grade point averages.

Predictive value of the DREEM in relation to academic achievement: the value of the DREEM as a predictive tool for identifying those students who are likely to be academic achievers within an institution and those at risk of poor academic performance has been explored.

The PHEEM (Roff et al 2005) has been used in several countries including the UK, New Zealand, Pakistan, Chile, Brazil and the Netherlands. It is being used for programme review and quality assurance by the Postgraduate Medical Council of Victoria, Australia (www.pmcv.com.au/education/pheem/lessons-learnedvicpheem). The Surgical Theatre Education Environment Measure (STEEM) was developed and tested in Scotland and has been found to be reliable in Canada (Kanashiro et al 2006). It has been distributed electronically to all 1500 Royal Australasian College of Surgeons trainees in Australia and New Zealand.

According to research publications listed in MEDLINE reporting use of the inventories, they can:

- Generate a profile of a particular institution or training site's strengths and weaknesses
- Identify perceived differences in the learning environment within the cohorts by variables such as gender, stage of curriculum and type of curriculum.
- Determine the correlation between academic results such as grade point averages and perceptions of the learning environment.
- Enable identification of dysfunctional learning sites and/or learners in order to target remediation of potential underachievers.
- Constitute part of the quality assurance process in order to identify dysfunctional learning sites and to triangulate 'broad brush' trainee surveys such as those conducted by the UK General Medical Council.
- Enable multi-site comparisons in distributed teaching/learning programmes.
- Enable multi-disciplinary comparisons in 'poly' professional programmes.
- Compare staff and student perceptions of the student experience in a new UK medical school.

An example of the impact of such inventories is reported by Herrera et al (2010), who conclude:

There is a significant variability between the six [Chilean] medical schools evaluated and two of these obtained significantly better scores than the rest. The identified positive and negative areas will orient the actions to improve the Educational Environment for undergraduate medical students.

Summary

The UK General Medical Council now surveys perceptions of the 'environment' for approved training sites which goes beyond the physical resources available. The U.S. Veterans Agency administered a Learners' Perception Survey over 5 years with responses from 6527 medical students and 16583 physician residents. They reported that factors influencing training satisfaction were similar for residents and medical students. The domain with the highest association with satisfaction was the learning environment (Cannon et al 2008).

Such inventories are probably best used as initial 'diagnostic' tools that quantify perceived elements of the educational environment. They usually need to be followed up with qualitative investigations in order to confirm the areas and types of intervention that will best remediate perceived deficiencies. Not all students want the same type of educational environment: some will find intense competitiveness motivating, but others will find it demotivating or dysfunctional. But we owe it to our learners to explore the dynamics of the educational environment in order to enhance their chances of successful learning in the healthcare professions.

References

Cannon GW, Keitz SQ, Holland GJ, et al: Factors determining medical students' and residents' satisfaction during VA-based training: findings from the VA Learners' Perception Survey, *Academic Medicine* 83(6):611–620, 2008.

Cross V, Hicks C, Parle J, Field S: Perceptions of the learning environment in higher specialist training of doctors: implications for recruitment and retention, *Medical Education* 40:121–128, 2006.

Feletti GI, Clarke RM: Review of psychometric features of the Medical School Learning Environment Survey, *Medical Education* 15:92–96, 1981.

Freiberg HJ: Measuring school climate: let me count the ways, *Educational Leadership* 56(1):22–26, 1998.

Genn JM: *AMEE Medical Education Guide No. 23: Curriculum, environment, climate, quality and change in medical education – a unifying perspective.* Dundee, 2001, Association for Medical Education in Europe.

Genn JM, Harden RM: What is medical education here really like? Suggestions for action research studies of climates of medical education environments, *Medical Teacher* 8(2):111–124, 1986.

Gerzina TM, McLean T, Fairley J: Dental clinical teaching: Perceptions of students and teachers, *Journal of Dental Education* 69(12):1377–1384, 2005.

Hart G, Rotem A: The clinical learning environment: Nurses' perceptions of professional development in clinical settings, *Nurse Education Today* 15(1):3–10, 1995.

Herrera C, Pacheco J, Rosso F, et al: Evaluation of the undergraduate educational climate in six medical schools in Chile, *Revista Médica de Chile* 138(6):677–684, 2010.

Homana G, Henry Barber C, Torney-Purta J: *School Citizenship Education Climate Assessment. National Centre for Learning and Citizenship.* Denver, 2005, Education Committee of the States.

Hutchins EB: The 1960 medical school graduate: his perception of his faculty, peers and environment, *Journal of Medical Education* 36:322–329, 1961.

Jefferys M, Elston MA: The medical school as a social organisation, *Medical Education* 23:242–251, 1989.

Kanashiro J, McAleer S, Roff S: Assessing the educational environment in the operating room – a measure of resident perception at one Canadian institution, *Surgery* 139(2):150–158, 2006.

Parry J, Mathers J, Al-Fares A, et al: Hostile teaching hospitals and friendly district general hospitals: final year students' views on clinical attachment locations, *Medical Education* 36:1131–1141, 2002.

Patel VL, Dauphinee WD: The clinical learning environments in medicine, paediatrics and surgery clerkships, *Medical Education* 19:54–60, 1985.

Pololi L, Price J: Validation and use of an instrument to measure the learning environment as perceived by medical students, *Teaching and Learning in Medicine* 12(4):201–207, 2000.

Postgraduate Medical Education and Training Board: What is curriculum? 2005. Available at: http://www.gmc-uk.org/PMETB_what_is_curriculum.pdf_30379314.pdf

Robins LS, Gruppen LD, Alexander G, et al: A predictive model of student satisfaction with the medical school learning environment, *Academic Medicine* 72(2):134–139, 1997.

Roff S, McAleer S, Harden RM, et al: Development and validation of the Dundee Ready Education Environment Measure (DREEM), *Medical Teacher* 19(4):295–299, 1997.

Roff S, McAleer S, Skinner A: Development and validation of an instrument to measure the postgraduate clinical learning and teaching environment for hospital-based doctors in the UK, *Medical Teacher* 27:326–331, 2005.

Rotem A, Godwin P, Du J: Learning in hospital settings, *Teaching and Learning in Medicine* 7(4):211–217, 1995.

Rothman AI, Ayoade F: The development of a learning environment: a questionnaire for use in curriculum evaluation, *Journal of Medical Education* 45:754–759, 1970.

Soemantri D, Herrera C, Riquelme A: Measuring the educational environment in health professions studies: A systematic review, *Medical Teacher* 32:947–952, 2010.

Wakeford RE: Students' perception of the medical school learning environment: a pilot study into some differences and similarities between clinical schools in the UK, *Assessment and Evaluation in Higher Education* 6(3):206–217, 1981.

Wangsaturaka D: Development of learning climate measures for Thai medical education, PhD thesis. Scotland, 2005, Faculty of Medicine, Dentistry and Nursing, University of Dundee.

Medical education research

J. Cleland, T. E. Roberts

Introduction

It has been said that in the past the practice of medicine was simple, safe and largely ineffective; today it is much more effective but complex, and potentially dangerous. More than ever, then, medical education needs to prepare and support students and doctors in their roles as providers of safe healthcare. Within the UK the amount of time spent as a trainee has changed dramatically within the last decade. Streamlining of medical training and the implementation of the European Working Time Directive has meant that education and training will need to be delivered differently, and knowledge and skills cannot be expected to osmose into trainees merely from them spending time within that discipline. Not only have major changes occurred during the trainee years but modern consultants and senior GPs are different too. There is recognition that mastery of a medical specialty is impossible and that the key to high-quality patient care is nested within continuous professional development and adopting an attitude of lifelong learning. All these changes have meant that medical education has achieved a new prominence and importance, and following the development of evidenced-based clinical practice it is becoming increasingly accepted that medical education should be evidence-based rather than founded on pragmatism, fashion and whim (Todres et al 2007).

Alongside this increasing acknowledgement of the importance of educating medical professionals has grown an interest in medical education research.

 Medical education research can be described as conducting and evaluating original enquiry and developing innovation, using appropriate theoretical and conceptual frameworks in order to achieve meaningful outcomes which advance the understanding and practice of medical education.

Until recently many individuals undertaking this research work have been interested amateurs,

clinician-teachers who have not undertaken formal training in the area of educational research but who may have a track record of research in their own clinical area. Others have a background in the social sciences, bringing their own research conceptualizations of learning but having to apply them to a very specialized and hitherto tightly collegiate, disciplined club that they do not always understand in-depth and by whose members they have been viewed with suspicion. Tensions have also arisen between those who have sought to undertake research into medical education for its own sake, the so-called 'research for researchers', and those who feel that research should inform practice: 'research for practice'.

In this chapter we propose that medical education research can be described as conducting and evaluating original enquiry and developing innovation, using appropriate theoretical and conceptual frameworks in order to achieve meaningful outcomes which advance the understanding and practice of medical education, and that this can be usefully thought of under the umbrella term of scholarship.

Medical education scholarship therefore should inform continued improvement of medical education locally and also seek to influence medical education policy and practice nationally and internationally. Thus, medical education scholarship is grounded in the real world of medical education practice and, in turn, medical education practice informs work undertaken under the heading of scholarship. This is analogous to applied research, where research yields actionable knowledge.

 Use your ideas and hunches from the real world of medical education practice to inform the work you undertake under the heading of scholarship.

The Leeds Institute for Medical Education (LIME) has developed a useful representation of this idea of scholarship (Fig. 49.1) (Kilminster & Roberts 2010, personal communication). Other colleagues, such as those at the Karolinska Institute in Finland, have independently developed similar concepts. The LIME model consists of two circles of activity. The 'internal' circle relates to work generated and undertaken in the educators' own institution for the benefit of its staff, students and trainees. The 'external' circle relates to activities undertaken outside the educators' institution such as disseminating good practice developed as part of their 'internal' circle work or undertaken in response to external issues or challenges.

Next, we provide examples of how this model has or might be used to structure the scholarly work undertaken by medical educators.

The internal circle

Accurate assessment of competence is fundamental to any medical education programme. Some years ago at one of our institutions concern was expressed about the reliability of the final assessments (identification of issues). Members of the medical education unit (MEU) undertook an analysis of these issues and reviewed the literature and examined theories of assessment to identify best practice (academic activities). The result of these activities was the use of item response theory to analyse question performance, the production of a number of workshops to address areas such as question, OSCE station construction, examiner and simulated patient training (outputs). These workshops were piloted, evaluated and, where appropriate, adopted into mainstream practice (local impact) and formed a very obvious example of scholarship-informed local medical education practice. Continued evaluation and further identification of new issues feed the continuation of the internal circle. These activities also fed into external work (Fig. 49.2).

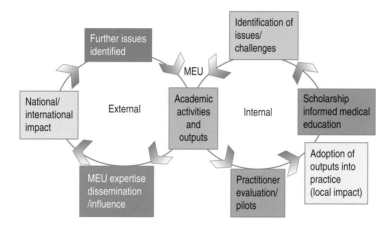

Fig. 49.1 The LIME (Leeds Institute of Medical Education) scholarship model (Kilminster & Roberts 2010, personal communication).

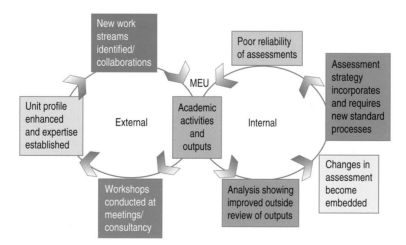

Fig. 49.2 Professionalism in medical school curricula.

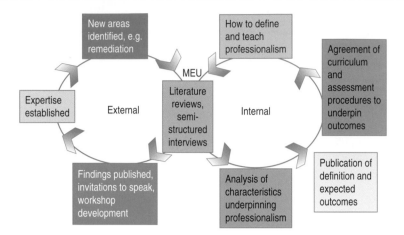

Fig. 49.3 The transition from medical student to first-year doctor.

It has become increasingly obvious that teaching, learning and assessment of the development of medical professionalism are as important as the development of medical knowledge and skills. Many of the referrals to regulatory bodies are related to medical professionalism issues. Work by Papadakis and colleagues (2008) has shown that doctors who were reported to state licensing bodies in the United States had often had professionalism issues when in medical school when their records were examined (identification of issues).

Improving the curricula in this area involved a series of academic activities. An initial literature search was undertaken to identify a definition of professionalism together with characteristics identified with the term professionalism. A separate literature search was undertaken to investigate methods of assessment of professionalism. Within the institution a series of semi-structured interviews were undertaken with a range of healthcare professionals and undergraduate students to identify characteristics associated with the individuals who would be considered excellent role models for professionalism. Using the results of the literature reviews and empirical research, a curriculum and associated assessment programme was devised, piloted (evaluation), refined and subsequently adopted (outputs; Fig. 49.3).

 Do not underestimate the importance of demonstrating the value of your work directly to your institutional practice locally.

In the UK there has been considerable criticism about the performance of medical graduates and their ability to function as doctors in the National Health Service (NHS). In national surveys new doctors have expressed the feelings that the education they received as part of their undergraduate studies did not 'prepare' them for the work they were expected to undertake. Employers, too, bemoaned the lack of 'preparedness' of new doctors (identification of the issues). In an effort to understand the issues and with recognition that these issues were seen in other groups of new workers and expressed by non-health-related employers, an extensive programme of research was undertaken, involving a series of academic activities. First, a literature search on the issues of transitions from education to the workplace not only in medical education but also in other areas such as engineering was carried out. Interviews were conducted with a range of different stakeholders, for example, newly qualified doctors, ward nurses, pharmacists, managers and senior doctors. Finally, a number of extensive periods of observations of new doctors in the workplace were conducted, covering a range of different times and places to look at actual learning practices. This study showed that 'performance' of newly qualified medical practitioners was related not only to personal attributes of the individual but also to the culture and support within the workplace and organization. It became obvious that learning about the local workplace culture was a very important aspect that influenced how well a new trainee was perceived as performing (outputs/analysis of characteristics). So, workplaces which specifically sought to induct new members into local practices produced environments where these incomers were more likely to feel able to perform well and to be seen as performing well. These times of transition were labelled 'critically intense learning periods' or CILPS. It was also clear that one-off inductions, usually consisting of a day of endless induction lectures to new organizations, were both inadequate and inappropriate.

The next stage of the research is to move the outputs into practice by developing work placement 'change laboratories' to help organizations recognize these CILPS and provide specific support for staff during this time and evaluating the acceptability and impact of this innovation.

Medical education research approaches

The examples provided above exemplify the use of a range of research frameworks, or methods, to advance the understanding and practice of medical education. Item response theory (as used in our assessment example; Fig. 49.2) is a psychometric paradigm for the design, analysis and scoring of tests and questionnaires measuring abilities, attitudes or other variables. It is based on the application of related mathematical models to test data. In contrast, semi-structured interviews and observations of doctors in practice (as used in our professionalism and transitions examples described above) are social science research tools, qualitative methodology used to explore and understand people's perceptions, thoughts, views and actions. Other scholarly work (not presented) from our respective institutions has included large-scale questionnaire surveys to explore medical students' career preferences and what influences these preferences, and focus groups to explore students' views and experiences of remote and rural undergraduate placements. In short, a wide range of methodological approaches are appropriate to advance the understanding and practice of medical education.

Research methodology falls into two main camps: quantitative and qualitative. Quantitative approaches are used to test a hypothesis, to answer questions about 'how much' or 'how many'. Qualitative approaches seek answers to the 'what', 'how' or 'why' of a phenomenon, exploring people's attitudes, behaviours, and so on. Quantitative methods tend to generate numerical data, while qualitative methods tend to generate language data (written or oral). In qualitative research, the research question is exploratory, while quantitative research is explanatory.

As alluded to earlier in this chapter, there is an ongoing 'paradigm' war (Gage 1989) in medical education. Clinicians working in medical education have been taught and trained in the scientific model. This is based on quantitative research: gathering empirical and measurable evidence through experiments, hypothesis testing (e.g. 'Is this treatment or intervention effective?'), controlling variables other than the one(s) under study so that any statistically significant difference must be a consequence of the treatment/intervention, and producing objective data which can be verified by other scientists reproducing the study. Randomized controlled trials (RCTs) are the gold standard research methodology of this paradigm. If one

believes science is the only reliable source of knowledge, then the scientific model is therefore the appropriate model for all research, including educational research. However, social scientists working in medical education have been taught and trained in quite a different model, one that focuses on the human social life and which requires quite a different approach to understand what people do and why. In methodological terms, social scientists argue that we cannot understand why people do what they do, or why particular institutions exist and operate in characteristic ways, without grasping how those involved interpret and make sense of their world: in other words, without understanding the distinctive nature of their perceptions, beliefs, attitudes. There is no gold standard methodology; rather, social scientists tend to use qualitative methods to explore the phenomenon under question. Because of the type of research questions under investigation in qualitative research studies, sample sizes are usually quite small but selected because they have certain characteristics.

Research methodology falls into two main camps: quantitative and qualitative. Quantitative approaches are used to test a hypothesis, to answer questions about 'how much' or 'how many'. Qualitative approaches seek to answers to the 'what', 'how' or 'why' of a phenomenon.

Both sides can lack understanding of the methods of the other. For example, social scientists working in medical education research view the RCT as inappropriate to the complex and multi-factorial environment of medical education (Norman 2003). Conversely, clinicians and natural scientists working in medical education view the work of social scientists as too situation-specific to produce any general conclusions. This schism is not helpful. Our own view is that both paradigms have strengths and hence both can be applied successfully to medical education scholarship, if done so guided by theory and reflection.

Remember that good-quality data relating to a significant problem furthers knowledge whatever the methodological or theoretical basis of the empirical work or stance of the researchers.

Theory-driven scholarship

There are debates in the wider literature as to whether theory is a product (the aim of the research) or a tool (something that helps explain what we are researching). For most of us, it will be the latter, something that helps us do our research and explain our findings. Thus, by theory-driven scholarship or research, we mean using theory as a tool to draw ideas together, make links and offer explanations (Bourdieu 1992). Using a theoretical or conceptual framework in your research can enable the following:

1. Discovering links between your own research and that of others
2. Synthesizing, analysing and generalizing
3. Abstracting ideas from your data and offering explanations
4. Clarifying how or why something might have worked or not worked (Cook et al 2008)
5. Having insights.

The following example shows how theory was used in practice in a medical education programme of research. Our early work showed that weak medical students were progressing, but then failing late in the programme, suggesting that 'failure to fail' was a local issue.

The wider literature suggested that difficulty in assessing students' clinical performance is an issue in the training of all healthcare professionals who undergo combined theoretical and practical professional training. However, the subject of failing medical students in clinical placements had received relatively little attention, particularly in the UK, where medicine is mostly an undergraduate degree.

Improving assessment in this area involved a series of academic activities. An initial literature search was undertaken to identify what was already known on this subject. This highlighted that there seemed to be a variety of determining factors, but the existing research was atheoretical and did not provide a fundamental understanding of what was going on. We used a well-researched behaviour change model, the elements of which seemed applicable to the research question, to underpin a qualitative study. Data collection involved focus groups with medical educators from two very different UK medical schools. Our data supported the use of the behaviour change theory to explore this phenomenon within a medical education context.

So what did the use of a theory add? It added that 'failure to fail' occurs for a variety of reasons – attitudes towards the individual students, attitudes and beliefs towards failing a student, what is expected by others, lack of skills or knowledge, self-efficacy and environmental constraints (e.g. time) – and that sometimes these different reasons conflict with each other. Thus, the use of the model clarified a complex phenomenon. It also facilitated a cumulative programme of research focusing on behaviour change (the particular theory has been used widely in areas other than medical education to assess how best to change people's behaviour). We used this wide literature to inform the next step: the development of a questionnaire to identify which of the six factors is most

important. Once piloted and evaluated, questionnaire data will inform what needs to be done to encourage accurate reporting of student underperformance. Thus, if skills and knowledge are the greatest barrier at our medical school, an intervention to address this will be developed, delivered and evaluated locally. It may be that barriers are different at different medical schools, so the theory-based questionnaire will enable individual schools to identify their own particular barriers, then address them appropriately.

This programme of scholarship fits with the LIME model, as it was firmly grounded in local issues (the internal circle). One of the papers from the qualitative work (Cleland et al 2008) was one of the top-10 accessed articles in the journal *Medical Education* for an extended period of time, indicating that the work resonated with medical educators nationally and internationally (the external circle of the LIME model).

In summary, theory strengthens the practice of research. Theory helps to identify the appropriate study question and target group; clarify methods and measurement issues; provide more detailed and informative descriptions on characteristics of the intervention and supportive implementation conditions (if, indeed, an intervention is the focus of the work); uncover unintended effects; and assist in analysis and interpretation of results.

Theory can be used as an 'umbrella' to aid generalization and abstraction, rather than your work, and you, standing alone.

 Consider using a theoretical or conceptual framework to strengthen your scholarship.

Using theory also addresses the thorny issue of mixed methods research. Mixed methods research is the systematic combination of qualitative and quantitative methods in research or evaluation. However, as discussed earlier, quantitative and qualitative methods are based on contrasting assumptions and ideologies about social phenomena and knowledge. Mixed methods research must address how these two approaches or methods can be meaningfully combined in a study while minimizing tensions and conflicts. To use the same analogy as above, a theoretical or conceptual framework can act as an 'umbrella' to allow qualitative and quantitative methods to use their strengths to make contributions to achieving the common goal and de-emphasizes their differences and incompatibilities (Chen 2006).

For example, using the same behaviour change model to underpin different steps in the 'failure to fail' programme of work enabled us to combine qualitative (focus groups) and quantitative (questionnaire development and survey) methodology in a complementary way.

The idea of applying and even engaging with 'theory' can be daunting for many medical educators, leading to reluctance to develop a theorized approach to scholarship. This is very understandable, particularly if you are tentatively setting out on the path of scholarly activity in medical education, and/or have not undertaken formal training in the area of educational research. If this is the case, look to collaborating with colleagues who work from a perspective which seems appropriate to address your question. This might be other medical educators or individuals working in other academic areas but with relevant theoretical expertise. We have collaborated successfully with, for example, health psychologists, statisticians and educationalists. There are also many opportunities for continuing professional development in medical education research, from reading journal articles and accessing the wider resources often found on journal websites (e.g. podcasts) to attending local, national and international conferences and seminars.

 Look for professional development and collaborative opportunities in medical education research skills and knowledge.

Reflection in scholarship

It is important that any scholar, whether in medical education or any other area of endeavour, is aware of his or her pre-conceptions and scientific assumptions and how these could be problematic as well as helpful.

Reflection is a skill, an attitude and a mental habit of consideration and analysis of the why, how and what-ifs of situations. Reflection is about standing in a different place and seeing things from a different perspective, and ultimately doing things differently, e.g. asking 'Why do I do things the way I do?' and 'Why do I think this?' It can be particularly useful to reflect on your own values, feelings, thinking and actions, as well as the context of a situation. In thinking of situations and people we encounter in our ordinary and professional lives, we consider our feelings and values, the context, and also the codes of practice that underpin our behaviour and attitudes. Reflection not only increases one's self-awareness but also can influence competence. You may well already use reflection in the context of thinking about your clinical practice.

Reflection is an important, and often neglected, element of scholarship. Reflection can help you decide if your assumptions are helpful in considering the issue in question. Do you see the issue? Do you regard it as important? Are you in conflict with others as to what should/could be done, and how? For example, can medical students who are taught solely by medical doctors be adequately prepared for working in a multi-professional health service? Do you see interprofessional education (IPE) as an important issue? If not, you are likely to come into conflict with colleagues who support IPE scholarship and who wish to, for example, develop and evaluate initiatives where medical students shadow practice nurses.

 Reflect on your stance in terms of research approach rather than acting reflexively.

Reflection can also help you consider how best to conduct an enquiry. If you reject the use of an experimental trial, reflection will help ensure that this is because such an approach was not appropriate to the question, not because you could not conduct one, did not know anyone who could conduct one, or did not even consider the possibility. However, reflection cannot in itself determine what are and are not productive working assumptions about the phenomena being investigated and how they can best be understood. To some extent, this must be decided in pragmatic terms, on the basis of using particular research strategies and reflecting on what they can achieve.

Summary

This chapter aims to give a practical guide to medical education research, or scholarship. We urge you to ground your research in local and significant issues, to collaborate as appropriate with others, to use theory to underpin your research and never to think of a research project as providing all the answers. Our experience is that any piece of research leads to new questions to explore, which is a big part of the enjoyment and stimulation of doing research.

References

Bourdieu P: *The Logic of Practice*. Cambridge, 1992, Polity Press.

Chen HT: A theory-driven evaluation perspective on mixed-methods research, *Research in the School* 13:75–83, 2006.

Cleland JA, Knight LV, Rees CE, et al: Is it me or is it them? Factors that influence the passing of underperforming students, *Medical Education* 42:800–809, 2008.

Cook DA, Bordage G, Schmidt HG: Description, justification and clarification: A framework for classifying the purposes of research in medical education, *Medical Education* 42(2):128–133, 2008.

Gage NL: The paradigm wars and their aftermath, *Educational Researcher* 18:4–10, 1989. (reprinted in Hammersley M, editor: Educational Research and Evidence-Based Practice, London, 2007, Sage.)

Norman G: Results confounded and trivial: the perils of grand educational experiments, *Medical Education* 37:582–584, 2003.

Papadakis MA, Arnold GK, Blank LL, et al: Performance during internal medicine residency training and subsequent disciplinary action by state licensing boards, *Annals of Internal Medicine* 148(11):869–876, 2008.

Todres M, Stephenson A, Jones R: Medical education research remains the poor relation, *BMJ* 335:333–335, 2007.

How to manage a medical college

H. Hamdy

Introduction

Medical colleges and health profession education institutions are complex organizations interacting with different systems at the micro college level and the macro university, healthcare, economic and political systems level. All this is embedded in a multi-ethnic and multi-professional culture with the values, beliefs and assumptions of faculty, students, patients and community at large.

Defining the deanship or the leadership of these institutions has always been an elusive task because this position lacks uniformity in content and function (Dupont 1968). Academic deans, although still charged with the intellectual leadership of their colleges, were also expected to be fiscal experts, fund raisers, politicians and diplomats (Tucker & Bryan 1988).

 "The Dean's role is somewhat anomalous. For success in the school, it must go up, down, across and out and each part of the school and university must feel that it is getting full value from the Dean."

Fagin 1997

Senior academics involved in managing a health professional education institution need to play several roles and exhibit many leadership traits. Role theory is commonly used to explain the relationship between the individual self and collective social structure of the society in general or organization in particular (Schuler 1975). His or her primary role evolved into the maintenance of balance between the various external and internal demands placed on the institution (Wolverton et al 2001). The difference between leadership and management in medical schools has been described by many as managers produce order and consistency in the organization and leaders produce change and movement (Northouse 2004). In practice, it is often the same person who operates in both capacities (Storey 2004).

A dean's challenge is to develop shared goals among a range of faculty, students and other groups who may frame the academic environment in varied ways (Lessor 2008). Aligning the various frames' 'schemata of interpretation' and adjudicating frame disputes can be described as frame amplification or frame transformation activities (Goffman 1974). A challenging task for deans is how to manage effectively the faculty in a manner that is congruent with the external demands for change. The dean seeks external support for college goals by framing them to resonate within the understanding of nonacademic audiences such as parents and donors while harmonizing faculty interests with those of other significant audiences (Snow 2006).

Managers of medical colleges are usually senior faculty selected to lead due to their clinical and/or scholarly reputation. They moved directly from faculty or modest administrative positions into the deanship and learned on the job. The complex issues faced by medical college leaders and managers are tangled up in priorities, emotions, rules, procedures and human relations.

This chapter describes and reflects on the cultural complexity of managing a medical college or a health professional education institution, the multiple roles and functions of senior managers, focusing on the 'dean', and gives practical examples from personal experience regarding which of its features could be applied in other contexts.

The roles of the dean

THE VISIONARY

The first task which a new dean encounters is to review the college vision, mission, goals and strategic direction. It is important to develop with all stakeholders a mission statement which is focused and could be translated into action. Mission statement clichés of 'excellence in education, research and service' are meaningless. Differentiating the institution in the light of a good SWOT analysis and developing a focused mission is the first important step a dean should take.

What's next is how to translate its meanings into a strategic direction. This necessitates involving different stakeholders – faculty, students, support staff, university officials and professionals – to share a common understanding of its meanings and implications and to develop among them a sense of ownership. An example of a focused mission is from the University of Sharjah, College of Medicine in the United Arab Emirates, stating, 'we differentiated ourselves in the full spectrum of medical education, undergraduate, postgraduate and continuing professional development'. This was translated over 4 years to a medical programme which is a student-centred, integrated and outcome-based curriculum. The main strategy of learning is problem-based learning (PBL) and team-based learning (TBL). While adopting and applying several new trends and innovations in medical education, a Masters and PhD programme in molecular medicine and translational research was developed in order to initiate and stimulate basic medical science research. A faculty development programme in medical education for clinical and basic medical science faculty was offered, supported and considered mandatory in order to prepare faculty for their educational role. A Clinical and Surgical Training Center for professional training was established. As it was a new medical college, like hundreds that have emerged all over the world during the last few years, differentiating the college in excellence in education was its primary overarching goal for the first 5 years of its inception. This does not mean that research was ignored; faculty have conducted and published several research papers in medical education, and strategic alliance with leading international research institutions was established, but this was done without losing focus on medical education.

THE LEADER–MANAGER AND MANAGER–LEADER

In medical colleges, the senior executive, i.e. dean, plays the dual roles of manager and leader. These positions are inter-related and inseparable – 'two sides of the same coin'. Leadership can be thought of as the process of influencing the activities of an organized group in its efforts towards goal setting and goal achievement (Stoghili 1950), and the leader can be regarded as a manager of meaning (Smircich & Morgan 1982). In medical colleges, today's deans need to change their manner of leadership from a transactional style, which comprises an exchange between leader and follower, to a transformational leadership, where the leader and followers share the same aspirations (Kotler 1996). Managing and leading a medical college require an adaptive, situational leadership style with a high degree of flexibility.

 "Transformational leadership is about strategy and people whereas transactional leadership revolves around systems and resources. Both are needed in an effective organization."

Kotler 1996

Situational leadership was defined by Gilbert (2005) as 'an approach based on the idea that there will be interactions in most situations between the leader's attitude, the tasks to be undertaken, the strengths and weaknesses of the team and the environment in which the leader and team have to operate'. Situational leadership is an adaptive model in which leaders adopt their stance to the situation (Peck et al 2006).

 "Transformational characteristics of a leader may be more appropriate in the earlier stages of a transition process with the transactional characteristics required to stabilize transformational change."

Peck et al 2006

It is not that one is more superior or inferior to the other but rather that effective leaders appear to be able to utilize many styles appropriate to the situation (Mc Kinnan & Swanwick 2010).

 "Less attention has been paid to the personal development of healthcare professionals, educational leadership, scholarship and organization development and changes."

Steinert et al 2006

The dean needs to be able to read and understand the implications of the 'topography' of the college, university and community landscape. He or she should anticipate problems and take appropriate actions at the appropriate time. Awareness and understanding of the complex medical college culture are important tasks for a medical dean.

The culture of an educational institution learning environment is made and reproduced over time. It affects all aspects and constituents in the college: students, faculty and staff. Sensitivity of the leader to the college's 'hidden curriculum' is an important task which can support or jeopardize the educational programme and the college mission (Hafferty 1998, Maudsley 2001). Medical colleges, with their multi-cultural, multi-ethnic students and faculty, are a fertile land for gossips and mistrust. Sometimes actions taken for the purpose of educational quality assurance (like faculty peer evaluation) can have a negative impact and create a culture of mistrust among faculty. This situation existed in one medical college, but the leadership changed it by suggesting that each faculty member ask a peer if they would observe his or her teaching and learning activities and give him or her constructive feedback. This led to the development of a culture of support, collegiality and trust. The fear from 'scratch my back and I scratch yours' was not observed.

THE CARING AND HUMAN LEADER

Another angle of the effective leader is his or her human and caring attributes. Whether they are part of the individual's personality or can be acquired is a debatable issue. Genuine caring about small things which may bother a staff member or a student can have a major impact on their satisfaction and loyalty to the institution, e.g. helping them to find a school for their children, housing, healthcare, etc.

THE EDUCATOR

Although research and clinical services in a medical college or other health professional educational institutions and its affiliated hospitals are important activities, still its raison d'être is to educate and graduate competent doctors or health professionals (nurses, physiotherapists, etc.). This means that the leader/manager of the medical college should understand the field of medical education in order to respond to the rapid changes in how medicine or health sciences are learned and taught and how curricula are developed, revised and renewed. They also need to understand how student performance is best assessed and how to ensure and maintain quality education. In an era of quality and standards, all deans are heavily involved in accreditation of their programmes. Deans need to maintain alignment between the college mission, goals, programme outcomes, learning and teaching strategies and student assessment. The gap between the declared curriculum, curriculum in action and learned curriculum (Coles & Grant 1985) to which I have added 'used curriculum' should be narrowed (Hamdy 2002).

The dean as 'guardian of the faith' should always keep asking self, faculty and students, 'Are we really doing and achieving what we claim to do? And if not, why, and what can we do about it?' Perhaps this could be considered a 'deficiency model of management'.

THE PROFESSIONAL

Football coaches were usually well-known, respected football players. The same applies to the dean's professional credibility (clinician or researcher) and how he or she is viewed in the eyes of peer faculty and professionals. A dean should have a good research track record. This is valued by faculty, as the dean will

be active in guiding them, looking into their performance and recommending their promotion and tenure. It is advisable, if possible, that the dean should continue with clinical and scholarly activities but at a reduced level. This way he or she can stay close to the field, receive firsthand information about how clinical teaching is implemented and hear what the faculty or students have to say: discussions in the theatre coffee room can be a valuable source of information.

THE RESOURCE MANAGER

A major responsibility of a manager of a medical college is the effective and efficient management of its human and financial resources. Balancing a dean's vision for the role of the medical school with the various conflicting demands on resources is a challenge. Priorities should be identified in the light of the school's mission and strategic plan.

An example of a common misconception in relation to introducing curriculum changes or new strategies of learning is that student-centred learning (PBL or TBL) is more expensive than traditional education. Several research studies and publications have shown that this may not be the case (Hamdy & Agamy 2011, Mennin & Martinez-Burrola 1986).

Faculty salaries constitute approximately 80% of the college operational budget (Hamdy & Agamy 2011). In an education-intensive medical college, faculty educational responsibilities should go beyond teaching, facilitation of learning, curriculum management, student's guidance and assessment and programme evaluation. This necessitates investing in faculty development, valuing their educational responsibilities, expanding scholarly activities to include excellence in education and reviewing promotion and tenure regulations.

The successful dean should be able to develop and use the educational experience of clinical faculty in teaching hospitals and expand their educational role in the different phases and activities of the medical programme. Residents in training are an unexplored asset and resource. The college needs to develop them and reward their involvement. They are the ones closer to the students, when they are in the hospitals, than the consultants and clinical faculty. Offering academic titles to clinicians is usually appreciated. It is not advisable to call them 'part-time' or even 'honorary' faculty, as it gives a sense of lesser commitment and distance. Titles such as clinical assistant, associate or professor as in the American system or clinical lecturer or senior lecturer as in the British system are more appropriate. Involving the clinicians should be handled through negotiation with the hospital and management. Different financial and healthcare arrangements should be established in order to create sustainable, realistic, clinician–educator involvement.

Internal motivation needs to be boosted by rewards including financial and accountability systems. Their performance needs to be evaluated and constructive feedback provided (Hamdy et al 2001).

THE NEGOTIATOR/POLITICIAN AND DIPLOMAT

Deans need to continuously answer, negotiate with and respond to different stakeholders inside the college from faculty, students and support staff to university administration. Outside the college, health authorities, corporate sponsors, funding agents, media and press are important players which a dean should have on his or her side. Knowing what to say, when to say it and how to say it is a skill which can be developed. An open, interactive and quality information system should be in place. The community and public need to know about health and about those who are providing healthcare.

An important responsibility of the dean includes building relationships and communicating effectively the needs of faculty, staff and students to central university administration. Representing the college reflects the need to communicate what is occurring within the college using both quantitative and qualitative data. The financial aspects of the dean's position have expanded beyond overseeing budgets to include securing new funds. This role change has come as a result of a change in how higher education is funded. Deans became advocates for external funds from private donors to keep technology up to date, establish skills labs, for research and sometimes to recruit and retain good faculty (Shuhan & Mihailidis 2007).

Recruiting and hiring faculty, appointing chairpersons and negotiating salaries and financial packages are all leadership and managerial responsibilities that take a good part of the dean's time, particularly when developing new medical colleges. Evaluating CVs, conducting interviews and deep probing into applicants' potential are skills which could be acquired through training.

Governance and organizational structure of the medical college

Systems of governance in a medical college should facilitate the accomplishment of its mission, programme outcomes and strategic plans. Educational organization structures have an ongoing, developmental nature (Fig. 50.1). The institution should be committed to an ongoing process of organizational critique consistent with the stated mission. The quality assurance processes should be a continuous activity, not only for the purpose of accreditation or re-accreditation but should be reflected on all review and reporting activities. In my college, the dean's annual reports are structured around the accreditation standard domains and achievements on the time line of the strategic plans.

These organizational principles and governance systems are usually relatively easier to establish and implement in new medical colleges with a small number of students and faculty. An annual intake of 100 students and approximately 60–100 full-time equivalent (FTE) faculty is a 'convenient size'.

The situation is different in old medical colleges with history, established organizational culture and university by-laws which apply to all its colleges. Most of the old colleges have student intakes of up to 800–1000 students and a large number of faculty, up to approximately 2000.

Introducing change and governance of such an organization is a real challenge, and the dean's job is more difficult but not impossible. Perhaps the first important step to be taken is to create among the faculty and students a sense of need to change by reviewing the college mission, which most probably has been forgotten over the year. Change should be by evolution and not revolution. Negotiating new by-laws and regulations with the university or higher authorities in order to introduce quality improvement in the curriculum is a battle which deserves to be fought. Creating a critical mass of followers and believers in the value of quality improvement movement is key for its success. The dean and the management team should think out of the box and find ways of turning obstacles and threats into opportunities, e.g. a large number of faculty with proper training in medical education can positively change the educational environment. Distributing the leadership at different levels of the college through functional productive committees, giving them responsibility and authority, is a good strategy.

Modern medical colleges adopting many of the current trends in medical education require an organizational structure which is responsive, ensures proper implementation of the curriculum, and is in alignment with its mission, outcomes and core values. The traditional organizational structure of a college council headed by the dean, associate/assistant deans for education, research and postgraduate studies and department chairs does not respond to a curriculum which is outcome based and integrated horizontally and vertically, whose main strategy of learning is student-centred (PBL/TBL), and that uses early introduction of clinical skills and balances clinical training between hospitals and community-based medical education. Although choosing the best organizational structure which ensures successful management of the college

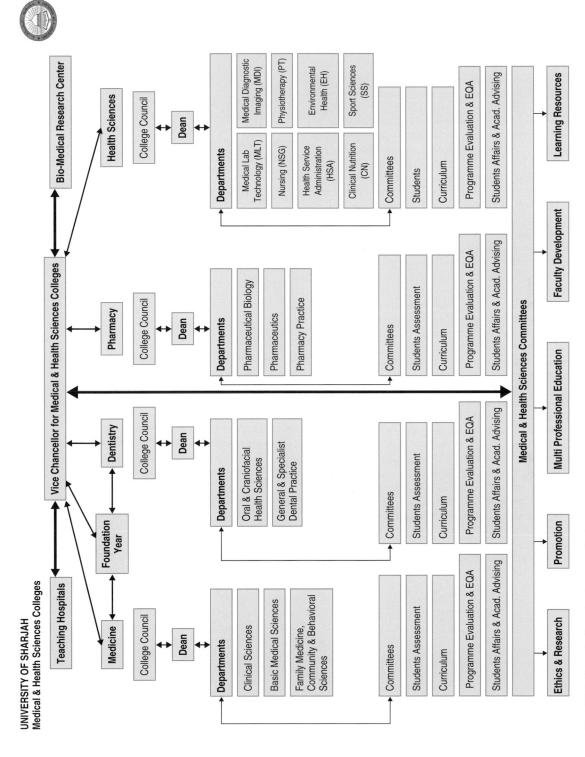

UNIVERSITY OF SHARJAH
Medical & Health Sciences Colleges

Fig. 50.1 Organization structure: medical campus.

is very much context related, it should still have some key features:

- Departments become the hub of subject matter expertise 'resources' which respond to the curriculum needs.
- Committees play a major role in planning, implementation, evaluation and programme renewal.

The responsibilities and terms of reference of programme administrators, department and conveners of committees should be clearly defined. In a modern medical curriculum which is outcome/competency-based, integrated and student-centred, the curriculum committee, student assessment committee, student advising and support committee, programme evaluation and educational quality assurance committees are responsible for development, implementation and evaluation of different aspects of the programme. Other important committees, like research and ethics, learning resources, multi-professional education, promotion and faculty development, could be in one college or between the colleges if more than one health profession education college is in the same university (nursing, dentistry, pharmacy, etc.). Having representation on these transverse committees from each college can increase their cohesiveness and efficiency by sharing resources and providing a practical model of teamwork, professional role identification and appreciation. This can influence the behaviour of the graduates and prepare them to work together as teams. Students' representation in different college committees creates a sense of partnership and helps students' personal development. They usually come up with solutions to implementation problems, which constantly arise.

The CEO of the school, dean and some senior faculty should create a strong link with the local health authorities, contribute to some of their committees and provide academic support to their activities, e.g. conduct collaborative population and health system researches and provide training and development of their staff. These initiatives support the college's social responsibility and create important strategic alliances.

Training, governing and self-development

As previously mentioned, most deans/heads of educational institutions come to the position without previous formal training. Experiential learning on the job is the main strategy used in the training of a dean. The leader of the institution should be a role model for the faculty of being a lifelong learner. Attending short courses on leadership, organizational culture, strategy, medical education and finance will definitely have an impact on the dean's management skills and the whole college. The dean of a health professions education institution needs to create learning opportunities for leadership development in an interprofessional context which should be offered to senior and junior faculty: grooming the young faculty for future leadership roles and to distribute leadership skills at all levels in the organization.

Selecting a dean

This chapter has highlighted the different roles, attributes and skills a leader/manager of a medical college should acquire in order to provide quality medical education. Still, selecting a dean or evaluating the performance of an existing one is a complex issue influenced by politics and interest groups' perceptions and expectations. Faculty usually evaluate the dean on what he or she has done for them. Selection based on elections may sound like a democratic process but should be carefully planned and evaluated to avoid turning it into a popularity context. Institutional goals should take priority over individual stakeholders' interest.

Summary

Managing a medical college is a heavy, demanding and challenging task. The complex nature of the medical college as an organization necessitates that its senior managers, deans, assistant deans and heads of departments should have acquired and developed leadership and managerial skills so they can respond to the rapid changes in medical practice and education. Senior managers should be aware of their different roles: vision, leader, manager, educator, professional, resource and finance manager and public figure. More in-depth management and leadership training is highly desirable and should be incorporated in faculty development programmes.

All these roles and responsibilities are embedded in organizational culture which the dean should consider in managing the college: 'doing the thing right and not only doing the right thing' (Schein 1990). Introducing new trends and changes requires the creation of an organizational structure which reflects the college's mission and strategic direction. Leadership of a medical college can be developed through training programmes and needs to be distributed at different levels of the college.

References

Coles CR, Grant JG: Curriculum evaluation in medical and healthcare education, *Medical Education* 19:405–422, 1985.

Dupont GE: The dean and his office. In Dibden AJ, editor: *The Academic Deanship and American Colleges and Universities*, Southern Illinois University Press, Carbondale and Edwardsville, IL, pp 4–27, 1968.

Fagin CM: *The Leadership Role of a Dean. New Directions for Higher Education, No. 98.* San Francisco, 1997, Jossey-Bass Publishers.

Hamdy H: *Quality measurement in medical education. PhD thesis.* The Netherlands, 2002, Groningon University.

Hamdy H, Agamy E: Is running a problem-based learning curriculum more expensive than a traditional subject-based curriculum? *Medical Teacher* 33:509–514, 2011.

Hamdy H, Williams R, Tekian A, et al: Application of 'VITALS': Visual indicators of teaching and learning success in reporting student evaluations of clinical teachers, *Education for Health* 14(2):267–276, 2001.

Hafferty F: Beyond curriculum reform: Confronting medicine's hidden curriculum, *Academic Medicine* 73:403–407, 1998.

Gilbert P: *Leadership: Being Effective and Remaining Human.* Lyon Regis, 2005, Russel House Publishing.

Goffman E: *Frame Analysis: An Essay on the Organization of Experience.* New York, 1974, Harper and Row.

Kotler J: *Leading Change.* Boston, MA, 1996, Harvard Business School Press.

Lessor RG: Adjudicating frameshifts and frame disputes in the new millennial university. The role of the Dean, *American Society* 39:114–129, 2008.

Maudsley R: Role models and the learning environment: Essential elements in effective medical education, *Academic Medicine* 76:432–434, 2001.

Mc Kinnan J, Swanwick T: *Educational leadership in understanding Medical Education: Evidence, Theory and Practice.* Sussex, UK, 2010, Wiley-Blackwell.

Mennin SP, Martinez-Burrola N: The cost of problem-based versus traditional medical education, *Medical Education* 20:187–194, 1986.

Northouse P: *Leadership: Theory and Practice*, ed 3, London, 2004, Sage.

Peck E, Dickinson H, Smith J: Transforming or transacting? The role of leaders in organizational transition, *British Journal of Leadership in Public Services* 2(3):4–14, 2006.

Schein EH: Organizational culture, *American Psychologist* 45:109–119, 1990.

Schuler RS: Role perceptions, satisfaction and performance. A partial reconciliation, *Journal of Applied Psychology* 60:683–687, 1975.

Shuhan MC, Mihailidis P: Deans of change, *American Journalism Review* 2007. Available at: http://www.ajr.org/article.asp?id=4412

Smircich L, Morgan G: Leadership: the management of meaning, *Journal of Applied Behavioural Science* 18:257–273, 1982.

Snow DA: Framing and social movements. In George R, editor: *Blackwell Encyclopedia of Sociology*, Oxford, UK, 2006, Blackwell, pp 1780–1784.

Steinert Y, Mann K, Carteno A, et al: A systematic review of faculty development initiatives designed to improve teaching effectiveness in medical education. BEME Guide No. 8, *Medical Teacher* 28(6):497–526, 2006.

Stoghili RM: Leadership, membership and organization, *Psychological Bulletin* 47:1–14, 1950.

Storey J: *Leadership on Organizations: Current Issues and Key Trends.* London, 2004, Rouledge.

Tucker A, Bryan RA: *The Academic Dean: Dove, Dragon and Diplomat.* New York, 1988, ACE and Macmillan.

Wolverton M, Gmelch WH, Montez J, Nies CT: The Changing Nature of the Academic Deanship, Vol 28. ASHE-ERIC Higher Education Report. San Francisco, 2001, Jossey Bass.

Index

Illustrations are comprehensively referred to from the text. Therefore, significant material in illustrations (figures and tables) have only been given a page reference in the absence of their concomitant mention in the text referring to that illustration.